CONTRAINDICATIONS
IN PHYSICAL REHABILITATION
Doing No Harm

CONTRAINDICATIONS IN PHYSICAL REHABILITATION

Doing No Harm

Mitchell Batavia, PhD, PT

New York University
Department of Physical Therapy, 380 Second Avenue,
Room 421, New York, New York 10010, (212) 998-9409,
mitchell.batavia@nyu.edu

SAUNDERS

ELSEVIER

SAUNDERS
ELSEVIER

11830 Westline Industrial Drive
St. Louis, Missouri 63146

CONTRAINDICATIONS IN PHYSICAL REHABILITATION: ISBN-13: 978-1-4160-3364-6
DOING NO HARM   ISBN-10: 1-4160-3364-5

Copyright © 2006 by Saunders, an imprint of Elsevier Inc.

Notice

ISBN-13: 978-1-4160-3364-6
ISBN-10: 1-4160-3364-5

Acquisitions Editor: Marion Waldmann
Developmental Editor: Annette Ferran
Publishing Services Manager: Julie Eddy
Project Manager: Andrea Campbell
Design Direction: Amy Buxton

Printed in the United States of America

Last digit is the print number: 9 8 7 6 5 4 3 2 1

To Evgenia and Michael.

TABLE OF CONTENTS

THE PURPOSE OF THIS REFERENCE BOOK

The primary aim of this reference book is to bring contraindication guidelines from various physical rehabilitation sub-specialties under "one roof." Currently, precautions and contraindications in patient care cannot be found easily in a single dedicated, portable source. Instead, they are scattered throughout the various subspecialties of physical rehabilitation—often buried deep within the pages of journal volumes and not-so-portable textbooks. Often, contraindications are not even indexed in the back of textbooks, making it challenging for readers to locate them. Having a pocket-size text devoted to this subject is therefore a convenience for the clinician.

A unique feature of this book is the compilation of contraindication from *multiple sources and experts* for a particular therapy. There are several advantages to including multiple sources in guidelines. First, the reader can begin to appreciate that guidelines (and opinions) may vary.[1-3] By juxtaposing guidelines, the reader can observe the range of opinions, the amount of agreement, and the degree to which concerns are voiced. Second, by including multiple sources, the reader has a better chance of seeing an issue that perhaps he or she did not previously entertain when assessing risk. Third, by including multiple sources with different professional affiliations, readers can determine to what extent guidelines relate to their professional practice.

Other features of this book include providing rationales for guidelines, suggesting alternative treatment strategies, and detailing complications of therapy. Complications (i.e., real stories) are included to help place safety concerns into proper perspective. This, in turn, may aid clinical reasoning by allowing readers to vicariously benefit from the insights and hindsight of others.

Finally, I include patient screening checklists at the end of the book for selected therapies because it is unreasonable to expect clinicians to memorize the numerous patient safety concerns.[a] This is particularly true as our knowledge base of treatments expands. Taken together, these features may enable clinicians to formulate safer care plans, help researchers identify risks when developing research protocols, and alert policy makers to inconsistencies in current guidelines.

Physical rehabilitation specialists such as physiatrists, physical therapists, occupational therapists, recreational therapists, and athletic trainers may find this resource useful. A secondary audience includes sports medicine physicians, orthopedists, neurologists, rehabilitation nurses, complementary/alternative medical practitioners, clinical researchers, and policymakers.

OVERVIEW. **In Part I,** the reader is offered a *birds-eye view* of contraindication guidelines in physical rehabilitation, using figures and a table. The figures present a summary of information, such as the total number of concerns or total number of (organ) systems needed to review for any given intervention. The table lists interventions by international classification of disease (ICD) categories. Markings (●) indicate areas of concern (ICD categories) for a given therapy in tabular form. In this manner, readers can quickly grasp areas to focus on during a patient screening. The table format also allows for direct comparisons between therapies. For example, although *thermotherapy* and *cryotherapy* share many safety issues, by using the tables, the reader can readily discern that thermotherapy lists concerns for neoplasms and pregnancy whereas cryotherapy does not. Similarly, although both *TENS* and *NMES* are forms of electrotherapy, NMES lists distinct issues about bleeding, circulatory problems, neoplasms, and infection whereas TENS does not.

In Parts II and III of the book, I briefly define therapies and other patient-related activities that raise safety concerns.a Contraindications and precautions are listed in tabular form (Table 1). These concerns vary in degree and span from a precautionary (P) to absolute contraindication (ACI). In general, concerns cited as absolute carry more weight than precautions. Also, concerns mentioned by several sources should, in general, give the reader more reason to pause than those mentioned by only one expert.

A source author's clinical affiliation/discipline (first author only) is identified to provide greater insight about their clinical perspective, the audience they address, and/or the population of patients they treat. For example, athletic trainers may see few debilitated patients with comorbidities (i.e., dementia, diabetes) and their guidelines may therefore fail to reflect these broader patient concerns. In an effort to be inclusive, I represent more than one discipline, when possible. When the source author's affiliation cannot be determined, I try to note their academic background.

Rationales are included under *Comments/Rationale* to offer readers some insight into the nature of a concern. These explications are provided by the source/s listing the concern (*not me*). The reader should know that sources often fail to explain their foreboding. A prime example is the condition *subcutaneous emphysema*; although fairly popular as a contra-indication among percussion sources, its rationale remains elusive—at least for this intervention.[b] When this is the case, white space (no text) "fills" the *Comments/Rationale* section. If possible, I address the rationale question under the heading *Note* with either physiologic or pathologic information offered by other sources or with my own commentary. In general, I only provide commentary in this textbook under the headings *Summaries* and/or *Notes*.

Adverse events (i.e., complications) from therapies are **bold** to help shed further light on what may happen when patients are not adequately screened or monitored during a therapy, and to offer possible support or evidence for a particular contraindication. The list is not exhaustive; it is a first approximation. As noted later in this section, minimizing complications during therapy is largely a matter of appropriate patient selection and/or treatment modification, that is, attending to contraindications and precaution guidelines. Alternative treatments, when suggested by sources, are included to expand readers' options in clinical decision-making. Adverse events are further detailed in a separate table.

In Part IV, checklists are provided to facilitate the screening of patients for selected therapies. These pages can be reviewed during the patient interview process. If any concern is checked off, the clinician can review the issue in more depth in the appropriate chapter. Although the screening forms are an added convenience, I recommend the reader rely on the full text as a more complete and detailed listing of concerns.

Finally, the Index is organized by diagnosis and provides a useful look-up tool for readers who wish to determine what therapies may be of concern for a particular patient ailment.

WHAT SOURCES ARE USED? I extracted guidelines from refereed English-language biomedical journals and established textbooks within the field of physical rehabilitation, giving preference to peer-reviewed journal articles. At least one source was cited for each therapy, but three or more were included whenever possible. Although preference was given to journal article sources, textbooks ironically served a larger role of communicating contraindications. Remarkably, journal articles frequently cited textbook sources rather than the reverse.

Journal articles and government/agency sites were searched using the following databases: MEDLINE, Embase, HealthSTAR, CINAHL, Cochrane reviews, Food and Drug Administration (FDA),[c] The Consumer Product Safety Commission (CPSC), Medical Device Agency (London), the National Guidelines Clearinghouse (www.guideline.gov), and Medical Malpractice Verdicts, Settlements and Experts.[d] In addition, I consulted bibliography (reference) lists and conducted manual searches. Key words used in the searches included: adverse event, adverse effect, complication, iatrogenic, safety, contraindication, precaution, danger, harm, risk, caution, physical rehabilitation, physiatry, physical therapy, occupational therapy, speech therapy, and type of intervention (e.g., thermotherapy).

Textbooks were included as sources if listed with more than 300 world wide library holdings in the Worldcat database.[e] The most recent editions were sought at the time of data collection.[f] If guidelines were not in wide circulation, then I sought publications in smaller circles. Often, this literature included specialty topics that attracted a limited audience (e.g., hydrotherapy, cranial-sacral therapy, myofascial release). Reference textbooks were usually avoided, and popular literature/magazines were eschewed.

I used the International Classification of Diseases (ICD-10) to categorize medical conditions and the Guide to Physical Therapy Practice as a general framework for chapter organization and terminology.[g] I added some supplementary categories to manage the data in this book, among them *Vulnerable Biological Tissues* and *Procedural Concerns*. These procedural concerns were included if they were either contained within a source's guidelines or were proximal to them and suggested a safety issue.

Information from the tables was generally graphed if three or more sources listed a set of CI guidelines. These graphs illustrated (1) source variability (i.e., the variability in the number of concerns voiced by different sources); (2) the proportion of concerns based on disease categories (i.e., ICD); and (3) the top safety concerns (i.e., the most frequently stated concerns). Although I use this approach to highlight "popular" concerns, readers should resist the temptation to rely exclusively on "top safety concerns" while ignoring other important, albeit less commonly cited, contraindications. The reader should also be aware that these graphs are based on non-randomly sampled data and therefore may not necessarily be generalized to other data sets such as a sample of different sources. Nevertheless, I believe these "pictures" can help to both summarize and highlight potentially important information contained in this text.

ASSUMPTIONS   *Common sense informs many safety concerns.* Examples include: (1) ensuring a safe patient environment (e.g., slippery floors; ungrounded electrical systems), (2) reading user manuals (e.g., poorly maintained or operated equipment); (3) having basic training in first aid; and (4) having sufficient skills, qualifications, and licensing to prescribe or administer a particular therapy (e.g., incompetence; this text is not a procedural manual). Of course, clinicians should always obtain informed consent from the patient before proceeding (i.e., involve patients in their own healthcare decisions).

DELIMITATIONS   *Type of Information*: (1) Data contained within this text are clinical guidelines and/or opinions of various experts and panels; they are not necessarily standards. (2) Some, and perhaps many guidelines are theoretically, rather than experimentally, derived. Evidence of harm can help to validate guidelines, and I have tried to include harm-related evidence for selected therapies whenever possible. Nevertheless, readers are cautioned that case reports, which are frequently used to describe harm in the rehabilitation field, are a *weak* form of evidence. (3) Incidence rates and risk magnitude (i.e., relative risk, numbers needed to harm) cannot be extracted from this text. That is, the number of adverse events reported in this book should not be confused with how frequently these events actually occur in the clinic. (4) As previously stated, data are limited primarily to English-language publications.

LIMITATIONS (1) *Potential for Bias*: I sampled purposefully, not randomly; selection biases may therefore exist. To address this concern, I established selection criteria, searched multiple databases, and included multiple expert opinions. Textbook selections, based on the number of library holdings, often enabled me to identify material that withstood some level of scrutiny. More importantly, purposeful sampling allowed me to collect data from highly cited sources. Examples include exercise testing guidelines promulgated by the American College of Sports Medicine or medical device alerts issued by the FDA. Using randomly selecting sources may have led to the wholly undesirable prospect of not including these important resources. (2) *Accessibility of Data*: I may have missed literature, particularly material published before 1966 or indexed idiosyncratically. Gleaning reference lists was extremely helpful in dealing with this challenge of finding relevant, and sometimes classic, important literature.

CLINICAL REASONING   *This text is not intended to be prescriptive.* Instead, clinicians should weigh at least three factors when prescribing therapies: <u>risks,</u> <u>benefits,</u> and <u>patient values.</u> *Risks* can be addressed by consulting epidemiologic studies, reviewing therapeutic complications reported in the literature, attending to alerts/warnings issued from various authoritative agencies such as the FDA, and by using clinical guidelines containing contraindications and precautions. Contraindications/precautionary guidelines, in turn, can help guide patient selection and/or treatment modifications to minimize the risk of complications. *Benefits* can be assessed by determining if a therapy is effective, usually based on well-designed studies such as randomized clinical trials (RCTs) and meta-analyses. Note that some therapies included in this textbook, although more or less common to the field of physical rehabilitation, may not necessarily possess a convincing degree of effectiveness (i.e., *P* values and effect sizes). Finally, *patient values* can be assessed by asking patients about their goals, financial concerns, and preferences (e.g., personal, cultural, religious). These factors, along with the clinician's *expertise* are "important players" in the prescription process.[4]

Clinical Decisions = Therapeutic Effectiveness + Risks + Patient Values

In the ideal world, one would like to prescribe an extremely effective treatment that carries no risks and has total patient compliance. Unfortunately, this scenario is a fiction; not all therapies have convincing efficacy; most therapies carry at least some minimal risk and even motivated athletes may be non-compliant. A therapy's benefits therefore need to be weighed against possible risks. Certainly it makes no sense to prescribe a risky intervention with no good evidence for improving the patient's condition (even useless therapies, considered "harmless," carry some risk such as the missed opportunity of receiving a more effective intervention, such as a cancer treatment, somewhere else). Nor should patients be exposed to undue risks if their condition is expected to resolve naturally and in a timely manner (e.g., administering cervical manipulation for headaches or a stiff neck in a high-risk population). For equally effective therapies, the one that carries the least risk should probably be tried first. *The ultimate goal is to promote recovery without interfering with healing.* By factoring in safety concerns, in conjunction with the therapy's effectiveness and the patient's particular wishes, the decision-making task can be made more manageable.

READING THE FIGURES

Graphs in this book summarize information contained in the tables. Brief explanations for the three types of graphs are included below, using **Therapeutic Massage** as an example.

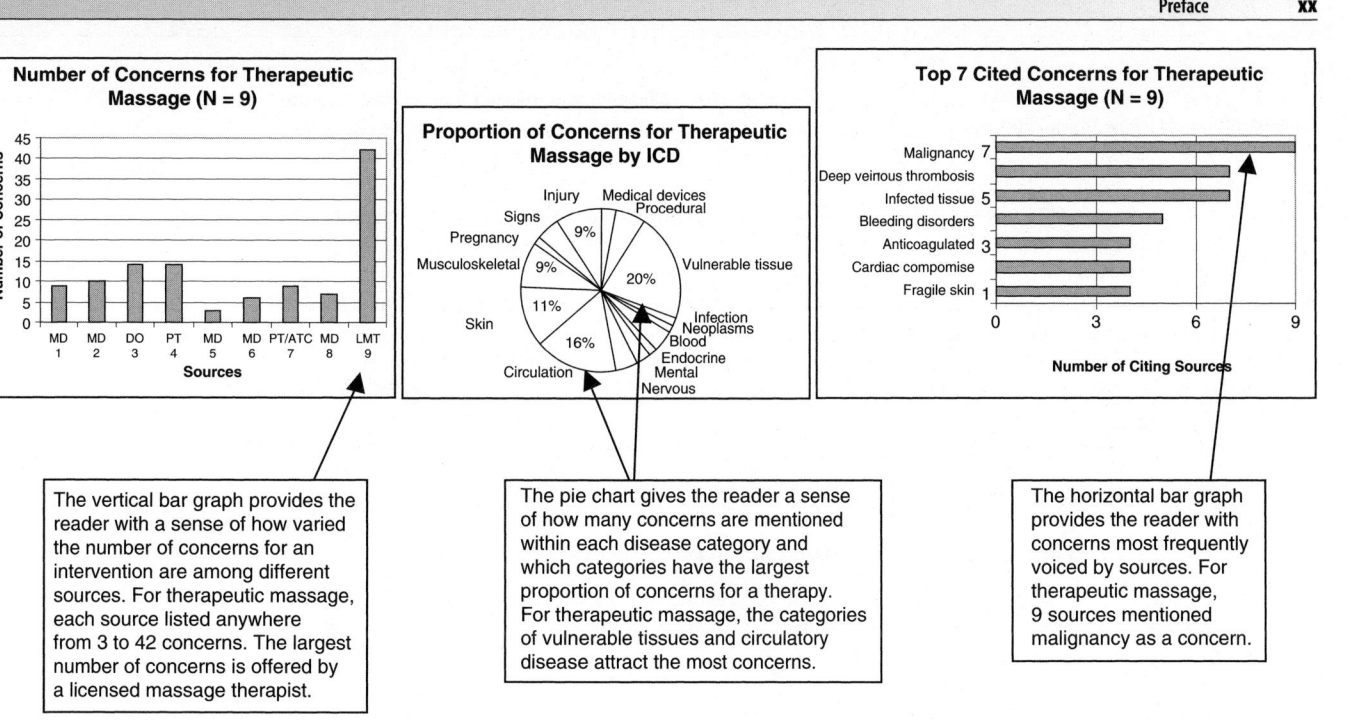

Number of Concerns for Therapeutic Massage (N = 9)

The vertical bar graph provides the reader with a sense of how varied the number of concerns for an intervention are among different sources. For therapeutic massage, each source listed anywhere from 3 to 42 concerns. The largest number of concerns is offered by a licensed massage therapist.

Proportion of Concerns for Therapeutic Massage by ICD

The pie chart gives the reader a sense of how many concerns are mentioned within each disease category and which categories have the largest proportion of concerns for a therapy. For therapeutic massage, the categories of vulnerable tissues and circulatory disease attract the most concerns.

Top 7 Cited Concerns for Therapeutic Massage (N = 9)

The horizontal bar graph provides the reader with concerns most frequently voiced by sources. For therapeutic massage, 9 sources mentioned malignancy as a concern.

There are two types of tables in this book. The first type contains information on contraindications/precautions and the second contains data on adverse events. Examples using Therapeutic Massage and Shiatsu follow.

CONTRAINDICATIONS AND PRECAUTIONS

Column 1 states the ISSUE of concern (contraindications and/or precautions) for a therapy.

Column 2 cites the LEVEL OF CONCERN (LOC). Note that several sources may be cited because different experts may cite varying levels of concern for a particular condition. For example, one source may document a condition as an absolute contraindication, whereas another may indicate only a precaution. As stated above, when making a clinical decision, readers should also rely on level of evidence for harm, clinical rationale, alternative therapies, their clinical expertise, patient preferences, treatment effectiveness, and any established standards in weighing the risk and benefits of the therapy in question.

The LOC used in this text are based on how experts generally document or phrase their concern. Note that sources rarely operationally define these terms, and some even fail to distinguish a contraindication from a precaution. Wherever possible, I used the source's own terminology or classification scheme to avoid "filtering out" the source's original intent. Some of this terminology is listed below.

DEFINITIONS

- **Absolute Contraindication (ACI):** If a source documents an absolute contraindication or reports that the procedure should *never* be performed. An example may be performing cervical manipulation on a person with active rheumatoid arthritis.
- **Relative Contraindication (RCI):** If the source documents a relative contraindication or reports that performing the procedure is *relative* to or *depends* on factors such as the required level of clinician expertise or the complexity of the patient presentation.

- **Contraindication (CI):** If the source documents a contraindication. A contraindication is defined as a medical condition that renders an intervention undesirable.[2,3] Occasionally a source invokes the term "contraindication" to indicate that the therapy will be of limited value for the condition in question. In other words, it is not indicated.
- **Precaution (P):** If the source documents a precaution when performing the procedure. A precaution is defined as a protective measure implemented in advance to minimize treatment complications.[2,3]
- **Contraindication/Precaution (CI/P):** If the source documents a Contraindication/Precaution (CI/P) but fails to distinguish between the two.
- **Advice:** If the source appears to offer a recommendation or share safety information without specifying a concern.
- **Recommendation:** If the source offers a guideline or if they state "recommend."
- **Avoid:** If the source suggests that you avoid doing something but does not specifically state a contraindication. The term "*Do not do*" is invoked when the source chooses those words.
- **Caution** or **Warning:** If specifically stated as such by a source such as the FDA.
- **Concern:** I use the term "concern" generally to mean any safety issue. That is, any of the 11 terms listed above expressed by a source would also be viewed as concern.

Column 3 indicates the SOURCES (authors) including the date of their guideline.

Column 4 identifies the sources AFFILIATION (Affil) such as their health-related or academic training.

Column 5 discusses RATIONALES/COMMENTS about the concern. Rationales may either be theoretical or grounded in experimental data, can foster understanding of the problem, and can help facilitate clinical decision-making.

The ICD 10 disease category for thrombophlebitis

CONTRAINDICATIONS AND PRECAUTIONS FOR MASSAGE

I00-99 DISEASES OF THE CIRCULATORY SYSTEM

Issue	LOC	Source	Affil	Rationale/Comment
Thrombophlebitis	CI	Geiringer and DeLateur, 1990[2]	MD	Mechanical stimulation of vessels and enhanced circulation may both cause a thrombus to detach and become an embolism. A coronary thrombosis is a CI because the shaking/vibration may aggravate the condition. **In a 1997 case report, Mikhail et al[11] described a 59-year-old male smoker with an aorto-bifemoral bypass graft who threw an embolus to his left kidney following wife's back massage (walking on his back).**
DVT	ACI	Braverman and Schulman,1999[3]	MD	
	CI	Knapp, 1968[5]	MD	
	CI	Cotter et al, 2000[6]	MD	
	CI	De Domenico and Wood, 1997[1]	PT	
	CI	Prentice and Lehn, 2002[8a]	PT/ATC	
	ACI	Wieting et al, 2005[4]	DO	

The condition of concern

A source offers a level of concern (i.e., ACI: Never massage over an area of a deep venous thrombosis.)

Indicates the source's clinical affiliation.

Notes are included to shed additional light on this topic or report, including a case report by Mikhail **(in bold typeface)** that offers some support for the concerns.

ADVERSE EVENTS

Evidence (i.e., published data) of adverse events from therapies provides readers with a richer understanding of the circumstances and context under which concerns of potential patient harm have occurred. Review of actual adverse events can serve as educational/training material in journal clubs and therapy/medical schools.

Because *the devil is often in the details*, it is important to read original sources (recommended). Specific information in these report such as comorbidities, level of practitioner expertise (certifications), and actual treatment parameters (equipment, dosage: intensity, duration, frequency) are often, but not always, present to help clarify why poor outcomes have occurred.

Column 1 SOURCE (authors, year), the DESIGN type, and the JOURNAL that published the report
- **Author:** informs reader of first and second authors
- **Year:** when the report was filed or published (older issues may no longer be a current relevant concern [e.g., newer cardiac pacemakers may be less susceptible to external interference than older models])
- **Journal Title:** suggest quality of the source and the type of audience (readership)
- **Design:** indicates overall strength and quality of the evidence (see below)

Quality of the Evidence: Although there are numerous methods of ranking a design's strength (i.e., I, IIa, IIb, etc.), I provided the raw data (see below) because it is intuitive and useful in capturing the entire spectrum of designs used to report harm in the field of physical rehabilitation. The levels of evidence, in order from weakest to strongest, range from opinions to randomized controlled experiments. Although rare, one would ideally rely on harm-related evidence drawn from experimental data; for ethical reasons, much of the evidence in the fields of physical rehabilitation is at the observational level, such as case reporting.

In addition to evidence of adverse events located in journals, warnings and alerts from agencies (i.e., FDA, CPSC) and outcomes from law suits are also reported. It is important to point out that outcomes from therapy-related litigation (determined by the court system) or device-related injuries (reported to the FDA) do not necessarily provide unequivocal proof of a causal link. For example, a device-related injury may be caused by user error in addition to equipment failure and court outcomes are often decided by the judgment of a jury or through some settlement.

Designs and Other Levels of Evidence: listed from strongest to weakest

- **Experiments**
  - Meta-analyses (quantitative summaries of experiments)
  - Randomized Clinical Trials; Pretest/Post-test Control Group Designs
  - Cross-over studies; Within-subjects designs
  - Animal studies (experiments)
- **Observational (Associational)**
  - Cohort studies (prospective; epidemiological)
  - Case control studies (retrospective, epidemiological)
  - Retrospective (chart reviews)
- **Observational (Descriptive)**
  - Descriptive (group data)
  - Case series
  - Case report
  - FDA reports
  - Litigation
- **Opinion/Theory (no evidence)**

Columns 2–5 Data from the report are read from left to right with DEMOGRAPHIC data on the left, therapeutic INTERVENTION in the middle, and OUTCOME, FOLLOW-UP and researcher's COMMENTS in the right columns.

- **Patient background:** Readers can determine to what extent the characteristics of the patient/s in the report generalize to their own patient.
- **Therapy:** Identify treatment parameters and the qualification of the practitioner who administered treatment.
- **Outcomes:** Note adverse effects *possibly attributed to* the therapy.
- **Remedial interventions:** Indicate what remedial actions the authors took following the adverse event.
- **Follow-up/Interpretation/Notes**
    - **Follow-up:** Refers to the time interval before the problem resolved itself. Knowledge of recovery rates from adverse events may be useful when developing consent forms for research.
    - **Interpretation:** Authors often offer a "take-home message" or recommendation.
    - **Notes:** Technical notes (i.e., design issues) may be noted by *me* to highlight some key issue or design weakness.

ADVERSE EVENT FROM SHIATSU TO THE NECK REGION

Source	Background	Therapy	Outcome	Follow-up/Interpretation
Shiatsu, neck, and paresis Tsuboi and Tsuboi, 2001 Case report Lancet	An 80-year-old man presented with a recent history of TIA, a right frontal lobe small infarct, and bilateral internal carotid artery stenoses. He was free of neurologic symptoms and was discharged following anticoagulation treatment.	That evening, he received a Shiatsu massage on his neck while prone for 10 minutes because of a mild headache with neck/shoulder stiffness.	After the massage, he noted a right visual field impaired (nasal half). At the hospital, slight left UE hemiparesis, retinal edema with multiple emboli in central retinal artery branches, and small infarctions of right frontoparietal lobe were noted. Dx: Cerebral and retinal artery embolism (stroke).	The patient's left paresis recovered after one week but ocular symptoms improved only minimally. The authors postulate that direct pressure over the extracranial carotid artery (neck region) may have led to the embolic event in this high-risk patient.

Closing Comments: a, Technical notes: (1) Although the range of topics covered in this text is fairly broad, I tried to limit them to *physical* interventions (as the title implies). In other words, pharmaceuticals are not included except for brief discussion on injection therapy concerns (i.e., corticosteroids) and potential drug interactions that are pertinent in rehabilitation. Excellent drug manuals are available in the literature. (2) For patients with activity restrictions because of conditions such as deep vein thrombosis, recent arthroplasty, recent fractures, or recent skin grafts, it would be wise to consult the appropriate specialist. Management protocols may vary locally or may need to be tailored to the particular circumstances of the patient.

b, It is possible that the rationale is similar to postural drainage concerns for patients with surgical emphysema. In postural drainage, dyspnea may occur when patients with this condition are tilted head-down.

c, FDA databases (http://www.fda.gov/cdrh/index.html) include Medical Device Reporting (MDR) and The Manufacturers, Users Facility, and Distributor Experience (MAUDE). *MDR* contains more than 600,000 reports from the Center for Device and Radiological Health's (CDRH) former database, the Device Experience Network database (DEN) (up to June 1993 voluntary;1984–1996 mandatory) on devices that may have malfunctioned, caused serious injuries, or caused death. *MAUDE* represents more recent reports of adverse events involving medical devices and includes voluntary reports (since June 1993), user facility reports (since 1991), distributor reports (since 1993), and manufacturer reports (since August 1996). The FDA notes that "reports regarding device trade names may have been submitted under different manufacturer names." In addition, MAUDE may not include all reports (e.g., those exempted).

d, Medical Malpractice Verdicts, Settlements & Experts (http://www.verdictslaska.com/) is a published newsletter reporting settlements and verdicts of medical malpractice. Begun in 1985, the database contains more than 36,000 cases. Although the AMA style guidelines were generally followed in the text, I chose to reference litigation using a format of Journal, Month, Year, Page, Location on page (e.g., Medical Malpractice Verdicts, Settlements and Experts, October, 1994, 45, 4) so as to document events rather than focus on the parties involved.

e, Worldcat (http://www.oclc.org/) is the union catalog for the Online Computer Library Center (OCLC). The OCLC is a non-profit organization founded in 1967; it is used by more than 53,000 libraries in 96 countries and territories to locate and lend library material.

f, I used Kisner and Colby's 3rd edition of *Therapeutic Exercise: Foundations and Techniques* at the time of data collection. Many of the therapeutic exercise concerns raised in the 4th edition appear to reiterate, and occasionally, expand on those issues culled from their 3rd edition.

g, Technical note: (1) Sources offered diverse classification schemes; some sources listed concerns by symptom (e.g., inflammation), whereas others used a diagnostic taxonomy (e.g., rheumatoid arthritis), and still others used both. Furthermore, some sources described disorders in general terms (e.g., cardiovascular disorder), and others were more specific (vertebral-basilar insufficiency). This variability presented a challenge in presenting the information to the reader. On the one hand, I wanted to be true to the source, but I also wanted to consolidate intolerable redundancy and allow for any patterns in the data to emerge. To ensure a complete and accurate record, however, I tried to retain all source concerns in their relatively "raw" form. To deal with idiosyncratic taxonomies (e.g., severe; uncontrolled; acute, fresh, recent), I footnoted source-specific information. (2) *The PT Guide to Professional Practice:* Although I used the physical therapy profession's guide as a starting point, there are instances when it was more helpful to depart from its structure in order to address diverse healthcare audiences, reflect shared terminology (i.e., FDA terms), and to avoid unnecessary redundancy.

REFERENCES

1. Houghton PE, Campbell KE. Choosing an adjunctive therapy for the treatment of chronic wounds. Ostomy/Wound Manag 1999;45(8)43-52.
2. Batavia M. Contraindications for superficial heat and therapeutic ultrasound: Do sources agree? Arch Physical Med & Rehabil 2004;85(6): 1006-12.
3. Batavia M. Contraindications for therapeutic massage: Do sources agree? J Bodywork Movement Ther 2004;8:48-57.
4. Straus SE, Richardson WS, Glasziou P, Haynes RB. Evidence-based medicine: How to practice and teach EBM, 3rd ed. Edinburgh: Churchill Livingstone, 2005.

ACKNOWLEDGMENT

Contraindications in Physical Rehabilitation was a massive undertaking—about 5 years in the making. I certainly had abundant guidance, encouragement, and stellar support along the way. I thank Marion Waldman, who was the Executive Editor at the time that I contracted the book with Elsevier and who saw the project through from its early Word file origins to the proofs. Also early on, Jacquelyn Merrell, Senior Development Editor, was instrumental in helping me decide on a much-needed tabular format for the book. Annette Ferran, Developmental Editor, adeptly walked me through the manuscript's growth spurts as Word files grew into mature, edited pages. Andrea Campbell, Production Manager, and Amy Buxton, Designer, at Elsevier stood up to the unique challenges of designing and producing a final product without the use of a one-size-fits-all roadmap. Finally, I wish to thank my NYU colleagues' ongoing encouragement and my wife's enduring tolerance for my frequent self-imposed exile into the world of libraries and databases these past years.

This text contains concerns for more than 100 interventions and 7 tests used in physical rehabilitation and related disciplines. This section provides an overview and an illustrative summary for many of these concerns.[a]

Table 1 gives a birds-eye view of interventions classified into 10 major categories[b]: therapeutic exercise, manual techniques, AAOPSP (equipment), airway clearance, wound care, injections, physical agents, mechanical modalities, electrotherapy (E stimulation), and complementary and alternative medicine (CAM). Concerns under an intervention are listed by disease categories (ICD-10). By identifying an intervention in the left column and then reading across the disease categories from left to right, the reader can identify categories that may be of concern for a particular intervention (noted by solid circles). For example, power mobility lists the eye disease category as a concern. By consulting the power mobility chapter, the reader will see blindness listed as a contraindication.

When interpreting the table, the reader should be aware of the types of conditions that may be listed under the various disease categories used by ICD-10. For example, "Medical Devices" may mean latex toys, contact lenses, an unstable joint arthroplasty, or equipment that emits electromagnetic interference. Vulnerable tissue may imply immature epiphyseal plates, superficial peripheral nerves, or unprotected eye exposure to ultraviolet radiation. Injury can include acute trauma, burns, and open wounds such as pressure ulcers. Blood usually implies bleeding but may also include immunological problems and sensitivities/allergies in some cases. A fuller description of these concerns can be found in each chapter.

Figure A lists the total number of concerns for 62 physical rehabilitation interventions in order of magnitude. On the left, two debridement procedures offer relatively few concerns, whereas on the far right, therapeutic massage contains more than 60 total concerns from various sources. Please note that individual sources typically list far fewer concerns (**see figure C**), suggesting that sources do not always agree on precautions.

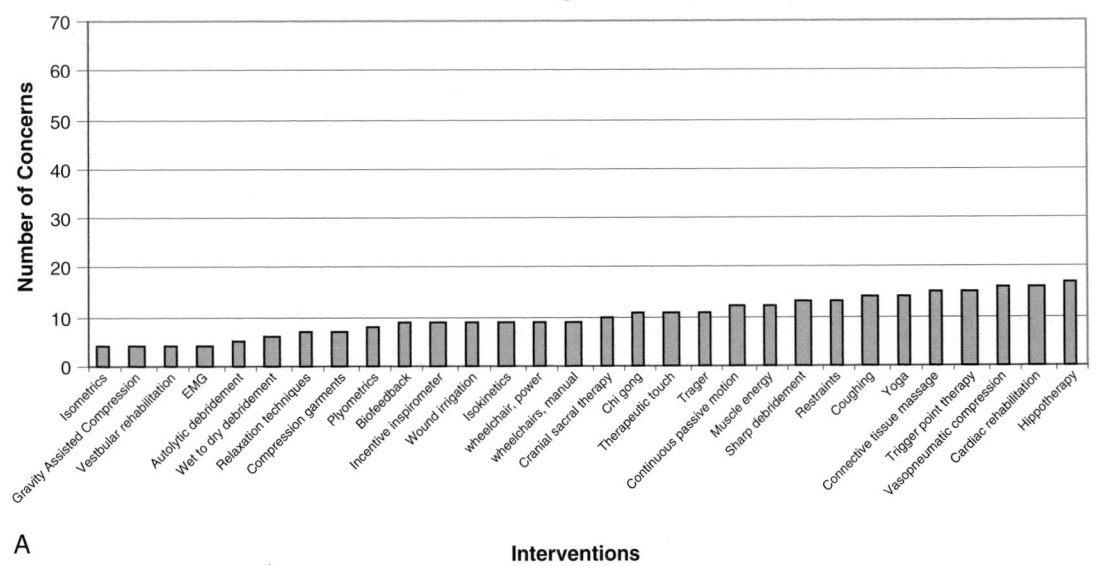

The Total Number of Concerns for Interventions, In Order of Magnitude (N = 62)

A

Interventions

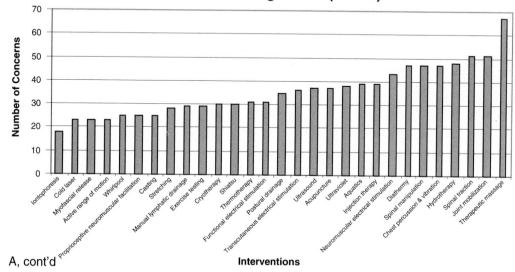

The Total Number of Concerns for Interventions, In Order of Magnitude (N = 62)

A, cont'd

Interventions

Figure B reorganizes the same information, but grouped by modality. In this way, the reader can get a sense of which interventions within each area of rehabilitation note the greatest number of patient concerns. For example, for physical agents, electrical stimulation and complementary and alternative medicine, hydrotherapy, neuromuscular electrical stimulation, and acupuncture list the greatest number of concerns, respectively.

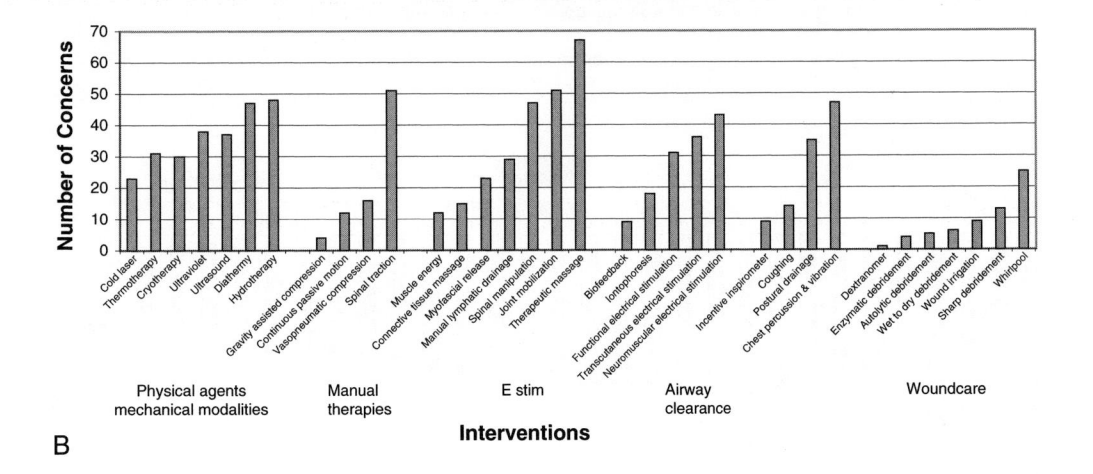

The Total Number of Concerns for Interventions, Grouped by Modality (n = 62)

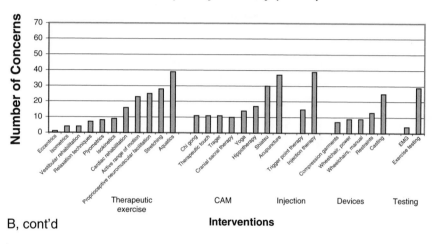

The Total Number of Concerns for Interventions, Grouped by Modality (n = 62)

B, cont'd

Figure C shows the *average* number of concerns for interventions, in order of magnitude. Average means that if one source lists 15 concerns and another lists five concerns, the average for this intervention will be 10. The reader will notice that the number of average concerns is far less than the total number presented in Figure A. For example, although the total number of concerns for hydrotherapy is more than 40 (Figure A), the average number per source is a little more than 20 (Figure C; second vertical bar on far right). The larger number of concerns under Figure A can be attributed to

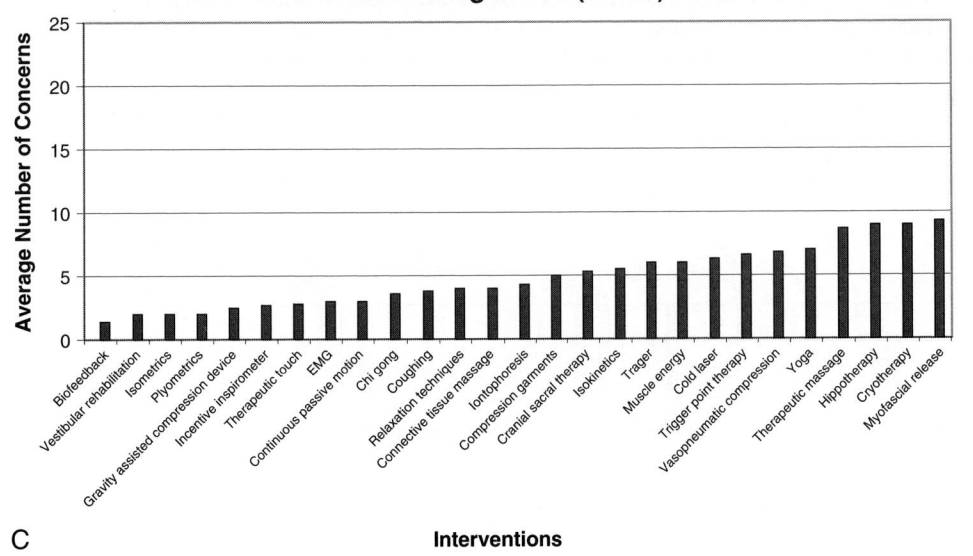

The Average Number of Concerns for an Intervention, In Order of Magnitude (n = 47)

C

Interventions

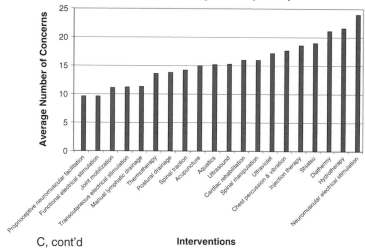

The Average Number of Concerns for an Intervention, In Order of Magnitude (n = 47)

C, cont'd

Interventions

individual sources contributing *somewhat different concerns* for a particular intervention that results in a larger list of guidelines overall.

Figure D lists the number of disease categories that may be a concern for a particular intervention. A useful way to think about this graph is to observe the number of systems a clinician may need to screen (i.e., systems review) when considering a patient for a particular intervention. For example, a clinician may only need to review three systems before dispensing a compression garment, but many more (16 systems) before prescribing neuromuscular electrical stimulation (NMES). Further reading and more graphs can be found at the end of this book in the Appendix.

The Number of Systems to Review Prior to Administrating an Intervention (N = 64)

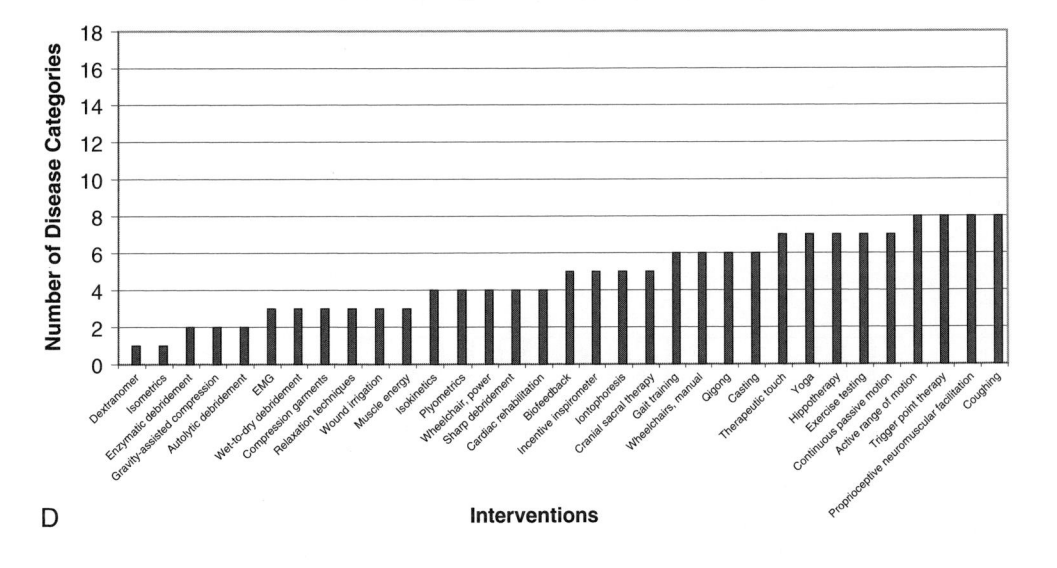

D

Interventions

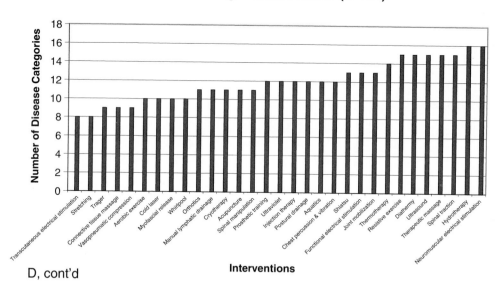

The Number of Systems to Review Prior to Administrating an Intervention (N = 64)

D, cont'd

Table 1

	Procedural	Vulnerable tissue	Infection A00-B99	Neoplasm B00-C97	Blood D50-D89	Endocrine E00-E90	Mental F00-F90	Nervous G00-G99	Eye H00-H59	Ear H60-H59	Circulatory I00-I99	Respiratory J00-J99	Digestive K00-K93	Skin L00-L99	Musculoskeletal M00-M99	Genitourinary N00-N99	Pregnancy O00-O99	Perinatal P00-P99	Congenital Q00-Q99	Symptoms R00-R99	Injury S00-T98	Medical Devices Y70-Y82
Therapeutic Exercise																						
Aerobics				•		•		•	•		•	•			•	•	•			•		
Aquatics	•		•				•	•			•	•	•	•		•				•	•	•
AROM	•										•			•	•		•			•	•	•
Balance exercise	•						•															
Cardiac rehabilitation						•					•				•					•	•	
Closed chain	•														•					•		
Eccentric exercise		•																				
Gait training	•										•			•					•		•	•
Isokinetics											•				•					•	•	
Isometrics											•											
Plyometrics	•														•					•	•	
PNF	•			•			•	•							•				•	•	•	
PREs		•									•	•										•
Relaxation technique	•						•				•											
Resistive exercise	•	•	•			•		•	•		•	•	•	•	•		•			•	•	•
Stretching	•		•	•	•										•					•	•	•
Vestibular rehab	•									•										•		

	Procedural	Vulnerable tissue	Infection A00-B99	Neoplasm B00-C97	Blood D50-D89	Endocrine E00-E90	Mental F00-F90	Nervous G00-G99	Eye H00-H99	Ear H60-H59	Circulatory I00-I99	Respiratory J00-J99	Digestive K00-K93	Skin L00-L99	Musculoskeletal M00-M99	Genitourinary N00-N99	Pregnancy O00-O99	Perinatal P00-P99	Congenital Q00-Q99	Symptoms R00-R99	Injury S00-T98	Medical Devices Y70-Y82
Drivers, older	●			●		●	●	●	●	●	●	●			●	●			●	●	●	

Manual techniques

	Procedural	Vulnerable tissue	Infection A00-B99	Neoplasm B00-C97	Blood D50-D89	Endocrine E00-E90	Mental F00-F90	Nervous G00-G99	Eye H00-H99	Ear H60-H59	Circulatory I00-I99	Respiratory J00-J99	Digestive K00-K93	Skin L00-L99	Musculoskeletal M00-M99	Genitourinary N00-N99	Pregnancy O00-O99	Perinatal P00-P99	Congenital Q00-Q99	Symptoms R00-R99	Injury S00-T98	Medical Devices Y70-Y82
CTM	●	●	●	●			●				●			●						●	●	
Joint mobilization	●		●	●			●	●			●	●			●		●		●	●	●	●
MLD	●	●	●	●		●					●	●	●			●	●					
MFR	●		●	●	●	●					●			●	●					●	●	
Muscle energy	●					●									●							
Therapeutic massage	●	●	●	●	●	●	●	●			●			●	●		●			●	●	●
Spinal manipulation	●			●	●	●	●	●			●				●		●		●	●		

AAOPSP

	Procedural	Vulnerable tissue	Infection A00-B99	Neoplasm B00-C97	Blood D50-D89	Endocrine E00-E90	Mental F00-F90	Nervous G00-G99	Eye H00-H99	Ear H60-H59	Circulatory I00-I99	Respiratory J00-J99	Digestive K00-K93	Skin L00-L99	Musculoskeletal M00-M99	Genitourinary N00-N99	Pregnancy O00-O99	Perinatal P00-P99	Congenital Q00-Q99	Symptoms R00-R99	Injury S00-T98	Medical Devices Y70-Y82
Casting	●						●	●			●			●	●					●	●	
Elastic bandages	●										●				●							
Manual wheelchairs							●	●	●						●						●	●
Orthotics (LE)	●	●					●	●			●	●	●	●	●					●	●	
Power mobility							●	●	●													●
Prosthetics	●					●	●	●	●		●	●		●	●				●	●	●	
Restraints	●																					

Continued

	Procedural	Vulnerable tissue	Infection A00-B99	Neoplasm B00-C97	Blood D50-D89	Endocrine E00-E90	Mental F00-F90	Nervous G00-G99	Eye H00-H59	Ear H60-H59	Circulatory I00-I99	Respiratory J00-J99	Digestive K00-K93	Skin L00-L99	Musculoskeletal M00-M99	Genitourinary N00-N99	Pregnancy O00-O99	Perinatal P00-P99	Congenital Q00-Q99	Symptoms R00-R99	Injury S00-T98	Medical Devices Y70-Y82
Pulmonary																						
Coughing	●		●					●	●		●	●			●						●	
Incentive spirometer	●						●					●								●		●
Percussion/vibration	●		●	●	●		●	●			●	●		●	●					●	●	●
Postural drainage	●			●	●		●	●	●		●	●	●		●	●					●	
Autolytic	●																				●	
Enzyme	●																				●	
Debridement																						
Wet-Dry	●				●																●	
Wound irrigation	●	●			●																	
Whirlpool	●						●	●			●		●	●	●	●				●	●	
Dextranomers	●																					
Sharp	●	●			●																	
Electrotherapy																						
Biofeedback	●						●	●							●							●
FES	●					●	●	●	●	●	●				●		●			●		
Iontophoresis	●							●							●						●	●
NMES	●	●	●	●	●		●	●			●				●			●	●	●	●	●
TENS	●	●					●	●							●			●			●	●

	Procedural	Vulnerable tissue	Infection A00-B99	Neoplasm B00-C97	Blood D50-D89	Endocrine E00-E90	Mental F00-F90	Nervous G00-G99	Eye H00-H59	Ear H60-H59	Circulatory I00-I99	Respiratory J00-J99	Digestive K00-K93	Skin L00-L99	Musculoskeletal M00-M99	Genitourinary N00-N99	Pregnancy O00-O99	Perinatal P00-P99	Congenital Q00-Q99	Symptoms R00-R99	Injury S00-T98	Medical Devices Y70-Y82
Physical Agents																						
Cold Laser	●	●		●	●		●	●			●			●			●			●		
Cryotherapy	●	●	●		●		●	●			●			●	●					●	●	
Diathermy	●	●		●	●	●	●	●			●			●	●	●	●			●	●	●
Hydrotherapy	●		●	●	●		●	●			●	●	●	●	●	●	●			●	●	●
Thermotherapy	●	●		●	●		●	●			●			●	●		●			●	●	●
Ultrasound	●	●	●	●	●	●	●	●			●			●	●		●			●	●	●
Ultraviolet	●	●		●		●	●				●	●		●		●				●	●	
Mechanical Modalities																						
CPM	●	●			●			●							●						●	●
GACD	●																					●
Mechanical traction	●			●	●		●	●	●		●	●	●		●		●		●	●	●	●
VCD		●		●		●	●	●			●	●		●							●	
CAM																						
Acupuncture	●	●	●	●	●	●	●				●				●		●			●		
Cranial sacral	●						●	●			●										●	

Continued

	Procedural	Vulnerable tissue	Infection A00-B99	Neoplasm B00-C97	Blood D50-D89	Endocrine E00-E90	Mental F00-F90	Nervous G00-G99	Eye H00-H99	Ear H60-H59	Circulatory I00-I99	Respiratory J00-J99	Digestive K00-K93	Skin L00-L99	Musculoskeletal M00-M99	Genitourinary N00-N99	Pregnancy O00-O99	Perinatal P00-P99	Congenital Q00-Q99	Symptoms R00-R99	Injury S00-T98	Medical Devices Y70-Y82
Hippotherapy					●		●	●			●				●				●	●		
Hypnosis	●						●															
Qi gong	●		●				●				●					●	●					
Shiatsu		●	●	●	●	●					●	●	●	●	●		●			●	●	
Therapeutic touch	●	●		●			●					●								●	●	
Trager				●	●		●	●			●				●		●			●	●	
Yoga	●								●	●	●		●		●				●			
Injections																						
Injections therapy	●		●	●	●	●		●			●	●			●	●					●	●
Trigger point therapy	●		●	●	●		●					●					●			●		
Test & Measures																						
EMG	●		●		●																	
Exercise testing	●		●			●	●				●						●			●		

a, (1) Table and figures illustrated here contain many but not all concerns that are listed in the text. Examples of items not included are communication, teaching, documentation issues, older driver concerns (>100 concerns), and concerns where averaging individual source contraindication (i.e., where sources do not offer a set of guidelines) would be inappropriate (e.g., aerobic exercise, resistive exercise). (2) Figure D (Review of systems) contains procedural and vulnerable tissue concerns, although these two categories are technically not ICD categories (see Preface). b, Also includes older drivers, tests and measures.

1 BLOOD PRESSURE ASSESSMENT

SPHYGMOMANOMETER

Concerns for sphygmomanometer use relate to circulatory occlusion in select patients and the possibility of cross-contamination from the cuff.

Issue	LOC	Sources	Affil	Rationale/Comment
Cross-contamination from sphygmomanometer cuff	Complication	Myers, 1978[1]	—	**In a 21-week longitudinal study of special care nurseries by Myers, a nosocomial infection rate of 21% was associated with blood pressure cuffs used by all infants with 46 of 248 infants at risk acquiring 52 infections.**
IV sites—above	Avoid	Pierson & Fairchild, 2002[2]	PT	Avoid applying a blood pressure cuff above the infusion site.
Shunts on upper arm	Avoid			Blood pressure measurements taken on the extremity with a shunt in kidney patients. Application of any occlusive item, such as a blood pressure cuff or restraint, to the upper arm of the extremity containing the shunt should be avoided.
Lymphedema—on involved limb	No	Lasinski, 2003[3]	PT	If measurements are taken on the involved limb, circulation may be compromised.

REFERENCES

1. Myers MG: Longitudinal evaluation of neonatal nosocomial infections: association of infection with a blood pressure cuff. Pediatrics 61(1):42-45, 1978.
2. Pierson FM, Fairchild SL: Principles & techniques of patient care, ed 3. Philadelphia: W.B. Saunders, 2002.
3. Lasinski B: The lymphatic system. In Goodman, Boissonnault WG, Fuller KS, eds: Pathology: Implications for the physical therapist. Philadelphia: W.B. Saunders, 2003.

2 ELECTRODIAGNOSTIC TESTING

2.1 Electrical Evaluation Tests

OVERVIEW. Nelson[1] identifies four CIs for all "traditional electrical evaluation tests," including reaction of degeneration, strength-duration curve and chronaxie, galvanic twitch-tetanus ratio, nerve excitability nerve conduction, evoked potentials, and electromyography (**Also see EMG**).

O00-O99 PREGNANCY, CHILDBIRTH, AND PUERPERIUM

Issue	LOC	Source	Affil	Rationale/Comment
Pregnancy—over abdomen	CI	Nelson, 1992[1,a]	PT	The effects of ES on developing fetus and on pregnant uterus have not been determined.

a, Should not be applied.

VULNERABLE BIOLOGICAL TISSUES

Issue	LOC	Source	Affil	Rationale/Comment
Carotid sinus—over	CI	Nelson, 1992[1,a]	PT	Electrical testing/stimulating patients over the carotid sinus may induce cardiac arrhythmia.
Heart—across	CI	Nelson, 1992[1,b]		Electrical testing/stimulating patients across heart may lead to cardiac arrhythmia or fibrillation. Place electrodes so path of current does not cross the heart.

a, Should not be used; b, Should not be placed.

Y70-Y82 MEDICAL DEVICES

Issue	LOC	Source	Affil	Rationale/Comment
Demand pacemakers	CI	Nelson, 1992[1,a]	PT	Electrical testing/stimulating patients who have demand pacemakers may lead to interference with the sensitivity of the device.

a, Should not be used.

REFERENCES

1. Nelson C: Electrical evaluation of nerve and muscle excitability. In Gersh MR, editor: Electrotherapy in rehabilitation. Philadelphia: FA Davis, 1992.

2.2 Electromyography

OVERVIEW. Electromyography (EMG) employs intramuscular needle electrodes to assess motor units, including the anterior horn cell, the axon, neuromuscular junction, and all associated muscle fibers.[1]

SUMMARY: CONTRAINDICATIONS AND PRECAUTIONS. Two sources (physician and PT) cited a total of four concerns for EMG that ranged from two to four per source. The greatest proportion of concerns was procedural and related to sterile technique. The most frequently cited concerns were testing patients with bleeding tendencies or with recurrent systemic infection (also see Electrical evaluation tests).

CONTRAINDICATIONS AND PRECAUTIONS

A00-B99 CERTAIN INFECTIONS AND PARASITIC DISEASES

Issue	LOC	Source	Affil	Rationale/Comment
Recurrent systemic infection—	CI	Kimura, 1989[2]	MD	In the presence of valvular disease or prosthetic values, bacteremia (transient) following needle
unusual susceptibility	CI	Nelson, 1992[3,a]	PT	EMG may lead to endocarditis. **In 1991, Nolan[4] reported that over a 6-week period, 6 patients who received EMG at one facility developed soft tissue infections (*Mycobacterium fortuitum*) at the site of needle insertion. The clinician disinfected but did not autoclave reusable needles.**

a, Great discretion.

D50-D89 DISEASES OF BLOOD AND BLOOD FORMING ORGANS AND CERTAIN DISORDERS

Issue	LOC	Source	Affil	Rationale/Comment
Bleeding tendency	CI	Kimura, 1989[2]	MD	In patients on anticoagulants or with coagulopathy (including hemophilia and thrombocytopenia), bleeding, partial thromboplastin, and prothrombin times must be tested. Local pressure may not be sufficient to counter minimal bleeding tendencies if platelet counts fall below 20,000 mm[2]. The following case highlights the possibility of small vessel punctures during needle EMG. **Farrell[5] described a 73-year-old man with suspected lumbar radiculopathy who underwent 26-gauge needle EMG and, several hours later, developed anterior compartment syndrome (possibly from small vessel wall puncture) that required a four-compartmental fasciotomy.**
	CI	Nelson, 1992[3,a]	PT	

a, Great discretion.

PROCEDURAL CONCERNS

Issue	LOC	Sources	Affil	Rationale/Comment
Never reuse needle electrodes	P/hazardous	Nelson, 1992[3]	PT	If transmission of pathogenic organism is likely (i.e., AIDS, hepatitis, Jakob-Creutzfeldt disease)—**see Nolan.**
Sterile technique	Strictly adhere to			**See Nolan.**

REFERENCES

1. Tan JC: Practical manual of physical medicine and rehabilitation: diagnostics, therapeutics, and basic problems. St Louis: Mosby, 1998.
2. Kimura J: Electrodiagnosis in diseases of nerve and muscle: principles and practice. Philadelphia: FA Davis, 1989.
3. Nelson C: Electrical evaluation of nerve and muscle excitability. In Gersh MR, editor: Electrotherapy in rehabilitation. Philadelphia: FA Davis, 1992.
4. Nolan CM, Hashisaki PA, Dundas DF: An outbreak of soft-tissue infections due to *Mycobacterium fortuitum* associated with electromyography. J Infect Dis 163(5):1150-1153, 1991.
5. Farrell CM, Rubin DI, Haidukewych GJ: Acute compartment syndrome of the leg following diagnostic electromyography. Muscle Nerve 27(3):374-377, 2003.

OVERVIEW. The risk of sudden death and morbidity from exercise stress testing, which is generally low, is greatly increased by failing to consider contraindications for testing.[1] The American College of Cardiology/American Heart Association (ACC/AHA),[2] American College of Sports Medicine (ACSM),[3] and the American Association of Cardiovascular and Pulmonary Rehabilitation (AACVPR)[4] generally agreed on concerns. The 3 sources cited a total of 29 concerns for Exercise Testing. The overwhelming proportion (70%) of concerns was circulatory. About half of the guidelines were considered ACIs, whereas the other half viewed as RCIs. These organizations also provide guidelines for terminating an exercise test.

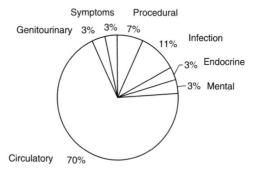

Proportion of Concerns for Exercise Testing Based on ICD

Symptoms 3%
Procedural 7%
Genitourinary 3%
Infection 11%
Endocrine 3%
Mental 3%
Circulatory 70%

CONTRAINDICATIONS AND PRECAUTIONS

A00-B99 CERTAIN INFECTIONS AND PARASITIC DISEASES

D50-D89 DISEASES OF BLOOD AND BLOOD FORMING ORGANS, AND CERTAIN DISORDERS

Issue	LOC	Sources	Affil	Qualification/Rationale/Comment
Acute infection	ACI	ACC/AHA[2,a] ACSM[3]	Org	
Chronic infectious disease	RCI	ACSM[3]	Org	(I.e., mononucleosis, hepatitis, AIDS)
Infection	ACI	AACVPR[4,a,b]	Org	The infection may affect exercise performance; exercise may aggravate the condition. Note: Exercise with fever stresses the cardiopulmonary system, the immune system, and may be further complicated by dehydration.[5]

a, Relative acute myocarditis or pericarditis; b, Also active endocarditis.
General note: Sources indicate that risk and benefits should be weighed for an RCI.

E00–E90 ENDOCRINE, NUTRITIONAL, AND METABOLIC DISEASES

Issue	LOC	Sources	Affil	Rationale/Comment
Electrolyte abnormalities	RCI	ACC/AHA[2] ACSM[3] AACVPR[4]	Org	(E.g., hypokalemia, hypomagnesemia) Note: Hypokalemia may clinically present as hypotension, arrhythmias, ECG changes, and cardiac arrest (with 2.5 mEq/L serum potassium). Hypermagnesemia may be seen in chronic renal failure and clinically presents as bradycardia, weak pulse, hypotension, heart blocks, and cardiac arrest. Hypomagnesemia may clinically present as arrhythmias, hypotension, or sometimes hypertension.[6]
Metabolic disease— uncontrolled	RCI	ACSM[3]	Org	The patient's condition may affect exercise performance; exercise may aggravate the condition, e.g., diabetes, thyrotoxicosis, myxedema.[7] Note: Hypoglycemia (<50 mg/dL) may clinically present as tachycardia, convulsions, and coma. Severe hyperglycemia (>300 mg/dL) is a life-threatening metabolic condition that can lead to diabetic ketoacidosis or hypoglycemic hyperosmolar nonketotic coma. In thyrotoxicosis, metabolism is elevated, sympathetic activity increased, and there is an increased risk of atrial fibrillations, congestive heart failure, and MIs.[7]

F00–F99 MENTAL AND BEHAVIORAL DISORDERS

Issue	LOC	Sources	Affil	Rationale/Comment
Mental impairment	RCI	ACC/AHA[2] AACVPR[4,a]		If leading to an inability to adequately exercise.

a, Inability to cooperate .

00-199 DISEASES OF THE CIRCULATORY SYSTEM

Issue	LOC	Sources	Affil	Rationale/Comment
Acute MI—within 2 days	ACI	AACVPR[4]	Org	Note: In an early post-MI, there may be activity restrictions. Uncomplicated cases are progressed in physical activity, starting with *gentle exercises* in conjunction with adequate rest periods, within the first 24 hours.[8]
Active endocarditis	ACI	AACVPR[4]	Org	Note: Endocarditis is an infection of the endocardium, heart valves, or a cardiac prosthesis; treatment includes bed rest.[8]
Angina—if unstable	ACI	ACC/AHA[2,a] ACSM[3] AACVPR[4,b]	Org	Note: If the patient presents with unstable angina, additional stress may induce an infarction.[9]
Aortic stenosis	ACI	ACC/AHA[2] ACSM[3] AACVPR[4,c]	Org	If severe and symptomatic.
Cardiac arrhythmias	ACI	ACC/AHA[2] ACSM[3] AACVPR[4]	Org	If uncontrolled, causing symptoms or hemodynamic compromise.[4] Note: Exercise may increase an arrhythmia or may induce one by increasing myocardial oxygen demand or increasing sympathetic tone.[8,9]
Dissecting aneurysm	ACI	ACSM[3] ACC/AHA[2,e]	Org	Known or suspected. Note: An aneurysm is an abnormal dilation of a vessel with a diameter $\geq$50% of normal. Weakness in the wall results in a permanent sac-like structure. A thoracic aortic aneurysm can rupture under the force of elevated blood pressure.[8,9]
Heart failure	ACI	ACC/AHA[2] ACSM[3] AACVPR[4,c]	Org	If uncontrolled and symptomatic.

Myocarditis or pericarditis—Acute	ACI	ACC/AHA[2] ACSM[3] AACVPR[4,f]	Org	Note: Pericarditis is an inflammation of the double-layered membrane—the pericardium—that surrounds the heart. In constrictive pericarditis, the fibrotic tissue compresses the heart, reduces CO, and leads to cardiac failure. One of the treatments is bed rest when fever is present (for acute idiopathic, post-MI and post-thoracotomy pericarditis).[8,9] Myocarditis is a focal or diffuse inflammation of cardiac muscle; treatment includes modified bed rest to reduce the workload of the heart.[8,9]
Pulmonary embolus or infarction—Acute	ACI	ACC/AHA[2] ACSM[3] AACVPR[4]	Org	
Resting ECG shows recent significant change	ACI	ACSM[3]	Org	If findings suggest an acute cardiac event such as an MI within 2 days. Note: ST displacement (on ECG) is the period between complete depolarization and beginning repolarization of ventricular musculature. It may be elevated or depressed in angina (transient muscle ischemia) or in muscle injury. Elevation may suggest the early stages of an MI (i.e., acute myocardial muscle damage).[8,9]
Arterial hypertension	RCI	ACC/AHA[2] ACSM[3] AACVPR[4]	Org	If severe (i.e., at rest systolic >200 mm Hg and/or diastolic >110 mm Hg).[4]
Atrial fibrillation	RCI	AACVPR[4]	Org	With an uncontrolled ventricular rate. Note: Atrial fibrillation is a chronic arrhythmia resulting in rapid irregular atrial myocardial contractions whereby blood remains in the atria. Blood flow is reduced; congestive heart failure and cardiac ischemia can develop.[8,9]

Continued

Issue	LOC	Sources	Affil	Rationale/Comment
Atrioventricular block	RCI	ACC/AHA[2] ACSM[3] AACVPR[4]	Org	If high-degree.
Bradyarrhythmias	RCI	ACC/AHA[2] ACSM[3] AACVPR[4]	Org	
Coronary stenosis	RCI	ACC/AHA[2] ACSM[3] AACVPR[4]	Org	Left main artery or its equivalent.[2-4]
Hypertrophic cardiomyopathy	RCI	ACC/AHA[2] ACSM[3] AACVPR[4]	Org	Note: Cardiomyopathy is a condition that involves myocardial muscle fiber impairment that presents similarly to CHF and can result in sudden death. Avoid risk by eliminating strenuous exercises (e.g., running, competitive sports).[8]
Other outflow tract obstructions	RCI	ACC/AHA[2] ACSM[3]	Org	
Stenotic valvular heart disease—Moderate	RCI	ACC/AHA[2] ACSM[3] AACVPR[4]	Org	Note: In severe aortic valvular heart disease, there is a low stress tolerance that is easily reached.[9]
Tachyarrhythmias	RCI	ACC/AHA[2] ACSM[3] AACVPR[4]	Org	
Ventricular aneurysm	RCI	ACSM[2]	Org	

a, If not stabilized previously by medical therapy; b, If high risk; c, If decompensated, symptomatic; d, Systolic BP >200 mm Hg and diastolic BP >110 mm Hg; e, Acute; f, Relative acute.

N00-N99 DISEASES OF THE GENITOURINARY SYSTEM

Issue	LOC	Sources	Affil	Rationale/Comment
Renal failure	ACI	AACVPR[4]	Org	This condition may affect exercise performance; exercise may aggravate condition.[4] Note: With renal failure, the concern is exacerbating the existing medical conditions with exercise. Check for physiological stability (e.g., potassium not >5 mEq/L).[10]

R00-R99 SYMPTOMS, SIGNS (ALSO POSSIBLY M00-M99 DISEASES OF THE MUSCULOSKELETAL SYSTEM AND CONNECTIVE TISSUE OR G00-G99 DISEASES OF THE NERVOUS SYSTEM)

Issue	LOC	Sources	Affil	Rationale/Comment
Physical impairment	RCI ACI	ACC/AHA[2] AACVPR[4,a]	Org	If resulting in an inability to adequately exercise.

a, If safe and adequate performance is precluded.

PROCEDURAL CONCERNS

Issue	LOC	Sources	Affil	Rationale/Comment
Disorders exacerbated by exercise	RCI	ACSM[3]	Org	If neuromuscular, musculoskeletal, rheumatoid.[3]
	ACI	AACVPR[4,a]		
Informed consent not obtained	ACI	AACVPR[4]	Org	

a, If acute non-cardiac disorder that can be exacerbated by exercise (infection, thyrotoxicosis, renal failure).
Abbreviations: ACC/AHA, American College of Cardiology/American Heart Association; ACSM, American College of Sports Medicine; AACVPR, American Association of Cardiovascular and Pulmonary Rehabilitation.

INDICATIONS FOR TERMINATING EXERCISE TESTING

I00-I99 DISEASES OF THE CIRCULATORY SYSTEM

R00-R99 SYMPTOMS, SIGNS, AND ABNORMAL CLINICAL & LABORATORY FINDINGS OF THE CIRCULATORY SYSTEM

Issue	LOC	Sources	Affil	Rationale/Comment
Systolic BP drop from baseline ≥10 mm Hg "despite increase workload, when accompanied by other evidence of ischemia"	AI	ACC/AHA[2,a] ACSM[3] AACVPR[4,a]	Org	
Angina—moderate to severe			Org	Grade 3-4.[4]
Signs of poor perfusion			Org	(Cyanosis, pallor).
Ventricular tachycardia—if sustained			Org	

"ST elevation ≥1.0 mm in leads without diagnostic Q-waves— other than V_1 or a V_R"			Org	
Systolic BP drop from baseline ≥10 mm Hg "despite increase workload, in absence of other evidence of ischemia"	RI	ACC/AHA[2,a] ACSM[3]	Org	
"ST or QRS changes such as excessive ST depression (>2 mm horizontal or down sloping ST-segment depression) or marked axis shift"		AACVPR[4]	Org	See **Resting ECG** above.
"Arrhythmias—other than sustained ventricular tachycardia"			Org	Arrhythmias such as multifocal PVCs, triplets of PVCs, supraventricular tachycardia, heart block, bradyarrhythmias.[3]
Chest pain increasing			Org	
Claudication			Org	
Development of a "bundle-branch block or intraventricular conduction delay, which can not be distinguished from ventricular tachycardia"	RI RI AI	ACC/AHA[2] ACSM[3] AACVPR[4,b]	Org	
Hypertensive response	RI	ACC/AHA[2] ACSM[3]	Org	Where systolic BP >250 mm Hg and/or diastolic BP >115 mm Hg when definitive evidence is lacking.[2]

a, >10 mm Hg; b, Only bundle-branch block mentioned.

R00-T98 SYMPTOMS, SIGNS, AND ABNORMAL CLINICAL & LABORATORY FINDINGS (NOT ELSEWHERE CLASSIFIED)

Issue	LOC	Sources	Affil	Rationale/Comment
Nervous systems symptoms increase	AI	ACC/AHA[2] ACSM[3] AACVPR[4]	Org	(E.g., ataxia, dizziness, near syncope) AACVPR CNS symptoms.[4]
Fatigue	RI	ACC/AHA[2] ACSM[3] AACVPR[4]	Org	
Shortness of breath **Wheezing** **Leg cramps**				

PROCEDURAL CONCERNS

Issue	LOC	Sources	Affil	Rationale/Comment
Technical difficulties monitoring— ECG, systolic BP	AI	ACC/AHA[2] ACSM[3] AACVPR[4]	Org	
Subject wishes to stop	AI	ACC/AHA[2] ACSM[3] AACVPR[4]	Org	

Abbreviations: ACC/AHA, American College of Cardiology/American Heart Association; ACSM, American College of Sports Medicine; AACVPR, American Association of Cardiovascular and Pulmonary Rehabilitation; AI, absolute indications for terminating; RI, relative indication.

REFERENCES

1. Richard D, Birrer R: Exercise stress testing [review]. J Fam Pract 26(4):425-35, 1988.
2. Gibbons RA, Balady GJ, Beasely JW, et al: ACC/AHA guidelines for exercise testing. J Am Coll Cardiol 30:260-315, 1997.
3. American College of Sports Medicine: ACSM's Guidelines for Exercise Testing and Prescription, ed 6. Philadelphia: Lippincott Williams & Wilkins, 2000.
4. American Association of Cardiovascular and Pulmonary Rehabilitation: American Association of Cardiovascular and Pulmonary Rehabilitation Guidelines for Cardiac Rehabilitation and Secondary Prevention Programs, ed 4. Champaign (IL): Human Kinetics, 2004.
5. Appendix B: Guidelines for Activity and Exercise. In Goodman CC, Boissonnault WG, Fuller KS, eds. Pathology: Implications for the physical therapist. Philadelphia: W.B. Saunders, 2003.
6. Goodman CC, Snyder TEK: Problems affecting multiple systems. In Goodman CC, Boissonnault WG, Fuller FS, eds. Pathology: Implications for the physical therapist. Philadelphia: W.B. Saunders, 2003. pp 85-119.
7. Goodman CC, Snyder TEK: The endocrine and metabolic systems. In Goodman CC, Boissonnault WG, Fuller KS, eds. Pathology: Implications for the physical therapist. Philadelphia: W.B. Saunders, 2003. pp 317-366.
8. Professional guide to diseases, ed 6. Springhouse (PA): Springhouse Corp., 1998.
9. Pagana KD, Pagana TJ: Mosby's Manual of Diagnostic and Laboratory Tests, ed 2. St. Louis: Mosby, 2002.
10. Boissonnault WG, Goodman CC: The renal and urologic systems. In Goodman CC, Boissonnault WG, Fuller FS, eds. Pathology: Implications for the physical therapist. Philadelphia: W.B. Saunders, 2003. pp 704-728.

4   SCREENING FOR FALLS IN OLDER PERSONS

Screening procedures may help to identify those older individuals more at risk for falls. Guidelines for fall prevention in older persons were jointly published by the (1) American Geriatric Society (AGS) on Falls in Older Persons, (2) British Geriatric Society (BGS), and (3) American Academy of Orthopaedic Surgeons (AAOS) Panel on Falls Prevention. Authors of the guidelines noted a possible synergism with falls increasing "dramatically" as the number of risk factors increase (see relative risks [RR] or odds ratio [OR] under Rationale).

Remarkably, of the 11 risk factors for falls, five factors are particularly relevant to physical rehabilitation specialists: muscle weakness, gait deviations, balance deficits, assistive devices, and impaired ADL.

PROCEDURAL ISSUES

If patient reports one fall in a year during routine care:

Issue	LOC	Source	Affil	Rationale/Comment
Observe patient do a "Get Up and Go" test (GUGT)	Guidelines[1]	AGS AAOS BGS	Org Org Org	The clinician needs to assess further if the patient is unsteady or has difficulty performing a GUGT (i.e., transferring from a chair, walking a designated distance <10 feet turning around, returning to the chair, and sitting down).

If GUGT is unsteady or difficult to perform:

Issue	LOC	Source	Affil	Rationale/Comment
Administer a falls evaluation that includes: • History of falls • Medications	Guidelines[1]	AGS AAOS BGS	Org Org Org	**Based on univariate analysis of 16 studies that examined most common risk factors for falls (i.e., mean RR or OR).** • Age >80 years = 1.7

- Acute medical problems
- Chronic medical problems
- Mobility level
- Vision
- Gait
- Balance
- LE joint function
- Neuro-evaluation
  - mental status
  - strength
  - peripheral nerve of LE
  - proprioception
  - reflexes
  - cortical functions
  - extrapyramidal cerebellar function
- Cardiovascular status (rate, rhythm, postural pulses, blood pressure, and carotid sinus stimulation if appropriate)

- History of falls = 3.0
- Particularly psychometric medications; taking >4 medications
- Impaired ADL = 2.3
- Visual deficits = 2.5
- Gait deviations = 2.9
- Balance deficits = 2.9
- Arthritis = 2.4
- Depression = 2.2; Cognitive impairment = 1.8
- Muscle weakness = 4.4 use of assistive devices = 2.6

REFERENCES

1. Guideline for the prevention of falls in older persons. J Am Geriatr Soc 49(5):664-672, 2001.

5   MOBILITY TESTING

NEURAL TENSION TESTING

Neural tension tests used to help determine what structure is causing symptoms (i.e., nerve versus musculoskeletal tissues). An example is the passive straight leg raise test. The test generally involves passively placing the neural structure in a lengthened position.

C00-C97 NEOPLASM

Issue	LOC	Source	Affil	Rationale/ Comment
Tumors	P	Monroe, 2003[1]	PT	

R00-R99 SYMPTOMS, SIGNS INVOLVING THE SYSTEM

Issue	LOC	Source	Affil	Rationale/Comment
Inflammatory conditions	P	Monroe, 2003[1]	PT	Neurological symptoms including weakness, reflex changes, loss of sensation, paresthesia/anesthesia, reflex sympathetic dystrophy.
Neurological symptoms	P			
Nerve root compression signs	P			
Pain, night	P			
Spinal cord symptoms	P			

RANGE OF MOTION ASSESSMENT, ACTIVE OR PASSIVE

The following concerns center around assessing range of motion (also see PROM; AROM)

D50-D89 DISEASES OF BLOOD & BLOOD FORMING ORGANS & CERTAIN DISORDERS

Issue	LOC	Source	Affil	Rationale/Comment
Hemophilia	P	Monroe, 2003[1]	PT	

M00-M99 DISEASES OF THE MUSCULOSKELETAL SYSTEM & CONNECTIVE TISSUE

Issue	LOC	Source	Affil	Rationale/Comment
Ankylosis—bony	P	Monroe, 2003[1]	PT	
Fragility—bone	P			Also osteoporosis.
Hypermobility—joint	P			Joint may be prone to subluxation (further instability).
Infection—joint	P			
Inflammation—joint	P			
Myositis ossificans	P			
Surgery to soft tissue—immediately after	CI			Surgeries to tendon, muscle, ligament, capsule, or skin.

R00-R99 SYMPTOMS, SIGNS INVOLVING THE SYSTEM

Issue	LOC	Source	Affil	Rationale/Comment
Hematoma	P	Monroe, 2003[1]	PT	

S00-T98 INJURY, POISONING, & CERTAIN OTHER CONSEQUENCES OF EXTERNAL CAUSES

Issue	LOC	Expert	Affil	Rationale/Comment
Dislocations—joint	CI	Monroe, 2003[1]	PT	
Fractures—unhealed	CI Extreme caution	Monroe, 2003[1] Schmitz, 2001[2]		Extreme caution if testing ROM in SCI patients with spinal instability because of the possibility of stressing the fracture site.[2]
Injury—immediately after	P	Monroe, 2003[1]		If disruption of soft tissue.

PROCEDURAL CONCERNS

Issue	LOC	Source	Affil	Rationale/Comment
Motion that disrupts healing	P	Monroe, 2003[1]	PT	The primary concern is motion that increases symptoms or intensifies a condition. Signs of undesirable motion are increase inflammation (i.e., increased pain, heat, redness).[1]
Pain medication	P			The patient may not respond appropriately to exercise if on pain medication.

REFERENCES

1. Monroe L: Motion restrictions. In Cameron MH, editor. Physical agents in rehabilitation: From research to practice. St. Louis, W.B. Saunders, 2003.

2. Schmitz TJ: Traumatic spinal cord injury. In O'Sullivan SB, Schmitz TJ, eds: Physical rehabilitation: Assessment and treatment, ed 4. Philadelphia: FA Davis, 2001.

6 PAIN ASSESSMENT

Pain assessment sometimes involves pressing a device into a patient's body part to evaluate responsiveness to pain. Two sources express concern of inflicting trauma or potentially spreading infection when applying pain assessment procedures.

PROCEDURAL CONCERNS

Issue	LOC	Sources	Affil	Rationale/Comment
Nail-bed pressure—"Pen push purpura"	FYI	Pierson, 1993[1]	MD	In 1993, Pierson described a 62-year-old comatose female with subarachnoid hemorrhage who sustained proximal nail-bed purpura of the left three middle digits of the hand from a physician who pressed a pen into her nails to elicit pain responses.
Pain-testing tools	Concern	Scott, 1969[2]	MD	The author posits the theoretical concern that non-disposable pain-testing tools (test pins, multi-pointed wheels, safety pins) may be able to transmit infection. He recommends disposable pins for use on every patient tested for pain.

REFERENCES

1. Pierson JC, Lawlor KB, Steck WD: Pen push purpura: Iatrogenic nail bed hemorrhages in the intensive care unit. Cutis 51(6):422-423, 1993.
2. Scott M: Infectious hazards of neurologic tests. N Engl J Med 280(16):904, 1969.

7   STRENGTH TESTING: ISOKINETIC TESTING & EVALUATION (CLASS II DEVICES)

This section reviews complications during isokinetic testing. Nine knee (or related) injuries were reported to the FDA from 5/28/97 to 6/25/99 in Maude and from 5/14/96 to 11/26/86 in MDR (also see **Exercise equipment** for injuries not specifically related to testing).[1]

Y70-Y82 MEDICAL DEVICES

Date	Device during Testing	Event
5/14/96	KIN-COM	A patient with an ACL surgery sustained a patella fracture during maximal strength testing. Note: No unit malfunction was noted.
9/05/95	VIDO ACTIVE	A 52-year-old female was 7 weeks post-op for a TKR and had received 4 weeks of PT. During testing, the patient felt something snap/move, resulting in extreme swelling and pain. Note: No unit malfunction was noted.
6/16/95	KINCOME	A 34-year-old female was s/p patella tendon graft for an ACL repair 14 weeks earlier. During a post-op evaluation, a loud pop was heard with the patella fracturing. No unit malfunction was found.
11/19/93	KINCOM II	During concentric and eccentric right knee testing, the actuator head moved, resulting in knee discomfort in the user.
5/10/93	KINCOM I	A man sustained a laceration to the lower leg during quadriceps testing at 80 degrees/sec in a concentric/eccentric mode when the unit's head tilted unexpectedly.

2/15/93	KINCOM 125 E+	During bilateral dual speed isokinetic knee flexion/extension testing at 100 degrees/sec, the actuator head, which was not locked, rotated and resulted in back strain in the user's muscles.
1/05/93	CYBEX 6000	During testing, the unit's adapter separated from the device, requiring additional left knee surgery in the user.
11/06/92	KINCOM II	During knee testing (comparison) at 180 degrees/sec in an eccentric mode, the user felt knee pain (no details).
2/10/92	ISOTECHNOLOGIES	A patient s/p rectal surgery re-injured a sphincter muscle during testing.

Note: FDA reports do not necessarily establish cause–effect relationships between equipment and injury. Incidences may be due to equipment or user error. Also, some reports are alleged by attorneys.

MANUAL MUSCLE TESTING

S00-T98 INJURY, POISONING, AND CERTAIN OTHER CONSEQUENCES OF EXTERNAL CAUSES

Issue	LOC	Sources	Affil	Rationale/Comment
SCI—Acute stage	Extreme caution/ Discretion	Schmitz[2]	PT	The patient may still have spinal instability that can be further stressed during manual muscle testing. An example is applying resistance to the low back and hip when testing persons with paraplegia or offering resistance to the shoulder when testing persons with tetraplegia.

REFERENCES

1. US Food and Drug Administration. Center for Device and Radiological Health. Available at: http://www.fda.gov/cdrh/mdr/. Accessed November 7, 2005.
2. Schmitz TJ: Traumatic spinal cord injury. In O'Sullivan SB, Schmitz TJ, eds: Physical rehabilitation: Assessment and treatment, ed 4. Philadelphia: FA Davis, 2001.

8   COORDINATION: COMMUNICATION AND DOCUMENTATION

8.1 Communication

To communicate means to inform or make known.[1] This section will address issues regarding (1) general communication principles, (2) communicating bad news, (3) humor and communication, (4) select patient population interactions, (5) physician telephone calls, and (6) interpreters.

GENERAL COMMUNICATION PRINCIPLES

Issue	LOC	Sources	Affil	Rationale/Comment
Actively listen	Advice	Reisfield and Wilson, 2004[2]	MD	People want to feel understood and value nonjudgmental listening. Don't think of next patient, etc.
Ambiguity				Ambiguity may be appropriate or ethically inappropriate (if patients do not want restricted information about their illness).
Attend to affective and cognitive aspects of speech				If the affective component is not addressed, underlying fears or guilt may not be adequately addressed.
Balance talking with listening				Patients get interrupted, don't always get to complete their statements (found not to take longer than 150 sec), and tend to have a hard time getting a word in or expressing their values.
Preferences				Explore what the patient's preference is for information and how they prefer it to be communicated. Do not make assumptions based on cultural factors.

DELIVERING BAD NEWS

Delivering bad news may be broken down into six steps. Baile,[3] who wrote to an oncology audience, describes a SPIKES approach (Setting up, Patient Perceptions, Invitation by the patient, providing Knowledge, Empathizing, Summary and Strategy).

Issue	LOC	Sources	Affil	Rationale/Comment
Prepare—for the discussion	Advice	Baile et al, 2000[3]	MD	Set up the environment: arrange for privacy, mentally rehearse, manage time
		Reisfield and Wilson, 2004[2,a]	MD	constraints, and arrange for interpreters.[3]
Find out what the patient knows				What are the patient's perceptions of his or her medical situation?[3]
Find out what the patient wants to know				Ask how the patient prefers to get information on a test.[3]
Tell the news—at appropriate level				Avoid technical words and excessive bluntness[3] (e.g., *spread*, not *metastasized*).
Respond				Provide an empathetic response[3] (e.g., "I know this is not what you wanted to hear").
Plan—for the future				If the patient is willing, discuss options.[3]

a, Reisfield's advice is based on a 1992 book by Buckman (*How to Break Bad News*), the second author in Baile's[3] 2000 SPIKE approach.

HUMOR TO COMMUNICATE

OVERVIEW. Humor can be viewed as an intervention to promote health and well-being, cope with stress and illness, or establish rapport by appreciating the incongruity in life's situations.

Four sources cited a total of seven concerns for humor when working with patients. Concerns ranged from one to three per source with nursing citing the largest number. The most frequently cited concern was making fun of others (cited by two sources).

Issue	LOC	Sources	Affil	Rationale/Comment
Abstract humor	CI	Vergeer and MacRae, 1993[4]	OT	Humor that requires abstract thought.
				Based on Vergeer and MacRae's qualitative phenomenological interviews with five occupational therapists who used humor therapeutically in practice
Inappropriate humor	CI	Crane, 1987[5]	Nurs	From clinicians: humor as an jokes or poorly timed (at the height of a patient's illness).
				From patients: Personal attacks or sexually aggressive remarks made by the patient. Don't encourage a patient's inappropriate humor. Instead consult with a social worker or psychologist to get at the root of the problem.
Incomprehensible humor	CI[a]	Vergeer and MacRae, 1993[4]	OT	Humor for those unable to understand the joke (i.e., unshared culture)
				Based on Vergeer and MacRae's[4] qualitative phenomenological interviews with five occupational therapists who used humor therapeutically in practice
Judging humor	Advice	Crane, 1987[5]	Nurs	Some patients use humor to cope with fear or a sense of loss. Don't judge it.
Making fun of others	CI	Vergeer and MacRae, 1993[4]	OT	Humor that makes fun of people affects confidence, destroys teamwork, and singles out
	Advice	Goodman, 1992[6]	EdD	people who are different.
				Based on Vergeer and MacRae's qualitative phenomenological interviews with five occupational therapists who used humor therapeutically in practice
Receptivity	Caution	Leiber, 1986[7]	Nurs	Assess patient's receptivity to humor.
Sarcasm	Advice	Crane, 1987[5]	Nurs	Sarcasm destroys a person's self-worth and dignity.

a, Jokes.

PATIENT INTERACTIONS

The following section contains suggestions for interaction with individuals with visual, hearing, mental retardation, cerebral palsy, and spinal cord injuries.

Visual Impairment, Person With

Issue	LOC	Sources	Affil	Rationale/Comment
Directing conversation	Advice	McConnell, 1996[8]	Nurs	Talk to the person, not the companion.
Doors and drawers	Advice			Keep doors completely open or closed, but keep dresser drawers closed.
Good-byes	Advice			Tell the person when you are leaving the room. Otherwise, they may think you are still present and continue talking to you.
Guide dog	Advice			Do not interfere with, excite, or feed a guide dog.
Introductions	Advice	King, 1995[9]	Nurs	Introduce yourself before speaking. Later introductions may be less necessary as person with visual
		McConnell, 1996[8]	Nurs	impairment becomes more familiar with the visitor.
Orientation	Advice	King, 1995[8]	Nurs	Orient the person to the room.
		McConnell, 1996[8]	Nurs	
Permissions	Advice	King, 1995[9]	Nurs	Ask permission before touching or performing a task (i.e., vital signs)
Return items	Advice	McConnell, 1996[8]	Nurs	Return all items to their original locations.
Seating arrangements	Advice	King, 1995[9]	Nurs	Used preferred and planned seating arrangements.
Voice tone	Advice			Speak in a normal tone. The person will not see better if you raise your voice.
Walking assistance	Advice	McConnell, 1996[8]	Nurs	If the individual needs help walking, have him or her take your arm. Do not grab the person. Do not drag the person around.

Hearing Impairment, Persons With

Issue	LOC	Sources	Affil	Rationale/Comment
Determine mode of communication	Advice	King, 1995[9]	Nurs	Inquire if sign language, an interpreter, lip reading, or writing will be used.
Directing communication	Advice			Speak to the person, not an interpreter; it is rude to speak to the interpreter.
Eye contact	Advice			
Gesture or sign to facilitate communication	Advice			Learn to sign a little.
Lip reading	Advice			Don't exaggerate lip movements; lip reading becomes more difficult.
Voice tone	Advice			Speak in a normal voice tone.
Voicing opinions	Advice			Encourage expression of opinion; have pen and paper available if necessary.

Cerebral Palsy, Persons With

Issue	LOC	Sources	Affil	Rationale/Comment
Communication boards	Advice	King, 1995[9]	Nurs	If a communication board is used, articulate word or letter loudly.
Difficulty understanding	Advice			If you cannot understand the person, ask him/her to spell the word or use a synonym.
Directing communications	Advice			Speak directly to the person. Do not assume he/she is deaf or has mental retardation.
Interpreters	Advice			A person with CP whose speech is unaffected serves as a possible interpreter for a person with CP whose speech is affected.

Mental Retardation, Persons With

Issue	LOC	Sources	Affil	Rationale/Comment
Assistance	Advice	King, 1995[9]	Nurse	Ask if the person needs assistance.
Directing communication	Advice			Speak directly to the person. Don't speak through a partner.
Eye contact	Advice			Maintain eye contact.
Voicing opinion	Advice			Allow the person to express opinions.
Voice tone	Advice			Speak in a normal voice tone.

Spinal Cord Injury, Persons With

Issue	LOC	Sources	Affil	Rationale/Comment
Accessibility—wheelchair	Advice	King, 1995[9]	Nurse	Arrange the room so that a wheelchair can easily maneuver around. Ensure that areas, parking, etc., are wheelchair accessible so person feels welcomed.
Conversation position	Advice			Sit at the level of the person (i.e., wheelchair level). Only stand to emphasize a point.
Voicing opinions[a]	Advice			Allow for expression of opinion.

a, I am not sure why the author includes this guideline, as this is such a highly vocal, productive patient population (in general).

PHYSICIANS—TELEPHONE INTERACTIONS

Issue	LOC	Sources	Affil	Rationale/Comment
Gather all data before call	Advice	Sperling, 2001[10,a]	Nurs	Gather all notes.
Organize your thoughts	Advice			Organize your thoughts so you don't forget to mention or request information.
Refresh physician's memory	Advice			Briefly give synopses of past days or week.
Recommendation and justify	Advice			Prepare to make your recommendation and defend it.
Behavior—professional	Advice			Treat office personnel professionally, as colleagues.
Indicate where to sign	Advice			If mailing documentation for signing, indicate where to sign.
Email	Advice			If the physician is accessible by email, use it.
For emerging patient problems, call, don't wait	Advice			If a patient concern emerges, call the physician, do not wait. Provide a direct phone number for returning a call. Do not use your voice mail number for returning calls.

a, Sperling's guide was written within the context of nurse-physician interaction.

TRANSLATORS

Issue	LOC	Sources	Affil	Rationale/Comment
Family members as translators	Advice	Rollins, 2002[11]	—	Avoid liability problems and safety concerns. Interpreters must have health care delivery experience and should have translation certification (e.g., Spanish). Note: It may be undesirable for children to serve as interpreters for their parents because of the inappropriate role reversal they're placed in, as well as exposure and access to confidential/inappropriate medical information.

ADVERSE EVENTS

Source	Background	Design	Outcome	Comments
Vergeer and MacRae, 1993[4] **Humor and CI** Qualitative (phenomenological; interview) Am J Occup Ther	Five occupational therapists were interviewed who used humor therapeutically in the San Francisco Bay area in a variety of settings.	16 themes, including contraindications to humor in therapy, were identified in the analysis.	Contraindications for humor included: (1) humor that makes fun of people, (2) humor that requires abstract thought, (3) humor for those unable to understand the joke (i.e., unshared culture).	Note: The authors did not elaborate on the rationale or specific incidents that led to formation of the stated contraindications.
Wells et al, 2003[12] **Writing questions for their doctors** Descriptive Clin Oncol	88 patients, mean age 60.5 years, were permitted to list questions and discussion topics on a pro forma prior to seeing their doctor in an outpatient oncology unit. Cancer diagnoses included breast (56), lung (9), anus (4), melanoma (4), thyroid (4), colon (3), sarcoma (3), esophagus (2), lip (1), lymphoma (1), and mesothelioma (1).	65 of the 88 listed one or more questions. 23 failed to write down any questions.	The authors suggest providing patients with the opportunity to list their own questions to doctors, which may be a useful aid to communication and should be studied further. Also, patients may be less likely to forget topics important to them if they write them down on paper. They argue that: (1) Using checklists can be seen as patronizing; and (2) Physicians and patients misunderstand each other without acknowledging it.	Note: The study examined only the use of a technique, not its effectiveness in improving understanding. Furthermore, the study was part of a correspondence, and the design was not reported in detail.

REFERENCES

1. Webster's third new international dictionary. Springfield, MA: Merriam-Webster, 1981.
2. Reisfield GM, Wilson GR: Communicating with patients and families. Clin Fam Pract 6:325-347, 2004.
3. Baile WF, Buckman R, Lenzi R, et al: SPIKE—A six step protocol for delivering bad news: Application to the patient with cancer. Oncologist 5:302-322, 2000.
4. Vergeer G, MacRae A: Therapeutic use of humor in occupational therapy. Am J Occup Ther 47(8):678-683, 1993.
5. Crane AL: Why sickness can be a laughing matter. RN 50:41-42, 1987.
6. Goodman JB: Laughing matters: Taking your job seriously and yourself lightly. JAMA 267(13):1858, 1992.
7. Leiber DB: Laughter and humor in critical care. Dimensions Crit Care Nurs 5(3):162-170, 1986.
8. McConnell EA: Caring for a patient who has a vision impairment. Nursing 26(5):28, 1996.
9. King EH: Health teaching for people with disabilities. Home Healthcare Nurse 13(6):52-58, 1995.
10. Sperling R: Communicating with physicians. Home Healthcare Nurse 19(8):463, 2001.
11. Rollins G: Translation, por favor. Hosp Health Netw 76(12):46-50, 2002.
12. Wells T, Falk S, Dieppe P: Let patients have their say: Reducing miscommunication [correspondence]. Clin Oncol 15(5):298, 2003.

8.2 Documentation

OVERVIEW. Documentation is an act of authenticating with factual or substantial support.[1] Guidelines for medical documentation of patient care have been collected from occupational therapy, physical therapy, and nursing sources and grouped under (1) content, (2) editing, (3) procedural, and (4) style issues.

SUMMARY: CONTRAINDICATIONS AND PRECAUTIONS. Seven sources cited a total of 32 concerns for medical documentation. Concerns ranged from 5 to 11 per source. Most concerns were content-related (what should be included within a document). The most frequently cited concern was how entry errors were to be corrected.

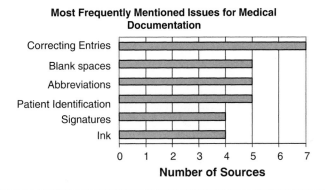

Most Frequently Mentioned Issues for Medical Documentation

CONTRAINDICATIONS AND PRECAUTIONS

Content of Entries

Issue	LOC	Sources	Affil	Rationale/Comment
Adverse incidents	Advice	Quinn and Gordon, 2003[2]	PT	Follow institutional policies for completing incident reports.
Appointments—Missed	Advice	Quinn and Gordon, 2003[2]	PT	Document missed appointments. Record if the patient missed a session.
Complete and objective entries	Advice	Pierson and Fairchild, 2003[3]	PT	Avoid incomplete, subjective entry, or inconsistent (left vs. right hip). Information should be sufficient for a new team to take over a case and pick up where the old team left off.[3] Use objective measures.[6]
		Smith, 2001[6]	Nurse	
Derogatory statements	Advice	Quinn and Gordon, 2003[2]	PT	Avoid derogatory statement about a patient: "Patient reports" instead of "Patient complains..."
Documenting actions	Advice	McConnell, 1999[4]	Nurse	Document actions taken, not just the problem. If a serious patient event occurs, document all actions, all reports to others (i.e., physician), and objective observations.
		Eggland, 1993[5]	Nurse	
Document communications	Advice	Smith, 2001[6]	Nurse	Document all calls and responses to primary care provider. For telephone conversations, record name, time, issue discussed, and action taken.[2]
		Quinn and Gordon, 2003[2]	PT	
Document facts only	Advice	Smith, 2001[6]	Nurse	Use patient's comments in quotes. Don't document assumptions or opinions.
		Eggland, 1993[5]	Nurse	
Home program chart	Advice	Pierson and Fairchild, 2003[3,a]	PT	Documentation should include: • Patient understood program • Required equipment or assistance • Precautions/Contraindications

				• Goals
				• How one knows goals were achieved
				• When/whether to terminate program
				• Contact information
				• Follow-up information
				Place program in the medical record.
Informed consent	Advice	Smith, 2001[6]	Nurse	Document patient informed and consented to procedures.
		Quinn and Gordon, 2003[2]	PT	Document that patient acknowledges an *understanding* of the procedure.[2]
Professional negligence—Suggesting	Advice	Smith, 2001[6]	Nurse	Do not suggest staffing problems or professional negligence in document.
Referral mechanism	Guideline	APTA, 2004[7,a]	Org	For physical therapy, document how service was initiated, e.g., self-referral, consultation.

a, PTA guidelines serve a general purpose only and are not designed to reflect unique requirements of specialty areas.

Editing Documents

Issue	LOC	Sources	Affil	Rationale/Comment
Amending someone's document	Advice	Smith, 2001[6]	Nurse	Do not amend someone else's document.
Backdating		Eggland, 1993[5]	Nurse	Don't backdate an entry; indicate "late entry" with date and time. Backdating
		Quinn and Gordon, 2003[2]	PT	is illegal.[2]

Continued

Issue	LOC	Sources	Affil	Rationale/Comment
Correcting entries	Advice	Pierson and Fairchild, 2003[3]	PT	Avoid tampering with, writing over, or whiting out words.
		Smith, 2001[6]	Nurse	• Correct entry by drawing a single line through inaccurate information that is still legible; date and initial the corrections.[7,8]
		McConnell, 1999[4]	Nurse	
		Eggland, 1993[5]	Nurse	• Add a note in the margin stating why correction was necessary.[3]
	Guideline	APTA, 2004[7]	Org	• Follow hospital policy for correcting documents.[6]
	Advice	Quinn and Gordon, 2003[2]	PT	• Write "mistaken entry," not "error."[4]
	Guideline	Clark et al, 2003[8]	Org	• Don't throw away a note.[5]
				• Date and note time of the corrected entry.[2]
Liquid correction	Guideline	Clark et al, 2003[8]	Org	Don't use liquid correction or erasures.

PROCEDURAL CONCERNS

Issue	LOC	Sources	Affil	Rationale/Comment
Confidentiality	Guideline	Clark et al, 2003[8]	Org	Comply with confidentiality standards.
How soon to chart?	Advice	McConnell, 1999[4]	Nurse	Chart as soon as possible after service is delivered. Information is still "fresh," and there is less chance of entering errors in chart.[2]
		Quinn and Gordon, 2003[2]	PT	
Patient ID	Advice	McConnell, 1999[4]	Nurse	Confirm you have the correct patient chart or computer record with patient's name on each page.
		Eggland, 1993[5]	Nurse	
		Quinn and Gordon, 2003[2,a]	PT	
	Guideline	APTA, 2004[7,a]	Org	
	Guideline	Clark et al, 2003[8]	Org	

Records: Storage and destruction	Guideline	Clark et al, 2003[8]	Org	Comply with laws or agency for storage and destruction of records.
Signing documents	Advice	Smith, 2001[6]	Nurse	Don't sign your name or cosign unless you provided the care or observed it.
		Quinn and Gordon, 2003[2,b,c]	PT	For students or graduates pending an unrestricted license, the supervisor cosigns.[7]
	Guideline	APTA, 2004[7,b]	Org	
	Guideline	Clark et al, 2003[8,b]	Org	
Technology		Clark et al, 2003[8]	Org	Adhere to technological standards (e.g., digital).
Type of document, OT, agency	Guideline	Clark et al, 2003[8]	Org	
When to chart	Advice	Smith, 2001[6]	Nurse	Chart *only after* servicing; not before. Do not document care before you provide the service.
		Eggland, 1993[5]	Nurse	

a, Have patient's name and ID number on each page; b, Sign full name, date, and professional designation; c, Signatures should be original.

Style Concerns

Issue	LOC	Sources	Affil	Rationale/Comment
Abbreviations	Advice	Pierson and Fairchild, 2003[3]	PT	Use accepted abbreviations. Check with approved symbols and abbreviations at your facility.[4]
		McConnell, 1999[4]	Nurse	
		Eggland, 1993[5]	Nurse	
		Quinn and Gordon, 2003[2]	PT	
	Guideline	Clark et al, 2003[8]	Org	

Continued

Issue	LOC	Sources	Affil	Rationale/Comment
Blanks or open spaces between entries	Advice	Pierson and Fairchild, 2003[3]	PT	Avoid blanks or open spaces between entries; blank lines can allow insertions. If an entry completes on part of a line, draw a horizontal line to the end of the line.[4] Draw a straight line through any open spaces.[2] Don't leave space between the end of entry and the signature.[8]
		Smith, 2001[6]	Nurse	
		McConnell, 1999[4]	Nurse	
		Eggland, 1993[5]	Nurse	
		Quinn and Gordon, 2003[2]	PT	
	Guideline	Clark et al, 2003[8]	Org	
Conciseness	Advice	Quinn and Gordon, 2003[2]	PT	Write concisely, using approved abbreviations and keeping your audience in mind with regard to professional jargon.
Ink	Advice	McConnell, 1999[4,a]	Nurse	Use ink. Avoid pencil or felt-tip markers.
		Eggland, 1993[5,a,b]	Nurse	
		Quinn and Gordon, 2003[2]	PT	
	Guideline	APTA, 2004[7]	Org	
Legibility	Advice	Pierson and Fairchild, 2003[3]	PT	Write legibly.
		Smith, 2001[6]	Nurse	
		Quinn and Gordon, 2003[2]	PT	
People-first language	Advice	Quinn and Gordon, 2003[2]	PT	Use people-first language: "A man with an above-knee amputation"; not "An amputee...."
Poor English	Advice	Smith, 2001[6]	Nurse	Avoid errors in grammar, spelling, and punctuation.
		McConnell, 1999[4]	Nurse	Start each sentence with a capital letter.[5]
Terminology	Guideline	Clark et al, 2003[8]	Org	Use accepted terminology for your setting.

a, Use black ink; b, Used prescribed ink for institution; c, Original signature in handwritten ink; maintain secure and confidential if electronic.

REFERENCES

1. Webster's third new international dictionary. Springfield, MA: Merriam-Webster, 1981.
2. Quinn L, Gordon J: Functional outcomes: Documentation for rehabilitation. St. Louis: W.B. Saunders, 2003.
3. Pierson FM, Fairchild SL: Principles and techniques of patient care. Philadelphia: W.B. Saunders, 2003.
4. McDonnell EA: Do's and don'ts: Charting with care. Nursing 29(10):68, 1999.
5. Eggland ET: Documentation do's and don'ts. Nursing 23(8):30, 1993.
6. Smith LS: Charting tips: Documentation do's and don'ts. Nursing 31(9):30, 2001.
7. American Physical Therapy Association. Guidelines for physical therapy documentation. Available at: http://www.apta.org/governance/HOD/policies; accessed November 23, 2004.
8. Clark GF, Youngstrom MJ, Brayman SJ: Commission on practice guidelines for documentation of occupational therapy (2003). Am J Occup Ther 57(6):646-649, 2003.

9   PATIENT INSTRUCTIONS

OVERVIEW. To instruct means to give special information, knowledge, or skill.[1] Two sources offer advice on instructing patients using auditory, cognitive, tactile, visual, and written methods. Ruholl[2] addresses the elderly patient's needs, whereas Balson[3] offers general advice on patient education from a pharmacist's perspective. Issue are organized by sensory modality, cognition, and written materials.

CONTRAINDICATIONS AND PRECAUTIONS

Auditory Considerations

Issue	LOC	Sources	Affil	Rationale/Comment
Do not shout	Advice	Ruholl, 2003[2]	—	
Hearing aids				Have patient wear hearing aid during the session. Assess problems: dead battery, poor fit, improper volume.
Face patient				Patients may compensate for a hearing loss by reading lips.
Level your mouth with their eyes				
Move closer to stronger ear				
Rephrasing				Ask patient to repeat or rephrase what they have learned.
Speak at lower pitch				
Speak at moderate pace				
Voice quality				Don't let your voice "fall off" at the end of sentences.

Cognitive Issues

Issue	LOC	Sources	Affil	Rationale/Comment
Active involvement of patient	Advice	Ruholl, 2003[2]	—	Have patient suggest location of an exercise program (i.e., at the mall).
Break down task				Have patient assist in the procedure, learn steps in a procedure by having them assist or by "clumping" to address short-term memory problems. Break down task into smaller steps.
Give an overview				First give an overview of teaching session.
Initiate the teaching session	Advice	Balson, 1995[3]	Pharm	Providers should initiate the teaching session. Patients may be reluctant to ask questions.
Limit amount of information provided				Patients forget much of the information. Adjust amount of information to individual need.
Open-ended questions				Ask open-ended questions to get more information. Ask, "How do you take your medications?" rather than, "Do you take your medications?"
Patient assisting in the procedure	Advice	Ruholl, 2003[2]	—	
Pause before changing topic				
Patient receptiveness				Avoid times when difficult to concentrate (medication, naps).
Simple language				Keep communication simple. Use active voice, few syllables, and short sentences.
Stick to small, discrete messages; avoid long lists of items				Don't hurry; allow time for the patient to process information.
				Cognitive processes decline with aging due to loss of neurons and reduced blood flow, leading to loss of abstract thinking. Watch for prolonged processing times, limited short-term memory, test anxiety, and afterimaging (fixating on an idea previously discussed).
Written tests				Avoid written tests of knowledge. Avoid test anxiety situations (try to not act like a "schoolteacher"). Instead, conduct verbal tests of what has been learned.

Tactile Considerations

Issue	LOC	Sources	Affil	Rationale/Comment
Type of material	Advice	Ruholl, 2003[2]	—	Avoid Styrofoam, slick paper, and lightweight plastic materials. These materials may be difficult to handle. Pressure, temperature, and texture sensitivity diminish with age.

Visual Issues

Issue	LOC	Sources	Affil	Rationale/Comment
Bright lighting	Advice	Ruholl, 2003[2]	—	Use bright overhead lighting. Desk lighting (at an angle) can cause glare. It is easier to read contrasting upper- and lowercase lettering. Note: The author uses theoretical notions and secondary references and textbooks throughout in citing evidence.
Demonstrate	Advice	Balson, 1995[3]	Pharm	Show as well as tell to enhance learning.
Eye contact				Maintain eye contact; show interest.
Pill—name or shape				Refer to pills by name or shape. Avoid identifying pills by color. Retinal changes lead to reduced color perception with age.

Written Material

Issue	LOC	Sources	Affil	Rationale/Comment
All capitals letters or italics	Advice	Ruholl, 2003[2]	—	Avoid written material with all capitals letters or italics. It is difficult to read.
Grade level	Advice	Ruholl, 2003[2] Balson, 1995[3,a]	— Pharm	Prepare handouts at or below the 5th-grade level. The elderly currently comprise one-third of the low-literacy population and read at a lower reading level. Most handouts are written at the 9th-grade level but need to be written at the 5th-grade level.
Highlighting	Advice	Balson, 1995[3]	Pharm	Highlighting as you speak personalizes the information.
Keep images simple	Advice	Ruholl, 2003[2]	—	Use uncluttered illustrations and pictures.
Large print				Recommend large-print labels on medications.
Literacy				Confirm literacy. If giving written information, make sure they can read it first.
Personalize instructions				The patient will feel they are "my instructions." Personalize the handout with the patient's name and fill in sections for specific instructions.
Small fonts				Avoid a font size smaller than 12 points. Consider Times New Roman, Courier, Geneva, Palatino, or Century Gothic—these fonts are easy to read.
Written material with verbal counseling	Advice	Balson, 1995[3]	Pharm	Do not just give written material. Use written material *in conjunction with* verbal counseling.

a, 3rd- to 5th-grade level

REFERENCES

1. Webster's third new international dictionary. Springfield (MA): Merriam-Webster; 1981.
2. Ruholl L: Tips for teaching the elderly. Med Econ 66(5):48-52, 2003.
3. Balson A: The do's and don'ts of patient education. Hosp Pharm 30(7):625-626, 1995.

10 INFECTION CONTROL

10.1 Guidelines for Hand Hygiene in Health-Care Settings

The Centers for Disease Control (CDC), Health Care Infection Control Practice Advisory Committee (HICPAC), Society for Healthcare Epidemiology of America (SHEA), Infectious Disease Society of America (DSA), and Association for Professionals in Infection Control (APIC) have made 2002 Hand Hygiene recommendations for the use of soap and water and alcohol-based rubs in the health care center.[1] Proper hand hygiene can help prevent the spread of antimicrobial-resistant infections, whereas poor hand hygiene may be a contributing factor in patient mortality. Compliance for hand hygiene is noted to be problematic among health care workers.[2]

Interestingly, the CDC/HICPAC recommendations address rehabilitation-related concerns such as hand hygiene management after lifting patients or touching equipment near patients. Along with guidelines below, additional recommendations for health care workers include keeping nail tips $< \frac{1}{4}$ inch length; not using same gloves on more than one patient; changing gloves when moving from a contaminated to an uncontaminated body site; wearing gloves if contacting blood, mucous membranes, non-intact skin or other infectious material; and not wearing artificial fingernails or extenders if one has direct contact with high-risk patients (e.g., ICU, operating rooms).

SOAP AND WATER

The CDC/HICPAC recommends you wash with *soap (non-antimicrobial or antimicrobial) and water* under the following circumstances.

Use soap (non-antimicrobial or antimicrobial) and water if:

Issue	LOC	Sources	Affil	Rationale/Comment
Hands are visibly dirty	Strongly recommended	CDC/HICPAC, 2002[1]	Org	Also if hands are visibly soiled with blood, other body fluids, or contaminated with proteinaceous material. Supported by well-designed studies.
Before eating	Strongly recommended			Supported by some studies and has a strong theoretical rationale.
After using the restroom	Strongly recommended			Supported by some studies and has a strong theoretical rationale.
Exposure to *Bacillus anthracis*— known or suspected	Suggested			Alcohol and other antiseptic activity against these spores are poor. Instead, the physical action of hand washing is recommended.

Procedure: Using Soap and Water

CDC/HICPAC recommends you wash with soap and water in the following manner: (1) Wet hands. (2) Apply amount of soap recommended by manufacturer. (3) Rub hands together vigorously for at least 15 seconds. (4) Rinse hands with water. (5) Dry hands thoroughly with a disposable towel. (6) Use towel to shut off faucet. (7) Avoid hot water (because repeated exposure increases risk of dermatitis). (8) If soap bar is used, drain soap on rack and use small bars. (9) Avoid multiple use of cloth towels (handing type; roll type)—they are not recommended in a health care setting.

ALCOHOL-BASED HAND RUB

The CDC/HICPAC recommends you use *alcohol-based hand rubs* under the following circumstances.

Use an alcohol-based hand rub if:

Issue	LOC	Sources	Affil	Rationale/Comment
Hands are not visibly dirty	Strongly recommended	CDC/HICPAC, 2002[1]	Orgs	Supported by well-designed studies.
Before direct patient contact if hands are not visibly dirty	Strongly recommended			Supported by some studies and has a strong theoretical rationale.
After patient contact (with their skin), if hands are not visibly dirty	Strongly recommended			For example, after lifting patients or taking blood pressures or pulses. Supported by some studies and has a strong theoretical rationale.
During patient care, when moving from a contaminated to a clean body area	Suggested			
After contacting inanimate objects	Suggested			For example, medical equipment in immediate area of patient.
After removing gloves	Strongly recommended			Supported by some studies and has a strong theoretical rationale.
Before inserting a central intravascular catheter with sterile gloves, if hands are not visibly dirty	Strongly recommended			Supported by some studies and has a strong theoretical rationale.

Before inserting a urinary catheter, peripheral vascular catheter, or other invasive device (not surgical procedures) if hands are not visibly dirty	Strongly recommended	Supported by some studies and has a strong theoretical rationale.
After contact with body fluids, excretions, mucous membranes, non-intact skin, wound dressing, if hands are not visibly dirty	Strongly recommended	Supported by well-designed studies.

Procedure: Using an Alcohol-Based Hand Rub

The CDC/HICPAC recommends the following technique for using alcohol-based hand rubs: (1) Apply the alcohol-based hand rub to one palm. Follow the manufacturer's recommended volume to use. (2) Rub hands together. (3) Cover all surfaces of your hands and fingers until hands are dry.

REFERENCES

1. Guidelines for Hand Hygiene in Health-Care Settings. MMWR Recommendation and Reports Oct 25, 2002/51 (RR16)/1-44.
2. Trampuz A, Widmer AF: Hand hygiene: A frequently missed lifesaving opportunity during patient care. Mayo Clin Proc 79(1):109-116, 2004.

10.2 Universal Precautions

The Centers for Disease Control (CDC) made 1987 recommendations for the prevention of HIV, hepatitis B virus, and other pathogens (blood-borne) transmission when providing health care or first aid.[1-3] These recommendations, known as Universal Precautions (or Universal Blood and Body Fluid Precautions), are briefly summarized below. For detailed guidelines of these and other precautions involving invasive procedures, dentistry, mortician services, dialysis, laboratories, and environmental considerations for HIV transmission (such as infection, housekeeping, decontamination of spills, and laundry) consult the CDC 1987[1] (and CDC 1988 supplement & clarification[3]) publications at http://www.cdc.gov/mmwr/preview/mmwrhtml/00023587.htm and http://www.cdc.gov/mmwr/preview/mmwrhtml/00000039.htm.

PROCEDURAL

Universal Precautions: Appropriate barrier precautions should be routinely used by all health care workers to prevent skin and mucous membrane exposure when contact with patient's blood or other body fluids is anticipated. Blood and body fluid precautions should be consistently used for *all* patients. Use gloves for touching blood, body fluids, mucous membranes, or non-intact skin of all patients, or when performing procedures for vascular access. Change gloves after contact with each patient. Use masks and protective eyewear or face shield if the procedure is likely to generate droplets of blood or fluids to prevent exposure of mucous membranes of mouth, nose, and eyes. Use gowns or aprons if procedure generates splash of blood or other body fluids. Wash skin surfaces (e.g., hands) immediately/thoroughly if contaminated with blood or other body fluids. Wash hands immediately after glove removal.	CDC, 1987[1-3]	Medical history and examination cannot reliably identify all patients infected with blood-borne pathogens or HIV.

Prevent injuries with sharp instruments (i.e., needles, scalpels). Do not recap needles or manipulate them with your hand. All sharp instruments and disposable syringes should be disposed of in puncture-resistant containers as close to the use area as practically possible.

Mouthpieces, resuscitation bags, and other ventilation devices should be available in areas anticipated. Even though saliva is not implicated in HIV transmission, minimize need for emergency mouth-to-mouth resuscitation.

Health care workers with exudative lesions or weeping dermatitis should refrain from all direct patient contact and equipment until condition is resolved.

Pregnant health care workers should be familiar with precautions to minimize risk of HIV transmission because of risk to the fetus from perinatal transmission.

REFERENCES

1. Centers for Disease Control and Prevention: CDC MMWR Supplements Recommendations for Prevention of HIV Transmission in Health-Care Settings. Aug 21, 1987/36(SU02). Available at: http://www.cdc.gov/epo/mmwr/preview/mmwrhtml/00023587.htm. Accessed May 17, 2005.
2. Centers for Disease Control and Prevention: Issues in Health Care Settings Universal Precautions for Prevention of Transmission of HIV and Other Bloodborne Infections. Available at: http://www.cdc.gov/ncidod/hip/Blood/universa.html/. Accessed May 17, 2005.
3. Centers for Disease Control and Prevention: Perspectives in Disease Prevention and Health Promotion Update: Universal Precautions for Prevention of Transmission of Human Immunodeficiency Virus, Hepatitis B Virus, and Other Bloodborne Pathogens in Health-Care Settings. MMWR Weekly 37(24):377-388, 1988. Available at: http://www.cdc.gov/mmwr/preview/mmwrhtml/00000039.htm. Accessed May 17, 2005.

10.3 Acquired Infections and Technologically-Dependent Children

The American Academy of Pediatrics, Committee on Injury and Poison Prevention, has made 2001 recommendations to protect technologically dependent children who tend to be more prone to acquiring infectious diseases.

Issue	LOC	Source	Affil	Rationale /Comment
Infection and technologically dependent children	Advice	AAP, 2001[1]	Org	Children who rely on technology may be at increased risk of acquiring infectious diseases. Caregivers should wash hands before and after providing direct care for patients (i.e., toileting, tracheostomy, gastrostomy care), employ universal precautions for blood-containing body fluids, and follow legal requirements of their state or OSHA regarding immunizations.

Note: For other rehabilitation-related infection concerns, see **Toys** (Exercise equipment), **Blood pressure cuffs** (Tests), and **Hydrotherapy**.

REFERENCES

1. American Academy of Pediatrics, Committee on Injury and Poison Prevention: School bus transportation of children with special health care needs. Pediatrics 108(2):516-518, 2001.

11   AEROBIC

11.1 Aerobic Exercises

OVERVIEW. Aerobic exercise involves submaximal, rhythmic, repetitive activity that uses large muscle groups and requires increasing uptake of oxygen.[1] The goal for aerobic exercise is improved fitness (cardiovascular function), endurance (prolonged work without fatigue), maximal oxygen uptake (improved efficiency), conditioning (increased energy capacity), adaptation (ability to satisfy energy requirements at increasing activity levels), and the avoidance of deconditioning.

Some equipment used during these repetitive exercises includes ergometers, treadmills, aquatics, pulleys, weights, hydraulics, elastic resistive bands, robotics, and mechanical devices.

SUMMARY: CONTRAINDICATIONS AND PRECAUTIONS. Aerobic exercise concerns chiefly center around cardiac disease (placing increasing O_2 demand on a stressed system), poorly controlled metabolic disorders (leading to potential cardiac complications), retinopathy (offending blood pressure and traction forces), orthopedic problems (if high impact on joints), neuropathies (sensory loss-related impact injuries; abnormal autonomic cardiac responses), renal/dialysis complications (poorly controlled comorbidities), and pregnancy (if mother or fetus are stressed).

Notes: (1) "Red flags " noted by one source[2] are conditions that may present with serious symptoms and signs during exercise—not just aerobic exercise. These conditions and associated signs suggest timely medical referral and/or management. (2) Aerobic exercise is a broad topic with diverse source backgrounds; some concerns may overlap with resistive exercise (also see **Resistive exercise**).

CONTRAINDICATIONS AND PRECAUTIONS

C00-C97 NEOPLASMS

Issue	LOC	Sources	Affil	Rationale/Comment
Spinal cord compression signs in persons with metastatic spinal lesions	Advice/red flag	Musnick and Hall, 2005[2]	MD	These patients may present with bone pain and new onset of neurological signs/symptoms. If neurological signs or bladder symptoms are noted, refer immediately. This condition may present with serious symptoms and signs during exercise.[2]

E00-E90 ENDOCRINE, NUTRITIONAL AND METABOLIC DISEASES

Issue	LOC	Sources	Affil	Rationale/Comment
Diabetes—hypoglycemia	Advice/red flag	Musnick and Hall, 2005[2]	MD	This condition may present with serious symptoms and signs during exercise. Ask to bring meter with strips to therapy in case hypoglycemic episode.[2] Note: Uncontrolled glucose levels can affect cardiovascular and neurological function. Hypoglycemia (<50 mg/dL), which may result from insulin overdose, exhaustive exercise, illness, or skipping meals, can clinically present as tachycardia, convulsions, and coma.[3]

Metabolic disease— uncontrolled	ACI	Neid and Franklin, 2002[4,a]	MD	Note[3,5]: Uncontrolled metabolic disease can affect cardiovascular function. Hypokalemia may clinically present as hypotension, arrhythmias, ECG changes, and cardiac arrest (with 2.5 mEq/L serum potassium), whereas hyperkalemia may present as tachycardia, bradycardia, ECG changes, and cardiac arrest (with >7.0 mEq/L serum potassium levels).
				In hyperthyroidism (also thyrotoxicosis), metabolism is elevated in most systems, with an increased risk of atrial fibrillations, congestive heart failure, and MI. Hypocalcemia can clinically present as arrhythmias and may be seen in renal failure. Hypernatremia can present as hypertension and tachycardia, whereas hyponatremia, which may be seen with liver cirrhosis, can present as hypotension, tachycardia, a thready pulse (reflects reduced stroke volume), and vasomotor collapse. Hypermagnesemia may be seen in chronic renal failure and clinically presents as bradycardia, a weak pulse, hypotension, heart block, and cardiac arrest. Hypomagnesemia may present as arrhythmias, hypotension, or sometimes hypertension.[3,5]
Obesity	P	Hoffman, 2005[6,b]	MD	If predisposed to injury, avoid weight-bearing activities to minimize the risk of musculoskeletal injuries.

a, Neid and Franklin specifically address aerobic exercises concerns in the elderly; b, Injury precautions: the risk of injury increases with rapid increase in participation, abnormal biomechanics, previous injury history, or weight-bearing exercises.

G00-G99 DISEASES OF THE NERVOUS SYSTEM

Issue	LOC	Sources	Affil	Rationale/Comment
Neuropathy—autonomic—diabetes	Advice	ADA, 2003[7]	Org	Vigorous exercise increases risk of a cardiovascular event.
	Advice	ACSM position[8]	Org	In autonomic neuropathy (diabetes type 2) increased resting heart rate, a depressed maximal heart rate and blood pressure, exercise-induced hypotension, and possible absent early warning indicators for ischemia may occur. Do low-level activities and stress test.[8]
Neuropathy—peripheral (significant)—diabetes (with loss of protective sensation) The following may be CI: • Treadmill • Prolonged walking • Jogging • Step exercise	Advice CI	ACSM position[8,a] ADA, 2003[7]	Org Org	In peripheral neuropathies (diabetes type 2), loss of distal sensation in lower leg and feet may result in infection and musculoskeletal injury. Repetitive exercises on insensitive feet can ultimately lead to ulceration and fractures.[7,8] Weight-bearing exercises should be limited if protective sensation is lost in significant peripheral neuropathies.[8] Participate in non–weight-bearing activities to reduce trauma.[8] Consider non–weight-bearing exercises such as swimming, bicycle riding, rowing, chair exercise, and arm exercises.[7]
Thermoregulation—diabetes	Advice	ADA, 2003[7]	Org	Individuals with diabetes may have difficulty with thermoregulation. Avoid activity in hot/cold environment; provide hydration.

a, Also use proper footwear while weight bearing, and conduct daily foot inspections.

H00-H59 DISEASES OF THE EYE

Issue	LOC	Sources	Affil	Rationale/Comment
Proliferative diabetic retinopathy	Avoid	ADA, 2003[7]	Org	Avoid anaerobic exercise and physical activity involving Valsalva maneuvers, straining, jarring. Strenuous activity may precipitate vitreous hemorrhage or traction retinal detachment.
	Caution	ACSM position stand[8]	Org	Supervised low-intensity aerobic activities are suggested in retinopathy; caution with activities that increase blood pressure such as head-down, jarring, and arm-overhead activities.[8]

I00-I99 DISEASES OF THE CIRCULATORY SYSTEM

Issue	LOC	Sources	Affil	Rationale/Comment
Cardiomyopathy	RCI	Neid and Franklin, 2002[4]	MD	Note: Cardiomyopathy is a condition that involves myocardial muscle fiber impairment and presents similarly to CHF. It may, rarely, result in sudden death. Because of this risk, strenuous exercises such as running and competitive sports are avoided.[9]
Cardiovascular disorders • Coronary artery • Heart valve • Cardiac tissue • Rhythm disturbance	Red flags	Musnick and Hall, 2005[2]	MD	These conditions may present with serious symptoms and signs during exercise.[2] The "profile" of an individual with the greatest risk of cardiovascular complications during exercise includes multiple myocardial infarction history, left ventricular function impairment (ejection fraction <30%), angina at rest or unstable, arrhythmias at rest (serious), multivessel atherosclerosis (significant) revealed on angiography, and low serum potassium (others may also experience complications).[2]

Continued

Issue	LOC	Sources	Affil	Rationale/Comment
				Note that a review of an individual's coronary risk factors helps in planning an exercise program (risk stratification).[10] For example, those deemed to be at moderate risk (e.g., having two or more risk factors[a] or satisfying age criteria[b]) would need a medical exam and exercise test before initiating vigorous exercise (see Exercise testing). Those at high risk[c] would need both exam and testing before starting moderate or vigorous exercise. Those with a recent coronary event might be under supervision in a cardiac rehabilitation program (see Cardiac rehab).[6]
Complex ventricular ectopy	RCI	Neid and Franklin, 2002[4]	MD	
Congestive heart failure—unstable	ACI			
Deep venous thrombosis	Red flag	Musnick and Hall, 2005[2]	MD	If DVT is suspected, refer to ER or physician within next few hours and walk minimally because of concern that the clot may break off from the vessel. This condition may present with serious symptoms and signs during exercise.[2] Note: DVT can lead to pulmonary embolism, a common cause of sudden death in hospitals.[11]
ECG changes or MI—recent	ACI	Neid and Franklin, 2002[4]	MD	Note: The ST segment is the period between complete depolarization and beginning repolarization of ventricular musculature It may be elevated or depressed in angina (transient muscle ischemia) or (cardiac) muscle injury. Elevation may suggest early states of an MI (acute myocardial muscle damage).[12] During an MI (heart attack) reduced blood flow to coronary artery leads to myocardial ischemia and necrosis. Treatment includes reducing the cardiac workload.[13]
Heart block—3rd degree	ACI			Note: A heart block is a disorder of the heart's conduction system that can present as fatigue, dizziness, and fainting and may require a pacemaker.[9]

Issue	LOC	Sources	Affil	Rationale/Comment
Hypertension—uncontrolled	ACI	Neid and Franklin, 2002[4]	MD	
Pulmonary embolism	Red flag	Musnick and Hall, 2005[2]	MD	If PE is suspected, send immediately to ED. This condition may present with serious symptoms and signs during exercise.[2] Note: A pulmonary embolism is a potentially fatal condition where blood supply to lung parenchyma is obstructed by a blood clot lodged in the pulmonary artery.[11]
Valve heart disease	RCI	Neid and Franklin, 2002[4]	MD	Note: In severe aortic valvular heart disease, stress tolerance is low.[12]

a, Family history of myocardial infarction, sudden death, or coronary revascularization; smoker (cigarettes); hypertension; hypercholesterolemia; impaired fasting glucose; obesity; sedentary; high serum HDL cholesterol. b, Men ≥45 years old; women ≥55 years old. c, Cardiovascular, pulmonary, or metabolic disease (known) or one or more sign/symptoms (pain-discomfort due to ischemia [i.e., anginal], SOB [with mild exertion or rest], syncope or dizziness; orthopnea or paroxysmal nocturnal dyspnea; ankle edema, palpitations, or tachycardia; intermittent claudication, unusual fatigue or SOB with usual activities; heart murmur [known]).[10]

J00–J99 DISEASES OF THE RESPIRATORY SYSTEM

Issue	LOC	Sources	Affil	Rationale/Comment
Allergies, exercise-related—reactions	Advice/red flag	Musnick and Hall, 2005[2,a]	MD	These allergy-related conditions may present with serious symptoms and signs during exercise.[2] Three types of reactions are (1) exercise-related hives. (2) angioedema, and (3) anaphylactic shock. If exercise-related anaphylactic shock history,[b] ask patient to bring in their epinephrine kit and have them exercise with someone.[2]
Asthma—active	Advice/red flag			This condition may present with serious symptoms and signs during exercise.[2] Encourage the patient to bring inhaler and peak flow meter to therapy (also see Sports).

Continued

Issue	LOC	Sources	Affil	Rationale/Comment
Pulmonary disease, chronic	Advice/red flag			These conditions may present with serious symptoms and signs during exercise.[2]
Upper respiratory tract infection	Advice/red flag			

a, Not necessarily limited to aerobic/endurance activities; b, Possibly induced by vigorous aerobic exercise.

M00-M99 DISEASES OF THE MUSCULOSKELETAL SYSTEM AND CONNECTIVE TISSUE

Issue	LOC	Sources	Affil	Rationale/Comment
Biomechanical abnormalities	Advice	Hoffman, 2005[6]	MD	Avoid weight-bearing activities to minimize injury risk because this condition may be predisposed to musculoskeletal injury.[6]
Fibromyalgia syndrome and chronic fatigue syndromes	Advice	Bennett, 2005[14]	PT	Relapse or symptom exacerbation can be caused by overexertion.[14]
Low back pain	Advice	Bezner, 2005[15]	PT	Choose activities that support the back.
Musculoskeletal fitness—inadequate	Avoid	Tan, 1998[16,a]	MD/PT	Activities of concern include contact sports, sports involving twisting, and high-impact activity if fitness is inadequate
Osteoarthritis—high-impact aerobic training	Avoid / Advice	O'Grady, 2000[17] / Bezner, 2005[15]	MD / PT	High-impact aerobic training with rapid application of loads is the concern for patients with osteoarthritis. The rate of joint loading may be important in producing pain and joint damage[17] (also see **Elderly—procedures**). Consider non–weight-bearing activities.
Osteoporosis	Advice	Bezner, 2005[16]	PT	During activities, choose postures that minimize risk of fracture (see **Resistive exercise**).
Meniscectomy—partial arthroscopic	P	Kisner and Colby, 1996[1]	PT	Progress cautiously when adding high-impact weight-bearing activities because of the concern of causing additional articular knee damage (e.g., jumping, jogging) .

a, If not well conditioned and not in good musculoskeletal condition.

Issue	LOC	Sources	Affil	Rationale/Comment
Exercising (high intensity) on dialysis days	P	Painter, 1995[18]	—	Exercise on non-dialysis days. Patients may feel fatigued and uncomfortable 1-2 hours following dialysis. The cardiovascular system will vasoconstrict to maintain blood pressure; exercise would counter this by causing vasodilation, possibly leading to hypotension. Stable patients (i.e., fluid and diets) may exercise at moderate intensities on dialysis days.
Exercising 1 to 2 hours following dialysis	P			
Hyperparathyroidism, renal osteodystrophy or other bone disease—long-standing, secondary	P Advice	Painter, 1995[18] Copley and Lindberg, 1999[19,a]	— —	The risk of orthopedic injuries increases in this population: avoid high-impact and heavy-resistance activities or increased grades on a treadmill (due to stress on Achilles tendon). Fractures and tendon ruptures due to weakness at the tendon-bone level have been reported. Copley suggests low-impact exercise to minimize orthopedic stress.[19] To minimize risks of exercise: (1) provide adequate dialysis, (2) control hypertension, (3) monitor and manage medical concerns (cardiac; glucose, potassium, calcium, phosphorus, parathyroid hormone, serum albumin levels). Note: Other exercise precautions are needed if the renal patient also has CAPD, diabetes, or cardiovascular disease.[19]
Weight gain (excessive) between dialysis treatments	P	Painter, 1995[18]	—	Avoid exercise immediately before dialysis if there is an excessive weight gain. The cardiac system is already stressed because of the extra fluid in the system.

Continued

Issue	LOC	Sources	Affil	Rationale/Comment
Shunt area—dialysis patient	Avoid	Pierson and Fairchild, 2002[20]	PT	Avoid excessive activity in the area of the shunt.
Nephropathy—diabetes type 2 activities that increase SBP	Avoid	ACSM position, 2000[8]	Org	With nephropathy, avoid activities that cause systolic BP to rise to 180-200 mm Hg such as a Valsalva, high-intensity aerobics, or strengthening. In later stages, perform low-intensity physical activities; undergo stress testing in advanced nephropathy and diabetes type 2 to establish safe exercise limits.[8]

a, Copley and Lindberg (1991) also offer the following advice for exercising with persons on dialysis: (1) Monitor weight and volume overload in end stage renal disease. Have frequent assessments of dry weight to avoid volume overload. (2) Manage comorbidities. These include metabolic bone disease, diabetes mellitus, arthritis, infection, anemia, hypertension. (3) Have a prolonged, adequate warm-up period to combat potential deleterious effects of plasma catecholamine increases associated with exercise. Engage in an adequate cool-down period to enhance venous return and reduce the possibility of postexercise hypotension and to combat the potential deleterious effects of plasma catecholamine increases associated with exercise.
Abbreviation: CAPD, continuous ambulatory peritoneal dialysis.

O00-O99 PREGNANCY, CHILDBIRTH, AND PUERPERIUM

Pregnancy: Issues When Aerobic Exercise Is CI

Issue	LOC	Sources	Affil
Anemia—severe	RCI	ACOG, 2002[21]	Org
Bleeding—persistent (second or third trimester)	ACI		
Bronchitis—chronic	RCI		

Cardiac arrhythmia—maternal (unevaluated)	RCI
Cervix/cerclage—incompetent	ACI
Diabetes type 1—poorly controlled	RCI
Heart disease—hemodynamically significant	ACI
Heavy smoker	RCI
Hypertension—poorly controlled	RCI
Hyperthyroidism—poorly controlled	RCI
Intrauterine growth restrictions in current pregnancy	RCI
Lung disease—restrictive	ACI
Multiple gestation at risk for premature labor	ACI
Obesity—extreme morbid	RCI
Orthopedic limitations	RCI
Placenta previa—after 26 weeks of gestation	ACI
Preeclampsia—pregnancy-induced hypertension	ACI
Premature labor—during current pregnancy	ACI
Ruptured membranes	ACI
Sedentary lifestyle—history (extreme)	RCI
Seizure disorder—poorly controlled	RCI
Underweight—extreme (BMI <12)	RCI

Pregnancy: Warning Signs to Terminate Exercise

Issue	LOC	Sources	Affil
Abdominal pain—unexplained	Terminate	ACSM, 2000[8]	Org
Amniotic fluid leakage	Terminate	ACOG, 2002[21]	Org
		ACSM, 2000[8,a]	Org
Calf pain or swelling	Terminate	ACOG, 2002[21,b]	
		ACSM, 2000[8,c]	
Chest pain	Terminate	ACOG, 2002[21]	
		ACSM, 2000[8]	
Dizziness	Terminate	ACOG, 2002[21]	
		ACSM, 2000[8] (or faintness; unexplained)	
Dyspnea prior to exertion	Terminate	ACOG, 2002[21]	
Fatigue—excessive	Terminate	ACSM, 2000[8]	
Fetal movement—decreased	Terminate	ACOG, 2002[21]	
Headache	Terminate	ACOG, 2002[21]	
		ACSM, 2000[8] (persistent, severe)	
Muscle weakness	Terminate	ACOG, 2002[21]	
Palpitations	Terminate	ACSM, 2000[8]	
Preterm labor	Terminate	ACOG, 2002[21]	
		ACSM, 2000[8,d]	
Pulse rate or blood pressure elevation that persists after exercise	Terminate	ACSM, 2000[8]	
Swelling (sudden) of ankle, hand, or face	Terminate	ACSM, 2000[8]	

Vaginal bleeding	Terminate	ACOG, 2002[21]	
		ACSM, 2000[8]	
Weight gain—insufficient (<1 kg/month during last two trimesters)	Terminate	ACSM, 2000[8]	

a, Premature rupture of membranes; gush of fluid from vagina (ACSM, 2000)[8]; b, Need to rule out thrombophlebitis; c, Phlebitis swelling, pain, or redness in the calf of one leg; d, Onset of premature labor—persistent contractions (>6-8/hour).

R00-R99 SYMPTOMS, SIGNS, AND ABNORMAL CLINICAL AND LABORATORY FINDINGS: FOR EXERCISE

Issue	LOC	Sources	Affil	Rationale/Comment
Fever and strenuous exercise	Avoid	Hoffman et al, 2005[6,a]	MD	The effects of exercise on an existing infection (i.e., viral respiratory infection) are poorly understood.[19] It is believed that myocarditis can develop when an individual exercises continuously in the presence of illness such as a respiratory infection.[6]
Glucose >250 mg/dL in diabetes	Red flag	Musnick and Hall, 2005[2]	MD	Do not start aerobic exercise at these levels as these are potentially serious lab value results to have during exercising. Note: Uncontrolled glucose levels can affect cardiovascular and neurological function. In severe hyperglycemia (>300 mg/dL), life-threatening metabolic conditions can develop such as diabetic ketoacidosis or hypoglycemic hyperosmolar nonketotic coma.[3]

Continued

Issue	LOC	Sources	Affil	Rationale/Comment
Heart rate • <50 bpm; or • Pause between beats >3 seconds or • 120 bpm 5 min following exercise • >140 bpm and chest pain[b]	Red flags			These are potentially serious signs and symptoms during exercise.[2]
Hemoglobin—low (<8 g/dL)	CI	Goodman and Kelly Snyder, 2003[22]	PT	Therapeutic interventions are contraindicated as the patient may present with fatigue, tachycardia, and poor exercise tolerance.
Myalgia and strenuous exercise	Avoid	Hoffman et al, 2005[6]	MD	
Platelet count—reduced (<15,000 to 20,000)	Advice	Goodman and Kelly Snyder, 2003[22]	PT	Reduced platelet counts suggests a serious potential for bleeding. Check with guidelines at your local facility regarding activity restrictions (e.g., only AROM, only ADL, only ambulation).
Potassium <3.2 mEq/L or >5.1 mEq/L	CI			Because of the possibility of arrhythmias and tetany, physical therapy is contraindicated.
Prothrombin time ≥2.5 times the reference range	CI			Because of the risk of spontaneous bleeding, PT and OT are contraindicated. (Note: These levels may be common in patients with mechanical valves.)
Respiration rate >20/min	Red flag/CI	Musnick and Hall, 2005[2]	MD	This is a potentially serious sign.[2] Unless there is a known chronic pulmonary condition, exercise is contraindicated.
Syncope	Red flag			This is a potentially serious sign. If non-vasovagal-related syncope occurs more than once, therapy should be terminated and the patient should be accompanied by someone to an ED.[2]

Systolic blood pressure **≥170 mm Hg**	Red flag/CI			This is a potentially serious sign. Exercise is contraindicated. Isometrics may be contraindicated if systolic pressure is >140.[2]
Systolic blood pressure **<85 mm Hg**	Red flag/CI			This is a potentially serious sign. Exercise is contraindicated.
White blood cell counts—low **(<5000/mm³ with fever)**	Suggest no exercise	Goodman and Kelly Snyder, 2003[22]	PT	As a general recommendation, low WBC counts suggest not exercising, but an individual determination should be made. Good hygiene is also important as the patient will be susceptible to opportunistic infections.

a, Illness precautions; b, Medical emergency.

S00-T98 INJURY, POISONING, AND CERTAIN OTHER CONSEQUENCES OF EXTERNAL CAUSES

Issue	LOC	Sources	Affil	Rationale/Comment
Previous injury	Advice	Hoffman, 2005[6]	MD	Avoid weight-bearing activities to minimize injury risk because this condition may be predisposed to musculoskeletal injury.[6]

PROCEDURAL CONCERNS

Issue	LOC	Sources	Affil	Rationale/Comment
Activity—gradually increase	Advice	Hoffman, 2005[6]	MD	To minimize injury risk.
Age—young • Exercise at lower intensity in hot environments • Give time to acclimate	Advice	Benzer, 2005[15]	PT	Children are less efficient at dissipating heat because of a higher threshold for sweating, lower rate of sweating, and higher level of metabolic heat generation for their size than adults.
Age—elderly • Low-impact activities	Advice			Activities that minimize impact on joints should be chosen for this population, such as water, bicycling, or stair-climbing activities.
Bicycling • Wear helmet • Comply with local laws	Advice			Note: Baby boomers have a higher number of emergency department-treated injuries associated with bicycling compared with 15 other popular sports (1998 data).[23]
Educate participants	Advice			Promote education to reduce complications from exercise.
Emergency plan	Advice			Have one to reduce complications during exercise.
Footwear, proper	Advice	Hoffman, 2005[6]	MD	To minimize injury risk.[6]
Impact activities, returning to— e.g., impact aerobics, jogging, sport-related jumping	Advice	Benzer, 2005[15]	PT	Progressively return to impact activities (i.e., "impact progression") to minimize chance of setbacks. Prerequisites for return include no swelling, full range of motion, and sufficient strength and endurance.
Intensity	Advice			Encourage mild to moderate exercise intensities initially to reduce complications during exercise.
Medical clearance/follow-up	Advice			To reduce complications from exercise, obtain clearance.

Monitoring • On-site medical supervision (if needed) • ECG monitoring (select patients)	Advice	Monitor to reduce complications from exercise.
Recreational games	Advice	Modify rules and minimize competition to reduce complications during exercise.
Screening/medical evaluation	Advice	Screening/medical evaluation is needed to determine if supervision is required during exercise. Note: See **Cardiovascular disorders** above.
Supervision	Advice	Maintain supervision during the recovery period to reduce complications from exercise.
Temperature of environment	Advice	Precautions in cold and heat (increased cardiac demands) to reduce complications during exercise.
Warm-up/cool-down	Advice	Emphasize these activities before and after vigorous exercise and stretches.

REFERENCES

1. Cameron MH: Physical agents in rehabilitation: From research to practice. St. Louis: W.B. Saunders, 2003.
2. Musnick D, Hall C: Red flags: Potentially serious symptoms and signs in exercising patients. Appendix 2. In Hall CM, Brody LT, eds: Therapeutic exercise: Moving toward function. Philadelphia: Lippincott Williams & Wilkins, 2005.
3. Goodman CC, Snyder TEK: The endocrine and metabolic systems. In Goodman CC, Boissonnault WG, Fuller KS, eds: Pathology: Implications for the physical therapist. Philadelphia: W.B. Saunders, 2003.
4. Neid RJ, Franklin B: Promoting and prescribing exercise for the elderly. Am Fam Phys 65(3):419-426, 2002.
5. Goodman CC, Snyder TEK: Problems affecting multiple systems. In Goodman CC, Boissonnault WG, Fuller KS, eds: Pathology: Implications for the physical therapist. Philadelphia: W.B. Saunders, 2003.
6. Hoffman MD, Sheldahl LM, Kraemer WJ: Therapeutic exercise. In: DeLisa JA, editor: Rehabilitation medicine and rehabilitation: Principles and practice, vol 1, ed 4. Philadelphia: Lippincott Williams & Wilkins, 2005.
7. American Diabetes Association: Physical activity/exercise and diabetes. Diabetes Care 26:S73-S77, 2003.

8. Albright A, Franz M, Hornsby G, et al: ACSM position stand: Exercise and type 2 diabetes. Med Sci Sports Exerc 32(7):1345-1360, 2000.

9. Goodman CC: The cardiovascular system. In Goodman CC, Boissonnault WG, Fuller KS, eds: Pathology: Implications for the physical therapist. Philadelphia: W.B. Saunders, 2003.

10. American College of Sports Medicine: ACSM's guidelines for exercise testing and prescription, ed 6. Philadelphia: Lippincott Williams & Wilkins; 2000.

11. Goodman CC: The respiratory system. In Goodman CC, Boissonnault WG, Fuller KS, eds: Pathology: Implications for the physical therapist. Philadelphia: W.B. Saunders, 2003.

12. Pagana KD, Pagana TJ: Mosby's manual of diagnostic and laboratory tests, ed 2. St. Louis: Mosby, 2002.

13. Professional guide to diseases, ed 6. Springhouse (PA): Springhouse, 1998.

14. Bennett K: Therapeutic exercise for fibromyalgia syndrome and chronic fatigue syndrome. In: Hall CM, Brody LT, eds: Therapeutic exercise: Moving toward function. Philadelphia: Lippincott Williams & Wilkins, 2005.

15. Bezner JR: Impaired aerobic capacity/endurance. In: Hall CM, Brody LT, eds: Therapeutic exercise: Moving toward function. Philadelphia: Lippincott Williams & Wilkins, 2005.

16. Tan JC: Practical manual of physical medicine and rehabilitation: Diagnostics, therapeutics, and basic problems. St. Louis: Mosby, 1998.

17. O'Grady M: Therapeutic and physical fitness exercise prescription. Rheum Dis Clin North Am 26:617-646, 2000.

18. Painter P, Blagg CR, Moore GE: Exercise for the dialysis patient. Madison (WI): The Life Options Rehabilitation Advisory Council Medical Education Institute, 1995.

19. Copley JB, Lindberg JS: The risks of exercise. Adv Renal Replac Ther 6(2):165-171, 1999.

20. Pierson FM, Fairchild SL: Principles and techniques of patient care, ed 3. Philadelphia: W.B. Saunders, 2002.

21. ACOG Committee Obstetric Practice: ACOG Committee opinion. Number 267, January 2002: Exercise during pregnancy and the postpartum period. Obstet Gynecol 99(1):171-173, 2002.

22. Goodman CC, Kelly Snyder TE: Laboratory tests and values. In Goodman CC, Boissonnault WG, Fuller KS, eds: Pathology: Implications for the physical therapist. Philadelphia: W.B. Saunders, 2003.

23. Consumer Product Safety Commission: Baby boomer sports injuries. April 2000. Available at: http://www.cpsc.gov/library/boomer.pdf. Accessed: October 26, 2005.

11.2 Aquatic Therapy

OVERVIEW. Aquatic therapy is a comprehensive approach to exercise in water that is designed to increase strength, flexibility, endurance, circulation, and relaxation[1] (also see **Hydrotherapy**).

SUMMARY: CONTRAINDICATIONS AND PRECAUTIONS. Five sources cited a total of 39 concerns for aquatic therapy. Concerns ranged from six to 24 per source, with a PT citing the largest number. The largest proportion of concerns related to digestive disease (e.g., aspiration risk, bowel incontinence) followed by medical devices (e.g., tracheostomy, catheters). The most frequently cited concerns were infectious diseases and cardiovascular patients who became worse following immersion. Understandably, there is overlap between concerns for patients during full-body immersion hydrotherapy and aquatic therapy.

In a 2003 survey of aquatic therapy and rehabilitation practitioners, Wykle[2] reported that facilities offering aquatic therapy do not have adequate staffing, appropriate rescue equipment, and communication systems.

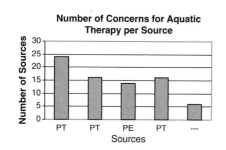

Number of Concerns for Aquatic Therapy per Source

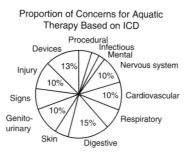

Proportion of Concerns for Aquatic Therapy Based on ICD

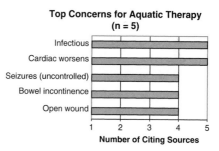

Top Concerns for Aquatic Therapy (n = 5)

CONTRAINDICATIONS AND PRECAUTIONS

A00-B99 CERTAIN INFECTIONS AND PARASITIC DISEASES

Issue	LOC	Sources	Affil	Rationale/Comment
Infectious diseases	CI	Giesecke, 1997[3,c]	PT	
	CI/P	McNeal, 1997[4,b]	PT	
	CI	Bates and Hanson, 1996[1,a]	PE	
	P	Petersen, 2004[5,d]	PT	
	CI	Haralson, 1985[6]	—	

a, Guidelines are CI for pool therapy; b, Rheumatoid disease populations; c, Spinal cord injury populations; d, Pediatric populations indicated similar concerns to adults.

F00-F99 MENTAL AND BEHAVIORAL DISORDERS

Issue	LOC	Sources	Affil	Rationale/Comment
Cognitive impairments	CI/P	McNeal, 1997[4]	PT	The concern is whether the client can safely enter/transfer into the pool.
	P	Bates and Hanson, 1996[1,a]	PE	

a, Requires supervision

G00-G99 DISEASES OF THE NERVOUS SYSTEM

Issue	LOC	Sources	Affil	Rationale/Comment
Autonomic dysreflexia	P	Giesecke, 1997[3]	PT	Monitor closely and begin with short sessions (15 minutes).
Seizures—uncontrolled	CI	Giesecke , 1997[3,a]	PT	
	CI	Petersen, 2004[5]	PT	
	CI/P	McNeal, 1997[4]	PT	
	CI	Bates and Hanson, 1996[1]	PE	
Sensory loss	P	Giesecke, 1997[3]	PT	Monitor for abrasions (i.e., feet dragging on bottom); consider protective pads for feet and knees.
Thermoregulation— poor in tetraplegia or high paraplegia	P	Giesecke, 1997[3]	PT	Monitor patient and temperature of water and air. These individuals with SCI have difficulty regulating temperature well, have decreased sweating and shivering ability below the level of their lesion, and are prone to heat prostration and hypothermia.

a, Also if recent seizure.

I00-I99 DISEASES OF THE CIRCULATORY SYSTEM

Issue	LOC	Sources	Affil	Rationale/Comment
Blood pressure—uncontrolled (high or low)	CI	Giesecke, 1997[3]	PT	
	CI/P	McNeal, 1997[4,a]	PT	
	CP	Bates and Hanson, 1996[1,b]	PE	

Continued

Issue	LOC	Sources	Affil	Rationale/Comment
Cardiac involvement	P	Giesecke, 1997[3]	PT	Monitor closely and start with short sessions (15 minutes).
Cardiovascular disease (severe)	P	Petersen, 2004[5]	PT	The concern is primarily for persons with CHF or cardiac involvement and
with symptoms exacerbated	CI/P	McNeal, 1997[4]	PT	their response to body immersion.
with immersion	CI	Haralson, 1985[6]	—	
	CI	Bates and Hanson, 1996[1]	PE	
	P	Giesecke, 1997[3]	PT	
Orthostatic hypotension	P	Giesecke, 1997[3]	PT	Monitor closely and start with short sessions (15 minutes).

a, Severe; b, Abnormal.

J00-J99 DISEASES OF THE RESPIRATORY SYSTEM

Issue	LOC	Sources	Affil	Rationale/Comment
Infectious respiratory event	P	Petersen, 2004[5]	PT	
Respiratory compromise—severely limited	P	Giesecke, 1997[3]	PT	
Vital capacity <1 L	CI	Giesecke, 1997[3]	PT	
	CI	Bates and Hanson, 1996[1,b]	PE	
	P	Petersen, 2004[5,a]	PT	

a, Severe respiratory compromise where respiratory symptoms are exacerbated when immersed; b, 900 to 1500 mL.

K00-K93 DISEASES OF THE DIGESTIVE SYSTEM

Issue	LOC	Sources	Affil	Rationale/Comment
Aspiration—history or aspiration precautions	P	Petersen, 2004[5]	PT	
Bowel incontinence— uncontrolled	CI	Giesecke, 1997[3]	PT	Manage with stool program and appropriate swim undergarment.[1]
	CI/P	McNeal, 1997[4]	PT	
	CI	Bates and Hanson, 1996[1]	PE	
	P	Petersen, 2004[5]	PT	
Diarrhea—persistent	CI	Petersen, 2004[5]	PT	
Gastrointestinal disorder	CI	Bates and Hanson, 1996[1]	PE	
Orofacial control—reduced	CI/P	McNeal, 1997[4]	PT	
Ostomies	P	Giesecke, 1997[3]	PT	

L00-L99 DISEASES OF THE SKIN AND SUBCUTANEOUS TISSUE

Issue	LOC	Sources	Affil	Rationale/Comment
Dry skin—area of skin folds	P	Giesecke, 1997[3]	PT	
Rashes	CI	Giesecke, 1997[3]	PT	Most of these authors express concern for contagious rashes.
	CI/P	McNeal , 1997[4]	PT	
	CI	Haralson 1985[6]	—	
	CI	Bates and Hanson, 1996[1]	PE	

N00-N99 DISEASES OF THE GENITOURINARY SYSTEM

Issue	LOC	Sources	Affil	Rationale/Comment
Bladder incontinence— uncontrolled	CI	Giesecke, 1997[3]	PT	
	CI/P	McNeal, 1997[4]	PT	
	CI	Bates and Hanson, 1996[1]	PE	
Bladder incontinence in children	P	Petersen, 2004[5]	PT	Until 3 years, accept child incontinence in the pool. Older children are expected to urinate before the aquatic therapy session.
Kidney disease	CI	Bates and Hanson, 1996[1]	PE	Where there is inability to adjust to fluid loss.
Urinary tract infections	CI	Haralson, 1985[6]	—	

R00-R99 SYMPTOMS, SIGNS, AND ABNORMAL CLINICAL AND LABORATORY FINDINGS (NOT ELSEWHERE CLASSIFIED)

Issue	LOC	Sources	Affil	Rationale/Comment
Fever	CI	Giesecke, 1997[3]	PT	Note: Exercise with fever stresses the cardiopulmonary and immune systems.[7]
	CI/P	McNeal, 1997[4]	PT	
	CI	Haralson, 1985[6]	—	
	P	Petersen, 2004[5,a]	PT	
	CI	Bates and Hanson, 1996[1,b]	PE	
Parent reports child "does not seem well"	P	Petersen, 2004[5]	PT	This may be the first signs of an illness.
Severely limited endurance	CI/P	McNeal, 1997[4]	PT	Monitor closely and start with short sessions (15 minutes).[3]
	P	Giesecke, 1997[3]	PT	

a, ≥100° F; b, If >100° F.

S00-T98 INJURY, POISONING, AND CERTAIN OTHER CONSEQUENCES OF EXTERNAL CAUSES

Issue	LOC	Sources	Affil	Rationale/Comment
Burns—acute stage	CI	Petersen, 2004[5]	PT	
Eardrum—perforated	CI	Bates and Hanson, 1996[1]	PE	
Orthopedic injuries—acute	P	Giesecke, 1997[3]	PT	Obtain orthopedic approval.[3]
	CI/P	McNeal, 1997[4,a]	PT	
Wounds—open without	CI	Petersen, 2004[5]	PT	Cover with waterproof dressing.[3]
bio-occlusive dressing	CI/P	McNeal, 1997[4,c]	PT	
	CI	Haralson, 1985[6,b]	—	
	P	Giesecke, 1997[3]	PT	

a, With instability; b, Open wounds; c, Also pressure ulcer.

Medical Devices

Issue	LOC	Sources	Affil	Rationale/Comment
Catheters—indwelling and	P	Giesecke, 1997[3]	PT	
condom catheters	CI/P	McNeal, 1997[4]	PT	
Gastrostomy tubes (G tube)—	P	Giesecke, 1997[3]	PT	
clamped	CI/P	McNeal, 1997[4]	PT	

Continued

Issue	LOC	Sources	Affil	Rationale/Comment
Nasogastric tubes	P	Petersen, 2004[5]	PT	
Suprapubic appliances— allowed with special handling	P	Giesecke, 1997[3]	PT	
Tracheostomy	CI	Giesecke, 1997[3]	PT	
	CI	Petersen, 2004[5]	PT	
	CI/P	McNeal, 1997[4]	PT	

PROCEDURAL CONCERNS

Issue	LOC	Sources	Affil	Rationale/Comment
Radiation treatment—last 3 months	CI	Bates and Hanson, 1996[1]	PE	
Stool program—ineffective	CI	Petersen, 2004[5]	PT	

Contraindications for Cardiac Clients in a Water Program

Issue	LOC	Sources	Affil	Rationale/Comment
Angina—unstable	CI	Congdon, 1997[8]	RN	
Cardiomyopathies	CI			
Congestive heart failure	CI			
High-grade ectopy (frequent) not medically corrected by medication, ablation, or AICD	CI			
Low ejection fraction (left ventricular failure)—symptomatic	CI			
Valve problems (aortic or mitral)—significant	CI			

Contraindications for Use of Hot Tub or Spa in People with Cardiovascular Disease

Issue	LOC	Sources	Affil	Rationale/Comment
Age—advanced (esp >70 years)	CI	Congdon, 1997[8]	RN	Due to reduced orthostatic responses and the extreme vasodilatory effect of hot tubs.
β-blockers—use of	CI			
Hypertensive drugs—use of other	CI			(That is, diuretics, angiotensin-converting enzyme inhibitors) because of massive interactions with the renin-angiotensin-vasopressin axis.)
Postural hypotension problems	CI			

REFERENCES

1. Bates A, Hanson N: Aquatic exercise therapy. Philadelphia: W.B. Saunders, 1996.
2. Wykle MO: Safety first. Rehab Manag 16(6):29-27, 50, 2003.
3. Giesecke CL: Aquatic rehabilitation of clients with spinal cord injury. In Ruoti RG, Morris DM, Coles AJ, eds: Aquatic rehabilitation. Philadelphia: Lippincott-Raven, 1997.
4. McNeal R: Aquatic rehabilitation of clients with rheumatic disease. In Ruoti RG, Morris DM, Coles AJ, eds: Aquatic rehabilitation. Philadelphia: Lippincott-Raven, 1997.
5. Petersen TM: Pediatric aquatic therapy. In Cole AJ, Becker BE, eds: Comprehensive aquatic therapy, ed 2. Philadelphia: Butterworth–Heinemann, 2004.
6. Haralson KM: Therapeutic pool programs. Clin Manag Phys Ther 5(2):10-13, 1985.
7. Appendix B, guidelines for activity and exercise. In Goodman CC, Boissonnault WG, Fuller KS, eds: Pathology: Implications for the physical therapist. Philadelphia: W.B. Saunders, 2003.
8. Congdon K: Aquatic rehabilitation of the client with cardiovascular disease. In Ruoti RG, Morris DM, Coles AJ, eds: Aquatic rehabilitation. Philadelphia: Lippincott-Raven, 1997.

11.3 Cardiac Rehabilitation

OVERVIEW. Cardiac rehabilitation is a supervised, interdisciplinary, goal-specific program used to restore persons with cardiac disease to achieve their optimal functional state (i.e., medical, physical, psychological, emotional, vocational). The program consists of four successive phases and incorporates education and lifestyle changes in addition to exercise.[1,2] Together, the ACSM and AACVPR have listed 16 conditions of concerns for cardiac rehabilitation, 75% of which are circulatory related.

E00-E90 ENDOCRINE, NUTRITIONAL, AND METABOLIC DISEASES

Issue	LOC	Source	Affil	Rationale/Comment
Diabetes—uncontrolled; resting blood glucose of >400 mg/dL	CI CI	ACSM, 2000[3] AACVPR, 2004[4]	Org Org	Note: In severe hyperglycemia (>300 mg/dL), life-threatening metabolic conditions such as diabetic ketoacidosis or hypoglycemic hyperosmolar nonketotic coma can develop.[5]
"Other metabolic conditions (such as acute thyroiditis, hypokalemia; hyperkalemia, hypovolemia, etc.)"[3]				Note: Hypokalemia can clinically present as hypotension, arrhythmias, ECG changes, and cardiac arrest (with 2.5 mEq/L serum potassium),[6] whereas hyperkalemia can clinically present as tachycardia, bradycardia (later), ECG changes, and cardiac arrest (with >7.0 mEq/L serum potassium levels).[6] In hyperthyroidism (also thyrotoxicosis) metabolism is elevated in most systems, sympathetic activity is increased, and there is an increased risk of atrial fibrillations, congestive heart failure, and MI.[5]

I00-I99 DISEASES OF THE CIRCULATORY SYSTEM

Issue	LOC	Source	Affil	Rationale/Comment
Angina—unstable	CI CI	ACSM, 2000[3] AACVPR, 2004[4]	Org Org	Note: With unstable angina, additional stress may induce an infarction.[7]
Atrial or ventricular arrhythmias— if uncontrolled				Note: Atrial or ventricular arrhythmias are characterized by automatic changes in heart rate and rhythm.[8] Exercise may increase an arrhythmia or may induce one because of increased myocardial oxygen demands or increased sympathetic tone.[9]

Continued

Issue	LOC	Source	Affil	Rationale/Comment
Congestive heart failure—if uncompensated	CI			
"Critical aortic stenosis (peak systolic pressure gradient of >50 mm Hg with an aortic valve orifice area of <0.75 cm² in an averaged size adult)"[3]				Note: Aortic stenosis is a progressive calcification of the heart valve that is associated with aging and presents with reduced cardiac output when stenosis becomes severe. Exercise testing may not provide useful information in patients with valvular disease.[9]
Embolism—recent				Note: A pulmonary embolism is a potentially fatal condition where blood supply to lung parenchyma is obstructed as a result of a blood clot lodged in the pulmonary artery.[10]
Orthostatic BP drop >20 mm Hg with symptoms				
Pericarditis (active) or myocarditis (active)				Note: Pericarditis is an inflammation of the double-layered membrane, the pericardium, which surrounds the heart. In constrictive pericarditis, the fibrotic tissue compresses the heart, reduces cardiac output, and leads to cardiac failure. One of the treatments for acute idiopathic (post-MI and post-thoracotomy types) is bed rest when fever is present.[8,9] Myocarditis is a focal or diffuse inflammation of cardiac muscle. The treatment includes modified bed rest to reduce the workload of the heart.[8]
Resting systolic BP >200 mm Hg; Resting diastolic BP >110 mm Hg— evaluated on a case-by-case basis				
ST segment displacement, resting (>2 mm)[a]				The ST segment is the period between complete depolarization and beginning repolarization of ventricular musculature. It may be elevated or depressed in angina (transient muscle ischemia) or muscle injury. Elevation may suggest early states of an MI (acute myocardial muscle damage).[8]

Sinus tachycardia (>120 beats/min, if uncontrolled)	CI			
Thrombophlebitis				Note: DVT can lead to pulmonary embolism, a common cause of sudden death in hospitals.[10]
Third-degree AV block—without pacemaker				Note: A heart block is a disorder of the heart's conduction system that can present as fatigue, dizziness, and fainting and may require a pacemaker.[9]

a, AACVPR—ischemic changes on resting ECG; b, AACVPR >10 mm Hg.

M00-M99 DISEASES OF THE MUSCULOSKELETAL SYSTEM AND CONNECTIVE TISSUE

Issue	LOC	Source	Affil	Rationale/Comment
Orthopedic conditions (severe) that would prohibit exercise	CI	ACSM, 2000[3]	Org	
	CI	AACVPR, 2004[4]	Org	

R00-R99 SYMPTOMS, SIGNS

Issue	LOC	Source	Affil	Rationale/Comment
Systemic fever or illness—acute	CI	ACSM, 2000[3]	Org	Note: Exercise with fever stresses the cardiopulmonary system and immune system, and may be further complicated by dehydration.[11]
	CI	AACVPR, 2004[4]	Org	

HEART TRANSPLANT AND EXERCISE TRAINING PRECAUTIONS

The following source provides exercise training precautions or contraindications with regard to exercise intensity, transient hypotension, resistance training, and glucocorticoid treatments in patients with heart transplants.

Issue	LOC	Source	Affil	Rationale/Comment
Enhanced glucocorticoid immunosuppression treatment for acute allograft rejection • **Discontinue exercise**	P	Braith, 1998[12]	Exercise science	Glucocorticoids increase the chance of a coronary event and also have catabolic effects on bone and muscle that may outweigh benefits of exercise (see below).
Exercise intensity in transplanted hearts	P			Transplant recipients have abnormal HR responsiveness to exercise, so it is difficult to use HR to guide exercise prescription. Suggested general guidelines: • Restrict intensity to HR ≤20 beats more than resting values • Use walking distance and pace as markers for prescription • Rate perceived exertion
Hypotension—transient	P			Hypotension may occur during resistance training and lifting above heart level (i.e., shoulder presses). It may be due to autonomic sympathetic denervation resulting in a reliance on preload to maintain systemic blood pressure. The source suggests the following to sustain venous return and prevent pooling of blood: • Alternating UE and LE exercise to prevent pooling • Walking 2 minutes between exercise or doing standing calf raises if symptomatic • Conclude sessions with 5-min cool-down on treadmill at low intensity
Resistance training if advanced osteoporosis	CI			There is a greater risk for fracture if bone mineral density is >2 SD from norm following transplantation due to glucocorticosteroid-induced osteoporosis. Manage the patient conservatively with initial resistance and progression of loads.

REFERENCES

1. Eisenberg MG: Dictionary of rehabilitation. New York: Springer, 1995.
2. Tan JC: Practical manual of physical medicine and rehabilitation: Diagnostics, therapeutics, and basic problems. St. Louis: Mosby, 1998.
3. American College of Sports Medicine: ACSM's guidelines for exercise testing and prescription, ed 6. Philadelphia: Lippincott Williams & Wilkins, 2000.
4. American Association of Cardiovascular and Pulmonary Rehabilitation: American Association of Cardiovascular and Pulmonary Rehabilitation guidelines for cardiac rehabilitation and secondary prevention programs, ed 4. Champaign (IL): Human Kinetics, 2004.
5. Goodman CC, Snyder TEK: The endocrine and metabolic systems. In Goodman CC, Boissonnault WG, Fuller KS, eds: Pathology: Implications for the physical therapist. Philadelphia: W.B. Saunders, 2003.
6. Goodman CC, Snyder TEK: Problems affecting multiple systems. In Goodman CC, Boissonnault WG, Fuller KS, eds: Pathology: Implications for the physical therapist. Philadelphia: W.B. Saunders, 2003.
7. Pagana KD, Pagana TJ: Mosby's manual of diagnostic and laboratory tests, ed 2. St. Louis: Mosby, 2002.
8. Springhouse: Professional guide to diseases, ed 6. Springhouse (PA): Springhouse, 1998.
9. Goodman CC: The cardiovascular system. In Goodman CC, Boissonnault WG, Fuller KS, eds: Pathology: Implications for the physical therapist. Philadelphia: W.B. Saunders, 2003.
10. Goodman CC: The respiratory system. In Goodman CC, Boissonnault WG, Fuller KS, eds: Pathology: Implications for the physical therapist. Philadelphia: W.B. Saunders, 2003.
11. Appendix B, Guidelines for activity and exercise. In Goodman CC, Boissonnault WG, Fuller KS, eds: Pathology: Implications for the physical therapist. Philadelphia: W.B. Saunders, 2003.
12. Braith RW: Exercise training in patients with CHF and heart transplant recipients. Med Sci Sports Exerc 30(10 Supp):S367-S372, 1998.

12   BALANCE AND COORDINATION

12.1   Balance Exercises

Balance exercises or training involves activities aimed at reducing instability/falls by improving patients' ability to maintain their center of gravity within their support base. Because balance training aims to challenge stability, it is important to structure patient activities at the appropriate level and to screen patients who may be exceedingly unsafe for these activities[1] (also see **Screening for Falls, Chapter 4; Gait and Locomotion Training, Chapter 14**).

CONTRAINDICATIONS AND PRECAUTIONS

F00-F99 MENTAL AND BEHAVIORAL DISORDERS

Issue	LOC	Sources	Affil	Rationale/Comment
Cognitive impairments	CI	Brody and Dewane, 2005[1]	PT	These individuals may be unable to understand the purpose or goal of the balance task.
Unsafe patients—inherently	CI			

PROCEDURAL CONCERNS

Issue	LOC	Sources	Affil	Rationale/Comment
Challenging tasks—appropriate level	Advice	Brody and Dewane, 2005[1]	PT	Choose challenging activities at an appropriate skill level.
Environment—remove obstacles	Advice			
Simple tasks—start	Advice			Begin with simple tasks.
Stabilizers—adequate	Advice			Use gait belt or parallel bars.

REFERENCES

1. Brody LT, Dewane J: Impaired balance. In: Hall CM, Brody LT, eds: Therapeutic exercise: Moving toward function. Philadelphia: Lippincott Williams & Wilkins, 2005.

12.2 Vestibular Exercises

Vestibular rehabilitation aims at addressing disequilibrium and dizziness symptoms related to peripheral vestibular pathology by using specific exercises to improve balance and reduce dizziness.[1] Unstable conditions listed below are CIs. For CRM, correct identification of semicircular canal involvement is necessary before treatment can be appropriately administered.

CONTRAINDICATIONS AND PRECAUTIONS

H60-H95 DISEASES OF THE EAR AND MASTOID PROCESS

Issue	LOC	Sources	Affil	Rationale/Comment
Perilymphatic fistula	CI	Schubert and Herdman, 2001[2]	PT	This is an unstable condition and is often treated with bed rest to allow membrane rupture between middle and inner ear to heal.
Ménière's disease	CI			This is an unstable condition.
Other unstable vestibular disorders	CI			

S00-T98 INJURY, POISONING, AND CERTAIN OTHER CONSEQUENCES OF EXTERNAL CAUSES

Issue	LOC	Sources	Affil	Rationale/Comment
Neck injuries—acute **Surgical procedures**	CI Observe	Schubert and Herdman, 2001[2]	PT	Individuals with neck injuries may not tolerate CRT or some gaze exercises. Discharge from the nose or ears may suggest leakage of cerebrospinal fluid.

R00-R99 SYMPTOMS, SIGNS

Issue	LOC	Sources	Affil	Rationale/Comment
Severe ringing in ear(s)	CI	Schubert and Herdman, 2001[2]	PT	
Sudden loss of hearing	CI			
Uncomfortable feeling of fullness or pressure in ear(s)	CI			

PROCEDURAL CONCERNS

Issue	LOC	Sources	Affil	Rationale/Comment
Correct identification of canal involvement—for CRM	Advice	Herdman and Tusa, 1996[3]	PT	Correct identification of canal involvement is necessary before CRM can be appropriately administered.

ADVERSE EVENTS

Source	Background	Therapy	Outcome	Follow-up/Interpretation
Herdman and Tusa, 1996[3] **Identifying correct canal involvement for CRM** Retrospective Arch Otolaryngol Head Neck Surg	85 patients with BPPV of the posterior canal (based on Hallpike-Dix maneuver) were treated.	All underwent canalith repositioning procedure (3 cases of female patients, ages 77, 66, and 27 years, described).	Of the 85 patients with posterior canal BPPV, 5 (6%) who remained symptomatic developed anterior canal ($n = 2$) or horizontal canal ($n = 3$) positional vertigo.	For patients not responding to initial canalith repositioning maneuver, observe nystagmus direction for correct canal involvement before administering treatment.
Kantner et al., 1982[4] **Seizure concern and vestibular stimulation** Quasi-experiment (within subject) Phys Ther	10 children ages 5 to 15 years presented with varied seizure history (stress, focal, petit mal, grand mal, psychomotor, vestibular, paroxysmal).	EEG measurements were taken before, during, and after exposure to warm and cold caloric vestibular stimuli.	Vestibular stimulation did not accentuate abnormal brain wave activity in these 10 seizure-prone children (6 children showed reduced paroxysmal activity; $p < .02$).	The authors suggest precautions for monitoring for photogenic seizures and hyperventilation while spinning patients during and shortly afterward. They also suggest restricting subjects' vision. Note: These authors *did not* physically spin patients as may be done in therapy. Also, the sample size was small and heterogeneous.

REFERENCES

1. Shumway-Cook A: Vestibular rehabilitation: What is vestibular rehabilitation? Available at: http://www.vestibular.org/rehab.html#rehabilitation. Accessed May 16, 2005.

2. Schubert MC, Herdman SJ: Vestibular rehabilitation. In O'Sullivan SB, Schmitz TJ, eds: Physical rehabilitation: assessment and treatment. ed 4, Philadelphia, 2001, FA Davis.

3. Herdman SJ, Tusa RJ: Complications of the canalith repositioning procedure. Arch Otolaryngol Head Neck Surg 122(3):281-286, 1996.

4. Kantner RM, Clark DL, Atkinson J, Paulson G: Effects of vestibular stimulation in seizure-prone children. An EEG study. Phys Ther 62(1):16-21, 1982.

12.3 Constraint-Induced Movement Therapy (Acute Rehabilitation Setting)

Constraint-induced movement therapy (CIMT, also called forced use) involves discouraging the use of the intact limb and encouraging active use of the hemiplegic one in order to maximize or restore function of the paralyzed upper limb.[1] Some animal studies suggest that introducing CIMT too early (during acute rehabilitation) may be harmful (see Kozlowski,[2] Humm,[3] and Risedal's[4] animal studies.)

Issue	LOC	Sources	Affil	Rationale/Comment
Compensatory technique— compromised (postulated)	Safety concern	Dromerick et al, 2000[1]	MD	If focus is on motor restoration rather than compensation, the technique may lead to excessive disability.
Frustration—increased (postulated)	Safety concern			Focusing on weaker limb may lead to increased frustration.
Overuse syndromes (postulated)	Safety concern			Use of the weaker limb could lead to a painful overuse syndrome.

| Very early CIMT may be harmful | Advice | Gratta et al, 2004[5,a,b] | MD | Animal studies of Kozlowski et al (1996),[2] Humm et al (1998),[3] Risedal et al (1999),[4] and Bland et al (2000),[6] suggesting that forced overuse, introduced early, may impede motor recovery of the affected limb and enlarge the volume of the lesion. Immediate forced and extreme overuse of affected forelimb in rats increased lesion volume that may be attributed to exercise-induced hyperthermia or excitotoxicity. |
| | Safety concern | Dromerick et al, 2000[1,a,c] | MD | |

a, Although source discussed these potential concerns, adverse events were not observed in source's human study; b, Source noted that many potential human subjects in the acute setting fail to qualify for CIMT; c, The treatment intensity for CIMT used in source's human study was less than that employed in reported animal studies.

REFERENCES

1. Dromerick, AW, Edwards DF, Hahn M: Does the application of constraint-induced movement therapy during acute rehabilitation reduce arm impairment after ischemic stroke? Stroke 31: 2984-2988, 2000.
2. Kozlowski DA, James DC, Schallert T: Use-dependent exaggeration of neuronal injury following unilateral sensorimotor cortex lesions. J Neurosci 16:4776-4786, 1996.
3. Humm JL, Kozlowski DA, James DC, et al: Use-dependent exacerbation of brain damage occurs during an early post-lesion vulnerable period. Brain Res 783:286-292, 1998.
4. Risedal A, Zeng J, Johansson BB: Early training may exacerbate brain damage after focal brain ischemia in the rat. J Cereb Blood Flow Metab 16:4776-4786, 1999.
5. Gratta JC, Noser EA, Ro T, et al: Constraint-induced movement therapy. Stroke 35[Suppl I]:2699-2701, 2004.
6. Bland ST, Schallert T, Strong R, et al: Early exclusive use of the affected forelimb after moderate transient focal ischemia in rats: functional and anatomic outcome. Stroke 31:1144-1152, 2000.

12.4 Neurodevelopmental Treatment

OVERVIEW. Neurodevelopmental treatment (NDT) is a neurological treatment approach that progresses individuals developmentally from a horizontal to a standing position. NDT has its roots in the reflex-based therapies of the 1950s, which relied heavily on the facilitation and inhibition of reflexes during treatment. The treatment is commonly administered to children with cerebral palsy.[1] Parette and Hourcade[2] raise a concern that this approach may limit a child's interactions or experiences with the environment that are needed for cognitive development.

Issue	LOC	Source	Affil	Rationale/Comment
Limited environment interactions	Conflict between philosophies[b] (cognitive and facilitation)	Parette and Hourcade, 1983[2]	Edu[a]	There is concern that a child with CP who is being treated with inhibitory techniques may have limited interaction with the environment. A potential conflict exists between the philosophies of motor development facilitation (using NDT inhibitory techniques) and interventions that focus on cognitive development (which requires child interactions with the environment).

a, Educators; b, Early intervention.

REFERENCES

1. Eisenberg MG: Dictionary of rehabilitation. New York: Springer; 1995.

2. Parette HP Jr, Hourcade JJ: Early intervention: A conflict of therapist and educator. Percept Motor Skills 57(3, Pt 2):1056-1058, 1983.

12.5 Proprioceptive Neuromuscular Facilitation

OVERVIEW.   Proprioceptive neuromuscular facilitation (PNF) is a hands-on therapeutic exercise technique used to improve mobility, stability, stamina, coordination, and range of motion. The clinician typically facilitates a contraction with the muscles initially placed on maximal stretch (to provide afferent input) and then offers maximal graded resistance to recruit additional muscle activity while having the patient move through diagonal and spiral patterns of the body part. During a session, patients may be subjected to various forces including manual resistance, repeated stretches, joint compressions, and distractions.[1]

SUMMARY: CONTRAINDICATIONS AND PRECAUTIONS.   Three sources cited a total of 25 concerns for PNF. Concerns ranged from five to 16 per source. The largest proportion of concerns were procedural (32%) and injury related (20%). The most frequently cited concern was the presence of a fracture.

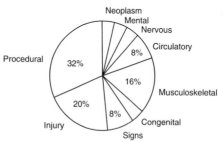

Proportion of Concerns for PNF
based on ICD

CONTRAINDICATIONS AND PRECAUTIONS

C00-C97 NEOPLASMS

Issue	LOC	Sources	Affil	Rationale/Comment
Malignancy	CI	Prentice, 2002[2]	PT	

F00-F99 MENTAL AND BEHAVIORAL DISORDERS

Issue	LOC	Sources	Affil	Rationale/Comment
Comprehension	CI	Adler et al, 2000[1]	PT	The patient must be able to follow instructions for rhythmic stabilization. Difficulties may be due to language, age, or cerebral dysfunction.

G00-G99 DISEASES OF THE NERVOUS SYSTEM

Issue	LOC	Sources	Affil	Rationale/Comment
Cerebellar involvement	CI	Adler et al, 2000[1]	PT	For rhythmic stabilization.

I00-I99 DISEASES OF THE CIRCULATORY SYSTEM

Issue	LOC	Sources	Affil	Rationale/Comment
Circulatory conditions	CI	Voss et al, 1985[3,b]	PT	
Cerebral vascular accident	CI	Voss et al, 1985[3,a]		When sustained effort against resistance is not permitted.

a, Repeated contraction; b, Rhythmic rotation (i.e., repeated rotation where limitation exists).

M00-M99 DISEASES OF THE MUSCULOSKELETAL SYSTEM AND CONNECTIVE TISSUE

Issue	LOC	Sources	Affil	Rationale/Comment
Bone disease	CI	Prentice, 2002[2]	PT, ATC	
Inflammatory arthritis	CI			
Instability, joint	CI/Great care	Adler et al, 2000[1,a,c]	PT	
Osteoporosis	CI	Adler et al, 2000[1,a,b]	PT	

a, Repeated stretch or repeated stretch through range; b, Unstable bone; c, Great care for traction and activating stretch reflex if joint is unstable.

Q00-Q99 CONGENITAL MALFORMATIONS, DEFORMITIES, AND CHROMOSOMAL ABNORMALITIES

Issue	LOC	Sources	Affil	Rationale/Comment
Bone deformity—Congenital	CI	Prentice, 2002[2]	PT, ATC	

R00-R99 SYMPTOMS, SIGNS, AND ABNORMAL CLINICAL & LABORATORY FINDINGS (NOT ELSEWHERE CLASSIFIED)

Issue	LOC	Sources	Affil	Rationale/Comment
Pain	CI	Adler et al, 2000[1,c]	PT	Pain inhibits coordinated performance. If techniques cause or increases pain, it is CI.[1]
		Voss et al, 1985[3,a]	PT	
Acute condition	CI	Voss et al, 1985[3,b]	PT	When active resistance is not permitted.

a, Maximal stretch; b, Reinforcement (i.e., resisting the stronger component); c, Repeated stretch or repeated stretch through range.

S00-T98 INJURY, POISONING, AND CERTAIN OTHER CONSEQUENCES OF EXTERNAL CAUSES

Issue	LOC	Sources	Affil	Rationale/Comment
Fractures	CI	Adler et al, 2000[1,a,i,j]	PT	With traction, there is danger of separating the bone fragments.
	CI	Prentice, 2002[2]	PT/ATC	
		Voss et al, 1985[3,a,c,d]	PT	
Muscle/tendon damage	CI	Adler et al, 2000[1,i]	PT	
Orthopedic conditions, acute	CI	Voss et al, 1985[3,b,d,e,f,h]	PT	

| Postoperative conditions | CI | Voss et al, 1985[3,a,c,d,e,g,h] | With manual contacts, when contact at the site is not permitted. |
| Wounds, open | CI | Voss et al, 1985[3,g] | |

a, Joint approximation; b, Contract-relax (also if active motion is present in the agonist), slow reversals (1. involves simultaneous isometrics; 2. also if agonist is not stimulated; 3. also applies to slow reversal-hold technique involving isometric and isotonics); c, Traction; d, Maximal stretch; e, Rhythmic rotation (i.e., repeated rotation where limitation exists); f, Maximal resistance; g, Manual contacts; h, Repeated contractions; i, Repeated stretch or repeated stretch through range; j, Unstable bone.

PROCEDURAL CONCERNS

Issue	LOC	Sources	Affil	Rationale/Comment
Coordinated pattern cannot be achieved, if	CI	Voss et al, 1985[3,e]	PT	Unless two hands are applied to the part.
Goal of technique not achieved, if	CI	Voss et al, 1985[3,d,g,h]	PT	During rhythmic stabilization, if the agonist is not stimulated.[3]
	CI	Adler et al, 2000[1,d]	PT	During hold-relax, if unable to perform an isometric movement.[3]
Muscle imbalances are favored from stimulation, if	CI	Voss et al, 1985[3,c]	PT	Unless the weaker pattern is stimulated upon reversal of the technique.
Passive movement is CI, if	CI	Voss et al, 1985[3,b]		
Range, full (of passive or resistive) not permitted, if	CI	Voss et al, 1985[3,j]		
Resistance is CI , if	CI	Voss et al, 1985[3,h,i]		
Sudden movement is hazardous, if	CI	Voss et al, 1985[3,a]		
Sustained effort is harmful, if	CI	Voss et al, 1985[3,c,f]		Note: Issues of cardiac precaution are not specifically addressed.

a, Quick reversals; b, Rhythmic initiation; c, Maximal resistance; d, Hold-relax (direct technique); e, Reinforcement (i.e., resisting the stronger component); f, Repeated contraction; g, Rhythmic stabilization; h, Slow reversal hold-relax in timing (i.e., superimposed on isotonics or isometrics) if any form of exercise is CI; j, Hold-relax-active (i.e., involves isometric, relaxation, and isotonics), also use more stimulating techniques instead when possible.

REFERENCES

1. Adler SS, Beckers D, Buck M, et al: PNF in practice: An illustrated guide, ed 2. Berlin: Springer; 2000.
2. Prentice WE: Proprioceptive neuromuscular facilitation techniques. In: Prentice WE, editor: Therapeutic modalities for physical therapists, New York: McGraw-Hill; 2002.
3. Voss DE, Ionta MK, Myers BJ: Proprioceptive neuromuscular facilitation: patterns and techniques, ed 3. Philadelphia: Harper & Row; 1985.

13   FLEXIBILITY EXERCISES

13.1   Passive Range of Motion

OVERVIEW. PROM is motion produced by an external force, without voluntary contraction, and within an unrestricted portion of a joint.[1] One of its chief purposes is to maintain (not increase) joint mobility.

SUMMARY: CONTRAINDICATIONS AND PRECAUTIONS. Four sources list a common contraindication.[1-4] PROM is contraindicated if it disrupts healing (i.e., condition intensifies). Complications from PROM are reported below and include (1) fractures/dislocations—in often fragile bone, (2) autonomic dysreflexia—in spinal cord patients, and (3) heterotopic ossification. In addition, overly vigorous techniques may have led to fractures in cases where family members or lay people administer PROM to infants.

Note: It is not always clear in the harm literature whether the injurious technique in question (often referred to as "passive") was truly that or perhaps a more forceful technique (i.e., stretching) (also see **Mobility testing; Devices; AROM section; Stretching**).

CONTRAINDICATIONS AND PRECAUTIONS

PROCEDURAL CONCERNS

Issue	LOC	Sources	Affil	Rationale/Comment
Active motion is possible and beneficial	CI	Pierson and Fairchild, 2002[4]	PT	If the patient can perform AROM and it is beneficial, then PROM is viewed as CI.
Motion that disrupts healing[a]	CI	Tan, 1998[2]	MD/PT	Signs of undesirable motion are increased inflammation (i.e., increased pain, heat, redness).
	CI	Brody, 2005[3]	PT	
	CI	Monroe, 1996[1,c]	PT	
	CI	Pierson and Fairchild, 2002[4,b]	PT	
Technique is indeed passive	Caution	Brody, 2005[3]	PT	If AROM is CI, then the patient should not be actively contracting muscle during PROM.

a, This guideline, while grounded in common sense, does not seem terribly useful in my opinion (e.g., any food that makes you fat is contraindicated for your weight-loss diet). More specific guidelines based on sound theoretical or reliable clinical outcomes may be helpful. Also see assessment recommendations[1] under mobility testing. b, If symptoms increase or the condition intensifies. c, Pertains to ROM (i.e., PROM and AROM are not distinguished).

ADVERSE EVENTS

Note: In some reports, it is unclear how PROM is defined.

Source	Background	Therapy	Outcome	Follow-up/Interpretation
Calenoff et al, 1979[5] **ROM and fracture in SCI** Case report Arch Phys Med Rehab	A 25-year-old man presented with C5-C7 quadriplegia due to fracture-dislocation from a fall (s/p decompression laminectomy and anterior cervical fusion). Some sensation in the LE and sacral pressure was preserved.	The patient had LE flexion spasticity and hip flexion contractures and added ROM exercises 11 months following his accident. During the exercise, he felt a "pop" in his back following 45-degree hip flexion that resulted in acute back flexion and an immediate sense of "heaviness" of the legs. He could not sense suppository during his bowel program. Also, skin ulcers on sacrum/buttocks developed in the following months.	Dx: Slice fracture (transverse fracture and posterior ligament rupture) of L4 body and a dislocation of L3 on L4 resulted in a new neurologic injury. Treatment: Surgical stabilization (Weiss spring). LEs became predominately flaccid; sensation not regained, bladder became hypotonic, and patient could not resume a bladder retraining program.	Proposed mechanism: Repetitive forces that may stress markedly demineralized bone coupled with an inability to feel pain (protective mechanism). The authors believed this rare event may be prevented if symptoms are properly interpreted (ranging patients in a restricted range when pain is not appreciated due to neurologic disease).
Crawford et al, 1986[6] JBCR	12 patients, ages 21 to 53, presented with severe burns (males and 1 female).	6 patients received PROM and assisted daily during their initial hospitalization, 2 received PROM, and 4 received active and AAROM in PT/OT.	Heterotopic ossification was noted in the posterior elbow joint with joint pain and sudden loss of range; onset 12 weeks (average).	Six cases spontaneously resolved within 6 months. Six required surgical excision.

ROM and HO in burn patients
Chart review
  1,066 records

The authors stated that the ossification progressed to ankylosis (requiring surgery) in patients receiving PROM beyond their pain-free range.

PROM and stretching are CI if HO suspected.

Handle these premature infants carefully.

PROM by parents, nurses, and PT should be done very gently.

Restrict chest physiotherapy to postural drainage and vibration to avoid rib fractures associated with vigorous chest PT.

Dabezies and Warren, 1997[7]
PROM, fractures, and rickets
Retrospective
Clin Orthop Rel Res

A chart review was conducted between Aug 1989 and Jan 1993 of 247 very low birth weight premature infants at a U.S. university medical center.

Rickets was diagnosed in 96 of 247 cases. Fractures occurred in 26 infants or 27.1% of infants with rickets.

Fractures involved the humerus (10), radius (13), ulna (8), metacarpal (4), clavicle (3), ribs (54), femur (5), and fibula (1).

Of the 26 infants with fractures, 9 who had received chest percussion therapy sustained a total of 54 rib fractures.

Long bone fractures were treated with simple splints (i.e., padded foam aluminum splint); all fractures healed.

Continued

Source	Background	Therapy	Ourcome	Follow-up/Interpretation
Daud et al, 1993[8] **Delayed ROM, heterotopic ossification, and SCI** Retrospective (chart review) Disabil Rehab	A chart review was conducted between Sept 1983 and 1989 of traumatic spinal cord injuries, at a National Spinal Injuries Centre. HO and date passive motion was started were collected.	Records of 91 patients, ages 15 to 77, were consecutively analyzed (median age 27 years; 61 male and 30 female; levels: 50 cervical, 34 thoracic, 7 lumbar). Clinical evidence of HO was noted in 10 (18%) and radiologic evidence noted in 12 (21%) of 56 patients who began passive motion 7 or more days following injury (as determined by discriminant analysis).	The time when passive movement is initiated may have played a role in HO development.	The authors suggest controlled passive movement in all parallel extremities from the first day of injury. Proposed mechanism: early ROM may keep the joint capsule supple whereas if contractures develop, passive motion may result in soft tissue tear, triggering HO development.
Helfer et al, 1984[9] **Fractures, PROM and infants**	A 7-month-old full-term male presented with no health problems.	PROM was provided at home.	Radiographs in the ER revealed dislocated left elbow; recent fractured bilateral radius, left ulna; left humeral fracture; a healing left tibia fracture. Later: Right humeral cloaking, bilateral chip fracture of the ankle.	The elbow was reduced and the fractures healed. The babysitter viewed the baby as handicapped, independently provided PROM, and used one ankle to roll the baby from supine to prone.

Case series J Pediatr	A 4-month-old male was born at 22 weeks' gestation.	The NICU staff taught PROM to the mother. The mother taught the father.	Outcome: fractured left femur; later: 9 fractured ribs, a skull fracture, periosteal callus bilaterally of the humerus and femurs, a chip fracture of the long bones.	The bones healed in 3½ months once PROM was discontinued. The parents applied PROM too vigorously. The father drank alcohol excessively while babysitting.
	A 28-week-gestation female presented with rickets of prematurity (healed).	PT taught PROM to the mother at the time of discharge from the neonatal ICU. The mother was not compliant with follow-up or PT appointments.	At 3 and 9 months, the mother reported tenderness and reduced use of the baby's right leg. Radiographs revealed a fracture of the left femur, cortical asymmetry of the right femur, fractured right humerus, cortical thickening of bilateral humeri, an avulsion fracture of the left ulna, bilateral metacarpal cloaking, and a right rib fracture.	PROM was discontinued. Injuries healed except for a bowing left leg due to an epiphyseal union. There were two corrective surgeries in the 2nd year. There was a history of vigorous PT provided primarily by mother's boyfriend.

Continued

Source	Background	Therapy	Outcome	Follow-up/Interpretation
	10-month-old, 28-week-gestation male with a history of ICH, RDS, pneumonia, bilateral pneumothoraces; 6 wk in NICU.	The NICU staff taught PROM to the mother because of hypertonicity. The mother taught the father.	A 4- to 6-week-old fracture of the left humerus was noted at 10 months during an evaluation of child abuse for a right eye injury.	PROM was discontinued. No evidence of child abuse was found.
London et al, 1984[10] **PROM, fracture, and cerebral palsy** Case report J Pediatr	A 10-month-old full-term female presented with cerebral contusion and left-sided hemiparesis at 4 months.	A PT provided PROM exercises at the patient's home.	She was brought to the ER with a 10-day history of a painful, swollen LLE. Radiographs: healing "bucket handle" fracture of distal femoral and proximal tibial metaphysis, and a right subdural effusion. No trauma was identified by the family.	A shunt was provided for the subdural effusion. Repetitive passive exercise to a compromised limb may have contributed to the fracture. The authors suggest the issue of an "overzealous" health care provider.
McGarry et al, 1982[11] **Autonomic hyperreflexia, ROM, SCI** Case series Phys Ther	A 21-year-old male presented with T1 paraplegia and complete anesthesia; s/p 5 months ago MVA.	The patient self-administered hip flexion SLR from 0 to 125 degrees bilaterally with ankles to ears. The following were noted: headache, bradycardia, sweating, and blood pressure increasing from 90/60 to 190/120.	Elevation of head to 90 degrees resulted in a fall in blood pressure to normal within 5 minutes. The patient was advised to perform SLR to 90-100 degrees, and no further symptoms occurred.	Autonomic hyperreflexia (e.g., increased blood pressure with bradycardia, sweating, and headaches) can occur in patients with severe upper thoracic and cervical spinal cord lesions and evoked by stimuli applied below the injury level, including passive hip joint stretching.

	A 31-year-old male with complete C5 quadriplegia due to MVA presented with episodes of hyperreflexia at 5 months related to bladder distension.	Episodes were noted when paralyzed legs were passively flexed at the hips to 90 degrees or more (120 degrees available). Blood pressure increased from 120/80 to 190/150 and headaches lasted 45 minutes.	Blood pressure fell after exercise ceased and normalized within 10 minutes. Passive hip flexion exercise was limited to <90 degrees with no further symptoms.	Mechanism: stretch of joint capsule or proximal leg muscles innervated by L4-5 and S1 stimulated the response.
	A 37-year-old man presented with C6 quadriplegia due to a MVA and s/p heterotopic bone formation in bilateral thighs at 3 months (ROM 0 to 65 degrees).	Passive hip flexion to 60 degrees caused sweating, a throbbing headache, and a rise in blood pressure from 110/70 to 170/110. Pulse rate dropped from 72 bpm to 52 bpm and lasted 5-10 minutes after exercise stopped.	No further episodes were noted following 0.1 mg reserpre/day.	CS Sherrington showed that hyperextension of the toes in spinal cat resulted in an abrupt rise in blood pressure.[11]
Merritt and Hunder, 1983[12]	26 New Zealand White rabbits were subjects in a study.	14 controls had 4 ml of monosodium urate injected into 1 knee.	Significantly increased intra-articular knee temperatures ($p < .01$) were noted in knees in experimental or controls.	In acute crystalline monosodium urate arthritis, PROM can increase the inflammatory response.

Continued

Source	Background	Therapy	Outcome	Follow-up/Interpretation
PROM and arthritis APMR Animal Study pretest posttest control design		6 experimental rabbits had both knees injected; PROM was administered 5 min/hr to 1 knee at 30, 90, 150, and 210 minutes.	Significantly increased leukocyte counts ($p < .05$) were observed in the PROM group compared to controls.	
Merkx and Freihofer, 1995[13] **Fracture and TMJ graft** Int J Oral Maxillofac Case report	A 32-year-old female with right TMJ "cracking sounds" presented with pain and restricted maximal interincisal opening; ventral disk luxation; failed surgical repositioning of disk; and failed condylectomy in conjunction with PT.	Reconstruction of the condyle and vertical dimension of the ramus using autogenous costochondral (rib) graft was undertaken at an oral/ maxillofacial surgical department.	A fracture of the graft occurred about 3 months after reconstruction during physical therapy.	The graft was not strong enough to withstand forces to mobilize TMJ. Note 1: Physical therapy was mentioned in abstract but not in body of text at the time of complication. Note 2: It is unclear what form of mobilization was administered in PT (i.e., ROM, joint mobilization, etc.).

Pickett, 1982[14] **ROM and fractures in arthrogryposis** Skeletal Radiol	A 33-week-gestation male infant presented with arthrogryposis, with bilateral contractures of the elbows, hips, and knees.	The infant received ROM and stretching 3× day (within first 2 days of life) by nursing staff at a hospital.	The infant sustained a corner fracture of the right proximal femoral metaphysis; "bucket-handle" fracture of the proximal tibia. Fractures were found only around joints treated by ROM and stretching and suggested that injuries were a result of this physical therapy technique.	Fractures closely resemble child abuse and should not be confused with this complication of physical therapy. The complication was attributed to periarticular ligaments being stronger than plates or bone in infants.
Simonian and Staheli, 1995[15] **ROM, fracture in immobilized patients** Case series	A male neonate with amyoplasia (a form of arthrogryposis multiplex congenital with associated skeletal fragility) presented with multiple LE contractures (hip flexion, knee hyperextension, equinovarus deformities).	After birth, both knees were manipulated from 15 degrees of hyperextension to 20 degrees of flexion (health care provider not mentioned) and casted in flexion.	One week later (prior to discharge), repeated radiographs revealed bilateral posterior fractures of the proximal tibial epiphyses.	The authors felt that (1) osteopenia played a large role in the increased susceptibility to periarticular fractures following immobilization; (2) PROM should never be painful; and (3) the knee joint is at particular risk because of its long level arm.

Continued

Source	Background	Therapy	Outcome	Follow-up/Interpretation
J Ped Orthop	An 11-year-old boy presented with a grade 1 open midshaft femoral fracture due to fall from a tree. He was treated with Kirshner wire fixation, traction, and spica cast. Patient had limited knee motion.	Physiotherapy noted knee motion from 0 to 55 degrees. During 1 session, flexion increased to 70 degrees and therapist reported "some adhesions had been broken." The patient experienced pain and therapy continued once pain decreased, but range became more limited at 45 degrees.	Six weeks following the episode, repeat radiographs revealed callus around a new fracture of the distal femur (47 degrees anterior angulation).	
Singleton, 1986[16] **Overzealous PT for contracture and fracture** Case report Curr Problem Diagn Radiol	Child with cerebral palsy.	Physiotherapy for treatment of contractures.	Fractures of proximal tibia and fibula. (Only radiograph and a figure description provided.)	"Overzealous physical therapy may also produce fractures." Note: The type of mobilization technique was not specified (i.e., ROM, stretching).

LITIGATION

State and date	Background	Therapy	Complication	Award and Comments
New York, 1998[17] **Calcification, PROM and elbow fracture**	A 38-year-old male stock broker s/p hairline fracture of left elbow radial head.	An orthopedist referred the patient to physical therapy; original order called for PROM therapy.	Calcification of soft tissue of elbow. The patient claimed the prescription of PROM led to calcification of soft tissues of elbow.	$500,000 verdict.

Note: Awards and settlements do not necessarily prove a cause-effect relationship between equipment or technique and injury.

REFERENCES

1. Monroe LG: Motion restrictions. In: Kisner C, Colby LA, eds: Therapeutic exercise: Foundations and techniques, ed 3. Philadelphia: FA Davis; 1996.
2. Tan JC: Practical manual of physical medicine and rehabilitation: Diagnostics, therapeutics, and basic problems. St Louis: Mosby; 1998.
3. Brody LT: Mobility impairment. In: Hall CM, Brody LT, eds: Therapeutic exercise: moving toward function. Philadelphia: Lippincott Williams & Wilkins; 2005.
4. Pierson FM, Fairchild SL: Principles and techniques of patient care, ed 3. Philadelphia: Saunders; 2002.
5. Calenoff L, Geimer PC, Rosen JS: Lumbar fracture-dislocation related to range of motion exercises. Arch Phys Med Rehab 60(4):183-184, 1979.
6. Crawford CM, Varghese G, Mani MM, et al: Heterotopic ossification: are range of motion exercises contraindicated? J Burn Care Rehabil 7(4):323-327, 1986.
7. Dabezies EJ, Warren PD: Fractures in very low birth weight infants with rickets. Clin Orthop Rel Res 335:233-239, 1997.
8. Daud O, Sett P, Burr RG, et al: The relationship of heterotopic ossification to passive movements in paraplegic patients. Disabil Rehab 15(3):114-118, 1993.
9. Helfer RE, Scheurer SL, Alexander R, et al: Trauma to the bones of small infants from passive exercise: a factor in the etiology of child abuse. J Pediatr 104(1):47-50, 1984.

10. London R, Noronha PA, Levy HB: Bone trauma caused by passive exercise. J Pediatr 105(1):172-173, 1984.

11. McGarry J, Woolsey RM, Thompson CW: Autonomic hyperreflexia following passive stretching to the hip joint. Phys Ther 62(1):30-31, 1982.

12. Merritt JL, Hunder GG: Passive range of motion, not isometric exercise, amplifies acute urate synovitis. Arch Phys Med Rehab 64(3):130-131, 1983.

13. Merkx MA, Freihofer HPM: Fracture of costochondral graft in temporo-mandibular joint reconstructive surgery: an unexpected complication. Int J Oral Maxillofac 24:142-144, 1995.

14. Pickett WJ III, Johnson JF, Enzenauer RW: Case report 192. Skeletal Radiol 8:85-86, 1982.

15. Simonian PT, Staheli LT: Periarticular fractures after manipulation for knee contractures in children. J Pediatr Orthop 15(3):288-91, 1995.

16. Singleton EB: Intentional and unintentional abuse of infants and children. Curr Problem Diag Radiol 15:277-280, 1986.

17. Malpractice verdicts, settlements, and experts. February 1998; p. 40; Loc 4.

13.2 Stretching

OVERVIEW.   Passive stretching is a therapeutic maneuver that involves applying an external manual or mechanical force to a passive patient.[1] The purpose is to lengthen shortened soft tissue in order to increase range of motion.

SUMMARY.   Eight sources contributed to a total of 28 concerns for stretching. The largest percentage of concerns was procedural and musculoskeletal. Three sources (two PTs and one MD/PT) were concerned about stretching recent fractures, osteoporotic bone tissue, or contractures, which would result in loss of function or stabilization. Stretching-related fractures (osteoporotic bone), soft tissue ruptures, graft ruptures, and autonomic dysreflexic responses (in persons with spinal cord injuries) have been reported in the literature (see below).

Note: Adverse events attributed to passive ranging in the literature may (*possibly*) reflect a more aggressively performed stretching technique (also see **Passive Range of Motion**).

CONTRAINDICATIONS AND PRECAUTIONS

A00-B99 CERTAIN INFECTIONS AND PARASITIC DISEASES

Issue	LOC	Sources	Affil	Rationale/Comment
Infectious process—in area	CI	Kisner and Colby, 1996[1]	PT	
	CI	Hall and Brody, 2005[4]	PT	

C00-C97 NEOPLASM

Issue	LOC	Sources	Affil	Rationale/Comment
Malignancy—bone	Extreme caution	Tan, 1998[2]	MD/PT	

D50-D89 DISEASES OF BLOOD AND BLOOD-FORMING ORGANS AND CERTAIN DISORDERS

Issue	LOC	Sources	Affil	Rationale/Comment
Hemophilia	Do not	Pauls and Reed, 2004[3]	PT	Do not force involved joints through ROM.

M00–M99 DISEASES OF THE MUSCULOSKELETAL SYSTEM AND CONNECTIVE TISSUE

Issue	LOC	Sources	Affil	Rationale/Comment
Bony block	CI	Kisner and Colby, 1996[1]	PT	Bone will limit additional motion.
Contractures that serve to increase stability or improve function	CI	Tan, 1998[2]	MD/PT	Tightness may serve as a useful substitute for structural stability or strength at times.
	P	Sumers, 1992[5,a]	PT	
	Caution	Pierson and Fairchild, 2002[9,a]	PT	
Immobilization—prolonged	Extreme caution	Tan, 1998[2]	MD/PT	Immobilized connective tissue may possess reduced tensile strength.
	P	Kisner and Colby, 1996[1]	PT	**In a 2001 Pennsylvania lawsuit,[6] a person with long-standing quadriplegia was awarded $65,000 in a settlement after his PT fractured his femur during stretching exercises.**
Hypermobility	CI	Tan, 1998[2]	MD/PT	
Hypermobility of associated joints	Extreme caution			I.e., excessive motion at neighboring joints.
Osteoporosis—known/suspected	Extreme caution	Tan, 1998[2]	MD/PT	**In 1979, Shulman and Grossman[7] described an inactive 11-year-old girl with severe dermatomyositis, long-term steroid use, and severe osteoporosis who sustained a complete fracture-dislocation of her right proximal tibia and died from massive fatty microthromboembolisms to the lungs, brain, and kidney following passive range of motion and gentle stretching to her legs.**
	P	Kisner and Colby, 1996[1,b]	PT	
	Caution	Hall and Brody, 2005[4]	PT	

| Weakness | Caution | Hall and Brody, 2005[4,c] | PT | Avoid overstretching weak muscles, especially muscles that support |
| | P | Kisner and Colby, 1996[1] | PT | body structures against gravity.[1] |

a, (1) Tenodesis grasp for persons with SCI[5,9]: Avoid extending fingers and wrist simultaneously as when weight bearing on palms during bed/mat activities, or during PROM exercise. Overstretching these long finger flexors in people with C7 lesions or higher results in the loss of a functional tenodesis grasp (i.e., ability to write or self-catheterize). Also, overstretching wrist extensor (through PROM or effects of gravity) can weaken the tenodesis mechanism. Consider splints with the wrist supported in extension. Educate the patient and family members. Avoid long sitting positions if hamstrings are tight (less than 90 SLR) or if it results in poor positioning while in a wheelchair (kyphotic posturing). (2) Transfers in persons with SCI: Mild back tightness permits motion to be transmitted from the head/upper limbs to the pelvis/legs. Overstretching these muscles (by stretching or poor wheelchair positioning) can result in difficulties moving the buttocks during transfers. Consider hamstring stretching while in supine and not in long-sitting.[5] b, Also: age, steroid use, prolonged bed rest. c, Very weak.

S00-T98 INJURY, POISONING, AND CERTAIN OTHER CONSEQUENCES OF EXTERNAL CAUSES

Issue	LOC	Sources	Affil	Rationale/Comment
Brachialis muscle—trauma	P	Kisner and Colby, 1996[1]	PT	Ossification is potential complication of stretching. Evaluate for myositis ossificans. If not present, progress carefully with stretching.
Fractures—after period of immobilization	Care/P			Until fracture site is radiologically healed (consult with physician), use care any time stress is placed distal to the fracture site (e.g., stretching, resistance, weight bearing).
Factures—newly united	P			United fracture sites need to be protected by stabilizing between the fracture site and the area of stretching.
Fracture—recent	CI	Tan, 1998[2]	MD/PT	
	CI	Kisner and Colby, 1996[1]	PT	
	Caution	Hall and Brody, 2005[4]	PT	

R00-R99 SYMPTOMS, SIGNS, AND ABNORMAL CLINICAL & LABORATORY FINDINGS (NOT ELSEWHERE CLASSIFIED)

Issue	LOC	Sources	Affil	Rationale/Comment
Pain—excessive	Extreme caution	Tan, 1998[2]	MD/PT	
	CI	Kisner and Colby, 1996[1]	PT	
Effusion	CI	Tan, 1998[2]	MD/PT	Edematous tissue is more susceptible to injury and can result in further pain and edema.
	P	Kisner and Colby, 1996[1]	PT	
Inflammation	CI	Tan, 1998[2]	MD/PT	
	CI	Hall and Brody, 2005[4,a]	PT	
Hematoma	CI	Tan, 1998[2]	MD/PT	
	CI	Kisner and Colby, 1996[1]	PT	

a, Acute.

Y70-Y82 Medical Devices

Issue	LOC	Sources	Affil	Rationale/Comment
Arthroplasty—total elbow	P	Kisner and Colby, 1996[1]	PT	To protect the reattachment of the triceps mechanism during the postop management of total elbow arthroplasty (i.e., during the maximal protection phase [3-5 days], avoid stretching the triceps).
Joint replacements—total	CI	Maihafer, 1990[8,a]	PT	
	Extreme caution	Tan, 1998[2]	MD/PT	

a, Forcible movement of a total joint replacement that leads to pain during the immediate postoperative stages.

PROCEDURAL CONCERNS

Issue	LOC	Sources	Affil	Rationale/Comment
Ballistic stretching—bouncing	Avoid P	Hoffman et al, 1998[10] Tan, 1998[2]	MD MD/PT	Ballistic stretches involve high-intensity, short-duration,[2] repetitive, bouncing movements and body momentum.[10] The risk of injury increases during ballistic stretching because more energy is absorbed by the musculotendinous unit, causing potential ruptures,[10] microtrauma, and stretch reflex activity.[2] Elderly sedentary individuals and those in the early healing stages of injuries are particularly at risk, and therefore ballistic type stretches are not advised during the early phase of rehabilitation.[9]
Elderly	Caution	Hall and Brody, 2005[4]	PT	This population presents with greater stiffness.[4]
Pain or soreness lasting >24 hours following stretching	P	Kisner and Colby, 1996[1]	PT	Normally, only transitory tenderness should be experienced.
Prolonged immobility, persons with	Caution	Hall and Brody, 2005[4]	PT	
Stretching—beyond a joint's normal range of motion	P	Kisner and Colby, 1996[1]	PT	The range of motion of a joint varies among individuals and has a limit, beyond which tissues may rupture. **In a 1997 New Jersey lawsuit,[11] a 55-year-old male was awarded $537,507 after his rotator cuff reruptured during allegedly aggressive physical therapy.** **In a 1982 case series, McGarry[12] describes three patients with SCI (levels: T1; C5; C6) who experienced autonomic hyperreflexia while stretching.**

Continued

Issue	LOC	Sources	Affil	Rationale/Comment
				In a 1996 Florida lawsuit,[13] a 32-year-old male with a healing Achilles tendon rupture was awarded $115,000 in a settlement after a PT, unfamiliar with the diagnosis, stretched and reruptured the tendon.
Stretching of elbow flexors— vigorous	P	Pierson and Fairchild, 2002[9]	PT	Vigorous stretching of the elbow flexors may cause internal trauma of these muscles and precipitate myositis ossificans, especially in children. Consider doing stretching gently and use active inhibition techniques.
Stretching of knee extensors— too vigorously	P	Pierson and Fairchild, 2002[9]	PT	Vigorous stretching at the knee extensors can traumatize the knee joint and cause edema. **In a 1999 Maryland lawsuit,[14] a 25-year-old female with an ACL reconstruction was awarded $890,068 after her PT allegedly hyperflexed patient's right knee, fracturing the bone plug, and rupturing the graft of the ACL.**
Stretching the metatarsal heads	P	Pierson and Fairchild, 2002[9,a]	PT	Overstretching the long arch of the foot may result in a rocker-bottom foot.

a, Excessive force against the heads of the metatarsal heads and stretching the long arch of the foot.

ADVERSE EVENTS

Source	Background	Therapy	Outcome	Follow up / Interpretation
McGarry et al, 1982[12] **Autonomic hyperreflexia, self-stretching, and SCI**	A 21-year-old male with T1 paraplegia due to a MVA presented 5 months ago with complete anesthesia.	He self-administered hip flexion SLR from 0 to 125 degrees bilaterally, moving ankles close to ears. He noted a headache, bradycardia, and sweating, and his blood pressure increased from 90/60 to 190/120.	Elevation of his head to 90 degrees resulted in a fall in blood pressure to normal within 5 minutes. The patient was advised to perform SLR to 90-100 degrees (i.e., and stop), and no further symptoms occurred.	Autonomic hyperreflexia (e.g., increased blood pressure with bradycardia, sweating, and headaches) can occur in patients with severe upper thoracic and cervical spinal cord lesions and can be evoked by stimuli applied below the injury level, such as passive hip joint stretching.
Case series Phys Ther	A 31-year-old male presented with complete C5 quadriplegia due to MVA. He had experienced episodes of hyperreflexia at 5 months related to bladder distension.	It was noted that when his paralyzed legs were passively flexed at the hips to 90 degrees or more (120 degrees available), blood pressure increased from 120/80 to 190/150 and headaches appeared that lasted 45 minutes.	Blood pressure fell after exercise ceased and normalized within 10 minutes. Passive hip flexion was limited to less than 90 degrees with no further symptoms noted.	Proposed mechanism: stretching of the joint capsule or proximal leg muscles that were innervated by L4-5 and S1 stimulated the response. CS Sherrington showed that hyperextension of the toes in spinal cat resulted in an abrupt rise in blood pressure.[12]

Continued

Source	Background	Therapy	Outcome	Follow up / Interpretation
	A 37-year-old man presented with C6 quadriplegia due to a MVA and heterotopic bone formation in bilateral thighs at 3 months (ROM 0 to 65 degrees)	Passive hip flexion to 60 degrees caused sweating, a throbbing headache, and a rise in blood pressure from 110/70 to 170/110. His pulse rate dropped from 62 to 52 bpm and continued for 5-10 minutes after exercise stopped.	No further episodes noted following 0.1 mg reserpre/day	
Shulman and Grossman, 1970[7] **Stretching, fracture and fatal embolism** Case report Am J Dis Child	An 11-year-old girl with severe dermatomyositis (proximal muscle tenderness/ weakness) presented with bilateral adrenalectomy and oophorectomy (to control disease progression), calcinosis universalis, severe osteoporosis and severe flexion contractures of her elbows and knees. She was on long-term steroid use (prednisone, hydrocortisone) from 1965 to 1968.	She was seen in physical therapy for bracing (to permit ambulation); On the 10th day, range of motion and hair combing improved. On day 17, the child complained of pain following passive range of motion and gentle stretching to her legs. She became semidelirious, dyspneic, tachypneic, and tachycardic. After 20 minutes, she turned pale, cyanotic, and comatose.	Chest x-rays revealed diffuse infiltrates in both lungs (R>L). She was given O_2 and 50 mg hydrocortisone, but she *died* within 4 hours from cardiorespiratory arrest. Postmortem exam revealed massive fatty microthromboembolisms to the lungs, brain, and kidney and a complete fracture-dislocation of her right proximal tibia with hemarthrosis.	Contributing osteoporotic factors offered by the author include immobilization, corticosteroids, dermatomyositis with calcinosis universalis, and estrogen and/or androgen (patient had undergone adrenalectomy and oophorectomy). The issue of vigorous physical therapy was also discussed.

Year State	History	Location	Therapy	Complication	Comments Award
2001 Pennsylvania[6] **Femoral fracture and SCI**	A person with quadriplegia over 25 years	Physical therapist—home care	Weekly ROM "stretching exercises." During one session, the patient's femur made an audible "crack."	A femur fracture requiring rod insertion and 5-day hospitalization.	$65,000 settlement.
1999 Maryland[14] **Hyperflexion and fractured bone graft**	A 25-year-old female presented with an ACL tear due to a fall and ACL reconstruction.	Hospital and physical therapist.	The physical therapist performed a prone flexion maneuver.	The therapist allegedly hyperflexed the patient's right knee, fracturing the bone plug, and rupturing the graft of the ACL.	The patient claimed the PT was negligent in hyperflexing the injured knee. Allegedly required three surgeries and anticipated three future surgeries including two knee replacement surgeries. $890,068 verdict.
1996 Florida[13] **Reruptured Achilles tendon**	A 32-year-old male s/p Achilles tendon rupture due to a flag football game in 1991 was treated with an 8-week cast and then referred to PT.	PT	A therapist unfamiliar with the case showed the treating therapist how to "stretch the muscles better." The foot was dorsiflexed while the leg was held straight in a raised position.	Immediate pain and verbal reaction followed. The tendon reruptured and required surgical repair.	It was claimed that the therapist stated, "Oops, I thought you were treating for a hamstring pull." $115,000 settlement.

Note: Awards and settlements do not necessarily prove a cause-effect relationship between equipment or technique and injury.

REFERENCES

1. Kisner C, Colby LA: Therapeutic exercise: foundations and techniques, ed 3. Philadelphia: FA Davis; 1996.
2. Tan JC: Practical manual of physical medicine and rehabilitation: diagnostics, therapeutics, and basic problems. St Louis: Mosby; 1998.
3. Pauls JA, Reed KL: Quick reference to physical therapy. Austin (TX): Pro-Ed; 2004.
4. Hall CM, Brody LT: Impaired range of motion and joint mobility. In: Hall CM, Brody LT, eds: Therapeutic exercise: moving toward function. Philadelphia: Lippincott Williams & Wilkins; 2005.
5. Sumers MF: Spinal cord injury: functional rehabilitation. Norwalk (CT): Appleton & Lange; 1992.
6. Medical malpractice verdicts, settlements and experts, September 2001, p 46, loc 1.
7. Shulman ST, Grossman BJ: Fat embolism in childhood. Review with report of a fatal case related to physical therapy in a child with dermatomyositis. Am J Dis Child 120(5):480-484, 1970.
8. Maihafer GC: Rehabilitation of total hip replacements and fracture management considerations. In Echternach JL, editor: Physical therapy of the hip. New York: Churchill Livingstone; 1990.
9. Pierson FM, Fairchild SL: Principles and techniques of patient care, ed 3. Philadelphia: W.B. Saunders; 2002.
10. Hoffman MD, Sheldahl LM, Kraemer WJ: Therapeutic exercise. In Delisa JA, Gans BM, eds: Rehabilitation medicine: principles and practice, ed 3. Philadelphia: Lippincott-Raven; 1998.
11. Medical malpractice verdicts, settlements and experts, September 1997, p 37, loc 3.
12. McGarry J, Woolsey RM, Thompson CW: Autonomic hyperreflexia following passive stretching to the hip joint. Phys Ther 62(1):30-31, 1982.
13. Medical malpractice verdicts, settlements and experts, February 1996, p 44, loc 2.
14. Medical malpractice verdicts, settlements, and experts, July 1999, p 42, loc 1.

OVERVIEW. Gait training is a technique of teaching walking skills. Deficient patterns are corrected by attending to muscle imbalances and the biomechanical components of walking during the stance and swing phase.[1] Preambulatory skills are often practiced in preparation for walking (mat activities that progress to a standing position). In this section, ambulation/gait training concerns are listed, followed by preambulatory issues.

SUMMARY: CONTRAINDICATIONS AND PRECAUTIONS. Sources contribute varied concerns for gait training. Major themes for gait training seem to center around (1) patient diagnoses—such as those with activity restriction, (2) environmental hazards, (3) inappropriate patient attire, and (4) hazardous tasks (also see *Chapter 29, Assistive Devices*, for proper use of equipment).

IMPORTANT NOTE. If the patient has activity-related restrictions (e.g., deep vein thrombosis; recent arthroplasty; recent fractures, recent skin grafts), it would be wise to consult with the appropriate specialist because management protocols can vary locally or may need to be tailored to the particular circumstances of the patient *(also applies to exercise)*.

GAIT TRAINING

CONTRAINDICATIONS AND PRECAUTIONS

I00-I99 DISEASES OF THE CIRCULATORY SYSTEM

Deep Venous Thrombosis (DVT)

Issue	LOC	Sources	Affil	Rationale/Comment
DVT: Ambulation as tolerated— patients treated with LMWH	Recommendation	ACCP, 2004[2]	Org	These 2004 ACCP recommendations are based on two randomized studies showing that patients on bed rest with anticoagulation did not have a reduced incidence of silent PE. Also, in another small randomized study, pain and swelling resolution rate were faster with early ambulation and leg compression as compared to bed rest. Furthermore, a low incidence of recurrent and fatal PE was noted in a study of 1289 patients with acute DVT involving walking exercises and compression bandages.
DVT restricted gait training and mobilization	Recommendation	Tan, 1998[3]	MD/PT	Restrict gait training and mobilization of affected limb until at least 1 to 2 days of therapeutic aPTT range have been attained while on IV heparin therapy. Until then, a bed rest regimen with affected limb elevated is recommended, and the patient is prohibited from moving it or walking.

Abbreviation: LMWH, low-molecular-weight heparin.

Peripheral Vascular Disease

Issue	LOC	Sources	Affil	Rationale/Comment
Dependency—Lower limb **Pain—At rest** **Pain—Increased over time**	Advice CI CI	Kisner and Colby, 1996[4]	PT	Avoid prolonged periods of standing still and sitting with legs in a dependent position. Patients experiencing resting pain should not participate in an ambulation or bicycling program. If leg pain increases rather than decreases over time, graded ambulation or bicycling should be discontinued.

Q00-Q99 CONGENITAL MALFORMATIONS, DEFORMITIES, AND CHROMOSOMAL ABNORMALITIES

Issue	LOC	Sources	Affil	Rationale/Comment
Osteogenesis imperfecta (moderate to severe)— need braces for ambulation	Recommend	Bleakney and Donahoe, 1994[5]	PT	Braces and splints are usually required for standing to protect weight bearing on *osteoporotic* bony deformities during the preschool period. Without adequate support, further bending of long bones may occur because of abnormal stresses acting on weakened structures.

L00-L99 DISEASES OF THE SKIN AND SUBCUTANEOUS TISSUE

Issue	LOC	Sources	Affil	Rationale/Comment
Cellulitis	CI	Helm, 1982[6]	MD	Ambulation is contraindicated if cellulitis is present.
Skin graft— new	Ambulation can be limited due to presence of new skin graft, i.e., LE graft, 5-10 days	Spires[7] Staley and Richard, 2001[8]	MD PT	Discontinue ambulation in patients with LE skin grafts until safe to resume.[8] In general, the patient is not permitted to place legs in a dependent position for up to 5-10 days. Begin ambulation once
	Discontinue ambulation			competent circulation is established in the graft and the risk of venous pooling, which can cause graft loss, is reduced.[7] Walking is resumed
	Resume 6-10 days	Helm, 1982[6]	MD	6 to 10 days after grafting.[6] Note: Protocols may vary.

S00-T98 INJURY, POISONING, AND CERTAIN OTHER CONSEQUENCES OF EXTERNAL CAUSES

Issue	LOC	Sources	Affil	Rationale/Comment
Foot burns—severe	CI	Helm, 1982[6]	MD	Ambulation is contraindicated if a severe foot burn is present.[6]
Fracture site—Distal stress	Care	Kisner and Colby, 1996[4]	PT	Until a fracture site is radiologically healed (consult with physician), use care any time stress is placed distal to the fracture site following the immobilization period (examples of stress are resistance, stretch, and weight bearing).[4]
Swelling of legs/feet—severe (in burn patients)	CI	Helm, 1982[6]	MD	Ambulation is contraindicated if severe swelling of the feet and legs are present in the burn patient.[6]
Tendons of joint capsule— Exposed (in burn patients)	CI			Ambulation is contraindicated if exposed tendons of the joint capsules are present in the burn patient.[6]

Issue	LOC	Sources	Affil	Rationale/Comment
Wound—i.e., diabetic; neuropathic	CI	Knight, 2001[9,a]	PT	Patients with ulcerations of the feet and wounds or fungal infections should not participate in a walking program.[4] Plantar wounds (i.e., diabetic, neuropathic) must be treated with pressure reduction (bed rest or non–weight-bearing gait patterns).[9]

a, Plantar diabetic wounds.

Y70-Y82 Medical Devices, General

(also see specific assistive device under **Devices**)

Issue	LOC	Sources	Affil	Rationale/Comment
Adjustment buttons—locations	P	Pierson and Fairchild, 2002[10]	PT	Check that spring adjustment buttons are securely in their holes.
Devices—inspect for damage	P			Inspect device for cracks or broken parts. Inspect wing nuts for adequate tensions. **See FDA reports under Devices: canes, crutches, walkers.**[11]
Grab bars	P			Safety grab bars should be attached to wall studs or the floor.
Infusion site (IV)—keep at heart level	Avoid			Ambulators are instructed to grasp the IV line support pole so the infusion site will be at their heart level. If the IV site remains in a dependent position, retrograde flow of blood into the IV line tubing may result. Similar procedures are observed when patients are treated in bed or on a treatment mat.
Patient appliances—tubes, dressings	P			Protect patient appliances during ambulation (e.g., drainage tubes, intravenous tubes, dressings).
Support tips (ambulatory devices)—inspect for wear	P			Inspect support tips of devices for wear or damage or dirt; moisture on support tips cause slips.
Wheelchair—preparation	Advice	Pierson and Fairchild, 2002[10]	PT	In preparation for standing to walk, stabilize wheelchair and place footrests in an upright position.

Y70-Y82 Medical Devices

(for assistive devices, see **Chapter 29**)

Total hip replacement[a]

Issue	LOC	Sources	Affil	Rationale/Comment
Weight bearing				
Hip arthroplasty—cemented	Advice	Brander and Stulberg, 2005[12,a]	MD	Weight-bearing status is commonly FWB or PWB (about 70% weight).
Hip arthroplasty—uncemented	Advice	Brander and Stulberg, 2005[12,a]	MD	Restricted weight-bearing (PWB or touch down [10-15% body weight])
	P	Maihafer, 1990[13]	PT	for 6-12 weeks after surgery.[12] (Uncemented implants that completely fill and fit femoral canal may be FWB).[12] Use an assistive device for longer time to allow bony ingrowth into prosthetic device (porous-coated arthroplasties) to occur.[13]
Hip arthroplasty—with trochanteric osteotomies	Gait training delayed or caution (PWB)	Maihafer, 1990[13]	PT	Treat osteotomies more conservatively because the trochanter is reflected before the prosthesis is installed. The trochanter is then internally fixated—thus the osteotomized bone can be damaged if stressed (i.e., forces generating by the gluteus maximus during gait).
Turning/pivoting				
Turning or pivoting on a lower extremity with a recent total hip replacement	ACI	Pierson and Fairchild, 2002[10]	PT	The patient must learn to pivot while bearing weight on the non-surgical lower extremity
	CI	Tan, 1998[3,b]	MD/PT	

a, Protocols are not standardized and are based on surgeon preference. Some conditions that may affect weight-bearing status for THR include the presence of fractures, trochanteric osteotomies, bone grafts, acetabular or femoral bone loss (significant), or other unusual circumstances. b, Leg-crossing concern.

Issue	LOC	Sources	Affil	Rationale/Comment
Guarding	Advice	Minor, 1999[14]	PT	<u>Ambulating advice</u>—stand behind, slightly to one side, and in stride with the patient. <u>Stair advice</u>—(ascending or descending)—position self below patient, stand in stride (to allow weight shifting), with one hand on gait belt (worn by the patient) and other hand on the stair rail (a stability point).
Instructions—patient and family	P	Pierson and Fairchild, 2002[10]	PT	Provide written instructions and precautions for the patient and family, especially if the patient uses an assistive device for maximal body support, such as in persons who are NWB on one lower extremity.
Monitor—physiologic responses	P			Monitor physiologic responses—vital signs, general appearance, mental alertness—and compare to normal values to determine patient's tolerance and response to activity.
Patients—unattended	P			Do not leave patient unattended while standing, because patients may be less stable than they appear.
Patient behaviors—unusual	P			Be alert to unusual patient behaviors or equipment problems, as the patient may slip or lose stability at any time. **In 1999, Goriganti[15] described a 79-year-old man with a left transtibial amputation who partially ruptured his pectoralis major while gait training with a walker, possibly due to the high UE loads.**

Continued

Issue	LOC	Sources	Affil	Rationale/Comment
Safety belts	P/Advice	Pierson and Fairchild, 2002[10]	PT	A safety belt is necessary during all initial level ground and functional gait activities until the patient is able to ambulate independently and safely.[10] **In a 1970 case report, James[16] described a**
	Advice	Minor, 1999[14]	PT	**54-year-old female who was awarded $18,312.50 in a lawsuit after the patient fell while walking with crutches due to PT's inadequate grasp of her. In a 1997 Wisconsin lawsuit,[17] a 6-year-old child with cerebral palsy was awarded $45,000 in a settlement after he sustained a fracture from a fall while a school PT stood behind him to hold his leg straight.**
Training— individualized	Advice	Tan, 1998[3]	MD/PT	Training is individualized, based on diagnosis, specific contraindications (e.g., weight-bearing status), and goals for the patient.

PROCEDURAL CONCERNS: CLOTHING

Issue	LOC	Sources	Affil	Rationale/Comment
Clothes—inappropriate use as a support	P	Pierson and Fairchild, 2002[10]	PT	Do not use patient's clothing, upper extremity, or personal belt for control, because it is not sufficiently strong or secure.
Footwear—fitting	P	Pierson and Fairchild, 2002[10]	PT	Avoid slippers or loose-fitting shoes, as patient may be less secure, leading to injury. In patients
	P	Kisner and Colby, 1996[4]	PT	with PVD, shoes must fit properly and should not cause sores or skin irritation blisters.[4]

PROCEDURAL CONCERNS: ENVIRONMENTAL

Issue	LOC	Sources	Affil	Rationale/Comment
Area rugs	P	Pierson and Fairchild, 2002[10]	PT	Loose and small area rugs threaten safety.
Floors—wet	P			Ambulation on wet floors can lead to slips.
Floors—waxed or polished	P			Waxed or polished floor surfaces threaten safety.
Furniture placement	P			Provide 36-inch-wide unobstructed pathways.
Real-world conditions	P			Grass; rough, uneven surfaces in crowded, busy stores; or sidewalk may be more challenging for the patient.
Thresholds, lips, overhangs	P			I.e., doorway thresholds, stair lips, stair tread overhang, or changes from one type of surface to different surface (linoleum to carpeted surface).
Walking area	P	Pierson and Fairchild, 2002[10]	PT	The walking area used for ambulation should be free of hazard-related obstructions such as equipment or furniture.
Weather/temperature—cold	P	Kisner and Colby, 1996[4]	PT	Avoid exercising a person with PVD in very cold weather.
Weather/temperature—hot		Simons, 1937[18]	MD	Avoid exercising persons with multiple sclerosis in hot weather/temperatures because it may lead to fatigue and a worsening of their symptoms **(also see Resistive exercise).**

PROCEDURAL CONCERNS: TASKS

Issue	LOC	Sources	Affil	Rationale/Comment
Turning by pivoting on a single extremity	Advice	Schmitz, 2001[19]	PT	The patient may potentially lose balance under the small base of one limb. Consider stepping in small circles instead.
Falling techniques	P	Pierson and Fairchild, 2002[10]	PT	Floor mats should be used to prevent injury.
Walking—backward Author suggested backward walking as CI if any of the following patient conditions exist: • Visual postural sway • History of falls • Obstacles; low friction surfaces • Poor reaction time • Poor protective reflexes • Neuromuscular disease • Impaired judgment/cognition • Lack of available assistance	CI	Thomas and Fast, 2000[20]	MD	**In 2000, Thomas and Fast[20] described two cases: (1) A 73-year-old male with hemiparesis walked backwards on a beam placed on the floor under close supervision of a PT. He fell, fractured his hip, and required an ORIF. (2) A 74-year-old female with LS radiculopathy, who was asked by the PT to walk backward, tripped over a treadmill and fell down; she required diskectomy and fusion due to an exacerbation of her condition.**

PREAMBULATORY ACTIVITIES

Prone-on-elbows position (POE)

I00-I99 DISEASES OF THE CIRCULATORY SYSTEM

J00-J99 DISEASES OF THE RESPIRATORY SYSTEM

G00-G99 DISEASES OF THE NERVOUS SYSTEM

M00-M99 DISEASES OF THE MUSCULOSKELETAL SYSTEM AND CONNECTIVE TISSUE

Issue	LOC	Sources	Affil	Rationale/Comment
Tolerance of posture— poor	Caution	Schmitz, 2001[20]	PT	The prone-on-elbows position may be difficult for some patients to tolerate. Examples include patients with low back pain (the lordotic curve required for this position may exacerbate pain); with stroke-related spasticity; with shoulder or elbow pathologies; with cardiac or respiratory compromise; or with hip flexor tightness. Consider using a wedge cushion to reduce load.

Sitting

M00-M99 DISEASES OF THE MUSCULOSKELETAL SYSTEM AND CONNECTIVE TISSUE				
Issue	LOC	Sources	Affil	Rationale/Comment
Long sitting—difficulties	Caution	Schmitz, 2001[20]	PT	Long sitting may be difficult to attain (due to tight low back or hamstrings) and can result in sacral sitting.

Standing—Assuming

I00-I99 DISEASES OF THE CIRCULATORY SYSTEM				
Issue	LOC	Sources	Affil	Rationale/Comment
Orthostatic hypotension—postural	Caution	Schmitz, 2001[20]	PT	Caution particularly if the patient has been on bed rest or in a wheelchair for a period of time.

Parallel Bar Activities

PROCEDURAL CONCERN				
Issue	LOC	Sources	Affil	Rationale/Comment
Axillary pressure	Caution	Schmitz, 2001[20]	PT	Take care not to exert pressure into the axilla; **see Assistive devices—crutches (Chapter 29.2).**
Gait belt	Caution/ Advice	Schmitz, 2001[20]	PT	Use a guarding belt while gait training in parallel bars because it helps to control loss of balance, improve patient safety, facilitate body mechanics, and address liability issues.

ADVERSE EVENTS

Source	Background	Therapy	Outcome	Follow-up/Interpretation
Thomas and Fast, 2000[20] **Falls and Backwards walking** Case series Am J Phys Med Rehab	A 73-year-old male with R hemiparesis and viral encephalitis was alert and oriented, independent in ambulation without device, had normal sensation, but could not stand unilaterally.	Referred to physical therapy for strength and balance training, the patient could stand 15 sec on RLE and 5 sec on LLE and tandem walk without support in parallel bars. In outpatient PT, the therapist asked him to walk backwards on a beam placed on the floor under close supervision.	Patient fell and fractured hip, requiring an ORIF.	Backward walking tasks eliminate visual cues. Authors suggest using suspension device.
	A 74-year-old female with a Dx of LBP with right LS radiculopathy, spinal stenosis, and disk herniation (L4/5) had undergone microdiskectomy without relief.	Referred to outpatient PT 6 weeks later, she was asked to walk backwards.	The patient tripped over a treadmill and fell down. A few hours later, LBP and radicular signs were exacerbated. An MRI scan revealed a recurrent hematoma in a right recess. She underwent diskectomy, decompression, and fusion when she did not respond to conservative treatment.	

Continued

Source	Background	Therapy	Outcome	Follow-up/Interpretation
Goriganti et al, 1999[15] **Muscle rupture and Gait training** Case report Arch Phys Med Rehab	A 79-year-old man with a recent left transtibial amputation had a PMHx of coronary artery disease, hypertension, MI, pacemaker, and severe right hip degenerative joint disease.	He received gait training for 1 week using a lightweight endoskeletal below-knee prosthesis and a standard walker. The next day, he reported acute pain and noted ecchymosis over left pectoral area.	Dx: Partial rupture pectoralis major (proximal portion). Treated with rest, ice, and analgesics, the patient's pain resolved in 1 week. Progressive isometrics were started, and prosthetic training resumed within 2 weeks.	The authors wish you to be aware of the high UE loads during walker ambulation, particularly for persons with musculoskeletal deficits and in age-related weakness.
Rafii et al, 1982[21] **Stress fractures and ambulation** Case report Arch Phys Med Rehab	A 17-year-old man with T8 paraplegia in October 1977 with GI, GU, and decubiti ulcer complications received bedside PT.	Upon eventual transfer to rehabilitation in May 1978, he began ambulation training with crutches.	At the end of August, serum alkaline phosphatase levels were found to be elevated and radiographs revealed a bilateral acetabular fractures. There were no reports of falls.	The authors believe the repetitive nature of ambulation using bracing and crutches and the lack of sensation contribute to these stress fractures.
James, 1970[16] **Fall and gait training** Case report (litigation) Phys Ther	A 54-year-old female (dx and history not reported) was escorted by a PT from a waiting room to treatment area.	The patient lost control of her crutches and slipped from the PT's grasp.	Patient fell, severely injuring her back. The PT admitted having an inadequate grasp on the patient's arm.	Verdict for the plaintiff: $18,312.50.

Brooks and Fowler, 1964[22] **Axillobrachial ischemia and axillary crutches** Case series J Bone Joint Surg	A 48-year-old male office worker used a single crutch on his right side since age 5 due to poliomyelitis. He complained of a sudden pain onset, numbness, and weakness of his RUE and hand for the past 5 days.	An ischemic RUE and absent axillobrachial pulse were noted.	Treatment included sympathetic blocks to decrease pain, and increase strength and a knee fusion to eliminate the need for a crutch. At 6 years, some RUE aching was reported with use.	If axillary crutches cause exertional pain in the extremity, discontinue crutches. Use forearm crutches to eliminate axillary pressure.
	A 50-year-old farmer used a single axillary crutch on the right side due to right LE paralysis in childhood. In December (1955) he developed a thorn-induced wound infection in his right ring finger.	1 month later, he developed numbness and tingling of the right forearm and hand which decreased when the crutch was not used. At 4 months, numbness, burning, and ischemia with ulceration of the ring finger were noted, as well as a reduced axillobrachial arterial pulse.	Dx: Gangrene. Treatment included sympathetic blocks and later removal of stellate and thoracic sympathetic ganglia. Infection persisted and amputation of the finger with follow-up amputation of the middle three rays of the hand and palmar structures were performed due to gangrene.	
	A 65-year-old man used one axillary crutch on his right side for 50 years due to poliomyelitis.	Sudden pain and numbness in the right forearm and hand was noted despite sympathetic blocks.	After 3 weeks he was hospitalized with an absent axillary pulse, and gangrene of his right hand. Treatment involved right mid-forearm amputation.	

LITIGATION

Year State	History	Location	Therapy	Complication	Comments/ Award
1997[17] Wisconsin **Fall and gait training**	A 6-year-old male s/p developmental disabilities, cerebral palsy.	School physical therapy.	The PT stood behind child to hold leg straight. The child fell face forward.	The child's leg was twisted and fractured. He was placed in a cast and hospitalized for 6 days.	It was claimed that the PT should have used a device or another method to stand with legs straight. $45,000 settlement.

Note: Awards and settlements do not necessarily prove a cause-effect relationship between equipment or technique and injury.

REFERENCES

1. Bottomley JM: Quick reference dictionary for physical therapy. Thorofare (NJ): Slack; 2000.

2. Agnelli G, Hull RD, Hyers TM, et al: Antithrombotic therapy for venous thromboembolic disease: the Seventh ACCP Conference on Antithrombotic and thrombolytic therapy. Chest 126(3, Suppl): 401S-428S, 2004.

3. Tan JC: Practical manual of physical medicine and rehabilitation: diagnostics, therapeutics, and basic problems. St Louis: Mosby; 1998.

4. Kisner C, Colby LA: Therapeutic exercise: foundations and techniques, ed 3. Philadelphia: FA Davis; 1996.

5. Bleakney DA, Donahoe M: Osteogenesis imperfecta. In: Campbell SK, Palisono R, Vander Linden, eds: Physical therapy for children. Philadelphia: W.B. Saunders; 1994.

6. Helm PA, Kevorkian CG, Lushbaugh M, et al: Burn injury: rehabilitation management in 1982. Arch Phys Med Rehab 63:6-16, 1982.

7. Spires MC: Rehabilitation of patients with burns. In: Braddom RL, editor: Physical medicine and rehabilitation, ed 2. Philadelphia: W.B. Saunders; 2000.

8. Staley M, Serghiou M: Casting guidelines, tips and techniques: proceedings from the 1977 American Burn Association PT/OT Casting Workshop. J Burn Care Rehab 19(3):254-260, 1998.

9. Knight CA: Peripheral vascular disease and wound care. In O'Sullivan SB, Schmitz TJ, eds: Physical rehabilitation and treatment, ed 4. Philadelphia: FA Davis; 2001.

10. Pierson FM, Fairchild SL: Principles and techniques of patient care, ed 3. Philadelphia: W.B. Saunders; 2002.

11. US Food and Drug Administration: Center for Device and Radiological Health. Available at: http://www.fda.gov/cdrh/mdr/.

12. Brander VA, Stulberg SD: Rehabilitation after lower limb joint reconstruction. In Delisa JA, editor: Physical medicine and rehabilitation: Principles and practices, vol 1. Philadelphia: Lippincott Williams & Wilkins; 2005.

13. Maihafer GC: Rehabilitation of total hip replacements and fracture management considerations. In Echternach JL, editor: Physical therapy of the hip, New York: Churchill Livingstone; 1990.

14. Minor MAD, Minor SD: Patient care skills, ed 4. Stamford (CT): Appleton & Lange; 1999.

15. Goriganti MR, Bodack MP, Nagler W. Pectoralis major rupture during gait training: case report. Arch Phys Med Rehab 80(1): 115-7, 1999.

16. James CA Jr: Medico-legal considerations in the practice of physical therapy. Phys Ther 50(8):1203-1207, 1970.

17. Medical Malpractice Verdict Settlement and Experts, January 1997, p 41, loc 2.

18. Simons DJ: A note on the effect of heat and of cold upon certain symptoms of multiple sclerosis. Bull Neurol Inst N Y 6:385-386, 1937.

19. Schmitz TJ: Preambulatory and gait training. In O'Sullivan SB, Schmitz TJ, eds: Physical rehabilitation and treatment, ed 4. Philadelphia: FA Davis; 2001.

20. Thomas MA, Fast A: One step forward and two steps back: the dangers of walking backwards in therapy. Am J Phys Med Rehab 79(5), 459-61, 2000.

21. Rafii M, Firooznia H, Golimbu C, et al: Bilateral acetabular stress fractures in a paraplegic patient. Arch Phys Med Rehab 63(5):240-241, 1982.

22. Brooks AL, Fowler SB: Axillary artery thrombosis after prolonged use of crutches. J Bone Joint Surg 46A(4):863-864, 1964.

15   RELAXATION TECHNIQUES (PROGRESSIVE MUSCLE RELAXATION)

OVERVIEW.   Progressive muscle relaxation (PMR) is a general method of relaxation by consciously contracting and then relaxing groups of muscles. The technique was originally developed by Jacobson, a Chicago physician, and has been used to reduce stress, reduce pain, and promote health.[1]

SUMMARY: CONTRAINDICATIONS AND PRECAUTIONS.   Two sources cited a total of seven concerns for relaxation techniques in the Jacobson tradition. Snyder, a nurse, cited six concerns, whereas Bernstein (PhD) cited one. About 70% of the concerns were procedural and related to eliciting hypotensive responses or potentiating medication effects. Other concerns relate to cardiac patients (performing isometric contractions) and chronic pain patients (focusing too much on pain).

CONTRAINDICATIONS AND PRECAUTIONS

F00–F99 MENTAL AND BEHAVIORAL DISORDERS/M00–M99 DISEASES OF THE MUSCULOSKELETAL SYSTEM AND CONNECTIVE TISSUE

Issue	LOC	Sources	Affil	Rationale/Comment
Chronic pain patients	P	Snyder et al, 2002[1]	Nurs	Tension and relaxation of muscles may heighten their awareness of their pain (pain intensification) following PMR.

Issue	LOC	Sources	Affil	Rationale/Comment
Cardiac patients	P	Snyder et al, 2002[1]	Nurs	When tensing and relaxing groups of muscles, an increased blood volume is placed into circulation at one time, placing an *undue* load on a damaged heart. Cardiac patients should avoid combining muscle groups (i.e., from 14 to 7) when tensing and relaxing groups of muscles.

PROCEDURAL CONCERNS

Issue	LOC	Sources	Affil	Rationale/Comment
Appropriate goal— relaxation	Advice	Bernstein and Borkovec, 1973[2]	PhD	Relaxation goals should not run contrary to other goals, i.e., if the goal is to strengthen (develop tension) rather than reduce it.
Expectation—unrealistic	Advice	Snyder, 1985[3]	Nurs	Avoid unrealistic expectation.
Hypotensive state— potential	P	Snyder et al, 2002[1]		Complete muscle relaxation can lead to a hypotensive state.
				Monitor blood pressure in some individuals after the session to determine those at risk. Sit for few minutes following session; gradually resume activities.
Medication— potentiating effects	P	Snyder et al, 2002[1]		Trophotropic reactions may occur (i.e., affecting the drug's pharmacokinetics) if the individual engages regularly in PMR. It can potentiate the effects of the medication. Lower dosage of medication may be needed if PMR is done regularly. Example: insulin.
Practice—narrow	Advice	Snyder et al, 2002[1]		Avoid narrowing practices that use only these techniques.

REFERENCES

1. Snyder M, Pestka E, Bly C: Progressive muscle relaxation. In: Snyder M, Lindquist R, eds: Complementary/alternative therapies in nursing, ed 4. New York: Springer; 2002.
2. Bernstein D, Borkovec TD: Progressive relaxation training: a manual for the helping professions. Champaign (IL): Research Press; 1973.
3. Snyder M: Independent nursing interventions. New York: Wiley; 1985.

16 STRENGTH, POWER, AND ENDURANCE TRAINING

16.1 Active Range of Motion

OVERVIEW. Active range of motion (AROM, also active assisted range of motion [AAROM]) is movement generated by active muscle contraction and produced within the unrestricted portion of a joint. In active-assisted range of motion, manual or mechanical assistance is provided by an outside force to assist the prime mover through the available joint range.[1,2] AROM concerns generally relate to acute cardiac or vascular conditions, stress to unstable or still fragile musculoskeletal or skin tissue (e.g., postop, injuries), or activities that further compromise a structure (e.g., spinal stenosis) (**also see ROM assessment**).

CONTRAINDICATIONS AND PRECAUTIONS

I00-I99 DISEASES OF THE CIRCULATORY SYSTEM

Issue	LOC	Source	Affil	Rationale/Comment
Cardiovascular status— unstable	CI/P	Tan, 1998[3]	MD/PT	During an MI, reduced blood flow to coronary artery leads to myocardial ischemia and necrosis. Initially, there may be some activity restrictions to reduce the cardiac workload **(also see Cardiac rehabilitation).**
	CI	Pierson and Fairchild, 2002[4,a]	PT	
Thrombophlebitis—acute	CI	Kisner and Colby, 1996[1]	PT	Life-threatening deep venous thrombosis can lead to pulmonary embolism. During the initial stages, the patient is usually on bed rest **(also see Gait training).**
Valsalva maneuvers	Caution	Pierson and Fairchild, 2002[4]	PT	Caution in an effort to prevent complications leading to stroke or death **(also see Resistive exercise).**

a, Cardiopulmonary dysfunction.

L00-L99 DISEASES OF THE SKIN AND SUBCUTANEOUS TISSUE

Issue	LOC	Source	Affil	Rationale/Comment
Skin grafts	Advice	Staley and Richard, 2001[5]	PT	To allow grafts to heal, discontinue AROM (and PROM) for 3-5 days if the patient just received a skin graft (reinstitution is determined by the surgeon).

M00-M99 DISEASES OF THE MUSCULOSKELETAL SYSTEM AND CONNECTIVE TISSUE

Issue	LOC	Source	Affil	Rationale/Comment
Spinal stenosis and extension	Avoid	Hall, 2005[8]	PT	Increased pain with extension activities may be attributed to a narrowing of the canal during spinal extension, rotation with extension, or anterior translation (i.e., swayback).
Spondylolysis/spondylolisthesis and lumbar extension	Avoid			Shear forces and lumbar extension should be avoided in this population.

O00-O99 PREGNANCY, CHILDBIRTH, AND PUERPERIUM

Issue	LOC	Sources	Affil	Rationale/Comment
Fire hydrant exercise—posture of male dogs urinating	Unsafe	Kisner and Colby, 1996[1]	PT	The sacroiliac (SI) joint can be excessively compressed when the hip is abducted and hip and knee are flexed during a fire hydrant exercise. This is particularly problematic if the patient has preexisting SI problems.[1]
One-legged activities	Unsafe			Unilateral weight-bearing activities can result in SI joint or pubic symphysis irritation (avoid if preexisting SI symptoms). One-legged balancing may be affected due to increased weight and changes in the patient's center of gravity during pregnancy.[1]
Quadruped (on all-fours) with hip extension	Unsafe			If the hip is extended beyond its available range, the pelvis can anteriorly tilt and hyperextend the lumbar spine.[1]
Straight leg raising—bilateral	Unsafe			Raising both legs places stress on abdominal muscles and low back and can result in back injuries or diastasis recti.[1]

R00-R99 SYMPTOMS, SIGNS INVOLVING THE SYSTEM

Issue	LOC	Sources	Affil	Rationale/Comment
Pain, joint or soft tissue	Caution	Pierson and Fairchild, 2002[5]	PT	E.g., acute RA, acute OA, hemophilia
Swelling, joint	Caution			

S00-T98 INJURY, POISONING, AND CERTAIN OTHER CONSEQUENCES OF EXTERNAL CAUSES

Issue	LOC	Sources	Affil	Rationale/Comment
Fracture, unhealed/unprotected	CI	Pierson and Fairchild, 2002[4]	PT	
Soft tissue trauma, severe	CI			
Surgical site, unhealed/unprotected	CI			

Y70-Y82 MEDICAL DEVICES

THR: Posterior lateral incisions/Approach

Issue	LOC	Sources	Affil	Rationale/Comment
Hip flexion (excessive), adduction past neutral, internal rotation	P/Avoid	Kisner and Colby, 1996[1]	PT	For posterior or lateral incisions: to protect against complications of a posterior dislocation.[6] For the first few days, avoid hip flexion past 45 degrees and adduction past neutral during ROM and ADL. By weeks 2 to 3 post-op, usually allowed hip flexion to 90 degrees (consult with surgeon).[1]
	Avoid	Brander and Stulberg, 2005[6,a]	MD	
	Avoid	Pierson and Fairchild, 2002[4,b]	PT	
	Avoid	Maihafer, 1990[7,c]	PT	

a, Hip flexion >90 degrees, adduction and internal rotation beyond midline; does not specify ROM by type (also see under **Anterior approach** [next] for additional prohibitions); b, Hip flexion >60 to 90 degrees, internal hip rotation, for posterior or posterolateral surgical approach; c, Hip flexion >90 degrees, internal rotation, adduction, surgical approach not specified.

THR: Anterior Lateral Incisions/Approach

Issue	LOC	Sources	Affil	Rationale/Comment
Hip hyperextension, adduction (past neutral), external rotation	Avoid	Kisner and Colby, 1996[1]	PT	
	Prohibited	Brander and Stulberg, 2005[6,a]	MD	
	Avoid	Pierson and Fairchild, 2002[4,b]	PT	

a, Anterior approach: hip external rotation and hip extension prohibited, does not specify ROM by type; b, Hip external rotation, anterior or anterolateral surgical approach.

THR with Trochanteric Osteotomy

Issue	LOC	Sources	Affil	Rationale/Comment
Hip abduction (active or resisted) to strengthen gluteus medius	Avoid	Maihafer, 1990[7]	PT	Treat osteotomies more conservatively. For THR with trochanteric osteotomy, the trochanter is reflected before the prosthesis is installed. It is then internally fixated. This osteotomized bone can be damaged if stressed (i.e., by the gluteals) during gait.

PROCEDURAL CONCERNS

Issue	LOC	Source	Affil	Rationale/Comment
Intensification of symptoms with improper technique during AROM[a]	Caution	Pierson and Fairchild, 2002[4]	PT	
Sit up, bend knees	CI/P	Hall, 2005[8]	PT	-if thoracic kyphosis, trunk flexion flexibility or short hip flexors
Sit up, straight leg	CI/P			-if disk pathology
Sit up, trunk curl	CI/P			-if thoracic kyphosis
Motion that disrupts healing	CI	Kisner and Colby, 1996[1]	MD/PT	Early controlled motion (within proper range, speed, tolerance) may be
	CI/P	Tan, 1998[3]	PT	beneficial in the acute stages (of tears, fractures, surgeries) if patient
	CI	Brody, 2005[9,a]	MD/PT	tolerance is monitored and no additional trauma is caused.[1]

a, Also AAROM.

REFERENCES

1. Kisner C, Colby LA: Therapeutic exercise: foundations and techniques, ed 3. Philadelphia: FA Davis; 1996.
2. Bottomley JM: Quick reference dictionary for physical therapy. Thorofare (NJ): Slack; 2000.
3. Tan JC: Practical manual of physical medicine and rehabilitation: diagnostics, therapeutics, and basic problems. St Louis: Mosby; 1998.
4. Pierson FM, Fairchild SL: Principles and techniques of patient care, ed 3. Philadelphia: Saunders; 2002.
5. Staley M, Serghiou M: Casting guidelines, tips and techniques: proceedings from the 1977 American Burn Association PT/OT Casting Workshop. J Burn Care Rehab 19(3):254-260, 1998.
6. Brander VA, Stulberg SD: Rehabilitation after lower limb joint reconstruction. In Delisa JA, editor: Physical medicine and rehabilitation: Principles and practices, vol 1. Philadelphia: Lippincott Williams & Wilkins; 2005.
7. Maihafer GC: Rehabilitation of total hip replacements and fracture management considerations. In Echternach, JL, editor: Physical therapy of the hip. New York: Churchill Livingstone; 1990.
8. Hall C: Therapeutic exercise for the lumbopelvic region. In: Hall CM, Brody LT, eds: Therapeutic exercise: moving toward function. Philadelphia: Lippincott Williams & Wilkins; 2005.
9. Brody LT: Impaired joint mobility and range of motion. In: Hall CM, Brody LT, eds: Therapeutic exercise: moving toward function. Philadelphia: Lippincott Williams & Wilkins; 2005.

16.2 Closed Chain Exercise

Closed chain (CC) exercises involve activities where an individual's proximal body part moves over his or her fixed (i.e., stabilized) distal segment. An example is performing an upper extremity push-up.[1] There is some concern for stressing joints, particularly at the knee, while performing squats (a closed chain activity) at certain angles following ACL injuries or repairs.

CONTRAINDICATIONS AND PRECAUTIONS

M00-M99 DISEASES OF THE MUSCULOSKELETAL SYSTEM AND CONNECTIVE TISSUE

Issue	LOC	Source	Affil	Rationale/Comment
Non–weight-bearing status	CI	Kisner and Colby, 1986[1]	PT	
Joint intolerance—for compressive forces	P	Lefever, 2005[2]	PT	
Joint effusion	P			
ACL repair—6-12 weeks	P	Kisner and Colby, 1996[1]	PT	Avoid closed chain squatting between 60 and 90 degrees of flexion, as it results in anterior tibial translation and can lead to graft disruption.

R00-R99 SYMPTOMS, SIGNS, AND ABNORMAL CLINICAL AND LABORATORY FINDINGS (NOT ELSEWHERE CLASSIFIED)

Issue	LOC	Source	Affil	Rationale/Comment
Pain	P	Lefever, 2005[2]	PT	

S00-T98 INJURY, POISONING, AND CERTAIN OTHER CONSEQUENCES OF EXTERNAL CAUSES

Issue	LOC	Source	Affil	Rationale/Comment
ACL injuries or repairs and lunges with knee in front of toes	Do not	Kisner and Colby, 1996[1]	PT	In anterior cruciate ligament deficiency, or in surgical repair of the knee, do not flex the knee forward of the toes when performing lunges because it increases shear forces and stress on the ACL.
ACL injuries and closed chain squatting exercises	P			Closed chain squatting between 60 and 90 degrees increases anterior translation of tibia and stresses to ACL. Do not perform exercise in these ranges with ACL injuries. Instead, do closed chain activities from 60 to 0 degrees.[1]
Patellar compression and closed chain knee flexion exercises	Advice			Patellar compression (between patella and femur) increases after 30 degrees of knee flexion; also when body weight is kept posterior to the knee. **Brownstein[3] describes a 23-year-old female with patella tendon ACL reconstruction who sustained a transverse patella fracture in week 7 of her rehabilitation during 105% body weight squat exercises.**

PROCEDURAL CONCERNS

Issue	LOC	Source	Affil	Rationale/Comment
Flat hard surfaces—exercising on	P	Lefever, 2005[2]	PT	Use proper footwear.
Footwear, appropriate	P			
Progression, gradation of exercise	P/Advice			Start submaximally and progress to functional goals. Watch out for substitutions in muscle action.

REFERENCES

1. Kisner C, Colby LA: Therapeutic exercise: foundations and techniques, ed 3. Philadelphia: FA Davis; 1996.
2. Lefever SL: Closed kinetic chain training. In Hall CM, Brody LT, eds: Therapeutic exercise: moving toward function. Philadelphia: Lippincott Williams & Wilkins; 2005.
3. Brownstein B, Brunner S: Patella fractures associated with accelerated ACL rehabilitation in patients with autogenous patella tendon reconstruction. J Orthopaed Sports Phys Ther 26(3):168-172, 1997.

16.3 Eccentric Exercise

Eccentric exercise is a form of dynamic resistive exercise that involves tension development while the muscle is lengthening.[1] Familiar functions involving eccentric activity of the lower limbs include sitting down or descending stairs. Sources identify delayed muscle soreness from microtrauma as a concern following eccentric work.[1,2] In more severe cases, rhabdomyolysis may occur.[3]

Note: Because joint movement occurs against resistance, other resistive exercise concerns may also apply.

CONTRAINDICATIONS AND PRECAUTIONS

Vulnerable Biological Tissues

Issue	LOC	Sources	Affil	Rationale/Comment
Muscle and connective tissue	P Caution	Kisner and Colby, 1996[1,a] Hall and Brody, 2005[2]	PT PT	Eccentric exercise may lead to delayed muscle soreness 24 to 48 hours after exercise that may be due to microtrauma to muscle and connective tissue.[2] Hall and Brody recommend moderate exercise during the recovery period.[2] **In 1999, Sayers[3] reported on two studies where 2 of 27 males and 6 of 204 males (3% incidence) experienced adverse response to eccentric exercise including rhabdomyolysis**.

a, Maximal effort eccentric exercise.

ADVERSE EVENTS

Source	Background	Therapy	Outcome	Comments
Sayers et al, 1999[3] **Eccentric exercise and muscle power loss** Case series Med Sci Sports Exerc	The authors report on two studies where 2 of 27 males and 6 of 204 males (3% incidence) experienced adverse response to eccentric exercise.	Protocols involved two sets of 25 maximal eccentric elbow flexion exercises (90 degrees) with 5-minute rest between sets. Contractions lasted 3 sec with 12 sec rests between actions.	Six reported cases, age range 21 to 30 years, experienced (1) profound swelling after 3 days which took up to 7 days to resolve; (2) prolonged loss of muscle force (up to 47 days); (3) elevated serum CK activity that was consistent with rhabdomyolysis symptoms.	Rhabdomyolysis occurs when integrity of skeletal muscle membrane is lost, causing CK-MM, aldolase, and myoglobin to leak into the circulation at the time of injury. CK is the most reliable indicator. The authors caution with regard to eccentric exercise protocols, especially if several muscles are exercised.

REFERENCES

1. Kisner C, Colby LA: Therapeutic exercise: foundations and techniques, ed 3. Philadelphia: FA Davis; 1996.
2. Hall CM, Brody LT: Impairment in muscle performance. In Hall CM, Brody LT, eds: Therapeutic exercise: moving toward function. Philadelphia: Lippincott Williams & Wilkins; 2005.
3. Sayers SP, Clarkson PM, Rouzier PA, Kamen G: Adverse events associated with eccentric exercise protocols: six case studies. Med Sci Sports Exerc 31(12):1697-1702, 1999.

16.4 Isometric Exercise

Isometric exercise is a static form of exercise whereby tension develops in the muscle but there is essentially no joint movement. The length of the muscle remains unchanged during the contraction. Three sources identify four cardiovascular concerns for isometric exercise that primarily center around the pressor (increased blood pressure) response (also see **Resistive exercise**).

100-199 DISEASES OF THE CIRCULATORY SYSTEM

Issue	LOC	Sources	Affil	Rationale/Comment
Cardiovascular problems	Caution	Tan, 1998[2]	MD/PT	Isometrics can cause arrhythmias and significantly increase blood pressure,
	CI	Kisner and Colby, 1996[1,a]	PT	particularly in person with a recent MI.[3]

Continued

Issue	LOC	Sources	Affil	Rationale/Comment
Cerebral vascular accident— vigorous isometrics	CI Caution	Kisner and Colby, 1996[1,b] Tan, 1998[2]	PT MD/PT	The concern is a pressor response in patients with cerebral vascular accidents during vigorous isometric contractions. Note: ICD 10 recognizes a CVA as a circulatory, not a neurologic disorder.
High blood pressure	Caution	Tan, 1998[2]	MD, PT	Caution the use of isometrics in persons with uncontrolled HTN[3] because of the pressor response risk.
Pressor response risk, persons with	Caution	Hall and Brody, 2005[3,c]	PT	

a, If vigorous isometrics; b, Precaution for other diagnoses; c, "High blood pressure after an aneurysm," p 82.

REFERENCES

1. Kisner C, Colby LA: Therapeutic exercise: foundations and techniques, ed 3. Philadelphia: FA Davis; 1996.
2. Tan JC: Practical manual of physical medicine and rehabilitation: diagnostics, therapeutics, and basic problems. St Louis: Mosby; 1998.
3. Hall CM, Brody LT: Impairment in muscle performance. In Hall CM, Brody LT, eds: Therapeutic exercise: moving toward function. Philadelphia: Lippincott Williams & Wilkins; 2005.

16.5 Isokinetic Exercise

Isokinetic exercise is a form of resistive exercise in which a rate-limiting device controls the movement speed of the joint.[1] The device is used both for strength testing and exercise. Two sources identified nine concerns for isokinetic exercise, with the largest proportion related to unhealed injuries. Joint and bone instability was a shared concern (see **Isokinetic testing, Exercise equipment for complications;** also see **Resistive exercise**).

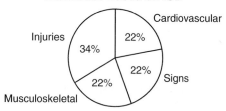

Proportion of Concerns for Isokinetics Based on ICD

I00-I99 DISEASES OF THE CIRCULATORY SYSTEM

Issue	LOC	Sources	Affil	Rationale/Comment
Cardiovascular compromise	Care	Perrin, 1993[2,a]	ATC	Slow and high-velocity isokinetic exercise of trunk and extremities places demands on the cardiovascular system. Slow isokinetics may increase intrathoracic/intraabdominal pressure if a Valsalva maneuver is used.
Cardiorespiratory compromise, unrelated	CI			If noted during maximal isokinetic resistance.

a, Protocols are based on muscle group, stage of progression, age, physical status of patient.

M00-M99 DISEASES OF THE MUSCULOSKELETAL SYSTEM AND CONNECTIVE TISSUE

Issue	LOC	Sources	Affil	Rationale/Comment
ROM restriction	CI RCI	Dvir, 1995[3]	Bioeng	Severely limited ROM. ROM limited.
Unstable joint	CI P	Dvir, 1995[3] Perrin, 1993[2]	Bioeng ATC	The clinician may need to limit range of motion for person with a surgically repaired recurrent shoulder dislocation.

R00-R99 SYMPTOMS, SIGNS INVOLVING THE SYSTEM

Issue	LOC	Sources	Affil	Rationale/Comment
Effusion	CI	Dvir, 1995[3]	Bioeng	Severe effusion
	RCI			Effusion
Severe pain	CI			

S00-T98 INJURY, POISONING, AND CERTAIN OTHER CONSEQUENCES OF EXTERNAL CAUSES

Issue	LOC	Sources	Affil	Rationale/Comment
Sprain or strain	CI	Dvir, 1995[3]	Bioeng	Acute stage
	RCI			Chronic third-degree
Unstable bone—fracture	CI	Dvir, 1995[3]	Bioeng	
	P	Perrin, 1993[2]	ATC	
Healing constraints—soft tissue	CI	Dvir, 1995[3]	Bioeng	

REFERENCES

1. Kisner C, Colby LA: Therapeutic exercise: foundations and techniques, ed 3. Philadelphia: FA Davis; 1996.
2. Perrin DH: Isokinetic exercise and assessment. Champaign (IL): Human Kinetics; 1993.
3. Dvir Z: Isokinetics: muscle testing, interpretation, and clinical applications. New York: Churchill Livingstone; 1995.

16.6 Open Chain Exercise

Open chain exercise is performed with the distal body part moving freely in space. Examples include cane exercises for the upper extremities or knee extension exercises while sitting for the lower extremities. One source lists several concerns related to stressing cruciate tissue with cruciate ligament injuries or repairs during open chain knee exercises (also see **Closed chain exercise**).

M00-M99 DISEASES OF THE MUSCULOSKELETAL AND CONNECTIVE TISSUE SYSTEM

Issue	LOC	Source	Affil	Rationale/Comment
ACL repair—0-6 weeks	P	Kisner and Colby, 1996[1]	PT	Avoid unsupported open chain terminal knee extension because it can cause shear forces from anterior tibial translation when the patella tendon graft is weakest and slightly necrotic (at 4-6 weeks).[1]
ACL repair—6-12 weeks	P	Kisner and Colby, 1996[1,a]	PT	Avoid open chain, resisted terminal knee extension (resisted at distal tibia) because it results in anterior tibial translation and can lead to graft disruption. The ligament must first be healed.[1]

a, Also applies to ACL injuries.

Issue	LOC	Source	Affil	Rationale/Comment
ACL injuries and resisted terminal knee extension exercises— open chain	P	Kisner and Colby, 1996[1]	PT	Open chain terminal knee extension (60 to 0 degrees) with resistance to the distal leg stresses to ACL due to increased tibial translation. Do not perform exercise in these ranges with ACL injuries. Instead, do open chain from 90 to 60 degrees.[1]
PCL injuries	P			Avoid open chain knee flexion exercise (isolated) as it increases posterior translation of the tibia and stresses the ligament.[1]

PROCEDURAL CONCERNS

Issue	LOC	Source	Affil	Rationale/Comment
Pendulum exercises (Codman's exercises)—**balance concerns**	P	Kisner and Colby, 1996[1]	PT	Patients may become dizzy after leaning over from this exercise. If balance is not good, do pendulum exercises in prone or while holding onto a nonmovable object (also see **Balance activities**).

REFERENCE

1. Kisner C, Colby LA: Therapeutic exercise: foundations and techniques, ed 3. Philadelphia: FA Davis; 1996.

16.7 Plyometrics

OVERVIEW. Plyometric training is high velocity, high intensity resistance exercise aimed at increasing muscle power and coordination. The individual performs a resisted eccentric contraction, which is then followed by a rapid concentric contraction.[1] The training is typically done toward the latter part of a patient's rehabilitation program.

SUMMARY: CONTRAINDICATIONS AND PRECAUTIONS. Three sources cited a total of eight concerns for plyometrics. Concerns ranged from one to six per source with a physical therapist/athletic trainer citing the largest number of concerns. The largest proportion of concerns (more than 60%) were procedural and focus around issues of patient selection and when the technique should be appropriately introduced to the patient.

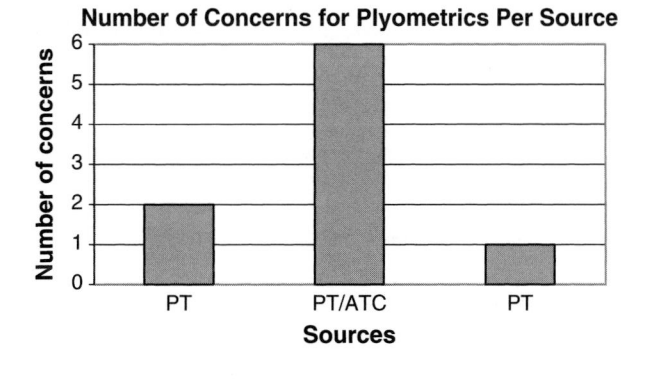

Number of Concerns for Plyometrics Per Source

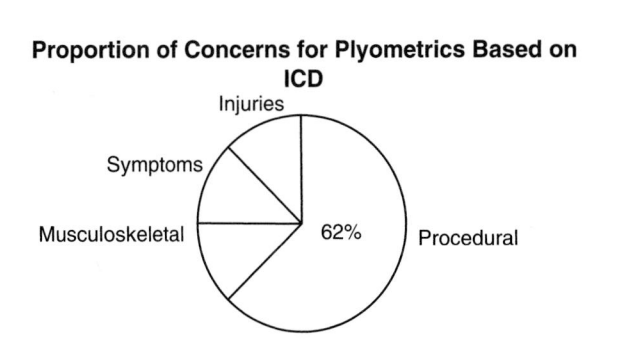

Proportion of Concerns for Plyometrics Based on ICD

CONTRAINDICATIONS AND PRECAUTIONS

M00-M99 DISEASES OF THE MUSCULOSKELETAL SYSTEM AND CONNECTIVE TISSUE

Issue	LOC	Sources	Affil	Rationale/Comment
Instability	CI	Houglum, 2001[2]	PT/ATC	Strength is a prerequisite and is needed to provide sufficient stability to the joint during plyometrics.

R00-R99 SYMPTOMS, SIGNS, AND ABNORMAL CLINICAL & LABORATORY FINDINGS (NOT ELSEWHERE CLASSIFIED)

Issue	LOC	Sources	Affil	Rationale/Comment
Inflammation—acute	CI	Houglum, 2001[2]	PT/ATC	Plyometrics may increase existing inflammation.

S00-T98 INJURY, POISONING, AND CERTAIN OTHER CONSEQUENCES OF EXTERNAL CAUSES

Issue	LOC	Sources	Affil	Rationale/Comment
Postoperative conditions	CI	Houglum, 2001[2]	PT/ATC	Tissues that poorly tolerate plyometrics are vulnerable to injury. **Brownstein[3] describes a 34-year-old male with an ACL repair who sustained a transverse patella fracture while performing plyometric exercises (jumps, hops, full weight bearing, and box jumps) on week 6 of an accelerated rehab program.**

PROCEDURAL CONCERNS

Issue	LOC	Sources	Affil	Rationale/Comment
Extended practice	P	Houglum, 2001[2]	PT/ATC	Avoid extended periods of plyometrics because high stresses are placed on the body.
Delayed onset muscle soreness (DOMS)	P			Caution patient about delayed onset muscle soreness (DOMS). DOMS is a common side effect. Note: Plyometrics involve vigorous eccentric activities.
Fatigue, late in session	P			Consider implementing early during a session, after the warmup, to avoid fatigue that may later set in.
Patient selection	Advice	Kisner and Colby, 1996[1] Hall and Brody, 2005[4]	PT	Selected patients who desire to return to high-demand functional activities.[1]
Stage of rehabilitation	Advice	Hall and Brody, 2005[4]	PT	Overuse-related tendon injuries may occur during this high-level activity. Introduce pylometrics in the advanced stages of rehabilitation.[4]

REFERENCES

1. Kisner C, Colby LA: Therapeutic exercise: foundations and techniques, ed 3. Philadelphia: FA Davis; 1996.

2. Houglum PA: Therapeutic exercises for athletic injuries. Champaign (IL): Human Kinetics; 2001.

3. Brownstein B, Brunner S: Patella fractures associated with accelerated ACL rehabilitation in patients with autogenous patella tendon reconstruction. J Orthopaed Sports Phys Ther 26(3):168-172, 1997.

4. Hall CM, Brody LT: Impairment in muscle performance. In Hall CM, Brody LT, eds: Therapeutic exercise: moving toward function. Philadelphia: Lippincott Williams & Wilkins; 2005.

16.8 Progressive Resistive Exercise

Progressive resistive exercise (PRE) is a form of resistive exercise involving a known, quantifiable load that is increased progressively over time and that is generated by some mechanical means (i.e., equipment). The approach is designed to increase muscle strength, endurance, and power and tends to stress individuals beyond what they are normally accustomed to.[1] Delorme's 1950s approach used exercise apparatus that included the use of straps.[2]

I00-I99 DISEASES OF THE CIRCULATORY SYSTEM

Issue	LOC	Sources	Affil	Rationale/Comment
Cardiac dysfunction	CI	Delorme and Watkins, 1951[2]	MD	Valsalva maneuver concern.

J00-J99 DISEASES OF THE RESPIRATORY SYSTEM

Issue	LOC	Sources	Affil	Rationale/Comment
Respiratory dysfunction	CI	Delorme and Watkins, 1951[2]	MD	Valsalva maneuver concern.

Y70-Y82 MEDICAL DEVICES

Issue	LOC	Sources	Affil	Rationale/Comment
Straps—equipment	Concern	Delorme and Watkins, 1951[2]	MD	Pressure-related straps concerns that may lead to minor skin abrasions.

Vulnerable Biological Tissues

Issue	LOC	Sources	Affil	Rationale/Comment
Ligament—possible microtrauma	Concern	Delorme and Watkins, 1951[2]	MD	**Possible microtrauma to ligaments, tendons, and joints.** A minor and temporary concern relating mostly to muscle injury.
Tendon—possible microtrauma	Concern			
Joint—possible microtrauma	Concern			
Skin—possible skin abrasions	Concern			**Possible skin abrasions.** A minor and temporary concern relating to skin disruption from strap pressure.

REFERENCE

1. Kisner C, Colby LA: Therapeutic exercise: foundations and techniques, ed 3. Philadelphia: FA Davis; 1996.
2. Delorme TL, Watkins AL: Progressive resistive exercises: technic and medical application. New York: Appleton-Century-Crofts; 1951.

16.9 Resistance Exercise: General

OVERVIEW. Resistance exercises are active exercises involving static or dynamic muscle contraction that is resisted by an outside force. When specific muscles are targeted for high intensity, high repetition, the activity is referred to as *resistance training*. The goal of resistive exercise, in general, is to increase strength, power, or endurance.[1] Concerns regarding this type of exercise may, in part, be attributed to its exercise-related complications, including rhabdomyolysis, compartmental syndrome, fatigue-related declines in neuromuscular patients, and Valsalva-related morbidity and deaths.

The Valsalva maneuver involves an expiratory effort while the glottis is closed. This maneuver, often unintentional, is one of the chief concerns for resistive exercise, particularly in patients with cardiovascular disease. Valsalva's (1666-1723) description[2] follows: "If the glottis be closed after a deep inspiration and a strenuous and prolonged expiratory effort to be then made such pressure can be extended upon the heart and intrathoracic vessels that the movement and flow of the blood are temporarily arrested."

Dawson[2] cites literature about a bandit who was captured and then committed suicide by performing the Valsalva maneuver in the presence, and to the surprise, of the Roman consul. In doing so, the bandit escaped cross-examination.

Note: Resistive exercise is a broad topic. Diverse sources have commented on disease-specific concerns below (also see **Aerobic; PREs, Isokinetics, Isometrics, Eccentrics, AROM** and **Sports Activities; Laboratory/clinical values [under Aerobic exercise]**).

A00-B99 CERTAIN INFECTIONS AND PARASITIC DISEASES

Issue	LOC	Sources	Affil	Rationale/Comment
Infection and resistive exercise	Caution	Hall and Brody, 2005[3]	PT	

E00-E90 ENDOCRINE, NUTRITIONAL, AND METABOLIC DISEASES

Issue	LOC	Sources	Affil	Rationale/Comment
Metabolic disease and fatigue Diabetes Alcoholism	Avoid	Hall and Brody, 2005[3]	PT	Fatigue and overtraining can lead to joint damage in this population.

G00-G99 DISEASES OF THE NERVOUS SYSTEM

Multiple Sclerosis

Issue	LOC	Sources	Affil	Rationale/Comment
Exercise to the point of fatigue	Caution	Tan, 1998[1]	MD/PT	Avoid overwork in this population due to fatigability (easy). Submaximal exercise intensities (low to moderate) that are balanced with rest periods are suggested. More frequent repetitions are necessary to get a training effect.[1]
Body temperature during exercise and Uthoff's symptom— an adverse reaction to heat	Advice	Erickson, 1989[4]	MD	Hot rooms, warm baths, fevers, and body temperature increases following exercise cause immediate, temporary fatigue and reduction in function. Consider exercising in the morning when body temperature is lowest. Air conditioning may be medically necessary.[4] **In a 1937 descriptive study of 21 patients with multiple sclerosis, Simons[5] reported that 62% became weaker, 24% remained unchanged, and 14% improved with heat.**

Myopathy

Issue	LOC	Sources	Affil	Rationale/Comment
Myopathy, acute—and resistive exercise	ACI	Hall and Brody, 2005[3]	PT	Permanent damage and stress can occur in a muscular system already compromised. E.g., neuromuscular disease, acute alcohol myopathy.
Myopathy, chronic—and resistive exercise	ACI			

Neurologic populations

Issue	LOC	Sources	Affil	Rationale/Comment
Fatigue/overtraining	Avoid	Hall and Brody, 2005[3]	PT	Fatigue and overtraining in neurologic populations can lead to joint damage.[3]

Neuromuscular

Issue	LOC	Sources	Affil	Rationale/Comment
Fatigue DMD	P	Kisner and Colby,1996[6]	PT	Vigorous fatiguing progressive resistive exercise is CI in most motor neuron diseases because it may lead to overuse weakness. There are possible detrimental side effects on muscle from exercise due to overwork weakness in DMD.[7]
Polio Guillain-Barré	Caution	Tan, 1998[1]	MD/PT	Strenuous exercise can impair muscle function in Guillain-Barré patients. Advancing too quickly can lead to a regression of strength that should alert clinician to reduce activity level. **In a 1970 case series, Bensman[8] described eight patients with Guillain-Barré who lost function following strenuous exercise.**

Continued

Issue	LOC	Sources	Affil	Rationale/Comment
				In 1915, Lovett[9] described children with poliomyelitis who were hospitalized with muscle power loss after resuming farm work at their homes. In 1953, Hyman[10] described a 10-year-old girl with poliomyelitis who was encouraged by her parents to exercise her legs as much as possible and subsequently suffered a relapse of weakness in her right leg. In 1953, Mitchell[11] described a 27-year-old with acute poliomyelitis who gained strength in rehabilitation, returned home where the patient used a flight of stairs, and subsequently lost the ability to climb stairs.

H00-H59 DISEASES OF THE EYE

Issue	LOC	Sources	Affil	Rationale/Comment
Eye surgery and Valsalva	P Avoid Avoid	Kisner and Colby, 1996[6] Hall and Brody, 2005[3,a] Tan, 1998[1]	PT PT MD/PT	There is a pronounced increase in blood pressure with the Valsalva maneuver. **In 2002, Obuchowska[12] described an 84-year-old female who developed a massive subarachnoidal hemorrhage when she had an unexpected Valsalva-induced cough during cataract surgery that resulted in sudden increased venous pressure and vessel wall rupture** (also see **Cough therapy**).
Proliferative diabetic retinopathy	Avoid	ADA, 2004[13]	Org	Strenuous activity may precipitate vitreous hemorrhage or traction retinal detachment. Avoid physical activity involving straining, jarring, or the Valsalva maneuver.

a, Recent surgery.

I00-I99 DISEASES OF THE CIRCULATORY SYSTEM

Issue	LOC	Sources	Affil	Rationale/Comment
Cardiopulmonary disease and Valsalva	Avoid	Hall and Brody, 2005[3]	PT	A Valsalva maneuver must be avoided especially in cardiac patients because of the subsequent fall in stroke volume.[1] **In a 1950 retrospective (chart review), McGuire[15] identified 11 patients (3 with known cardiac or vascular histories) who died during or immediately following the use of a bed pan (a Valsalva-related activity).**
Cerebral vascular accidents	P	Kisner and Colby, 1996[6,a]	PT	
	Caution	Delorme and Watkins, 1951[14]	MD	
		Tan, 1998[1,b]	MD/PT	
Hypertension—uncontrolled	Caution	Tan, 1998[1,b]	MD/PT	
Myocardial infarction	P	Kisner and Colby, 1996[6]	PT	
	CI	Delorme and Watkins, 1951[14]	MD	
	Caution	Tan, 1998[1]	PT	

a, If cardiovascular problems exist; b, Strengthening exercises.

J00-J99 DISEASES OF THE RESPIRATORY SYSTEM

Issue	LOC	Sources	Affil	Rationale/Comment
Cardiopulmonary disease and Valsalva	Avoid	Hall and Brody, 2005[3]	PT	
	CI	Delorme and Watkins, 1951[14]	MD	
Pulmonary disease and fatigue	P	Kisner and Colby, 1996[6,a]	PT	People with pulmonary disease are easily fatigued.[1]
	Caution	Tan, 1998[1,a]	MD/PT	

a, Cardiopulmonary dysfunction.

K00-K93 DISEASES OF THE DIGESTIVE SYSTEM

Issue	LOC	Sources	Affil	Rationale/Comment
Abdominal surgery	Caution	Tan, 1998[1]	MD/PT	Stress on the abdominal wall system can elevate intraabdominal pressure and lead to
	P	Kisner and Colby, 1996[6]	PT	herniation.
	Avoid	Hall and Brody, 2005[3,a]	PT	
Hernia—abdominal	Caution	Tan, 1998[1]	MD/PT	Patients with abdominal surgery or existing herniations are at risk.[6]
wall	P	Kisner and Colby, 1996[6]	PT	

a, Avoid Valsalva if recent abdominal surgery.

L00-L99 DISEASES OF THE SKIN AND SUBCUTANEOUS TISSUE

Issue	LOC	Sources	Affil	Rationale/Comment
Skin grafts—burn patients	Advice	Spires, 2000[16]	MD	Inspect graft area regularly because there is a risk that exercise may disrupt wound healing of grafts,
Wounds, during exercise— burn patients	Advice			particularly in cases of deep partial-thickness and full-thickness burns that are located over joint areas.

M00-M99 DISEASES OF THE MUSCULOSKELETAL SYSTEM AND CONNECTIVE TISSUE

Issue	LOC	Sources	Affil	Rationale/Comment
Degenerative joint disease, severe and fatigue	Avoid	Hall and Brody, 2005[3]	PT	Fatigue and overtraining can lead to additional joint damage in this population.[3]
Inflammation—muscle, joint	CI	Kisner and Colby, 1996[6]	PT	Exercise can lead to more swelling and damage in the presence of inflammation.
	Caution	Hall and Brody, 2005[3,a]	PT	Low-intensity isometrics, called muscle setting, are suggested with inflammation
	CI	Tan, 1998	MD/PT	if pain does not increase,[6] and when done gently.[1] Carefully monitor mode and dosage if inflammation or infection is present.[3]
Inflammatory conditions, acute—polymyositis	Caution	Tan, 1998[1]	MD/PT	
Intravertebral disc surgery (recent) and Valsalva	Avoid	Hall and Brody, 2005[3]	PT	Elevated intraabdominal pressure can lead to herniation.
Pain	Caution	Hall and Brody, 2005[3]	PT	
Osteoporosis and intensity level	P	Kisner and Colby, 1996[6]	PT	Modify program: low impact, low intensity, very gradually adding resistance; with no "explosive twisting."
	Caution	Tan, 1998[1]	MD/PT	
Osteoporosis and flexion exercises	Caution	Sinaki and Mikkelsen, 1984[17]	MD	**In a 1984 nonrandomized experiment of postmenopausal spinal osteoporotic women, Sinaki and Mikkelsen[17] found that fractures were significantly greater ($P < .001$) in the flexion and flexion/extension exercise groups as compared to the extension group. 89% of postmenopausal osteoporotic women who engaged in a flexion exercise program had sustained spinal fractures.**

Continued

Issue	LOC	Sources	Affil	Rationale/Comment
Rheumatoid arthritis (acute inflammation) **and exercise**	P/CI Caution	Kisner and Colby, 1996[6] Tan, 1998[1]	PT MD/PT	These individuals may need rest as they can fatigue more easily. Medications and steroids can cause osteoporosis and ligamentous laxity, so avoid excessive stress to bones and joints during exercise. Maximal resistive exercise is CI because it can result in joint compression and increased irritability, thus increasing the potential for joint surface damage.[6]
Rheumatoid arthritis, juvenile Atlantoaxial subluxation and exercise	CI	Scull, 1994[18]	PT	Identify subluxation with radiographs. Cervical collars are recommended for car travel to avoid deceleration injuries if there is an accident.

a, Not specific to structure.

O00-O99 PREGNANCY, CHILDBIRTH, AND PUERPERIUM (ALSO SEE AEROBIC EXERCISES, AROM, AND POSITIONING)

High-Risk Pregnancy[a]

Issue	LOC	Sources	Affil	Rationale/Comment
Pregnancy and abdominal exercises	P	Kisner and Colby, 1996[6]	PT	Some exercises, especially abdominal exercises, may stimulate uterine contractions and need to be modified or discontinued.
Pregnancy and Valsalva	P/avoid			Avoid increasing intraabdominal pressure.

a, High risk is defined as preterm rupture of membrane, premature labor onset, incompetent cervix, placenta previa, pregnancy-related hypertension (preeclampsia), multiple gestations, or diabetes. The medical goal is to prevent preterm delivery, typically through bed rest, restriction of activity, and medications.[6]

R00-R99 SYMPTOMS, SIGNS, AND ABNORMAL CLINICAL AND LABORATORY FINDINGS

See **Aerobic exercise for clinical and laboratory values** for exercise.

S00-T98 INJURY, POISONING, AND CERTAIN OTHER CONSEQUENCES OF EXTERNAL CAUSES

Issue	LOC	Sources	Affil	Rationale/Comment
Fracture site—distal stress	Care	Kisner and Colby, 1996[6]	PT	Following immobilization, and until the fracture site is radiologically healed (consult with physician), use care any time stress is placed distal to the fracture site (resistance, stretch, weight bearing).[6]
Tendon—exposed (i.e., burn patients)	Avoid	Helm et al., 1982[19]	MD	Exercises involving graft sites are initiated about day 5-10 and longer if graft is over bony prominences.[19]

Y70-Y82 MEDICAL DEVICES

Issue	LOC	Sources	Affil	Rationale/Comment
THR with trochanteric osteotomy (also see AROM, PROM, Positioning for THR)	Avoid	Maihafer, 1990[20]	PT	The concern is resisted hip abduction strengthening exercises for the gluteus medius muscle. For THR with trochanteric osteotomy, the trochanter is reflected before the prosthesis is implanted. It is then internally fixated. This osteotomized bone can be damaged if stressed (e.g., forces generated by gluteus maximus during ambulation). Treat more conservatively.

Vulnerable Biological Tissue

Issue	LOC	Sources	Affil	Rationale/Comment
Epiphyseal sites in children/ adolescents Adolescent and preadolescents should avoid CSMF • Body building • Power lifting • Maximal lifts • Competitive weight lifting	Care Avoid	Hall and Brody, 2005[3,a] AAP, 2001[21]	PT Org	The concern is stress on immature epiphyseal sites: stress should be minimized. Develop a balanced training program (i.e., to avoid muscle imbalances).[3] Case reports raise concern about epiphyseal injuries at the wrist and apophyseal injuries at the spine from weight lifting in skeletally immature individuals. Also **NEISS[22] data estimated 25,000 weight-lifting–related injuries in persons under 21 years (2004 data).** Avoid these activities until physical and skeletal maturity is reached.[21]

a, Children and adolescents and resistive programs.

PROCEDURAL CONCERNS

Issue	LOC	Sources	Affil	Rationale/Comment
Delayed onset muscle soreness	P Advice	Kisner and Colby, 1996[6] Hall and Brody, 2005[3]	PT PT	Delayed onset muscle soreness is reported after vigorous eccentric exercise that can lead to 5 to 7 days of stiffness and tenderness following exercise. Theorized causes include (1) waste accumulation or (2) microtrauma (see **Sayer[23]** below).

Exercise recovery	P	Kisner and Colby, 1996[6]	PT	Recovery requires about 3 to 4 minutes to replenish energy stores, oxygen, glycogen, and remove lactic acid and allow for long-term physical improvement.
Fatigue in neuromuscular and cardiopulmonary dysfunction	P Caution	Kisner and Colby, 1996[6] Tan, 1998[1]	PT MD/PT	There is noted fatigability in persons with MS, PVD, and cardiac or pulmonary disease.[1]
Overtraining	Advice	Hall and Brody, 2005[3]	PT	Overtraining can lead to reduced performance.
Overwork	P	Kisner and Colby, 1996[6]	PT	Slowly adjust intensity, duration, and progression of exercise to avoid overwork. **In 1989, Tietjen and Guzzi[24] described a 25-year-old white male who took a required Army physical fitness test, became symptomatic, and was subsequently hospitalized for acute renal failure attributed to myoglobinuria and postexercise rhabdomyolysis.**
	Advice	Hall and Brody, 2005[3]	PT	**In 1996, Klondell[25] described a 23-year-old with insulin-dependent diabetes who played basketball for 13 hours and subsequently developed bilateral compartment syndrome that required fasciotomies.**
				In 2003, Springer and Clarkson[26] described a 22-year-old female college student who was hospitalized with rhabdomyolysis after her personal trainer at a health club encouraged her to exercise until exhaustion despite her wish to stop.
Severe pain during or lasting more than 24 hours after exercise	CI	Kisner and Colby, 1996[6]	PT	**In 1999, Sayers[23] reported six cases from studies involving eccentric exercise where subjects experienced profound swelling 3 days after exercise that required up to 7 days to resolve.**

Continued

Issue	LOC	Sources	Affil	Rationale/Comment
Substitution	P	Kisner and Colby, 1996[6]	PT	Substitution occurs with weakness, paralysis, or pain. Stabilize and apply an appropriate level of resistance.
The Valsalva maneuver	P	Kisner and Colby, 1996[6]	PT	The Valsalva maneuver can lead to a pronounced pressor response (increase in blood pressure), stress on the abdominal wall, and stress to the cardiovascular system that is especially noted during isometric or heavy resistance exercise. Suggested strategies include exhaling during motion; avoid holding one's breath; counting out loud; or breathing in rhythm during exercise. **In 1985, Katz and Carmody[27] described a 23-year-old weight lifter who sustained a subperiosteal orbital hematoma during a prolonged and repeated Valsalva maneuver while spending the afternoon bench pressing.** **In 1968, Schartum[28] described a 66-year-old patient where syncope (loss of consciousness) occurred during defecation (Valsalva-related).**
	Avoid	Hall and Brody, 2005[3]	PT	
	CI	Delorme and Watkins, 1951[14]	MD	
	Avoid	Tan, 1998[1]	MD/PT	

ADVERSE EVENTS

Source	Background	Therapy	Outcome	Follow-up/Interpretation
Bennett and Knowlton, 1958[29] **Overwork and denervated muscle** Clin Ortho	A 16-year-old presented with C5 C6 spinal cord injury.	Finger flexor power was absent but tested well for wrist extensors. The patient was provided with a tenodesis splint.	After 6 weeks of use with the splint, weakness and paralysis of wrist extensors developed.	The splint was discontinued, but only minimal gains in active wrist extension were noted.
Bensman, 1970[8] **Excessive activity, Guillain-Barré, and function** Case series JAMA	The author reports on the exercise response in eight patients with Guillain-Barré from 1961 to 1970.	All eight patients were negatively affected by excessive activity. (Note: patient and exercise characteristics not reported.)	• Three patients temporarily lost function following strenuous exercise. • Three patients became weak, paretic, and lost function soon after strenuous exercise. They improved with bed rest and limited activity but relapsed with fatigue. • Two patients were rehospitalized 1 year after initial onset but improved with carefully controlled activity.	The author recommends: • Short periods of nonfatiguing activity commensurate with strength. • Monitor condition with MMT and NCV testing. • If decrease in function noted, return to bed until symptoms stabilize. • Avoid fatiguing exercise for 1 year with gradual return to sports and more strenuous activity.

Continued

Source	Background	Therapy	Outcome	Follow-up/Interpretation
Duane, 1973[30] **Valsalva hemorrhagic retinopathy and reflex spasm of the airway** A case from a series Personal communication Am J Ophthalmol	Case 3 A 36-year-old man presented with a repair to the extensor surface of the "distal metacarpal" of his fifth finger and trauma to his right eye with old choroiditis secondary to being hit by a fist. (Note: Two separate events occurred.)	The patient underwent a tendoplasty of his lacerated extensor digitorum communis but during anesthesia induction for surgery, he experienced a reflex spasm of the trachea and bronchial tree.	After surgery, he complained of disturbed vision in both eyes. Examination revealed 6/18 (right eye) and 6/60 (left eye) with a large preretinal hemorrhage in the macula of each eye. He was diagnosed with Valsalva hemorrhagic retinopathy. Over a period of 5 months, abnormalities resolved.	The author stated that the vision in patients with pure Valsalva hemorrhagic retinopathy will usually return to normal. In a personal communication, the author recalls a conversation with W.F. Hoyt, who discussed three cases of Valsalva-induced hemorrhagic retinopathy involving the preretinal and vitreous regions: A boy who performed bench presses with 175-lb weights A girl who held her breath as she was flipped by a wave while waterskiing A woman who assisted a neighbor with carrying a refrigerator down a flight of stairs

Giunta, 1999[31] **Cervical exercise and referred dental pain** Case report J Mass Dent Soc	A 73-year-old female in generally good health received physical therapy for a neck spasm.	One exercise involved flexing the head toward the chest. The patient went to her dentist, complaining of pain around tooth 18. Two weeks later, she returned again to her dentist with the same complaint.	Her diagnosis was dental pain of nonodontogenic origin. The dentist recommended she stop her cervical exercises, and the pain subsequently disappeared.	The author speculates that the pain had a neuroanatomic basis. Cervical level pain impulses entered into the dorsal horn (Lissauer's tract), mix with spinal tract V and nucleus, which could be interpreted as dental pain. Fibers (some) of spinal tract V may also descend to cervical segments 3 and 4. Thus, the tooth pain was referred from an exercise- induced neck spasm.
Gross and Schuch, 1989[32] **Postpolio and isokinetic exercise** Case report Phys Ther	A 59-year-old active, ambulatory man presented with postpolio syndrome (polio contracted at age 16). He had reduced strength and endurance and wanted a strengthening program.	An aggressive 6-week, 3×/week isokinetic knee exercise program involved 2 sets of 10 maximal contractions at 60 deg/sec with 2-minute rests followed by 2 sets at 180 deg/sec.	Peak torque before and during exercise and at 6 and 22 weeks' follow-up revealed no appreciable loss of ability to exert torque or appreciable increase in strength.	Authors indicated no deleterious effects due to the exercise program and suggest more research on efficacy of exercise in this population.

Continued

Source	Background	Therapy	Outcome	Follow-up/Interpretation
Hyman, 1953[10] **Polio and post exercise weakness** Case report Lancet	A 10-year-old girl presented with poliomyelitis.	She was hospitalized to improve strength and walking. At 5 weeks, her parents encouraged her to get out of bed and when in bed, to exercise her legs as much as possible.	A rapid relapse (weakness) was noted in her right leg (from grade 3 to 0) in the posterior tibialis, anterior tibialis, extensor hallux, digitorum longus, and gastrocnemius muscles.	Her calf remained paralyzed. Other muscles subsequently recovered 2 to 3 grades (about 7 months later).
Katz and Carmody, 1985[27] **Valsalva-induced subperiosteal orbital hematoma and bench pressing** Case report Am J Ophthalmol	A 23-year-old weight lifter spent the afternoon bench pressing.	After exercising, pain and puffiness around the left orbit and binocular vertical diplopia occurred that was worse on upward gaze.	The diagnosis was subperiosteal orbital hematoma. A hemorrhage occurred during a prolonged and repeated Valsalva maneuver. It resolved without intervention.	The authors postulated that increased abdominal and intrathoracic pressure against a closed glottis was transmitted to the orbital veins (which lack valves). Orbital congestion and secondary hyperemia then led to a rupture of the subperiosteal vessels, resulting in hematoma.

Klondell et al, 1996[25] **Prolonged exercise and compartment syndrome** Case report Am Surg	A 23-year-old African-American presented with insulin-dependent diabetes.	The individual played basketball about 13 hours the previous day. Later, the following symptoms were noted: bilateral leg pain (awoke from sleep), calves firm and tender, nonpalpable pedal pulses, intense calf pain with dorsiflexion, and diminished light touch and two-point discrimination.	The diagnosis was bilateral compartment syndrome: anterior (left 75 mm Hg; right 42 mm Hg), superficial posterior (left 55 mm Hg; right 56 mm Hg), lateral compartment (left 41 mm Hg; right 26 mm Hg). Urine was positive for myoglobin and creatine kinase isoenzymes (= 13,600 level). Treatment consisted of four compartmental fasciotomies and debridement of ischemic muscle.	The authors state that permanent deficits occur 6 to 12 hours after the beginning of symptoms.
Line and Rust, 1995[33] **Intense exercise and rhabdomyolysis** Case series Am Fam Phys	A 24-year-old man completed an intense 2-hour weight lifting session using heavy weights.	Tenderness of pectoral, biceps, and triceps muscles was noted, as well as pain and swelling of his arms and chest. The CK level was 13,758 IU/L. He was hospitalized and vigorously hydrated.	CK levels peaked at 50,200 IU/L before slowly returning to normal over the next 6 days.	

Continued

Source	Background	Therapy	Outcome	Follow-up/Interpretation
	A 32-year-old physically active (running 30 miles/week) physician ran a marathon.	The marathon took place on a warm day (85° F/29° C).	He collapsed after 9 miles with severe calf and thigh pain. CK levels peaked at 108,000 IU/L, and he required dialysis and treatment for compartmental compression syndrome of the thighs and calves. He fully recovered after 6 months.	
	A 37-year-old male sedentary emergency care physician exercised in a health facility.	His personal trainer instructed him on 10-12 repetitions of three sets of four exercises on a rowing machine; three sets of bicep curls, three sets of dumbbell curls, and low back and abdominal exercise.	He vomited after the session and experienced extreme soreness the following day. At 1 week, he returned and exercised chest and triceps (in same manner as the previous week but was unaccustomed to the exercise). The next day, he could not bend his arm. At 48 hours, he noted dark urine and he forced fluids, suspecting rhabdomyolysis. (CK was 19,746 U/L at 96 hours, 70,158 U/L 24 hours later, and 45,461 U/L the following day.)	A nephrologist recommended fluids and bicarbonate. He also took creatine supplements.

Lovett, 1915[9] **Polio and over work weakness** Case report JAMA	Children with a diagnosis of poliomyelitis.	Children were hospitalized for treatment if they presented with infantile paralysis.	After discharge, they returned to their homes (farms) where they resumed work on the farm.	These children were readmitted to hospitals within 4 weeks with muscle power loss.
Marshall and King, 1973[34] **Exercise, communication, and CVA** Quasi experiment (crossover; single blind) J Speech Hear Res	16 adults (15 males; ages 36-66) with mild to severe aphasia diagnosed 4 to 96 months earlier participated in an exercise program.	A physical therapy program of exercise and rest in the uninvolved knee for 15 minutes and then the involved knee consisted of knee flexion and extension (on a Cybex) for 10 reps at 30 deg/sec with a 1-minute rest.	Of the 16 subjects, 14 scored lower on the Porch Index of Communication Ability (PICA) (i.e., verbal and graphic scales) following exercise as compared to scores when at rest.	The authors suggest scheduling language therapy before physical exercise. Note: Although the title suggests fatigue may have played a role in the reduced PICA scores, fatigue was not measured.
McGuire et al, 1950[15] **Bed pan deaths** Retrospective (chart review)	The author reviewed bed pan deaths and their autopsies in patients at Cincinnati Hospital from 1936 to 1946.	11 patients, ages 6 to 72, were identified who died during or immediately following the use of a bed pan. The precise mechanism was determined in 4 cases.	A 60-year-old male ruptured a dissecting aortic aneurysm. A 52-year-old female had a cerebral and subarachnoid hemorrhage.	McGuire's proposed mechanism involved a sharp rise in intraarterial and intravenous blood pressure during bed pan strain, followed by a marked change in the heart rate and rhythm.

Continued

Source	Background	Therapy	Outcome	Follow-up/Interpretation
Am Pract Dig Treat			A 45-year-old female with a cardiac history had an MI. A 72-year-old female s/p old MI had a pulmonary embolism.	The majority of individuals with bed pan deaths had serious organic heart disease.
Mitchell, 1953[11] **Polio and over work weakness** Case report Lancet	A 27-year-old presented with acute poliomyelitis.	The patient was hospitalized for treatment of weakness. At 4 weeks post onset, the patient was able to ascend a shallow step, foot drop improved, and quadruped strength increased.	The patient was discharged to home (bedroom on 2nd floor). After 2 weeks at home, however, the patient could not climb steps, walk without assistance, abduct the hip, or dorsiflex the ankle.	The author stated that overactivity in the early convalescence stage of acute poliomyelitis (climbing stairs) may have led to weakness. Note: Need for carefully controlled progressive resistive exercise.
Riddle, 1932[35] **Intensive radio exercise and death** Case report Dallas Med J	A 39-year-old female vigorously cleaned her house. On the following morning, she participated in an exercise broadcast over the radio (to lose weight) and performed "rather strenuous movements" while lying down.	Later that day she looked pale. That evening she had hunger pains, became nauseated, vomited 1 quart of bright red blood, and passed dark bloody stools. On day 1 post exercise, her condition looked good.	Her diagnosis was enlarged veins noted at the cardiac end of her stomach. No stomach or intestinal lesions were found. The physician believed bleeding occurred where the veins entered the cardiac end of her stomach and speculated that a vein anomaly in her stomach ruptured during severe exercise.	The take-home message was to gradually increase daily amounts of exercise. The author recommended that radio announcers caution listeners to start with mild exercise and gradually increase the amount.

| On day 2, she vomited blood and passed tarry stools. On day 3, her pulse was 100 bpm, and she vomited small dark blood and had a little lightly bloody tarry stools. On day 4, she did not vomit blood but *died* at end of the day. | | | | Note: This case was published in the 1930s (radio exercises) and the duration or type of exercises involved was unclear. |
| Sinaki and Mikkelsen, 1984[17]
 Spinal osteoporosis and flexion exercises
 Experiment | 59 postmenopausal spinal osteoporotic women, ages 49-60, were given exercise prescription (physician's choice) from 1969 to 1981.
 Note: No history of steroid use or secondary causes for osteoporosis. | Patients were followed for 1.4 to 2 years with radiographs.
 Exercise groups:
 9 patients: flexion exercises (sit-ups and sitting, reaching hands to floor)
 25 patients: performed extension exercise | Wedging and compression fractures occurred in the flexion (89%), extension (16%), combination (53%), and no exercise (67%) groups.
 Fractures were significantly greater ($P < .001$) in the flexion and flexion/extension groups as compared to the extension group. | Sinaki and Mikkelsen caution that if an exercise program is provided, extension or isometric back/abdominal exercises may be more appropriate than flexion. |

Continued

Source	Background	Therapy	Outcome	Follow-up/Interpretation
Pretest posttest control group design (no randomization)		19 patients: combined flexion and extension		
Arch Phys Med Rehab		6 patients: no exercise		
Schartum, 1968[28] **Valsalva-induced syncope and defecation** Case Report Acta Med Scand	The case involved a 66-year-old patient	Syncope (loss of consciousness) occurred during defecation.	The Valsalva maneuver (a respiratory maneuver) that simulates stool straining was characterized by QRS widening and deformation and an A-V block, followed by ventricular asystole (4.6 sec) and then loss of consciousness.	Vagal cardiosensitivity and atrioventricular conduction disturbances were noted. The author postulated that myocardial hypoxia (ventricular standstill and loss of consciousness) results from reduced blood pressure. The maneuver may cause syncope due to ventricular arrest in susceptible individuals.
Simons, 1937[5] **Heat, multiple sclerosis, and strength** Descriptive Bull Neurol Inst N Y	The author reported on the effects of heat and cold on 21 patients with multiple sclerosis.	For heat: Of 21 cases, 13 (62%) became weaker, 5 (24%) were unchanged, and 3 (14%) improved with heat.	No other patterns were noted for spasticity, numbness, or bladder symptoms with either heat or cold application.	Note: Age, gender, and severity were not noted.

| Tietjen and Guzzi, 1989[24] **Fitness test and renal failure** Case report Milit Med | A 25-year-old white male in generally good health but with limited physical conditioning underwent a required Army physical fitness test (APFT) that involved the following: 2-mile run, push-ups, and sit-ups using the most repetitions or lowest time as the goal. | No overt symptoms were reported immediately after the test. At 6 hours, nausea, malaise, severe low back pain and vomiting episodes occurred. At 14 hours, he had not urinated and was diagnosed with nephrolithiasis (kidney stone) at the ER. The following day, symptoms did not improve and at 30 hours post exercise, he was not hydrating, only voided 40 mL, and experienced tenderness over his erector spine muscles bilaterally. | He was hospitalized, where lab tests revealed oliguric acute renal failure due to acute tubular necrosis (attributed to myoglobinuria and postexercise rhabdomyolysis; peak BUN = 42 mg/dL and peak creatinine = 6.4 mg/dL). He gradually responded to treatment of vigorous fluid resuscitation and IV furosemide. | The authors suggest a prospective study to determine the risk to renal function from the APFT. |

LITIGATION

Year, State	History	Location	Therapy	Complication	Comments	Award
1997, New Jersey[36] Rotator cuff re-injury	A 55-year-old male presented with a ruptured rotator cuff from falling 18 ft off a ladder during work (furniture delivery).	Orthopedic surgeon	Physical therapy (no details)	The rotator cuff reruptured during physical therapy; required a second surgery.	The patient contended surgeon did not monitor PT and allowed it to be too aggressive. He further claimed permanent injury with severe movement restriction, an inability to return to work.	$537,507 verdict

Note: Awards and settlements do not necessarily prove a cause-effect relationship between equipment or technique and injury.

REFERENCES

1. Tan JC: Practical manual of physical medicine and rehabilitation: diagnostics, therapeutics, and basic problems. St Louis: Mosby; 1998
2. Dawson PM: An historical sketch of the Valsalva experiment. Bull Hist Med 14:295-320, 1943.
3. Hall C, Brody LT: Impairment in muscle performance. In: Hall CM, Brody LT, eds: Therapeutic exercise: moving toward function. Philadelphia: Lippincott Williams & Wilkins; 2005.
4. Erickson RP, Lie YR, Chiniger MA: Rehabilitation in multiple sclerosis. Mayo Clin Proc 64:818-828, 1989.
5. Simons DJ: A note on the effect of heat and of cold upon certain symptoms of multiple sclerosis. Bull Neurol Inst N Y 6:385-386, 1937.
6. Kisner C, Colby LA: Therapeutic exercise: foundations and techniques, ed 3. Philadelphia: FA Davis; 1996.
7. Nelson MR: Rehabilitation concerns in myopathies. In: Braddom RL, editor: Physical medicine and rehabilitation, ed 2. Philadelphia: W.B. Saunders; 2000.

8. Bensman A: Strenuous exercise can impair muscle function in Guillain-Barré patients. JAMA 214:468-469, 1970.

9. Lovett RW: The treatment of infantile paralysis: preliminary report, based on a study of the Vermont epidemic of 1914. JAMA 64:2118-2123, 1915.

10. Hyman G: Poliomyelitis. Lancet 1:852, 1953.

11. Mitchell GP: Poliomyelitis and exercise. Lancet 2:90-91, 1953.

12. Obuchowska I, Mariak Z, Stankiewicz A: [Massive suprachoroidal hemorrhage during cataract surgery: case report]. [Polish]Klin Oczna 104(5-6):406-410, 2002.

13. American Diabetes Association: Physical activity/exercise and diabetes. Diabetes Care, 2004.

14. Delorme TL, Watkins AL: Progressive resistive exercises: technic and medical application. New York: Appleton-Century-Crofts; 1951.

15. McGuire J, Green RS, Hauenstein V, et al: Bed pan deaths. Am Pract Digest Treat 1:23-28, 1950.

16. Spires MC: Rehabilitation of patients with burns. In: Braddom RL, editor: Physical medicine and rehabilitation, ed 2. Philadelphia: W.B. Saunders; 2000.

17. Sinaki M, Mikkelsen BA: Postmenopausal spinal osteoporosis: flexion versus extension exercises. Arch Phys Med Rehab 65:593, 1984.

18. Scull SA: Juvenile rheumatoid arthritis. In: Campbell SK, Palisono R, Vander Linden DW, eds: Physical therapy for children. Philadelphia: Saunders; 1994.

19. Helm PA, Kevorkian CG, Lushbaugh M, et al: Burn injury: rehabilitation management in 1982. Arch Phys Med Rehab 63:6-16, 1982.

20. Maihafer GC: Rehabilitation of total hip replacements and fracture management considerations. In: Echternach, JL, editor: Physical therapy of the hip. New York: Churchill Livingstone; 1990.

21. American Academy of Pediatrics Committee on Sports Medicine and Fitness: Strength training by children and adolescents. Pediatrics 107(6):1470-1472, 2001.

22. U.S. Consumer Product Safety Commission, National Electronic Injury Surveillance System. Available at: http://www: cpsc.gov/library/neiss.html, Accessed December 16, 2005.

23. Sayers SP, Clarkson PM, Rouzier PA, et al: Adverse events associated with eccentric exercise protocols: six case studies. Med Sci Sports Exerc 31(12):1697-1702, 1999.

24. Tietjen DP, Guzzi LM: Exertional rhabdomyolysis and acute renal failure following the Army Physical Fitness Test. Mil Med 154(1):23-25, 1989.

25. Klodell CT Jr, Pokorny R, Carrillo EH, et al: Exercise-induced compartment syndrome: case report. Am Surg 62(6):469-471, 1996.

26. Springer BL, Clarkson PM: Two cases of exertional rhabdomyolysis precipitated by personal trainers. Med Sci Sports Exerc 35(9):1499-1502, 2003.

27. Katz B, Carmody R: Subperiosteal orbital hematoma induced by the Valsalva maneuver. Am J Ophthalmol 100(4):617-618, 1985.

28. Schartum S: Ventricular arrest caused by the Valsalva maneuver in a patient with Adams-Stokes attacks accompanying defecation. Acta Med Scand 184(1-2):65-68, 1968.

29. Bennett RL, Knowlton GC: Overwork weakness in partially denervated skeletal muscle. Clin Orthop 12:22-29, 1958.

30. Duane TD: Valsalva hemorrhagic retinopathy. Am J Ophthalmol 75(4):637-642, 1973.

31. Giunta JL: Neck exercises triggering dental pain. J Mass Dent Soc 48(1):38-39, 1999.

32. Gross MT, Schuch CP: Exercise programs for patients with post-polo syndrome: a case report. Phys Ther 69(1):72, 1989.

33. Line RL, Rust GS: Acute exertional rhabdomyolysis. Am Fam Phys 52(2):502-506, 1995.

34. Marshall RC, King PS: Effects of fatigue produced by isokinetic exercise on the communication ability of aphasic adults. J Speech Hear Res 16(2):222-230, 1973.

35. Riddle P: Fatal gastric hemorrhage after radio exercise. Dallas Med J 18:20, 1932.

36. Medical malpractice verdict settlement, and experts, September, 1997, p 37, loc 3.

17   ACTIVITIES OF DAILY LIVING (BASIC)

In the following sections, bed activities, transfer, feeding (aspiration), carrying, and lifting concerns will be listed. These concerns are activity (dynamic) related. (For static issues, see Positioning.)

17.1   Bed Activities

For bed activities, some safety issues to keep in mind include vertigo/syncope with position changes, unstable joint/prosthetic positions, and shear force effects on skin.

CONTRAINDICATIONS AND PRECAUTIONS

L00-L99 DISEASES OF THE SKIN AND SUBCUTANEOUS TISSUE

Issue	LOC	Sources	Affil	Rationale/Comment
Friction and shear forces	Avoid	AHCPR, 1992[3]	Agency	These forces can lead to skin damage.

M00-M99 DISEASES OF THE MUSCULOSKELETAL SYSTEM AND CONNECTIVE

Issue	LOC	Sources	Affil	Rationale/Comment
Low back trauma—logroll	Advise	Pierson and Fairchild, 2002[1]	PT	Turn in a logroll fashion rather than segmentally for less discomfort.

Y70-Y82 MEDICAL DEVICES

Issue	LOC	Sources	Affil	Rationale/Comment
THR—hip abduction	Advice	Pierson and Fairchild, 2002[1]	PT	Maintain operated limb in abduction when moving from side to side.
THR—hip rotation	Advice			Avoid twisting upper body on a fixed lower extremity because it rotates the hip indirectly (i.e., some reaching activities while in bed).
THR—log rolls	Advice	Maihafer, 1990[2]	PT	Transfers and log rolls should be performed away from the operative side with leg supported by a staff member. Note: rolling toward the involved leg indirectly internally rotates it, which is not desirable.

PROCEDURAL CONCERNS

Turning/Rolling

Issue	LOC	Sources	Affil	Rationale/Comment
Space to roll— Adequate	Advice	Pierson and Fairchild, 2002[1]	PT	Instruct patient to determine position on bed mat before any rolling attempted. Depending on the bed's width, the patient may need to adjust position. Note: that is, the patient should not get dangerously close to the bed's edge.

Supine to Sitting

Issue	LOC	Sources	Affil	Rationale/Comment
Position changes	Advice	Pierson and Fairchild, 2002[1]	PT	Do not allow patient to sit unattended or without support, even briefly. Some patients may experience vertigo or syncope when moved quickly from supine to sitting; others may lack sufficient strength or balance.

REFERENCES

1. Pierson FM, Fairchild SL: Principles and techniques of patient care, ed 3. Philadelphia: W.B. Saunders; 2002.
2. Maihafer GC: Rehabilitation of total hip replacements and fracture management considerations. In: Echternach, JL, editor: Physical therapy of the hip. New York: Churchill Livingstone; 1990.
3. AHCPR. Pressure ulcers in adults: prediction and prevention. Clinical Practice Guideline Number 3, AHCPR Pub. No. 92-0047, May 1992.

17.2 Carrying

Carrying is defined as the act of moving something from one place to another place and is applied below within the context of UE activity.[1] Upper limb prosthetic concerns and ergonomic issues are listed below.

Y70-Y82 MEDICAL DEVICES

Issue	LOC	Sources	Affil	Rationale/Comment
Total elbow arthroplasty—heavy loads	P	Kisner and Colby, 1996[2]	PT	Avoid using the operated arm for lifting and carrying heavy objects as it may result in loosening of the prosthetic components.

PROCEDURAL CONCERNS

Issue	LOC	Sources	Affil	Rationale/Comment
One-handed carrying	Don't	Pearson and Fairchild, 2002[3]	PT	Carry a one-handed object (e.g., one grocery bag) in upper extremities alternately.

REFERENCES

1. Webster's third new international dictionary. Springfield (MA): Merriam-Webster; 1981.
2. Kisner C, Colby LA: Therapeutic exercise: foundations and techniques, ed 3. Philadelphia: F.A. Davis; 1996.
3. Pierson FM, Fairchild SL: Principles and techniques of patient care, ed 3. Philadelphia: W.B. Saunders; 2002.

17.3 Feeding/Swallowing Problems (Dysphagia)

OVERVIEW. Aspiration of vomitus involves the inhalation of regurgitated gastric contents into the pulmonary system.[1] It may be unsafe to have patients feed by mouth if they are at *high* risk for aspiration. Signs of a person with high risk for aspiration include decreased alertness, decreased responsiveness, absent swallow, absent protective cough, difficulty handling secretions (excessive cough, choking), copious secretions, a wet gurgling voice quality, or a decreased movement (range and strength) of oral, pharyngeal, and laryngeal areas.[2]

Aspiration precautions, particularly in persons with neurological impairments, are listed below. Nevertheless, it is important to note that sources in the literature do recommend an individual approach to managing swallowing problems. In other words, not all patients will respond well to one particular positioning intervention to ensure a safe swallow.

PROCEDURAL CONCERNS

High Risk for Aspiration

Issue	LOC	Sources	Affil	Rationale/Comment
Nothing by mouth (NPO)	P	Tan, 1998[2]	MD/PT	Nothing by mouth for individuals at high risk for aspiration.

Aspiration Precaution for Neurologically Impaired Patients with Dysphagia

Issue	LOC	Sources	Affil	Rationale/Comment
Posture	Guidelines	Horner and Massey, 1991[3]	PhD	Sit fully upright in bed or chair while eating.
Bolus size				Take small bites and sips. A small bolus size is a "common sense" approach.
Textures				Thick liquids and pudding textures are often better than clear liquids, although it may vary for each patient.
Monitor				(1) Lung sounds, (2) wet voice quality, (3) upper airway congestion, (4) temperature, (5) hydration, (6) weight

Reflux refers to an abnormal return or backward flow of fluids. In gastroesophageal reflux, there is a backflow of contents from the stomach to the esophagus.[1] Homer and Massey[3] list some reflux precautions for neurologically impaired patients with dysphagia below.

Reflux Precautions for Neurologically Impaired Patients with Dysphagia

Issue	LOC	Sources	Affil	Rationale/Comment
Timing	Guidelines	Horner and Massey, 1991[3]	PhD	Have meals at least 1 hour before lying down. Do not exercise too soon after eating.
Sleeping				Elevate head of bed; use extra pillows.
Foods				Avoid spicy, acidic foods.
Liquids				Limit intake of coffee, tea, alcohol, and colas.

REFERENCES

1. Anderson K, Anderson L, Glanze WD: Mosby's medical, nursing, and allied health dictionary, ed 5. St. Louis: Mosby; 1998.
2. Tan JC: Practical manual of physical medicine and rehabilitation: diagnostics, therapeutics, and basic problems. St. Louis: Mosby; 1998
3. Horner J, Massey EW: Managing dysphagia: special problems in patients with neurologic disease. Postgrad Med 89(5):203-213, 1991.

17.4 Moving and Lifting: Body Mechanics (Moving Heavy Items or Patients)

This section lists recommendations on basic body mechanics while lifting and moving loads. Four sources (two physical therapists and two nurses) mentioned 19 do's and don'ts for moving heavy items (such as patients) that ranged from five to seven per source. The most frequently mentioned recommendation is to keep the load (patient) close to the therapist.

DO'S

Issue	LOC	Sources	Affil	Rationale/Comment
Ask for help if needed	Do	McConnell, 2002[1]	Nurs	Assess situation; ask for help if needed.
		Pearson and Fairchild, 2002[2]	PT	Know your limitations.
Back—keep straight	Do	Rantz and Courtial, 1981[3]	Nurs	While working or lifting, keep back straight.
Base of support—appropriate	Do	Minor and Minor, 1999[4]	PT	Have your base of support appropriately wide for the task to maintain balance.
Base of support—one foot forward	Do	Rantz and Courtial, 1981[3]	Nurs	To provide a wider base of support.
Height—comfortable	Do			Place work at a comfortable height level.
Legs and hips—use	Do			Use the hips and legs for lifting.[b]
Load (patient) close to therapist	Do	Minor and Minor, 1999[4]	PT	Keep load (patient) close to therapist.
		McConnell, 2002[1]	Nurs	Move COG of patient near therapist. Don't reach to lift. Carry children waist
		Pearson and Fairchild, 2002[2]	PT	high, near COG.[1] Keep load close to midline.[2]
		Rantz and Courtial, 1981[3]	Nurs	
Parallel forces to surface	Do	Pearson and Fairchild, 2002[2]	PT	Apply force parallel to surface when pushing or pulling.
Plan your action	Do	Rantz and Courtial, 1981[3]	Nurs	

Push, pull, or roll objects instead of lift	Do	McConnell, 2002[1]	Nurs	
		Rantz and Courtial, 1981[3,a]	Nurs	
Stable footstool—use	Do	Pearson and Fairchild, 2002[2]	PT	Use stable footstool/ladder to reach above shoulder level.

a, Also drag.

DON'TS

Issue	LOC	Sources	Affil	Rationale/Comment
Bending back	Don't	Minor and Minor, 1999[4]	PT	Keep back straight; don't bend back.
		McConnell, 2002[1]	Nurs	
Carrying—one-handed carrying	Don't	Pearson and Fairchild, 2002[2]	PT	Carry one-handed object in upper extremities alternately.
Pulling when you can push	Don't	McConnell, 2002[1]	Nurs	
Extending back	Don't	Minor and Minor, 1999[4]	Nurs	To keep back in a constant position, preferably erect.
				Do not extend back to lift. Lift with legs as these are large, strong muscles.
Long lever arms	Don't	Pearson and Fairchild, 2002[2]	PT	Avoid long lever arms when lifting, pushing, pulling, reaching, and carrying.
Shoes—slippery or high heeled	Don't	McConnell, 2002[1]	Nurs	Wear nonslip, flexible, low heels.
Simultaneous trunk bending and rotation	Don't	Pearson and Fairchild, 2002[2]	PT	Avoid trunk bending and rotation simultaneously.
Twisting spine	Don't	Minor and Minor, 1999[4]	PT	During transfers do not twist spine; instead, rotate entire body.
		Rantz and Courtial, 1981[3,b]	Nurs	

REFERENCES

1. McConnell EA: Using proper body mechanics: Clinical do's and don'ts. Nursing 32(5):17, 2002.
2. Pierson FM, Fairchild SL: Principles and techniques of patient care, ed 3. Philadelphia: W.B. Saunders; 2002.
3. Rantz MR, Courtial D: Lifting, moving, and transferring patients: a manual, ed 2. St. Louis: Mosby; 1981.
4. Minor MAS, Minor SD: Patient care skills, ed 4. Stamford (CT): Appleton & Lange; 1999.

17.5 Transfer Training

Transfer refers to the movement of someone from one surface to another one. The advice below is organized by type (general concerns, stretcher, stand-pivot, sliding board, floor) and by diagnosis (hemiplegia, spinal cord injury, burns). Complications such as falls have occurred during transfers from wheelchairs, plinths, and while in hydrotherapy (**see also Mechanical lift**).

CONTRAINDICATIONS AND PRECAUTIONS

TRANSFERS: GENERAL

Issue	LOC	Sources	Affil	Rationale/Comment
Body mechanics	Advice	McConnell, 1995[1]	Nurs	The assistors should keep their backs as straight as possible during the transfer.
Caster wheels—on wheelchair	Advice	Pierson and Fairchild, 2002[2]	PT	The wheelchair is less stable when the patient moves toward the front portion of the seat. Do not direct casters backward during transfers from wheelchair.
Environmental hazards				Clear environment of hazards such as unneeded equipment.
Equipment—protect bandages				e.g., casts, drainage tubes, IV tubes, dressings, and bandages.

Falling	Advice	McConnell, 1995[1]	Nurs	If patient starts to fall, ease to nearest surface. Otherwise, the provider may lose balance or injure self.
Footrests—on wheelchair	Advice			Don't leave footrests of wheelchair down. They interfere with the transfer.
Footwear	P	Pierson and Fairchild, 2002[2]	PT	Use proper shoes for standing transfers. No sandals, smooth leather-soled shoes, slippers, or socks only.
	Advice	McConnell, 1995[1]	Nurs	
Friction and shear forces	Avoid	AHCPR, 1992[3]	Agency	If risk of ulcer.
Patient capabilities	P	Pierson and Fairchild, 2002[2]	PT	Assess patient's capabilities.
Plan transfer		Pierson and Fairchild, 2002[2]	PT	
• Preplan the activity mentally				
Safety belts				Use safety belt on patient to protect patient during transfer.
Unusual events that may occur				Be alert and on guard.
Wheelchair brakes:	Advice	Minor and Minor, 1999[4]	PT	If pneumatic tires are not inflated enough, brakes may not work properly.
• Must be engaged during transfers		McConnell, 1995[1]	Nurs	

TRANSFERS: BY TYPE

Stretcher to Bed (and Reverse)

Issue	LOC	Sources	Affil	Rationale/Comment
Lock two surfaces	Advice	Pierson and Fairchild, 2002[2]	PT	Stretcher and bed should be locked or secured so the two surfaces will not separate during the transfer.
		McConnell, 1995[1]	Nurs	
Do not drag patients	Recommendations	AHCPR, 1992[3]	Agency	Friction is a common cause of superficial skin injuries. Use lifting devices such as linen or trapeze bars to lift and move rather than drag patients when transferring.

Pivot Standing Transfers (Assisted)

Issue	LOC	Sources	Affil	Rationale/Comment
Footwear	P Advice	Pierson and Fairchild, 2002[2] McConnell, 1995[1]	PT Nurs	Use proper shoes for standing transfers.
Footstools during standing transfers • Instruct to push down with foot and not push forward to avoid sliding or tipping the footstool.	Caution	Pierson and Fairchild, 2002[2]	PT	Occasionally it may be necessary for person with short stature to use a footstool.
Moving patient quickly	Don't	McConnell, 1995[1]	Nurs	The patient's cardiovascular system may not have sufficient time to adjust.
Patient's clothing belt • To lift patient		Pierson and Fairchild, 2002[2]	PT	Clothing belts can cause patient discomfort, tear clothing, or unbuckle. Use safety belt or grasp under buttocks if patient consents.
Use of upper extremity or clothing • As point of control during transfer	Don't			Clothing or an upper limb are insecure points of control.

Sliding Board Transfer

Issue	LOC	Sources	Affil	Rationale/Comment
Twisting injury of helper	Danger	MDA 1996[5]	Agency	

Wheelchair to Floor Transfers

Issue	LOC	Sources	Affil	Rationale/Comment
Paralyzed (or inactive) with osteoporosis	Caution	Pierson and Fairchild, 2002[2]	PT	Inactive or paralyzed patients may have osteoporosis in lower extremities and vertebral bodies. Some transfer methods may be unsafe. For example, floor reaction forces during wheelchair to floor transfers (e.g., dropping onto knees) may cause a fracture in weakened bone. Patient may need assistance to go down to floor.

TRANSFERS: BY DIAGNOSIS

Hemiplegia

Issue	LOC	Sources	Affil	Rationale/Comment
Pulling arm	Special precautions	Pierson and Fairchild, 2002[2]	PT	Pulling on involved or weakened extremities (i.e., unstable joints) should not be used to control or move patient. Note: The involved shoulder may also be subluxed in this population.

Burns

Issue	LOC	Sources	Affil	Rationale/Comment
Sliding across surfaces	P	Pierson and Fairchild, 2002[2]	PT	Avoid sliding or dragging patient across the surface of the burn wound graft site or harvested area. Sliding creates shear forces and can disrupt healing.

Spinal cord injury

Issue	LOC	Sources	Affil	Rationale/Comment
Injuries, recent—avoid distracting and rotational forces	Special precautions	Pierson and Fairchild, 2002[2]	PT	Log roll patients; do not pull lower extremities downward.
Supine to sitting	Special precautions			Blood pressure may be unstable.
Osteoporosis, long-standing	Special precautions			Osteoporosis may be present. Mild to moderate stress on these bones may lead to fracture in a person with a long-standing spinal cord injury.

Total hip replacement

Issue	LOC	Sources	Affil	Rationale/Comment
Pivots and leg movements	P	Pierson and Fairchild, 2002[2]	PT	Special precautions during transfers will be in place, especially the initial 2 weeks after surgery. Do not pivot on the extremity (operated) when standing. Avoid excessive hip flexion, trunk flexion, or hip adduction during transfers.
Pivot and involved side	P	Maihafer, 1990[6]	PT	Transfers and log rolling should be performed away from the operative side with the leg supported by a staff member.
Transfers to cars: low motor vehicles or bucket seats	Special care	AMA, 2003[7]	Org	The low sitting positioning may result in excessive hip flexion (greater than 90 degrees).

ADVERSE EVENTS

Source	Background	Therapy	Outcome	Follow-up/Interpretation
Illman et al, 2000[8] **SCI and hypotension during therapy** Observational— prospective Spinal Cord	14 of 17 patients with acute SCI were evaluated for the first 10 minutes of 10 physiotherapy sessions involving transitions to sitting or standing in a South Australian hospital and rehabilitation center.	10 tetraplegic and 4 paraplegic persons (10 male, 4 female); age range 16 to 46 years. Protocol: All patients wore anti-embolic stockings, and abdominal binders were worn in persons with complete motor tetraplegia. Transitions were performed slowly from supine to sitting or standing.	Blood pressure dropped in 73.6% of treatments (95 of 129 treatments). Signs and symptoms were noted on 58.9% of the occasions and occurred within 3 minutes of standing or being raised >60 degrees on the tilt table. (Mean fall in systolic = 21 mm Hg; mean fall diastolic = 7.2 mm Hg; mean rise in heart rate = 14.9 bpm; O_2 saturations: little change.)	Authors recommend monitoring signs and symptoms of orthostatic hypotension during treatment involving positioning changes in acute SCI patients. Stated patients with tetraplegia had higher occurrence of OH than paraplegic patients. Note: This study was descriptive; no inferential statistics were used.
James, 1970[9] **Fall from wheelchair** Case report (potential litigation) Phys Ther	A 15-year-old wheelchair-dependent female with cerebral palsy attended PT at a hospital. As PT stepped from the front to the rear of wheelchair to move patient into the treatment area, the patient fell face forward out of the wheelchair.	The patient dislodged an upper front tooth, broke the adjoining capped tooth, bruised his nose severely, and blackened both eyes.	The parents initiated legal action against the hospital but dropped the case later because of the excellent rapport between the parents, patient, and PT.	The PT's insurance company paid $424.43 in dental and other expenses. (Note: No information was provided about the seatbelt.)

LITIGATION

Year, State	History	Location	Therapy	Complication	Comments/Award
1995, Tennessee [10] **Patient dropped during transfer**	A 69-year-old female presented with a PMHx of 8 surgeries in 12 years due to arthritis and had sustained a fractured arm and leg due to a MVA.	Hospital physical therapy.	A physical therapy technician had dropped her.	She fractured her other leg, requiring the use of a walker. Her injury was described as an "uncorrectable broken leg."	The hospital failed to have a physical therapy procedure identifying patients who are "at risk." $375,000 verdict (patient $275,000; husband $100,000).
1994, Missouri [11] **Fall in hydrotherapy**	Plaintiff (no details) with arthritis in legs.	Physical therapy department.	Receiving whirlpool treatment.	The patient slipped, fell, and fractured patella while exiting whirlpool with assistance; injuries required surgery and eventual removal of patella.	It was contended that staff was negligent in provided assistance. Verdict: $47,773.90

Note: Awards and settlements do not necessarily prove a cause-effect relationship between equipment or technique and injury.

REFERENCES

1. McConnell EA: Transferring a patient from bed to chair. Nursing 25(11):30, 1995.
2. Pierson FM, Fairchild SL: Principles and techniques of patient care, ed 3. Philadelphia: Saunders; 2002.
3. AHCPR: Pressure ulcers in adults: prediction and prevention. Clinical Practice Guideline Number 3, AHCPR Pub. No. 92-0047, May 1992.
4. Minor MAS, Minor SD: Patient care skills, ed 4. Stamford (CT): Appleton & Lange; 1999.
5. Medical Devices Agency: Moving and transferring equipment: a comparative evaluation. DEA A19. London: Medical Devices Agency; 1996.
6. Maihafer GC: Rehabilitation of total hip replacements and fracture management considerations, In Echternach, JL, editor: Physical therapy of the hip. New York: Churchill Livingstone; 1990.

7. American Medical Association: Physician's guide to assessing and counseling older drivers [2003] Available at: http://www.ama-assn.org/ama/pub/category/10791.html. Accessed November 7, 2005.
8. Illman A, Stiller K, Williams M: The prevalence of orthostatic hypotension during physiotherapy treatment in patients with an acute spinal cord injury. Spinal Cord 38(12):741-747, 2000.
9. James CA: Medico-legal considerations in the practice of physical therapy. Phys Ther 50(8):1203-1207, 1970.
10. Medical malpractice verdict settlement, and experts, June 1995, p 27, loc 1.
11. Medical malpractice verdict settlement, and experts, December 1994, p 45, loc 4.

17.6 Wheelchair Activities

Pierson and Fairchild 2002[1] offer advice on safely managing a manual wheelchair in order to avoid tips, falls, and injuries. Most advice is directed toward the helper/attendant when assisting the user on curbs, stairs, and escalators.

Issues	LOC	Sources	Affil	Rationale/Comment
Chest belt as a restraint	Advice	Pierson and Fairchild, 2002[1]	PT	Comply with federal and state regulations concerning the use of belts or straps as restraints.
Curbs—Ascending forward	Advice			Footrest may hit the front of the curb with the user subsequently falling out of wheelchair.
Curbs—Descending backwards	Advice			Maintain wheelchair in a reclined position (i.e., caster up) until casters and front rigging clear the curb.
Curb cut outs—approaching	Advice			The wheelchair's footplate may bang into the cutout surface.

Continued

Issues	LOC	Sources	Affil	Rationale/Comment
Escalators	Extreme care			Use extreme care to prevent possible injury because escalator use is not viewed as an ordinary activity. Two people are recommended to control the chair, one in front and one behind.
Lifting wheelchair—e.g., on stairs; into car	Advice			Do not lift the chair using any of the removable components such as the armrests or front rigging because these components may detach from the chair during the lift (i.e., they are not a stable contact point).
Reaching for objects—in front of wheelchair	Advice			The wheelchair may tip forward onto its footplates when the user lifts object (e.g., 5-10 lbs) from the floor in front of the chair. It may be safer for the user to reach for objects when at side and parallel to object. Alternatively, rotate caster wheels to a forward position in order to increase the wheelchair's base of support.
Read the wheelchair owner's manual	Advice			For properly maintaining wheelchair.
Stairs—ascending and descending backwards, multiple levels	Advice			Stair activities require a two- or three-person assistance (i.e., for large or severely involved patient). Do not grasp detachable items of chair during the assist.
Tipping wheelchair backwards	Advice			Warn the user who is being pushed before tipping chair.

REFERENCE

1. Pierson FM, Fairchild SL: Principles and techniques of patient care, ed 3. Philadelphia: Saunders; 2002.

The ADA Checklist is used in complying with Title III requirements of removing architectural barriers in public areas of existing facilities when removal can be achieved without much expense or difficulty. The goal is to make existing facilities more usable by the disabled communities. Establishments that must meet requirements are places that serve the public such as **doctors' offices**, hotels, restaurants, theaters, stores, and schools. The checklist items included here contain information on the dimensions, clearances, or usability of pathways (routes), entrances, ramps, doors, rooms, stairs, elevators and lifts.[1,2]

Route (Pathway)[1,2]

Issue	Rationale/Comment
Elevation	Route that does not require stairs.
Clearance	Route is 36 inches wide.
Protruding objects	Visually disabled able to detect protruding objects in route's path using a cane.
Curbs	Curbs at drives, parking, and drop-off points have curb cuts.

Entrances[1,2]

Issue	Rationale/Comment
Door clearance	Door with at least 32 inches of clearance.
Door-pull clearance	18 inches of clear wall space on pull side of door.

Continued

Issue	Rationale/Comment
Opening indoor door	Can open indoor door with little force (5 pounds).
Mats and carpets	Mats and carpets no more than $1/2$ inch high to minimize tripping hazard.
Edge of carpet/mats are secured	
Door handles	
Door with closers	Door with closers take at least 3 seconds to close.
Automatic doors	Automatic doors—force to stop movement is not greater than 15 pounds.
Handle height is 48 inches or less	

Ramps[1,2]

Issue	Rationale/Comment
Rise between landings	Rise is no more than 30 inches between landings.
Landing areas	5-foot level landing at top and bottom of ramp for every 30 feet of horizontal ramp length.
Incline—height/length	Incline not greater than 1 inch height for every 1 foot of ramp length.
Non slip ramps	
Rails	Rails on both sides if ramp longer than 6 feet.
Rail dimensions	Rails are sturdy and between 34 and 38 inches in height.

Doors[1,2]

Issue	Rationale/Comment
Clearance	Clearance: at least 32-inch opening.
Wall space near door	Wall space near pull side of door, next to handle, is at least 18 inches so wheelchair or person using crutches can approach in order to open the door.
Handle height	Handle height is 48 inches or less.
Handle operation	Can operate handle with a closed fist.
Door threshold	Door threshold edge is $1/4$ inch high or less ($3/4$ inch or less if beveled).
Opening force	Can open indoor door with little force (5 pounds).

Rooms[1,2]

Issue	Rationale/Comment
Pathways clearance	Pathways and aisles at least 36 inches wide.
Turning clearance	To adequately turn: 5 foot circle or "T"-shaped space.
Carpet type	Low pile, tightly woven carpet.
Carpet edges	Carpet secured along edges.

Stairs[1,2]

Issue	Rationale/Comment
Surface	Nonslip surface on treads.
Stair rails	Continuous rails on both sides of stairs.
Rail dimensions	Rails extend beyond top and bottom of stairs.

Elevators[1,2]

Issue	Rationale/Comment
Indicators	Indicators visible and auditory when door opens and closes.
Call button	Call button no higher than 42 inches.
Controls for visually challenged	Controls with raised lettering/Braille.
Emergency intercom	Emergency intercom used with voice and identified with raised letters/Braille.

Lifts[1,2]

Issue	Rationale/Comment
Type of operation	Can be operated without assistance or have a call button.
	Controls located between 15 and 48 inches high.
	30×48 inches of clear space so able to use lift with a wheelchair and can operate controls.

ADVERSE EVENTS

Sweeney et al (1989) identified six safety concerns for portable ramps.[3]

Source	Background	Therapy	Outcome
Sweeney et al, 1989[3] **Portable ramp safety** Descriptive questionnaire Br J Occup Ther	Wheelchair users, ambulatory disabled persons, and their attendants in the UK evaluated the use and safety of portable commercial ramps (used for temporary access into buildings and vehicles).	45 respondents, ages 16 to 91 years, with wide range of orthopedic, neurologic, chronic impairments evaluated ramps (users of manual w/c, power w/c, attendants, three ambulatory persons).	Safety concerns: (1) Several trapped fingers were reported due to the folding and telescopic mechanism of ramps. (2) Dull aluminum color of most ramps is difficult for partially sighted patients to see. (3) Low-set footrests on wheelchairs push and interfere with ramps that are designed with high lips. (4) Some narrow ramps tip when wheels of chair hit against the inner lip of the ramps. (5) There is a risk of tipping when pushing wheelchair up or down a ramp because of the alignment bars (designed to prevent ramp movement). (6) Central portion of ramp must be supported by a firm surface when in use.

REFERENCES

1. Americans with Disabilities Act checklist for readily achievable barrier removal: checklist for existing facilities, version 2.1, August 1995, Adaptive Environments Center, Inc, for the National Institutes on Disability and Rehabilitation Research.
2. Checklist for readily achievable barrier removal. Available at: http://www.usdoj.gov/crt/ada/checktxt.htm. Accessed November 7, 2005.
3. Sweeney GM, Clarke AK, Harrison RA, et al: An evaluation of portable ramps. Br J Occup Ther 52(12):473-475, 1989.

19   SPORT ACTIVITIES

Sports—or to make oneself "merry"—is a pastime that serves as a pleasing or amusing diversion.[1] Concerns for sports participation for individuals with physical disabilities are listed below by sport and then by diagnosis. The American Academy of Pediatrics[2] has issued recommendations for children and preadolescents with medical conditions that affect sports participation; some require further evaluation of risk. Adams' recommendations,[3] although somewhat dated, offer insightful guidelines on game and sport participation for physically challenged individuals from a recreational perspective.

CONTRAINDICATIONS AND PRECAUTIONS

By Sport

Issue	LOC	Sources	Affil	Rationale/Comment
Archery	Cerebral palsy	Adams et al, 1975[3]	RT[a]	CI when the neuromuscular disorder is more than mild and is the predominate feature.
	Rheumatoid arthritis			Do not shoot longbow if joints are inflamed. If severely involved, they can use crossbow.
Badminton	Rheumatoid arthritis			Quick reversal movement of wrist and elbow may cause further pain and damage to involved joints—needs individual evaluation.
Bowling	Cardiac			Needs medical clearance; monitor for fatigue and dyspnea; stop if circulatory embarrassment exists.
Boxing: contact/ collision sports	No boxing	AAP, 2001[2]	Org	Boxing is the one contact/collision sport not recommended by the AAP.

Fencing	COPD caution	Adams et al, 1975[3]	RT	COPD: issue of heat and breathing through a wired mask.
	CV disorder			CV disorders need clearance for fencing because of the competitive nature of the sport.
	RA need clearance			RA needs clearance because of the need to avoid aggravating major joints.
Horseback riding (also see Hippotherapy)	Asthma	Adams et al, 1975[3]	RT	Allergy precaution to avoid dusty riding areas and horse hair.
	Cardiovascular disease			Avoid undue fatigue and possible frightening experiences. Requires medical clearance.
	Cerebral palsy			Depends on strenuousness of the ride.
	Hip disorders			Western saddle recommended because it provides a more secure base for riding compared to the English hunter saddle (places person at a forward incline).
	Rheumatoid arthritis			Generally not offered due to danger of injury or aggravating condition. Although non–weight-bearing, the hip joint is still loaded. Avoid this activity if joints are inflamed and range of motion is restricted.
Ice hockey	Body check concern	AAP, 2001[2]	Org	AAP recommends limiting the amount of body checking permitted in 15-year-olds or younger who play hockey.
Ice skating	Cardiovascular	Adams et al, 1975[3]	RT	Monitor pulse during pauses to assess stress level.
	Rheumatoid arthritis			Not if joints are inflamed due to the impact nature of skating.
	Cerebral palsy			Not in the presence of athetosis or severe LE spasticity.
				Caution: most individuals will need 1:1 attention; high-top footwear; and possibly, stabilization of the ankle.
Scuba diving	Asthma CI	Weiss and van Meter, 1995[4]	MD	**Two asthmatic patients sustained cerebral air emboli while taking scuba class in a swimming pool.[4]**
Swimming	Epilepsy	Kemp and Sibert, 1993[5]		Swim with friend in a lifeguard-supervised pool.
	Epilepsy—uncontrolled			Uncontrolled epilepsy—higher supervision is needed. Evaluate individually.

a, RT = recreational therapist.

By Diagnosis/Disability

Issue	LOC	Sources	Affil	Rationale/Comment
Arthroplasty—total hip replacement	Avoid high-impact recreational activities (jumping or resisted movements).	Schamerloh and Ritter, 1977[6]	PT	Heavy rotational forces on the limb contribute to loosening and failure of hip replacements.
Asthma	Most children can participate with proper management. Properly medicate and educate.[2] If severe asthma exists, modify participation.[2]	Adams et al, 1975[3] AAP, 2001[2]	RT Org	Note that exercise-induced asthma can occur during or 15-20 minutes after activity. In severe asthma, avoid sports with body contact.
Atlantoaxial instability (C1 C2)	Requires evaluation for sport participation.	AAP, 2001[2]	Org	
Auditory impairment— hard of hearing	Advice/precautions	Adams et al, 1975[3]	RT	Remove hearing aid during vigorous activity and use a buddy system to warn of instructions. Teach special signs. Avoid lengthy explanations and constant rule changes. Precaution: (1) Limit climbing activities if balance disturbances due to impaired SSC function are evident. (2) If there is a history of ENT problems, avoid low temperature, excessive water or wind exposures. If exposure is required, wear protective plugs.
Bleeding disorders	Requires evaluation.[2] Swimming okay, but avoid diving (i.e., hemophilia).	AAP, 2001[2] Adams et al, 1975[3]	Org RT	

Carditis	No participation	AAP, 2001[2]	Org	The heart is inflamed and sudden death may occur with exertion.
Congenital heart disease	If moderate to severe or patient had surgery, evaluation is required.			
Cystic fibrosis	Salt tablets during vigorous activity, especially outdoors during hot weather.[3]	Adams et al, 1975[3]	RT	
	Hydrate and acclimatize to reduce heat illness.	AAP, 2001[2]	Org	There is a risk of heat illness. During a graded exercise test, oxygenation should be adequate.
Diabetes mellitus	Can play all sports if proper attention to blood glucose, hydration, insulin, and diet.	AAP, 2001[2,a]	Org	Monitor blood glucose every 30 min during continuous exercise and at 15 min after exercise.
Diarrhea	Qualified no			No participation unless mild because of risk of dehydration and heat illness.
DMD	Never lift the child from under the armpits. Watch for signs of fatigue.	Adams et al, 1975[3]	RT	Precaution: Avoid exercise when child may be tired, i.e., immediately after school, late at night.
Down syndrome	Atlantoaxial instability evaluation	AAP, 2001[7]	Org	Controversial issue: look at radiographic evidence of atlantoaxial instability or subluxation at 3 to 5 years (preschool). Radiographs may be required for Special Olympics and are important if patient is symptomatic or plans to participate in contact sports.

Continued

Issue	LOC	Sources	Affil	Rationale/Comment
Dysrhythmia—irregular cardiac rhythm	Requires evaluation in presence of symptoms (e.g., chest pain, dizziness, shortness of breath) or evidence of mitral regurgitation.	AAP, 2001[2]	Org	
Emphysema and chronic bronchitis	Avoid highly competitive activities, i.e., in emphysema.	Adams et al, 1975[3]	RT	Nervous excitement can lead to forceful efforts at breathing, squeezing airway shut.
Enlarged liver	If acutely enlarged, avoid participation.	AAP, 2001[2]	RT	There is a risk of rupture. Need to evaluate other enlargements (i.e., chronic) for contact and collision sports.
Enlarged spleen	If acutely enlarged, avoid participation.	AAP, 2001[2] Adams et al, 1975[3]	Org RT	There is a risk of rupture. Need to evaluate other enlargements (i.e., chronic) for contact and collision sports.
Fever	No participation			Fever increases cardiopulmonary effort, reduces exercise capacity, increases likelihood of heat illness and orthostatic hypertension, and it may be associated rarely with some infections that are dangerous with exercise (e.g., myocarditis).
Heart murmur (if not innocent)	Requires evaluations if murmur is not innocent (i.e., if it indicates heart disease).			
Hernia	During recovery from surgery, avoid strenuous exertion, exercise, and heavy lifting until medically cleared.			

Hypertension— significant, essential, unexplained	Avoid weight and power lifting, body building and strength training.	AAP, 2001[2]	Org	Other HTN (i.e., severe essential HTN; secondary HTN [e.g., identified disease]) requires evaluation.
Juvenile RA	No football, trampoline, unmodified tennis (due to stress on knees), or power volleyball.	Adams et al, 1975[3]	RT	Physical activities are restricted to those that will not damage joints and depends on degree of involvement.
Low back pain— persistent	Curtail activities such as: hand ball, tennis, bowling, golf.	Adams et al, 1975[3] AAP, 2001[2]	RT	Note: these sports appear to have a prominent rotational component.
Nephritis—chronic	If unilateral kidney involvement, many physicians recommend exclusion from contact sports.	Adams et al, 1975[3]	RT	There is a concern for possible injury of the remaining organ.
Obesity	Acclimatization and hydration are required. Precaution			There is a heat illness risk. Monitor blood pressure before and after exercise. **(See also Aerobic exercise.)**
Osteogenesis imperfecta	Avoid contact sports such as football, soccer, or baseball.	Bleakney and Donahoe, 1994[9]	PT	Bones are brittle.
Otitis media	If perforated eardrum, no swimming.	Adams et al, 1975[3]	RT	Water and bacteria can enter the middle ear canal (i.e., fluid exudate is present in a cavity that normally only contains air— middle ear infections). Children are susceptible due to a shorter and wider eustachian tube.

Continued

Issue	LOC	Sources	Affil	Rationale/Comment
Seizure (convulsive) disorders	If poorly controlled seizures, avoid the following noncontact sports: archery, riflery, swimming, weight or power lifting, strength training, sports involving heights. Know first aid measures. If aura, assist child to a quiet area and lie down to prevent falls.	AAP, 2001[2] Adams et al, 1975[3]	Org RT	These noncontact sports may place patient or others at risk. Other activities (i.e., contact, collision) require evaluation.[2]
Sickle cell disease	Avoid overheating, dehydration, and chilling.[2] No high exertion, collision, and contact sports. Avoid fatigue, weakness. Precaution—avoid bruising and cuts.	AAP, 2001[2] Adams et al, 1975[3]	Org RT	Requires individual assessment. May lead to infection.
Skin disorders—herpes simplex, boils, impetigo, scabies, molluscum contagiosum	If contagious, no participation in martial arts, wrestling, other collision or contact sports, or gymnastics using mats.	AAP, 2001[2]	Org	
Spina bifida	Empty urine bag before entering pools. Examine for skin ulcers before and after brace use or physical activity.	Adams et al, 1975[3]	RT	These children may have impaired sensation and poor circulation. Note: also see **Latex allergies**.

Vision/Eyes	Requires individual assessment.	AAP, 2001[2]	Org	Requires individual assessment.
One functional eye, detached retina, loss of eye; previous eye surgery or serious eye injury		Adams et al, 1975[3]	RT	Protective eye gear (approved by the American Society for Testing and Materials) and equipment may permit participation in most sports, but decision should be made on an individual basis.
Visual impairment				Precaution: Children who wear glasses to correct vision should use a glass guard for protection during vigorous physical activities or, alternatively, be excused from the activity.

REFERENCES

1. Webster's third new international dictionary. Springfield (MA): Merriam-Webster; 1981.
2. American Academy of Pediatrics Committee on Sports Medicine and Fitness and Committee on School Health: Medical conditions affecting sports participation. Pediatrics 107(5):1205-1209, 2001.
3. Adams RC, Daniels AN, Rullman L: Games, sports, and exercise for the physically handicapped. Philadelphia: Lea & Febiger; 1975.
4. Weiss L, Van Meter K: Cerebral air embolism in asthmatic scuba divers in a swimming pool. Chest 107(6):1653-1654, 1995.
5. Kemp AM, Sibert JR: Epilepsy in children and the risk of drowning. Arch Dis Child 68(5):684-685, 1993.
6. Schamerloh C, Ritter M: Prevention of dislocation or subluxation of total hip replacements. Phys Ther 57:1028, 1977.
7. American Academy of Pediatrics, Committee on Genetics: Health supervision for children with Down's syndrome. Pediatrics 107(2): 442-449, 2001.
8. Bleakney DA, Donahoe M: Osteogenesis imperfecta. In: Campbell SK, Palisono R, Vander Linden DW, eds: Physical therapy for children. Philadelphia: Saunders; 1994.

20 OLDER DRIVERS WITH ACUTE OR CHRONIC MEDICAL CONDITIONS (INCLUDES NONCOMMERCIAL MOTOR VEHICLES, EXCLUDES COMMERCIAL DRIVERS)

The primary guideline for assessing and counseling older drivers is set forth by the American Medical Association (AMA)[1] in conjunction with the National Highway Traffic Safety Administration (NHTSA). Older drivers are at greater risk for fatal crashes because of their fragility. Three important areas that tend to decline in function in older drivers are (1) vision, (2) cognition, and (3) motor function.[2]

More than 100 medical conditions or situations identified by the AMA may affect the older driver. The largest proportion of concerns are diseases of circulation (25%), the nervous systems (15%), the eye (13%), or the musculoskeletal system (13%), or are medication related (13%).

**Proportion of Medical Concerns for Older Drivers from AMA
Classified by ICD & Miscellaneous Categories
(n= 104 conditions / situations)**

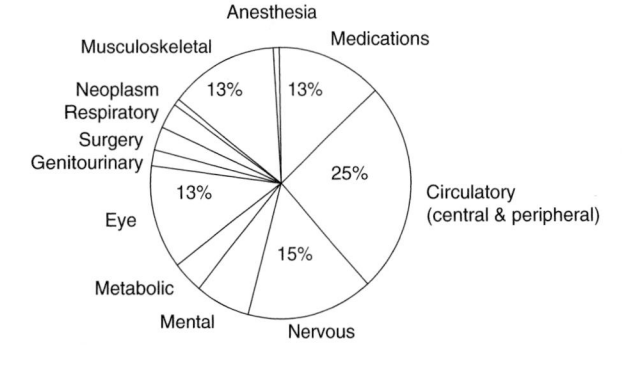

Red flags (listed below) indicate a medical condition in need of further evaluation or management. These concerns may be observed from patient behavior, witnessed during acute events, or noted in a patient's medical history.[1] The complete list of medical concerns with detailed explanations can be found at the AMA web site (http://www.ama-assn.org/ama/pub/category/1079.html).

Additional physician driver evaluation recommendations and signs of unsafe driving from the Association for Driver Rehabilitation Specialists (ADRS), the American Geriatric Society (AGS), and the Alzheimer's Association (AA) are also included below.

RED FLAGS AND CONTRAINDICATIONS FOR DRIVING

E00-E90 ENDOCRINE, NUTRITIONAL, AND METABOLIC DISEASES

Issue	LOC	Sources	Affil	Rationale/Comment
Hypoglycemic attack	Red flag	AMA/NHTSA, 2003[1]	Org	During an acute event, counsel not to drive. A medical condition having unpredictable episodic events is noted in the medical history.
Metabolic diseases (chronic) including: Diabetes mellitus (type I and II) Hypothyroidism				Chronic medical conditions as noted in a medical history suggest a need for formal assessment to determine their impact on functional level.

F00-F99 MENTAL AND BEHAVIORAL DISORDERS

Issue	LOC	Sources	Affil	Rationale/Comment
Delirium—from any cause	Red flag	AMA/NHTSA, 2003[1]	Org	An acute event can impair driving; counsel the patient about driving restriction, assessment, and rehabilitation prior to discharge from ED or hospital.
Psychiatric conditions (chronic) including: Alcohol/substance abuse Anxiety disorders Dementia Mood disorders Personality disorders Psychotic illness	Red flag			Chronic medical conditions as noted in a medical history suggest a need for formal assessment to determine their impact on functional level.

G00-G99 DISEASES OF THE NERVOUS SYSTEM

Issue	LOC	Sources	Affil	Rationale/Comment
Neurologic conditions (chronic) including: Multiple sclerosis Parkinson's disease Peripheral neuropathy Stroke (residual)	Red flag	AMA/NHTSA, 2003[1]	Org	Chronic medical conditions as noted in a medical history suggest a need for formal assessment to determine their impact on functional level.

| Seizure | During an acute event, counsel not to drive. A medical condition having unpredictable episodic events is noted in a medical history. Counsel patient about driving restriction, assessment, and rehabilitation prior to discharge from ED or hospital. |
| Sleep attack or cataplexy | During an acute event, counsel not to drive. A medical condition having unpredictable episodic events is noted in a medical history. |

H00-H59 DISEASES OF THE EYE

Issue	LOC	Sources	Affil	Rationale/Comment
Chronic diseases affecting vision including: Cataracts Diabetic retinopathy Field cuts Glaucoma Low visual acuity—even after correction Macular degeneration Retinitis pigmentosa	Red flag	AMA/NHTSA, 2003[1]	Org	Chronic medical conditions as noted in a medical history suggest a need for formal assessment to determine their impact on functional level.

H60-H95 DISEASES OF THE EAR AND MASTOID PROCESS

Issue	LOC	Sources	Affil	Rationale/Comment
Vertigo	Red flag	AMA/NHTSA, 2003[1]	Org	An acute event can impair driving; counsel patient about driving restriction, assessment, and rehabilitation prior to discharge from ED or hospital.

I00-I99 DISEASES OF THE CIRCULATORY SYSTEM

Issue	LOC	Sources	Affil	Rationale/Comment
Angina **Cardiovascular conditions (chronic), especially when related to cognitive deficits, syncope, or presyncope, including:** Arrhythmias Congestive heart failure Coronary syndrome (unstable) Hypertrophic obstructive cardiomyopathy Valvular disease	Red flag	AMA/NHTSA, 2003[1]	Org	During an acute event, counsel not to drive. A medical condition having unpredictable episodic events is noted in the medical history. Chronic medical conditions as noted in a medical history suggest a need for formal assessment to determine their impact on functional level, especially if these conditions are associated with cognitive deficits, presyncope, or syncope.

Myocardial infarction—acute	An acute event can impair driving; counsel patient about driving restriction, assessment, and rehabilitation prior to discharge from ED or hospital.
Presyncope	During an acute event, counsel not to drive. A medical condition having unpredictable episodic events is noted in the medical history.
Stroke—acute	An acute event can impair driving; counsel patient about driving restriction, assessment, and rehabilitation prior to discharge from ED or hospital.
Syncope	During an acute event, counsel not to drive. A medical condition having unpredictable episodic events is noted in the medical history. Counsel patient about driving restriction, assessment, and rehabilitation prior to discharge from ED or hospital.
Transient ischemic attack	During an acute event, counsel not to drive. A medical condition having unpredictable episodic events is noted in the medical history.

J00-J99 DISEASES OF THE RESPIRATORY SYSTEM

Issue	LOC	Sources	Affil	Rationale/Comment
Respiratory conditions (chronic) including: Chronic obstructive pulmonary disease Obstructive sleep apnea	Red flag	AMA/NHTSA, 2003[1]	Org	Chronic medical conditions as noted in a medical history suggest a need for formal assessment to determine their impact on functional level.

M00-M99 DISEASES OF THE MUSCULOSKELETAL SYSTEM AND CONNECTIVE TISSUE

Issue	LOC	Sources	Affil	Rationale/Comment
Musculoskeletal conditions (chronic) including: Arthritis Foot abnormalities	Red flag	AMA/NHTSA, 2003[1]	Org	Chronic medical conditions as noted in a medical history suggest a need for formal assessment to determine their impact on functional level.

N00-N99 DISEASES OF THE GENITOURINARY SYSTEM

Issue	LOC	Sources	Affil	Rationale/Comment
Renal failure—chronic	Red flag	AMA/NHTSA, 2003[1]	Org	Chronic medical conditions as noted in a medical history suggest a need for formal assessment to determine their impact on functional level.

S00-T98 INJURY, POISONING, AND CERTAIN OTHER CONSEQUENCES OF EXTERNAL CAUSES

Issue	LOC	Sources	Affil	Rationale/Comment
Medications	Red flag	AMA/NHTSA, 2003[1]	Org	Medication with strong potential of affecting driving performance.
Anticholinergics				
Anticonvulsants				
Antidepressants				
Antiemetics				
Antihistamines				
Antihypertensives				
Antiparkinsonians				
Antipsychotics				
Benzodiazepines				
Other sedatives; anxiolytics				
Muscle relaxants				
Narcotic analgesics				
Stimulants				
Surgery[a]	Red flag			An acute event can impair driving; counsel patient about driving restriction, assessment, and rehabilitation prior to discharge from ED or hospital.
Traumatic brain injury	Red flag			An acute event can impair driving; counsel patient about driving restriction, assessment, and rehabilitation prior to discharge from ED or hospital.

a, For driving restrictions following some orthopedic surgeries, additional factors such as steering (i.e., power) and transmission type (automatic or manual) are considered.[1]

R00-R99 SYMPTOMS, SIGNS

Issue	LOC	Sources	Affil	Rationale/Comment
Review of Systems	Red flag	AMA/NHTSA, 2003[1]	Org	Symptom condition in which driving safety should be addressed because it may impair driving performance.
Fatigue—general				
Weakness				
Headaches (HEENT)				
Vertigo				
Visual changes				
Head trauma				
Muscle weakness—musculoskeletal				
Muscle pain				
Joint stiffness/pain				
Reduced range of motion				
Shortness of breath—respiratory				
Chest pain				
Dyspnea on exertion				
Palpitations				
Sudden loss of consciousness				
Loss of consciousness—neurologic				
Feeling of faintness				
Seizures				

Weakness/paralysis

Tremors

Loss of sensation

Numbness

Tingling

Depression—psychiatric

Anxiety

Memory loss

Confusion

Psychosis

Mania

PROCEDURAL CONCERNS

Issue	LOC	Sources	Affil	Rationale/Comment
Concern: patient or family member expresses a driving safety concern	Red flag	AMA/NHTSA, 2003[1]	Org	Symptoms condition in which driving safety should be addressed because it may impair driving performance.
Licensing authority	Advice	Kakaiya, 2000[3]	MD/PT	The licensing authority makes the ultimate decision.
Medical compliance—excellent	Recommendation	Tan, 1998[4]	MD/PT	Patients should be compliant with medication and be aware of side effects.

Continued

Issue	LOC	Sources	Affil	Rationale/Comment
On-road tests "The on-road test is the ultimate evaluation of driving safety"	Advice	Kakaiya, 2000[3]	MD	
Physician role is advisory but can be influential	Advice			There may also be a legal reporting requirement in your state. Contact state's department of motor vehicles. Contact state attorney general's office. Go to www.carbuyingtips.com/driver-licenses.htm Go to www.povertylaw.org/links/statlink.htm Ask: What are state requirements for drivers with medical conditions? What are legal reporting requirements of physicians?
Under regular care of a physician	Recommendation	Tan, 1998[4]	MD/PT	The patient should be cared for on a regular basis by a physician.

DANGER SIGNS OF UNSAFE DRIVING

Issue	LOC	Source	Affil
Inappropriate driving speed—too fast/too slow	Danger signs	ADRS[5]	Org
		AA[6]	Org
Need instructions/help from passengers		ADRS[5]	Org
Does not observe signs or signals		ADRS[5]	Org
Stopping when there is no sign		AA[6]	Org
		AGS[7]	Org

Slow or poor decisions—i.e., judging distance	ADRS[5]	Org
	AA[6]	Org
Easily frustrated or confused	ADRS[5]	Org
	AA[6]	Org
Pattern of getting lost—even in familiar areas	ADRS[5]	Org
	AGS[7]	Org
	AA[6]	Org
Accidents or near misses	ADRS[5]	Org
	AGS[7,a]	Org
Drifting into other lanes of traffic	ADRS[5]	Org
Stopping at green light	AGS[7]	Org
Stopping in the middle of an intersection		
Confusing the gas pedal for the brake pedal		
Running red lights and stop signs without realizing it		
Moving into another lane without looking		

a, Without realizing it.
Abbreviations: ADRS, Association for Driver Rehabilitation Specialists; AGS, American Geriatric Society; AA, Alzheimer's Association.

TIPS ON PREVENTING A PERSON WITH ALZHEIMER'S FROM DRIVING

Tip	Source	Affil
Ask a doctor to write a "do not drive" prescription	AA[6]	Org
Control access to car keys		
Disable the car by removing the battery or distributor cap		
Park the car in a neighbor's driveway or on another block		
Substitute a license with a photo ID and make car inaccessible		

REFERENCES

1. American Medical Association: Physician's guide to assessing and counseling older drivers [2003]. Available at: http://www.ama-assn.org/ama/pub/category/10791.html. Accessed November 7, 2005.

2. American Medical Association: Why are older drivers at risk? Available at: http://www.ama-assn.org/ama/pub/category/9115.html. Accessed November 7, 2005.

3. Kakaiya R, Tisovec R, Fulkerson P: Evaluation of fitness to drive: The physician's role in assessing elderly or demented patients. Postgrad Med 107(3):229-236, 2000.

4. Tan JC: Practical manual of physical medicine and rehabilitation: diagnostics, therapeutics, and basic problems. St Louis: Mosby; 1998.

5. Association for Driver Rehabilitation Specialists: Home page. Available at: http://www.driver-ed.org. Accessed November 7, 2005.

6. Alzheimer's Association (AA): Home page. Available at http://search.alz.org/. Accessed November 7, 2005.

7. American Geriatric Society: The patient education forum: safe driving for seniors. Available at: http://www.americangeriatrics.org. Accessed November 7, 2005.

21 MANUAL LYMPHATIC DRAINAGE

OVERVIEW. Manual lymphatic drainage (MLD) is a gentle manual technique that involves mild, *suprafacially* applied mechanical stretches of the lymphatic collectors' walls to enhance activity in intact lymph vessels, improve lymph circulation, and treat lymphedema.[1,2] MLD is viewed as one component in a comprehensive approach to address lymphedema.[1] It is important to note that MDL does not involve kneading—it is not viewed as massage.[3]

SUMMARY: CONTRAINDICATIONS AND PRECAUTIONS. Three sources cite a total of 29 concerns for MLD. The greatest proportion of concerns is contained under the procedural category (almost 30%) and they relate to force level and correct technique.

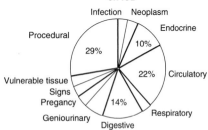

Proportion of Concerns for MLD Based on ICD

Other prominent categories where MLD presents a concern are patients with circulatory, digestive, and endocrine problems. These latter concerns are generally local and depend on *where* the technique is applied (e.g., the neck area in carotid sinus hypersensitivity or thyroid conditions).

CONTRAINDICATIONS AND PRECAUTIONS

A00-B99 CERTAIN INFECTIONS AND PARASITIC DISEASES

Issue	LOC	Sources	Affil	Rationale/Comment
Infection	CI	Benjamin and Tappan, 2005[2]	LMT	

Abbreviation: LMT, licensed massage therapist.

C00-C97 NEOPLASMS

Issue	LOC	Sources	Affil	Rationale/Comment
Malignant tumors	CI	Benjamin and Tappan, 2005[2]	LMT	

E00-E90 ENDOCRINE, NUTRITIONAL, AND METABOLIC DISEASES

Issue	LOC	Sources	Affil	Rationale/Comment
Diabetes	CI	Kelly, 2002[4]	PT	**For abdominal treatment:** Caution because some blood vessels become sclerotic.
Hyperthyroidism	CI	Kelly, 2002[4]	PT	**For neck treatments[4]:** The condition may be aggravated with increased circulating fluid.[2] Notes:
	Caution	Benjamin and Tappan, 2005[2]	LMT	Perhaps this endocrine concern is also related to stroking or stimulating the diseased thyroid
Hypothyroidism	CI	Kelly, 2002[4]	PT	(see **Tachi, 1990,** under **Massage[5]**). Hyperthyroidism (also thyrotoxicosis) is a condition with
	Caution	Benjamin and Tappan, 2005[2]	LMT	excessive thyroid hormone secretion that elevates metabolism in most systems, resulting in heat
				intolerance and sensitivity to light, and increases sympathetic activity, with increased risk of atrial
				fibrillations, congestive heart failure, and MI. Hypothyroidism is a deficiency of thyroid hormone
				characterized by slowed metabolism, fatigue, mild sensitivity to cold, and fluid retention.[6]

I00-I99 DISEASES OF THE CIRCULATORY SYSTEM

Issue	LOC	Sources	Affil	Rationale/Comment
Aneurysm—aortic (or suspected)	CI	Kelly, 2002[4]	PT	**For abdominal treatment[4]:** Note: an aneurysm is an abnormal dilation of a vessel with a diameter greater or equal to 50% of normal, resulting in a permanent sac-like structure. A thoracic aortic aneurysm can rupture under the force of elevated blood pressure.[7]
Cardiac arrhythmia	CI	Kelly, 2002[4]	PT	**For neck treatments[4]:** Stimulating stretch receptors in neck may lead to an arrhythmia[4] **(see Carotid sinus hypersensitivity).**

Continued

Issue	LOC	Sources	Affil	Rationale/Comment
Cardiac problems, major	CI	Benjamin and Tappan, 2005[2]	LMT	
Carotid sinus hypersensitivity	CI	Kelly, 2002[4]	PT	**For neck treatments[4]:** The neck region has stretch receptors that respond to longitudinal massage and static pressure on the carotid artery and can result in cardioinhibition (ventricular asystole), vasodepression (reduced SBP of at least 50 mm Hg), or both. Individuals with carotid sinus hypersensitivity may experience syncope.[8]
Deep vein thrombosis	CI	Kelly, 2002[4]	PT	**For lower extremity treatment[4]:** Avoid deep strokes. Practice patterns vary from waiting 2 weeks to 6 months for symptom resolution before beginning MDL. Check with physician.[4]
	CI	Benjamin and Tappan, 2005[2,b]	LMT	
Phlebitis or thrombophlebitis	CI	Kelly, 2002[4]	PT	**For lower extremity treatment.[4]**
	CI	Benjamin and Tappan, 2005[2,a]	LMT	

a, Phlebitis; b, Thrombosis.

J00-J99 DISEASES OF THE RESPIRATORY SYSTEM

Issue	LOC	Sources	Affil	Rationale/Comment
Asthma	Caution	Benjamin and Tappan, 2005[2]	LMT	

K00-K93 DISEASES OF THE DIGESTIVE SYSTEM

Issue	LOC	Sources	Affil	Rationale/Comment
Abdominal pain—undiagnosed	CI	Kelly, 2002[4]	PT	
Abdominal surgery—recent	CI			**For abdominal treatment[4]:** Check with physician.
Crohn's disease	CI			**For abdominal treatment[4]:** Note: Crohn's disease is an inflammatory bowel disease affecting any segment and all layers of the intestinal tract. The patient may present with long-term steroid effects as well as osteoporosis.[9]
Diverticulitis	CI			**For abdominal treatment.**

N00-N99 DISEASES OF THE GENITOURINARY SYSTEM

Issue	LOC	Sources	Affil	Rationale/Comment
Kidney conditions	Caution	Benjamin and Tappan, 2005[2]	LMT	The condition may be aggravated with increased circulating fluid.[2]
Menstrual period	RCI	Kelly, 2002[4]	PT	**For abdominal treatment[4]:** The condition may be aggravated by increased circulation of fluid.[2] Note: obviously not a disease.
	Caution	Benjamin and Tappan, 2005[2]	LMT	

O00-O99 PREGNANCY, CHILDBIRTH, AND PUERPERIUM

Issue	LOC	Sources	Affil	Rationale/Comment
Pregnancy	CI	Kelly, 2002[4]	PT	**For abdominal treatment.**

R00-R99 SYMPTOMS, SIGNS

Issue	LOC	Sources	Affil	Rationale/Comment
Chronic inflammation, fibrosis—due to radiation therapy	CI	Kelly, 2002[4]		**For abdominal treatment[4]:** This is an abdominal region complication of radiation therapy.

VULNERABLE BIOLOGICAL TISSUE

Issue	LOC	Sources	Affil	Rationale/Comment
Upper arm, inner area— don't massage	Advice	MacDonald, 2001[10]	Bodywork	Do not use deep pressure that causes skin to redden and don't massage the inside of the upper arm in patients with breast cancer who are at risk for lymphedema.[9]

Issue	LOC	Sources	Affil	Rationale/Comment
Age	CI	Kelly, 2002[4]	PT	**For neck treatments[4]:** Arteries and veins often become sclerotic with age (i.e., over age 60 years).
Chemotherapy, receiving	Caution	Benjamin and Tappan, 2005[2]	LMT	The condition may be aggravated with increased fluid circulation.[2]
Circulation—if condition worsens with increased circulation	Caution	Benjamin and Tappan, 2005[2]	LMT	Note: See kidney, thyroid, menstruation, asthma, and chemotherapy.
Force level of manual lymph massage	P Advice	Foldi, 1995[3,a] MacDonald, 2001[10]	MD Bodywork	Description of force level: "extremely gentle manner so as to increase lymphangiocontractile activity by smoothly stretching the wall of the lymphangions and later to push out edema fluid into unaffected lymphatics where it can be reabsorbed. A premature sudden increase of the lymphatic load in these watersheds with preparation should be avoided; it can cause an iatrogenic dynamic insufficiency with trapped edema."[1] MacDonald suggests that deep pressure that causes skin to redden should not be used.[9] **In a 1995 animal study, Eliska[11] showed that forceful massage with external pressure using two fingers in the direction of lymph flow (70–100 mm Hg) resulted in lymphatic damage after 10 minutes in dogs.**
Stroke away from the heart	Advice (Don'ts)	MacDonald, 2001[10]	Bodywork	Don't stroke away from the heart or backwards.

Continued

Issue	LOC	Sources	Affil	Rationale/Comment
Moving fluid directly into areas with nodal involvement	Advice (Don'ts)			Finish UE work at the upper trapezius area rather than clavicle. The clavicle area is often the treatment field for breast cancer patients and may be scarred.[10]
Exaggerated stretches or twists	Advice (Don'ts)			
Position the affected limb hanging off the table	Advice (Don'ts)			

a, Foldi's one concern is not included in descriptive statistics.

ADVERSE EVENTS

Source	Background	Therapy	Outcome	Follow-up/Interpretation
Eliska and Eliskova, 1995[11] **Forceful massage** Pretest Post test Lymphology	Subjects included dogs with experimental lymphedema, men without edema, and men with post-thrombotic venous edema.	Forceful massage with external pressure using two fingers in the direction of lymph flow (70–100 mm Hg) applied for 1, 5, and 10 minutes at 25 strokes/min to the hind paw of dogs and the feet of men. Evaluated with electron microscopy.	After 10 minutes, lymphatic damage noted with fewer changes noted in healthy men. First affected endothelial lining and later lymphatic collectors were altered. Also loosening of subcutaneous connective tissue and release of lipid droplets into lymphatics in lymphedema.	

MacDonald, 2001[10] **Lymphedema following massage** Anecdote/case series	1. A woman s/p breast cancer treatment returned to massage therapist for previous regimen that she had been doing for years. The following morning, the arm swelled, requiring months of MLD by a trained practitioner to reverse.
	2. A patient with a history of cancer and lymphedema was experiencing slight fullness in affected arm (sign of early-stage lymphedema); a body worker massaged gently but the patient asked for deeper pressure on the back of the affected side. The therapist pulled the patient's arm behind the back to access scapular muscles. The following day, lymphedema returned.
	3. A woman treated for breast cancer and several episodes of swelling (hand mostly) received a massage at a well-known resort. The therapist was careful with the arm but massaged her back on the affected side deeply. That night, the client did not feel well; her hand and abdomen became swollen.

REFERENCES

1. Lasinski B: The lymphatic system. In: Goodman CC, Boissonnault WG, Fuller KS, eds: Pathology: implications for the physical therapist, ed 2. Philadelphia: Saunders; 2003.
2. Benjamin PJ, Tappan FM: Handbook of healing massage techniques: classic, holistic, and emerging methods, ed 4. Upper Saddle River (NJ): Pearson Prentice Hall; 2005.
3. Foldi M: Massage and damage to lymphatics [editorial]. Lymphology 28:1-3, 1995.
4. Kelly DG: A primer on lymphedema. Upper Saddle River (NJ): Pearson Prentice Hall; 2002.
5. Tachi J, Amino N, Nyaik K, et al: Massage therapy on neck: a contributing factor for destructive thyrotoxicosis. Thyrology 2(1):25-27, 1990.
6. Goodman CC, Snyder TEK: The endocrine and metabolic systems. In: Goodman CC, Boissonnault WG, Fuller KS, eds: Pathology: implications for the physical therapist, ed 2. Philadelphia: Saunders; 2003.
7. Goodman CC: The cardiovascular system. In: Goodman CC, Boissonnault WG, Fuller KS, eds: Pathology: implications for the physical therapist, ed 2. Philadelphia: Saunders; 2003.
8. Strasberg B, Sagie A, Erdman S, et al: Carotid sinus hypersensitivity and the carotid sinus syndrome. Prog Cardiovasc Dis 31(5):379-391, 1989.

9. Goodman CC: The gastrointestinal system. In: Goodman CC, Boissonnault WG, Fuller KS, eds: Pathology: implications for the physical therapist, ed 2. Philadelphia: Saunders; 2003.

10. MacDonald G: Cancer, radiation, and massage: the benefits and cautions. Massage Bodywork 16(4):7,12,16, 2001.

11. Eliska O, Eliskova M: Are peripheral lymphatics damaged by high pressure manual massage? Lymphology 28(1):1-3, 1995.

22   CONNECTIVE TISSUE MASSAGE (BINDEGEWEBSMASSAGE)

OVERVIEW. Connective tissue massage (CTM, also called Bindegewebsmassage) is a deep massage technique of the fascia or connective tissue aimed at enhancing blood supply by affecting autonomic nervous system (ANS) activity. The technique attempts to affect ANS activity by targeting organs with associated dermatomal innervations.[1,2]

SUMMARY: CONTRAINDICATIONS AND PRECAUTIONS. Four sources cited a total of 15 concerns for CTM. Concerns ranged from two to six per source, with a physical therapist citing the largest number. The largest proportion of concerns, cited by one source, were procedural (almost 40%) and related to undesirable autonomic responses attributed to excessive treatment.[3] The most frequently cited concerns were the treatment of patients with TB and cancer (cited by two sources). Mental illness was also mentioned as a concern by two sources.

Note: Older guidelines from Dick's manual of reflexive therapy viewed all mental illness and virulent tumors as strict contraindications for CTM. In a subsequent 1978 edition, the staging of illness had become an important consideration in selecting patients for CTM. More advanced stages or less acute forms of disease were being considered for CTM.[4]

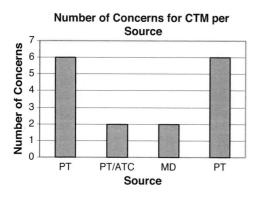

Number of Concerns for CTM per Source

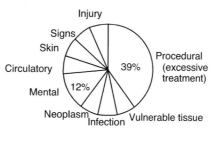

Proportion of CTM Concerns Based on ICD

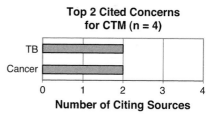

Top 2 Cited Concerns for CTM (n = 4)

A00-B99 CERTAIN INFECTIONS AND PARASITIC DISEASES

Issue	LOC	Source	Affil	Rationale/Comment
Tuberculosis	CI	De Domenico and Wood, 1997[2]	PT	No rationale provided.
	CI	Prentice and Lehn, 2002[5]	PT/ATC	

C00-C97 NEOPLASMS

Issue	LOC	Source	Affil	Rationale/Comment
Cancer	CI	De Domenico and Wood, 1997[2]	PT	
	CI	Prentice and Lehn, 2002[5,a]	PT/ATC	

a, Tumors.

F00-F99 MENTAL AND BEHAVIORAL DISORDERS

Issue	LOC	Source	Affil	Rationale/Comment
Acute psychosis	Inappropriate	Schliack, 1978[4]	MD	
Mental illness	CI	Prentice and Lehn, 2002[5]	PT/ATC	Psychological dependence.

I00-I99 DISEASES OF THE CIRCULATORY SYSTEM

Issue	LOC	Source	Affil	Rationale/Comment
Cardiac conditions—some	CI	De Domenico and Wood, 1997[2]	PT	Unspecified conditions.

L00-L99 DISEASES OF THE SKIN AND SUBCUTANEOUS

Issue	LOC	Source	Affil	Rationale/Comment
Skin conditions—of the back	CI	De Domenico and Wood, 1997[2]	PT	Generalized skin conditions of back (i.e., psoriasis).

R00-R99 SYMPTOMS, SIGNS

Issue	LOC	Source	Affil	Rationale/Comment
Acute illness—catastrophic	Inappropriate	Schliack, 1978[4]	MD	Examples include acute MI, acute pneumonia, acute fit, acute sciatica, or acute Sudeck's atrophy.

S00-T98 INJURY, POISONING, AND CERTAIN OTHER CONSEQUENCES OF EXTERNAL CAUSES

Issue	LOC	Source	Affil	Rationale/Comment
Wound—open	CI	De Domenico and Wood, 1997[2]	PT	Open wounds, sores, or lesions over area of treatment.

VULNERABLE BIOLOGICAL TISSUE

Issue	LOC	Source	Affil	Rationale/Comment
Hair	CI	De Domenico and Wood, 1997[2]	PT	CTM may be irritating and cause pain in persons with very hairy skin on their backs.

PROCEDURAL CONCERNS

Excessive Technique Leading to Undesirable Responses

Issue	LOC	Source	Affil	Rationale/Comment
ANS—labile (very)	Danger signs	Ebner, 1985[3]	PT	These patients can experience serious disturbance such as palpitations, a sense of general collapse, and headaches. Have the patient lie down immediately.[3] Note: As a general matter, other sources caution the clinician not to have the patient lie down if the problem is autonomic dysreflexia because of the associated high blood pressure (**see Autonomic dysreflexia).**
Headaches and nausea	Danger signs			When treating the shoulder and neck regions, you may activate the vagal reflex, which can lead to headaches and nausea. Apply strokes on anterior regions (forehead, upper clavicle) for relief.
Hypotension	Danger signs			Treatment may result in extensive vasodilation in some sensitive individuals with low blood pressure.

Painful stroking	Avoid	Circulatory disturbances may result from painful stroking because pain can lead to vasoconstriction (a sympathetic, defensive response), which counteracts the goals of treatment. Note: Strokes applied to healthy tissue are normally described as very slight scratching or cutting sensations (not painful).
Palpitations/dyspnea	Danger signs/Avoid	Palpitations or dyspnea symptoms may occur when treating dermatomes of the back (i.e., when applying short strokes to sides of thoracic spine that are associated with preganglion fibers). Intersperse stokes on anterior chest and subcostal area that are associated with postganglion fibers.
Transference of tension	Danger signs	E.g., treating the back will sometimes lead to sudden tension increased on the anterior body portion of the body. Treat the anterior body part to relieve this tension.

REFERENCES

1. Geiringer SR, Kincaid CB, Rechtien JJ: Traction, manipulation, and massage. In: Delisa JA, editor: Rehabilitation medicine: principles and practices. Philadelphia: J.B. Lippincott; 1988.
2. De Domenico G, Wood EC: Beard's massage, ed 4. Philadelphia: W.B. Saunders, 1997.
3. Ebner M: Connective tissue manipulations: Theory and therapeutic application. Malabar (FL): Krieger; 1985.
4. Schliack H: General indications, contraindications, and prescription. In: Dick E, Schliack H, Wolff A, eds: A manual of reflexive therapy of the connective tissue, "Bindegewebsmassage." Scarsdale (NY): Sidney Simon; 1978.
5. Prentice WE, Lehn C: Therapeutic massage. In Prentice WE, editor: Therapeutic modalities for physical therapist. New York: McGraw-Hill; 2002.

23 THERAPEUTIC MASSAGE (INCLUDES WESTERN TECHNIQUES, SWEDISH, CLASSIC; EXCLUDES EASTERN TECHNIQUE, SHIATSU)

OVERVIEW. Therapeutic massage (also called Western, Swedish, or classic) is a "hands-on," rhythmical application of pressure and stretching-type soft tissue stimulation that has been used to relieve pain, reduce edema, break up adhesions, stretch fascia, stretch skin scars, decrease muscle tightness and spasm, and increase sedation (relaxation).[1]

TYPES OF MASSAGE. Massage comprises both Western and Eastern techniques: Western massage includes classic (therapeutic) massage of effleurage, kneading, tapotement, friction, deep friction massage, connective tissue massage, and soft tissue mobilization. Rolfing involves very deep soft tissue massage. Urut is a regional practice involving abdominal massage. Mechanical devices can also administer massage (see vibratory device). Eastern approaches include Shiatsu, acupressure, and reflexology. These finger pressure techniques subscribe to a theoretical framework (e.g., Chi, energy) foreign to Western thinking and will be covered elsewhere (see Shiatsu). The present section will largely address therapeutic (Western) massage concerns.

Therapeutic massage's actions are mechanical (physiologic, reflexive) and psychological in nature.[1] Note: Because massage mobilizes fluid and exerts force on soft tissue, the potential exists for irritating skin, spreading infection, dislodging clots and malignancies, and causing compression-type injuries to pressure-sensitive tissues such as superficial nerves.

SUMMARY: CONTRAINDICATIONS AND PRECAUTIONS. Nine sources expressed a total of 67 therapeutic massage concerns that ranged from 3 to 42 per source, with a licensed massage therapist (LMT) source noting the most concerns. The largest proportion of concerns were contained under vulnerable tissues (endangerment sites such as the neck), circulatory, skin, musculoskeletal, and injury categories. Massaging over malignancies, DVTs, and infected tissue or in patients with bleeding/anticoagulation, compromised cardiac systems, or fragile skin were the seven most frequently cited concerns. More than one source cited ACIs.

Note: De Domenico and Wood[1] used the term *usually contraindicated (UCI)* to classify some concerns.

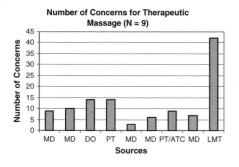

Number of Concerns for Therapeutic Massage (N = 9)

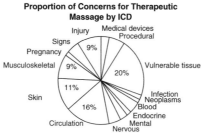

Proportion of Concerns for Therapeutic Massage by ICD

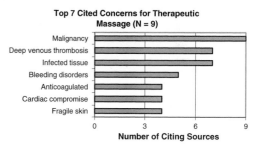

Top 7 Cited Concerns for Therapeutic Massage (N = 9)

CONTRAINDICATIONS AND PRECAUTIONS

A00-B99 CERTAIN INFECTIONS AND PARASITIC DISEASES

Issue	LOC	Source	Affil	Rationale/Comment
Infected tissue	CI	Geiringer and deLateur, 1990[2]	MD	Massage can break down barriers, allowing infections to spread. Stretching fibrous connective tissue may interrupt encapsulated infection. Enhancing lymphatic flow may also increase the rate of infectious agents carried throughout the body.[3]
	ACI	Braverman and Schulman, 1999[3,a]	MD	
	UCI	De Domenico and Wood, 1997[1]	PT	
	ACI	Wieting et al, 2005[4]	DO	
	CI	Knapp, 1968[5]	MD	

a, Active bacterial, viral or fungal infection, cellulitis lymphagitis, impetigo herpes simplex, tinea pedis, abscess, systematic febrile illness. Note: also see Skin Infection and Signs and Symptoms.

C00-C99 NEOPLASMS

Issue	LOC	Source	Affil	Rationale/Comment
Malignancy—over	CI	Geiringer and deLateur, 1990[2]	MD	Enhanced circulation may increase metabolic rate and lead to increase tumor growth
	RCI	Braverman and Schulman,1999[3]	MD	and metastases.[b] Note: Terminally ill patients may derive pain relief from massage.
	CI	Cotter et al, 2000[6]	MD	Exercise caution in patients with bony metastases that may be prone to fracture.[7]
	CI	Knapp, 1968[5]	MD	Also concern for spreading the condition.[4,9]
	UCI	De Domenico and Wood, 1997[1]	PT	
	Avoid	Weiger et al, 2002[7]	MD	
	CI	Prentice and Lehn, 2002[8]	PT/ATC	
	ACI	Wieting et al, 2005[4]	DO	
	CI/caution	Benjamin and Tappan, 2005[9,a]	LMT	

a, Malignant melanoma.

D50-D89 DISEASES OF BLOOD AND BLOOD FORMING ORGANS AND CERTAIN DISORDERS

Issue	LOC	Source	Affil	Rationale/Comment
Anticoagulant therapy	CI	Geiringer and deLateur, 1990[2]	MD	Avoid high-pressure massage techniques for drugs that affect clotting.[9]
	Caution	Weiger et al, 2002[7]	MD	
	RCI	Wieting et al, 2005[4]	DO	
	CI/caution	Benjamin and Tappan, 2005[9,b]	LMT	

Bleeding, bleeding disorders, blood vessel damage	ACI	Braverman and Schulman, 1999[3]	MD	Pressure may encourage the development of hematomas.
	CI	Cotter et al, 2000[6]	MD	(E.g., ecchymoses, petechiae, hemophilia.) Weiger cautions practitioners to avoid deep abdominal massage in hypocoagulable patients (i.e., thrombocytopenia).[4]
	Caution	Weiger et al, 2002[7]	MD	
	RCI	Wieting et al, 2005[4]	DO	
	CI/caution	Benjamin and Tappan, 2005[9,a]	LMT	
Compromised immune systems	CI/caution	Benjamin and Tappan, 2005[9]	LMT	For the patient's protection, exercise adequate hygiene in persons with depressed immunity (i.e., in persons with organ transplants, AIDS, chronic fatigue syndrome, or those taking immune-suppressing medications).[9]

a, Also bruising; b, Also aspirin.

E00-E90 ENDOCRINE, NUTRITIONAL AND METABOLIC DISEASES

Issue	LOC	Source	Affil	Rationale/Comment
Compromised nutritional status—of skin	P/Avoid	Kessler and Hertling, 1996[10]	MD	For friction massage.

F00-F99 MENTAL AND BEHAVIORAL DISORDERS

Issue	LOC	Source	Affil	Rationale/Comment
Chronic pain	Caution	Wieting et al, 2005[4]	DO	This issue is of patient dependency. Consider establishing an "end point" for treatment.[4]
Medications/alcohol/ recreational drugs	CI/caution	Benjamin and Tappan, 2005[9]	LMT	Medications/alcohol/recreational drugs are a concern if they alter judgment, mood, or sensation, or mask pain that can alter patient feedback and the ability to communicate.[9]

G00-G99 DISEASES OF THE NERVOUS SYSTEM

Issue	LOC	Source	Affil	Rationale/Comment
Hyperesthesia	CI	De Domenico and Wood, 1997[1]	PT	For shaking/vibration and tapotement/percussion.[1] The patient who is ticklish may respond to deeper pressure.[9]
	CI/caution	Benjamin and Tappan, 2005[9]	LMT	
Sensation, decreased	CI/caution	Benjamin and Tappan, 2005[9]	LMT	Exercise care with amount of pressure provided. The patient may not be capable of providing feedback on pressure tolerance and present with abnormal vasomotor responses.[9]
Spasticity	CI	De Domenico and Wood, 1997[1]	PT	For shaking/vibration and tapotement/percussion techniques. Stimulation may increase spasticity or increase discomfort.[1]

Issue	LOC	Source	Affil	Rationale/Comment
Arrhythmia or carotid bruit	CI/caution	Benjamin and Tappan, 2005[9]	LMT	Avoid the neck (anterior or lateral portion).[9]
Arteriosclerosis	CI	Prentice and Lehn, 2002[8]	PT/ATC	Concern for spreading the condition (i.e., plaque).[4]
	ACI	Wieting et al, 2005[4]	DO	
	CI/P	Benjamin and Tappan, 2005[9,b]	LMT	
Cardiac disease—	RCI	Braverman and Schulman,1999[3]	MD	Massage can increase intravascular volume and venous return, and challenge/stress
compromised	CI	Cotter et al, 2000[6]	MD	the heart.[3] Edema (fluid off-loaded into the periphery) in the legs is a means by which the cardiovascular system reduces load on the impaired heart. Also, percussion techniques may aggravate the condition.[1]
	CI	De Domenico and Wood, 1997[1]	PT	Be aware of the effect of medications on the patient.[9]
	CI/caution	Benjamin and Tappan, 2005[9,d]	LMT	
Lymphangitis	CI/caution	Benjamin and Tappan, 2005[9]	LMT	Lymphatics are inflamed and appear red on the skin. Massage could spread the "blood poisoning" through the circulation.[9]
Thrombophlebitis	CI	Geiringer and deLateur, 1990[2]	MD	Mechanical stimulation of vessels and enhanced circulation may both cause
DVT	ACI	Braverman and Schulman,1999[3]	MD	a thrombus to detach and become an embolism. Also, for shaking/vibration
	CI	Knapp, 1968[5]	MD	and tapotement/percussion techniques, coronary thrombosis is a CI because
	CI	Cotter et al, 2000[6]	MD	the shaking/vibration may aggravate the condition. **In a case report,**
	CI	De Domenico and Wood, 1997[1]	PT	**Mikhail et al[11] (1997) describe a 59-year-old male smoker with an**

Continued

Issue	LOC	Source	Affil	Rationale/Comment
	CI	Prentice and Lehn, 2002[8,a]	PT/ATC	**aorto-bifemoral bypass graft who threw an embolus to his left kidney**
	ACI	Wieting et al, 2005[4]	DO	**following wife's back massage (walking on his back).**
Hypertension—severe	CI	De Domenico and Wood, 1997[1]	PT	For shaking/vibration and tapotement/percussion techniques, massage may
	CI/caution	Benjamin and Tappan, 2005[9]	LMT	increase blood pressure.[1]
Hypotension	CI/caution	Benjamin and Tappan, 2005[9]	LMT	Patients may be susceptible to fainting following massage.
				Get up slowly. **In 2000, Palmer[12] recounted a story of a caller on a radio who described a client in the gym who received a massage in a sitting position, fainted, and was caught just before she collapsed to the floor.**
Pulmonary embolism—	CI	De Domenico and Wood, 1997[1]	PT	For shaking/vibration techniques, massage may aggravate the condition.
acute	CI	Prentice and Lehn, 2002[8]	PT/ATC	
Stroke	CI/caution	Benjamin and Tappan, 2005[9]	LMT	Avoid neck area. Caution with pressure-related technique if patient takes blood thinners.[9]
Varicose veins	CI	Cotter et al, 2000[6]	MD	Massage may produce local damage to vessel or free an embolus.
	P	De Domenico and Wood, 1997[1]	PT	
	CI	Prentice and Lehn, 2002[8,b]	PT/ATC	
	CI/caution	Benjamin and Tappan, 2005[9,c]	LMT	
Vascular response— impaired	P/Avoid	Kessler and Hertling, 1996[10]	MD	For friction massage, in patients with long-term high-dose steroid drug therapy or known peripheral vascular disease, the weakened tissue may not tolerate localized pressure.

a, Thrombosis; b, Severe; c, Atherosclerotic plaque; d, Cardiovascular disorder (general), did not specify compromised system.

Issue	LOC	Source	Affil	Rationale/Comment
Allergies to oils/lotions	CI/caution	Benjamin and Tappan, 2005[9,a]	LMT	Take a history of allergies to oils; watch for any skin reactions.
Cellulitis	CI	Prentice and Lehn, 2002[8]	PT/ATC	
Scar—new	CI	De Domenico and Wood, 1997[1]	PT	For tapotement/percussion, the technique may stimulate the overproduction
	RCI	Wieting et al, 2005[4,b]	DO	of scar tissue.[1]
Skin—fragile	CI	Geiringer and deLateur, 1990[2a]	MD	Braverman suggests using light pressure and a suitable medium to reduce friction.
	RCI	Braverman and Schulman,1999[3]	MD	Collagenous weakness may exist particularly in long-term steroid use, skin grafts,
	RCI	Wieting et al, 2005[4,c]	DO	partially healed scars, diabetes.[3] Also avoid deep pressure, forceful stretching,
	CI/caution	Benjamin and Tappan, 2005[9,d]	LMT	wringing, skin rolling if patient is taking medications such as corticosteroids that
				may compromise skin integrity.
Skin—graft	RCI	Wieting et al, 2005[4]	DO	
Skin—infection	CI	Prentice and Lehn, 2002[8]	PT/ATC	See Infections (also abscess concern: a collection of pus buried within a tissue).[8]
	CI/caution	Benjamin and Tappan, 2005[9]	LMT	Don't touch contagious skin ailments such as herpes simplex, impetigo, athlete's
				foot, and rashes that may spread from massage.[9]
Skin, inflamed—acute	CI	Geiringer and deLateur, 1990[2]	MD	
	ACI	Braverman and Schulman,1999[3]	MD	
Therapies—surgery or radiation	Avoid	Weiger et al, 2002[7]	MD	Surgery or radiation therapy can cause further tissue damage.

a, Grafted, atrophic skin; b, Unhealed; c, Atrophic; d, Compromised skin integrity due to corticosteroid use.

M00-M99 DISEASES OF THE MUSCULOSKELETAL SYSTEM AND CONNECTIVE TISSUE

Issue	LOC	Source	Affil	Rationale/Comment
Calcified tissue	CI	Geiringer and deLateur, 1990[2]	MD	Massage may facilitate the spread of deposits to other areas and lead to myositis ossificans.
	RCI	Wieting et al, 2005[4]	DO	**In a 1988 case report, Antao[13] describes a 23-year-old male soccer player with a game injury who received vigorous massage for 3 months and subsequently developed myositis ossificans.**
				In a case report, Danchik et al[14] describe a 20-year-old male college hockey player who was struck on the lateral right thigh by an opponent's knee, received vigorous massage, and developed a huge amorphous radiopaque mass, which subsequently ossified.
				In a chart review, Mohan[15] noted that 29% of posttraumatic stiff elbows in outpatient departments had radiologic evidence of myositis ossificans, with most of these having a history of massage.
Dermatomyositis	RCI	Braverman and Schulman,1999[3]	MD	Whole body massage may increase serum creatine phosphokinin, lactate dehydrogenase, and myokinase in individuals with dematomyositis.[3]
Fragile ribs	CI	De Domenico and Wood, 1997[1]	PT	For shaking/vibration and tapotement/percussion, the techniques can damage underlying lung tissue (especially ribs with brittle bone, metastatic bone cancer).
Osteoporosis	CI/caution	Benjamin and Tappan, 2005[9,a]	LMT	Avoid deep pressure or vigorous movement in persons with osteoporosis or at high risk because of the fracture concern.
Spinal fusion— recent	CI	De Domenico and Wood, 1997[1]	PT	For shaking/vibration and tapotement/percussion, the techniques can damage underlying lung tissue (especially ribs with brittle bone, metastatic bone cancer).
Synovitis	CI	Prentice and Lehn, 2002[8]	PT/ATC	

O00-O99 PREGNANCY, CHILDBIRTH, AND PUERPERIUM

Issue	LOC	Source	Affil	Rationale/Comment
Abdominal massage—during pregnancy	CI CI	Braverman and Schulman,1999[3] Cotter et al, 2000[6]	MD MD	**In 1971, Thambu[16] reported on a 30-year-old pregnant woman who received abdominal massage (Urut) and subsequently developed severe abdominal pain, shock, a tense abdomen, a ruptured uterus, and a dead fetus.** Also, the supine position may place too much pressure on the patient's descending aorta or vena cava.

R00-R99 SIGNS AND SYMPTOMS

Issue	LOC	Source	Affil	Rationale/Comment
Distress, severe	CI/caution	Benjamin and Tappan, 2005[9]	LMT	These patients can present with fever, severe pain, or a recent injury, or they can look physically ill. Swollen lymph glands (i.e., swollen glands) indicate the body's (immune system's) attempt to remove pathogens. Massage may drain this area and cause further spread of the organism.[9]
Edema, several forms	CI/caution			Edema due to acute trauma, infection, lymphatic blockage (e.g., parasites), deep venous thrombosis, the "general edema" due to cardiac, liver, or kidney disease, and the fragile tissue associated with pitting edema are all CI for massage.[9]
Inflammation—acute	CI RCI CI/caution	Prentice and Lehn, 2002[8] Wieting et al, 2005[4] Benjamin and Tappan, 2005[9,a]	PT/ATC DO LMT	

a, May include phlebitis—avoid; rheumatoid arthritis (avoid traction to joints; caution when not acute); appendicitis—avoid as it may spread infection.

S00-T98 INJURY, POISONING, AND CERTAIN OTHER CONSEQUENCES OF EXTERNAL CAUSES

Issue	LOC	Source	Affil	Rationale/Comment
Burns	CI/caution	Benjamin and Tappan, 2005[9]	LMT	
Foreign bodies—over	CI	De Domenico and Wood, 1997[1]	PT	Rubbing over the area may cause additional damage (massage should not be given). (e.g., embedded glass and dirt.)
Fractured rib;	CI	De Domenico and Wood, 1997[1]	PT	For shaking/vibration and tapotement/percussion, the techniques can damage underlying
Flail chest	CI/caution	Benjamin and Tappan, 2005[9,a]	LMT	lung tissue (especially ribs with brittle bone, metastatic bone cancer).[1]
Surgeries, recent	CI/caution	Benjamin and Tappan, 2005[9]	LMT	The concern is working over the site unless trained in scar management.[9]
Trauma, acute	CI/caution			Avoid massage over an acutely injured area (i.e., whiplash) for the first 24-48 hours.[9]
Wounds—recent; open	CI	Geiringer and deLateur, 1990[2]	MD	Massage may damage delicate cellular and fibrinous networks and possibly delay healing.[3]
	ACI	Braverman and Schulman,1999[3]	MD	
	CI	Cotter et al, 2000[6]	MD	

a, Any fracture.

Y70-Y82 MEDICAL DEVICES

Issue	LOC	Source	Affil	Rationale/Comment
Contact lenses	CI/caution	Benjamin and Tappan, 2005[9,a]	LMT	Avoid lens pressure or dislodging them; remove contacts.[9]
Hearing aid	CI/caution			Take care not to dislodge the device or create annoying noise during massages near the head.[9]
Stent or prosthetic	Avoid	Weiger et al, 2002[7]	MD	Stent displacement is possible.[7] Also, know range of motion restrictions for joint replacements.[9]
device—over	CI/caution	Benjamin and Tappan, 2005[9,a]	LMT	**In a case report, Kerr[17] reports a 51-year-old woman s/p ureteral stent placement who became incontinent to urine when a deep massage (Rolfing) displaced her stent.**

a, Joint replacement.

VULNERABLE BIOLOGICAL TISSUE: ENDANGERMENT SITES

Areas Containing Biological Tissue Susceptible to Damage with Excessive Force; Adjust Pressure Appropriately

Issue	LOC	Source	Affil	Rationale/Comment
Abdomen	Avoid	Weiger et al, 2002[7]	MD	Avoid deep abdominal massage. Associated internal bleeding may occur. **In a case report by Trotter,[18] a 39-year-old woman received a deep body massage of the abdomen and right upper quarter and subsequently developed a hematoma in the right hepatic lobe**.
Abnormal structures	Caution	Benjamin and Tappan, 2005[9]	LMT	Abnormal structures are potential endangerment sites and should be investigated before subjecting to massage.[9] **Kalinga et al[19] describe a 16-year-old schoolboy who developed an pseudoaneurysm from repeated massage over an exostosis on the medial thigh popliteal area**.

Continued

Issue	LOC	Source	Affil	Rationale/Comment
Axilla	Caution			The axilla houses several vulnerable structures, including the axillary artery and vein, cephalic vein, and brachial plexus.[9]
Elbow	Caution			The medial epicondyle region houses the ulnar nerve. The brachia vein and artery, median cubital vein, and medial nerve are located at the anterior fold of the elbow.[9]
Eye	Caution			Avoiding slipping into the eyeball during facial massage; only provide very light pressure on eyelids.[9] **Tang et al[20] reported a 44-year-old man with recurrent sinus congestion who self-administered a powerful AC-powered massaging device over his eyes and developed a traumatic cataract**.
Inguinal area	Caution			The groin area contains the femoral artery and the great saphenous and femoral veins. Exercise great care when working on the iliopsoas muscle.[9]
Kidney	Caution			Only provide very light pressure during percussion techniques.[9]
Neck, anterior	Caution			The anterior triangle of the neck, along with the sternal notch, contains sensitive structures such as the carotid artery, jugular vein, vagus nerve, larynx, and thyroid gland.[9] **In a 1990 case report, Tachi et al. described a 57-year-old woman with prior Hashimoto's thyroiditis who received vigorous massage over her neck, which led to goiter enlargement. The authors believed mechanical manipulation of the thyroid caused thyroid follicle injury and stimulated antigen release and antibody production in autoimmune thyroiditis.** In an unfortunate freakish accident, Deidiker[22] reported a 56-year-old Asian woman who was strangled when her blouse became entangled in an electric roller-type massage device used near her neck area.
Popliteal fossa	Caution			This unprotected area contains the popliteal artery, vein, and tibial nerve.[9]

Thoracic cage	Caution			Over the xyphoid; if it breaks off, it can penetrate the underlying liver; also avoid heavy pressure over the anterior lateral surface in the elderly.[9]
Umbilicus	Caution			The descending aorta and abdominal aorta lie beneath the umbilicus.[9]
Veins (major) of extremities	Caution			Deep effleurage applied improperly can damage vein valves. Always apply this technique in the direction of flow that opens the valves (i.e., distal to proximal, toward the heart).[9]
Vertebral column	Caution		LMT	Avoid thrusting or percussion over the spinous processes.[9]
Bony prominences— over	Avoid	AHCPR, 1992[23]		The recommendation[23] is based on postmortem biopsies that reveal maceration in areas exposed to massage. Following massage around bony prominences, skin blood flow and skin temperature are reduced.

PROCEDURAL CONCERNS

Issue	LOC	Source	Affil	Rationale/Comment
Edema that increases in tissue with massage	RCI	Wieting et al, 2005[4]	DO	Conditions where tissue is susceptible to increased edema accumulation when circulation is promoted is viewed as a RCI.
Scuba diving, recent	CI	Cotter et al, 2000[6]	MD	Following *scuba diving,* Cotter states to delay massage 24 hours because of the danger of releasing nitrogen bubbles within the circulation during massage.[6]
Worsens, if condition	CI	Wieting et al, 2005[4]	DO	Massage that worsens a condition or results in undesired tissue destruction is CI.
Vigorous technique, excessively	CI	Geiringer and deLateur, 1990[2]	MD	**In 1994, Ram et al[24] reported on a 1-day-old male neonate who received**
	Avoid	Benjamin and Tappan, 2005[9,a]	LMT	**a traditional massage to his testes using a warm sand bag to reduce hydrocele size and subsequently developed a blood clot.**

a, Heavy pressure should be avoided around superficially located or unprotected nerves, lymph vessels, or blood vessels.

ADVERSE EVENTS

Source	Background	Therapy	Outcome	Follow-up/Interpretation
Antao, 1988[13] **Hematoma, myositis ossificans, and massage** Am J Sports Med Case report	A 23-year-old male soccer player presented with right hip pain due to a game-related injury. He continued to play but complained of hip strain. An osteopath provided vigorous massage for 3 months.	He eventually went to a sports medicine clinic with c/o hip pain and difficulty playing soccer (problems kicking, decelerating, landing, changing direction, and sitting cross legged). Examination revealed a 10-degree hip flexion deformity, terminal 10-degree limitations in internal rotation, abduction, and adduction, only 30 degrees of external rotation, and a non-pulsating hard mass palpated under his rectus femoris and sartorius muscles.	He was diagnosed with myositis ossificans circumscript, based on radiographs. Treatment involved excision, immobilization for 3 weeks (Thomas splint), and non–weight-bearing for another 6 weeks. After 9 weeks, exercise gradually began. At 20 weeks, he began soccer playing. At 2 years, radiographs were normal.	"Massage can be detrimental." The authors believe the osteopath's vigorous massage played a role in hematoma intensification. The hematoma was a necessary prerequisite for myositis. The authors also believe the patient's joint should have been immobilized until the soft tissue (pain, inflammation) was healed.
Danchik et al, 1993[14] **Ossification and massage, other treatment** Case report J Manipulative Physiol Ther	A 20-year-old male college hockey player was struck on the lateral right thigh by an opponent's knee.	The health care worker provided vigorous massage, active stretching of the quadriceps, hot packs, analgesic cream, and elastic bandage; the patient was allowed to return to play until pain became too severe.	After the game, he was treated with ice at the college infirmary. At about 4 hours post injury, a "huge amorphous radiopaque mass" was noted on x-ray. Three months following the injury, complete ossification was noted. At 5 to 7 months, radiographs revealed resorption.	The authors attribute the patient's mass to an inappropriate treatment of hot packs, analgesic cream, massage, and elastic wrap.

Deidiker, 1999[22] **Strangulation and massage device** Case report J Forens Med Pathol	A 56-year-old Asian woman (no medical history reported) applied an electric roller type massage to the back of her neck.	She lay supine over the machine one evening. The husband reported her fine at 10:30 PM but found her blouse entangled in the roller device and constricted around her neck at 3:00 AM. She was pulseless and cool to touch.	The diagnosis was accidental death due to ligature strangulation.	The author states that a protective guard that covered the roller mechanism was not in use.
Kalinga et al, 1996[19] **Pseudoaneurysm, and massage** Case report Singapore Med J	A 16-year-old schoolboy presented with distal medial right thigh pain and swelling and osteochondroma.	The region over the osteochondroma area was rubbed with some force repeatedly after applying herbal medicine using traditional Chinese medicine.	Initially, pain was relieved, but on the third session-swelling commenced. On the fifth session the pain became intolerable and he was referred to a hospital for femoral artery angiography, which revealed aneurysm of the popliteal artery.	After removal of the exostosis and reconstruction of the arterial area (with a reverse long saphenous vein graft), recovery was noted. The authors speculate that repeated massage led to erosion of vessels near the tip of the exostosis.
Kerr, 1997[17] **Stent displacement and Rolfing** Case report Wis Med J	A 51-year-old woman presented with flank pain due to a ureteral stricture and calculi. She was s/p ureteral stent placement.	She underwent Rolfing (a deep body massage) to the abdomen, pelvis, and low back for relaxation and pleasure by a certified Rolfer.	The patient experienced severe left flank pain and urinary incontinence toward the end of the session. A radiograph revealed a distal migration of the stent.	Pain was relieved following proximal repositioning of the stent and ketorolac injection. The authors state that posterior pelvic tilting with pelvic traction and moderate epigastric pressure could have resulted in stent displacement.

Continued

Source	Background	Therapy	Outcome	Follow-up/Interpretation
Mikhail et al, 1997[11] **Embolism and walking-on-back massage** Case report Nephrol Dial Transplant	A 59-year-old male smoker (40 cigarettes/day) presented with LBP from lifting and an aortobifemoral bypass graft for severe claudication 18 months earlier.	His wife performed back massage at home by walking on her husband while he was in a prone position.	In the afternoon, he vomited twice and developed left loin pain that radiated to his groin. He was diagnosed with an embolus to the left kidney from an aortic thrombus following back massage.	At 4 months, after anticoagulation and a new aortobifemoral graft, no left kidney defect was noted.
Mohan, 1972[15] **Myositis ossificans, elbow trauma, and massage** Retrospective (chart review) Int Surg	The author reviewed 700 cases of posttraumatic stiff elbows in outpatient departments from an Institute of Medical Sciences and Safdarjang Hospital, New Delhi, from 1963 to 1971.	Of the 700 posttraumatic elbow cases, 200 had radiologic evidence of myositis ossificans, "nearly all" of which had a history of massage.		The authors believe that massage further aggravated traumatic ossification.
Ram et al, 1994[24] **Hydrocele, blood clot, and massage** Case report Trop Doctor	A 1-day-old male neonate (3500 g) presented as a vertex delivery at home.	He received a traditional massage to his testes bilaterally using a warm sand bag to reduced hydrocele size.	The neonate later presented with bilateral asymmetrical tense testicular swelling (of the scrotum). Fluid surrounding the testes consisted of a large blood clot, which was subsequently evacuated.	Note: Details of the traditional massage are absent.

Tang et al, 2003[20] **Cataract and massage device** Case report J Cataract Refract Surg	A 44-year-old man presented with a history of recurrent sinus congestion.	He self-administered a powerful AC-powered **massaging device** over his **eyes** to relieve sinus congestion.	He stopped using the device when visual acuity began to decline (right eye from 20/20 to 20/40 to 20/60). A 2+ anterior subcapsular opacification suggested traumatic cataract.	Low-velocity repetitive trauma from vigorous ocular massage led to proliferation of lens epithelium. Note: The device manual warned against use near eyes. The device was capable of delivering several thousand "patting" movements per minute.
Tachi et al, 1990[21] **Thyroiditis and neck massage** Case report Thyroidology	A 57-year-old woman presented with Hashimoto's thyroiditis 12 years earlier.	She had received vigorous massage over her neck and shoulder for muscle stiffness.	Ten days after the massage, an enlarged goiter was noted. The patient experienced palpitations, hot feelings, finger tremors, and mental instability.	After 6 months, serum thyroxine levels returned to normal. Hashimoto's destructive thyroiditis was probably due to vigorous mechanical stimulation over the cervical goiter.
Thambu, 1971[16] **Dead fetus and Urut** Case report Med J Malaya	A 30-year-old pregnant woman presented with a history of gravida 7, para 3, and stillbirth 3.	She was not progressing in her pregnancy, so an untrained kampong bidan administered Urut (massage). The patient subsequently developed severe abdominal pain.	She was admitted to a hospital in shock with a tense abdomen and a diagnosis of a ruptured uterus. Laparotomy revealed a dead fetus (7 lb, 2 oz) in her peritoneal cavity.	Urut (abdominal massage) has been used to induce bleeding, induce abortion, or hasten labor. Urut carried out in late pregnancy or during labor for the purpose of delivering is dangerous.

Continued

Source	Background	Therapy	Outcome	Follow-up/Interpretation
Trotter, 1999[18] **Hepatic hematoma and abdominal massage** Case report N Engl J Med	A 39-year-old woman presented with no history of liver or bleeding problems.	She received deep body massage of the abdomen and right upper quarter.	At 24 hours, nausea, abdominal discomfort, and right shoulder pain developed. At 72 hours, she went to a hospital where an abdominal CT scan revealed a 14×18 cm (large) hematoma in the right hepatic lobe.	She was treated with 2 units of packed red cells. Over the next 6 months, she developed low-grade fevers and a 23-lb weight loss due to nausea. She eventually recovered (recovery date not reported). Note: Practitioner and type of massage not revealed.

REFERENCES

1. De Domenico G, Wood EC: Beard's massage, ed 4. Philadelphia: WB Saunders; 1997.
2. Geiringer SR, deLateur BJ: Physiatric therapeutics 3. Traction, manipulation, and massage. Arch Phys Med Rehab 71(4-S):S264-266, 1990.
3. Braverman DL, Schulman RA: Massage techniques in rehabilitation medicine. Phys Med Rehab Clin North Am 10(3):631-649, 1999.
4. Wieting JM, Andary MT, Holmes TG, et al: Manipulation, massage, and traction. In: Delisa JA, editor: Physical medicine and rehabilitation: Principles and practice, ed 4 (vol 1). Philadelphia: Lippincott Williams & Wilkins; 2005.
5. Knapp ME: Massage. Postgrad Med 44 (1):192-195, 1968.
6. Cotter AC, Bartoli L, Schulman RA: An overview of massage and touch therapies. Phys Med Rehab State Art Rev 14(1):43-64, 2000.
7. Weiger WA, Smith M, Boon H, et al: Advising patients who seek complementary and alternative medical therapies for cancer. Ann Intern Med 137:889-903, 2002.

8. Prentice WE, Lehn C: Therapeutic massage. In Prentice WE, editor: Therapeutic modalities for physical therapist. New York: McGraw-Hill; 2002.

9. Benjamin PJ, Tappan FM: Handbook of healing massage techniques: classic. holistic, and emerging methods, ed 4. Upper Saddle River (NJ): Pearson Prentice Hall; 2005.

10. Kessler RM, Hertling D: Friction massage. In: Kessler RM, Hertling D, eds: Management of common musculoskeletal disorders: Physical therapy principles and methods, ed 3. Philadelphia: Lippincott; 1996.

11. Mikhail A, Reidy JF, Taylor PR, Scoble JE: Renal artery embolization after back massage in a patient with aortic occlusion. Nephrol Dial Transplant 12(4):797-798, 1997.

12. Palmer D: What just happened? Massage Bodywork 15(3):76-81, 2000.

13. Antao NA: Myositis of the hip in a professional soccer player: a case report. Am J Sports Med 16(1):82-83, 1988.

14. Danchik JJ, Yochum TR, Aspegren DD: Myositis ossificans traumatica. J Manipulative Physiol Ther 16(9):605-614, 1993.

15. Mohan K: Myositis ossificans traumatica of the elbow. Int Surg 57(6):475-478, 1972.

16. Thambu JAM: Rupture of the uterus: Treatment by suturing the tear. Med J Malaya 25(4):293-294, 1971.

17. Kerr HD: Ureteral stent displacement associated with deep massage. Wis Med J 96(12):57-58, 1997.

18. Trotter JF: Hepatic hematoma after deep tissue massage. N Engl J Med 341(26):2019-2020, 1999.

19. Kalinga MJ, Lo NN, Tan SK: Popliteal artery pseudoaneurysm caused by an osteochondroma—a traditional medicine massage sequelae. Singapore Med J 37(4):443-445, 1996.

20. Tang J, Salzman IJ, Sable MD: Traumatic cataract formation after vigorous ocular massage. J Cataract Refract Surg 29:1641-1642, 2003.

21. Tachi J, Amino N, Miyai K: Massage therapy on neck: a contributing factor for destructive thyrotoxicosis? Thyroidology 2:25-27, 1990.

22. Deidiker RD: Accidental ligature strangulation due to a roller-type massage device. Am J Forens Med Pathol 20(4):354-356, 1999.

23. AHPCR: Pressure ulcers in adults: Prediction and Prevention Clinical Practice Guideline No 3, AHCPR Pub. No. 92-0047, May 1992.

24. Ram SP, Kyaw K, Noor AR: Haematoma testes due to traditional massage in a neonate. Trop Doctor 81-82, 1994.

24   MYOFASCIAL RELEASE

OVERVIEW. Myofascial release (MFR) is a manual therapy involving deep friction and stroking of the body's fascia in order to improve its ability to move and deform within the body. The aim is to eliminate pain, reduce structural imbalances, and ultimately, improve functional ability.[1]

SUMMARY: CONTRAINDICATIONS AND PRECAUTIONS. Three physical therapy sources cited a total of 23 concerns for MFR. Concerns ranged from 3 to 17 per source. The largest proportions of concerns were circulatory, and to a lesser extent, musculoskeletal and integumentary. The most frequently cited concerns were malignancy, hematomas, aneurysms, open wounds, and acute rheumatoid arthritis. Malignancy, aneurysms, and acute RA were considered an ACI by one source.

Note: MFR sources offer few rationales for their contraindications. Because MFR incorporates stroking (massage-like) and pressure (mobilization-like) forces, it is likely that many of the same concerns and rationales described by those manual therapies also apply here.

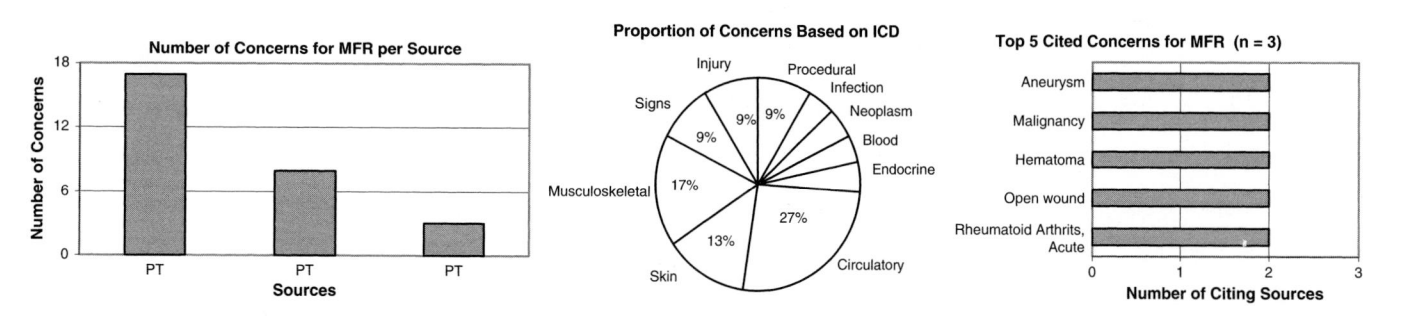

CONTRAINDICATIONS AND PRECAUTIONS

A00-B99 CERTAIN INFECTIONS AND PARASITIC DISEASES

Issue	LOC	Sources	Affil	Rationale/Comment
Infection—systemic or localized	CI	Ramsey, 1997[2]	PT	

C00-C97 NEOPLASMS

Issue	LOC	Sources	Affil	Rationale/Comment
Malignancy	CI	Ramsey, 1997[2]	PT	
	ACI	Barnes, 1990[3]	PT	

D50-D89 DISEASES OF BLOOD AND BLOOD FORMING ORGANS AND CERTAIN DISORDERS

Issue	LOC	Sources	Affil	Rationale/Comment
Anticoagulant therapy	CI	Ramsey, 1997[2]	PT	

E00-E90 ENDOCRINE, NUTRITIONAL AND METABOLIC DISEASES

Issue	LOC	Sources	Affil	Rationale/Comment
Diabetes—advanced	CI	Ramsey, 1997[2]	PT	

I00-I99 DISEASES OF THE CIRCULATORY SYSTEM

Issue	LOC	Sources	Affil	Rationale/Comment
Aneurysm	CI	Ramsey, 1997[2]	PT	Note: An aneurysm is an abnormal dilation of a vessel (diameter ≥50% of normal)
	ACI	Barnes, 1990[3]	PT	that results in a permanent sac-like structure, is weak, and can rupture (e.g., the force of elevated blood pressure can rupture a thoracic aortic aneurysm).[4]
Carotid pulse differences and vigorous head/neck movements	CI	Manheim and Lavett, 1989[1,a]	PT	If there are significant differences between the two carotid pulses, vigorous head and neck movements are contraindicated. If there is a significant difference in pulse strength, consider referring to physician before initiating MFR.
Circulatory conditions—acute	CI	Ramsey, 1997[2]	PT	
Edema—obstructive	CI			
Femoral pulses absent and lower limb treatment	CI	Manheim, 1994[5]	PT	If femoral pulses are absent, lower extremity treatment is CI. Refer to physician.
Vertebral artery disease and vigorous head/neck movements	CI	Manheim and Lavett, 1989[1]	PT	Vigorous head and neck movements are CI in VAD. If the vertebral artery test is positive, consider referring to physician.

a, Source's recommendations from two textbook editions are included in these tables.[2,5]

L00-L99 DISEASES OF THE SKIN AND SUBCUTANEOUS TISSUE

Issue	LOC	Sources	Affil	Rationale/Comment
Cellulitis	CI	Ramsey, 1997[2]	PT	
Hypersensitivity—of skin	CI			
Sutures	CI			

M00-M99 DISEASES OF THE MUSCULOSKELETAL AND CONNECTIVE TISSUE

Issue	LOC	Sources	Affil	Rationale/Comment
Degenerative changes—advanced	CI	Ramsey, 1997[2]	PT	
Osteoporosis	CI			Note: Osteoporosis (porous bone) is a condition characterized by reduced bone mass and an increased susceptibility to fractures, particularly vertebral compression fractures. This type of fracture is not typically associated with severe trauma.[6]
Osteomyelitis	CI			Note: Osteomyelitis is an inflammation of bone, usually due to bacterial infection, and is characterized by bone destruction, abscess formation, and reactive formation of new bone. Avoid any technique such as massage that may mechanically spread infection.[6]
Rheumatoid arthritis—acute	CI	Ramsey, 1997[2]	PT	
	ACI	Barnes, 1990[3]	PT	

R00-R99 SYMPTOMS, SIGNS, AND ABNORMAL CLINICAL AND LABORATORY FINDINGS (NOT ELSEWHERE CLASSIFIED)

Issue	LOC	Sources	Affil	Rationale/Comment
Febrile	CI	Ramsey, 1997[2]	PT	
Hematoma	Regional CI	Barnes, 1990[3]	PT	
	CI	Ramsey, 1997[2]	PT	

S00-T98 INJURY, POISONING, AND CERTAIN OTHER CONSEQUENCES OF EXTERNAL CAUSES

Issue	LOC	Sources	Affil	Rationale/Comment
Fracture—healing	Regional CI	Barnes, 1990[3]	PT	
Wounds—open	CI	Ramsey, 1997[2]	PT	
	Regional CI	Barnes, 1990[3]	PT	

PROCEDURAL CONCERNS

Issue	LOC	Sources	Affil	Rationale/Comment
Comprehensive history and evaluation	Advice	Barnes, 1990[3]	PT	Comprehensive history and evaluation is recommended prior to administering MFR.
Organic disease	Advice			A physician should rule out organic disease prior to administering MFR.

REFERENCES

1. Manheim CJ, Lavett DK: The myofascial release manual. Thorofare (NJ): Slack; 1989.
2. Ramsey SM: Holistic manual therapy techniques. Primary Care Clin Off Pract 24(4):759-786, 1997.
3. Barnes JF: Myofascial release: the search for excellence. A comprehensive evaluatory and treatment approach. John F. Barns PT and Rehabilitation Services; 1990.
4. Goodman CC: The cardiovascular system. In: Goodman CC, Boissonnault WG, Fuller KS, eds: Pathology: implications for the physical therapist, ed 2. Philadelphia: Saunders; 2003.
5. Manheim CJ: The myofascial release manual, ed 2. Thorofare (NJ): Slack; 1994.
6. Brashear HR Jr, Raney RB Sr: Shand's handbook of orthopaedic surgery, ed 9. St. Louis: C.V. Mosby; 1978.

25 | JOINT MOBILIZATION (ARTICULATION, NONTHRUST TECHNIQUE; NONIMPULSE TECHNIQUE)

OVERVIEW. Joint mobilization (also called articulation, non-thrust) is a manual technique directed to the patient's joint whereby the clinician imparts passive movements such as glides and distractions. The technique is characterized by low-velocity movements (i.e., rather than high-velocity thrusts) and is generally slow enough for the patient to stop. The goal is to relieve pain or improve range of motion by improving joint play and restoring the roll and glide arthrokinematics of the joint.[1]

SUMMARY: CONTRAINDICATIONS AND PRECAUTIONS. Seven sources cited a total of 51 concerns for joint mobilization. Concerns ranged from four to 18 per source. All seven sources were physical therapists. The largest proportion of concerns were musculoskeletal (>40%). The most frequently cited concern was neoplasm followed by recent fracture and hypermobility.

Several absolute CIs were also listed. Notes: Grieve,[2] Kisner and Colby,[1] and Sprague[3] address spinal mobilization, peripheral joint mobilization, and the cervical spine concerns, respectively. Harris and Lundgren[4] address pediatric concerns with nervous system disorders.

ADVERSE EVENT. Michaeli,[5] in a 1993 descriptive study, reported on a 75-year-old man who suffered a minor CVA with aphasia a day or two following an occipito-atlantal and atlantoaxial joint mobilization with a forceful rotatory component. No premanipulative screening was conducted.

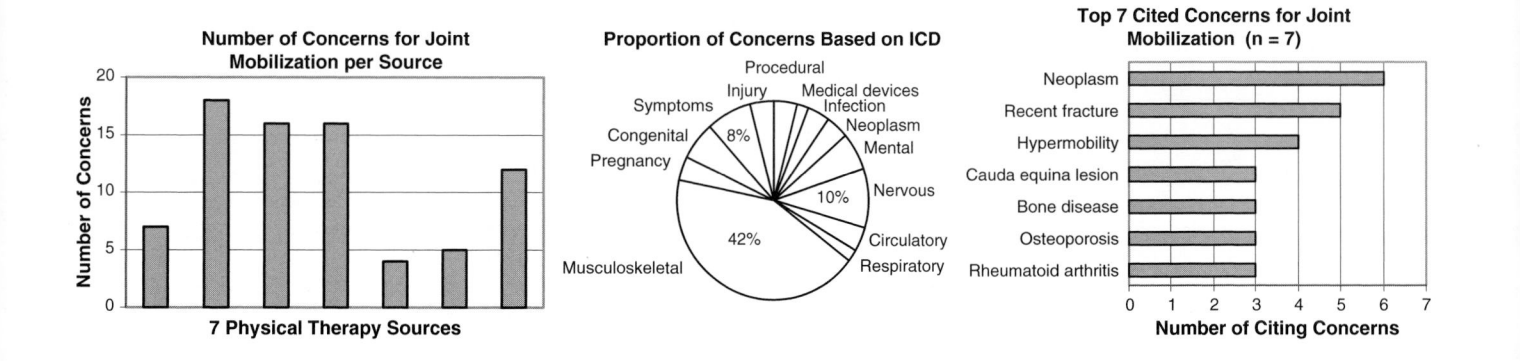

Number of Concerns for Joint Mobilization per Source

Number of Concerns / 7 Physical Therapy Sources

Proportion of Concerns Based on ICD

Procedural, Injury, Medical devices, Infection, Neoplasm, Mental, Symptoms, Congenital, Pregnancy, 8%, 10%, Nervous, Musculoskeletal, 42%, Circulatory, Respiratory

Top 7 Cited Concerns for Joint Mobilization (n = 7)

Neoplasm
Recent fracture
Hypermobility
Cauda equina lesion
Bone disease
Osteoporosis
Rheumatoid arthritis

Number of Citing Concerns

CONTRAINDICATIONS AND PRECAUTIONS

A00-B99 CERTAIN INFECTIONS AND PARASITIC DISEASES

Issue	LOC	Source	Affil	Rationale/Comment
Infection	ACI	Hertling and Kessler, 1996[6,a]	PT	
	ACI	Grieve, 1989[2,b]	PT	
Tuberculosis	ACI	Paris, 1979[7]	PT	Bacterial infection can affect bone and soft tissue.
	CI	Cookson, 1979[8]	PT	

a, Bacterial concerns; b, Infective arthritic concerns.

C00-C97 NEOPLASMS

Issue	LOC	Source	Affil	Rationale/Comment
Malignant tissue (previous)— non-spinal	Care	Grieve, 1989[2]	PT	For spinal mobilization, if there is a previous history of a malignant tumor (non-spinal), one must "reasonably" exclude metastases to the spine.
Neoplasm	ACI	Hertling and Kessler, 1996[6]	PT	There may be undiscovered metastasis to bone.
	ACI	Grieve, 1989[2,b]	PT	
	ACI	Paris, 1979[7]	PT	
	CI	Cookson, 1979[8]	PT	
	CI	Sprague, 1983[3,a]	PT	
	Extreme care	Kisner and Colby, 1996[1,c]	PT	

a, Primary or secondary malignancy; b, Malignancy involving vertebral column; c, Extreme care if patient's response and signs are favorable.

F00-F00 MENTAL AND BEHAVIORAL DISORDERS

Issue	LOC	Source	Affil	Rationale/Comment
Developmental delay—generalized of unknown etiology (with hypotonia and ligamentous laxity)	CI	Harris and Lundgren, 1991[4]	PT	The patient may exhibit hypotonia and ligamentous laxity.
Neurosis—severe	Caution	Cookson, 1979[8]	PT	
Psychologic pain	CI	Sprague 1983[3]	PT	

G00-G99 DISEASES OF THE NERVOUS SYSTEM

Issue	LOC	Source	Affil	Rationale/Comment
Cauda equina lesions with bowel and bladder disturbance	ACI	Grieve, 1989[2]	PT	Note: Cauda equina syndrome presents as flaccid paralysis of the lower limbs bilaterally, paralysis of the rectal and bladder sphincter, and anesthesia of the buttocks, perineum, and posterior legs and feet.[9]
	CI	Cookson, 1979[8]	PT	Evaluate evidence of neural compression such as a positive Babinski, nonsegmental paresthesia, or spastic weakness resulting in spastic gait.[8]
	CI	Sprague, 1983[3,a]	PT	Evaluate compression of 4th sacral root with signs of sexual impotence, impaired bowel and bladder, saddle area pain, and paraesthesia.[8]

Cerebral palsy—athetoid or ataxic	Strongly CI	Harris and Lundgren, 1991[4]	PT	Neck movements (rapid, repetitive) in athetoid cerebral palsy can accelerate progression of cervical instability.
Neurological signs	Care	Grieve, 1989[2]	PT	**See Manipulation.**
Spasticity and older children with joint restrictions	Caution and conservative use	Harris and Lundgren, 1991[4]	PT	Reasons: First, immature growth plates are vulnerable to linear and torsional shears during growth spurts, which may be a particular issue with younger children. Second, children with CNS involvement may not adequately provide a history. Third, clinicians need the competence to differentiate capsular tightness from spasticity. Perform gentle oscillations and avoid techniques that cause pain or reactive muscle spasms. Avoid quick stretches to muscle surrounding joints in children with spasticity because of the concern for temporarily increasing spasticity.
Spinal cord involvement of more than one spinal nerve root on one side or two adjacent roots in one limb only	ACI	Grieve, 1989[2]	PT	

a, Spinal cord compression.

I00-I99 DISEASES OF THE CIRCULATORY SYSTEM

Issue	LOC	Source	Affil	Rationale/Comment
Circulatory disturbance	Caution	Cookson, 1979[8]	PT	If signs of circulatory disturbances are noted, consider the use of gentler techniques.[8] Inquire about drop attack history, calcification of large blood vessels on x-ray; dizziness, visual disturbance related to neck posture, or vertebral artery disease of the cervical spine (i.e., vertebral artery occlusion; advanced arteriosclerosis).[8] **Also see Michaeli.[5]**
Dizziness aggravated by neck rotation or extension	Care	Grieve, 1989[2]	PT	Note: This maneuver is a component of the vertebral artery test, and dizziness may suggest circulatory embarrassment of the vertebral artery and a potential hazard for cervical techniques.

J00-J99 DISEASES OF THE RESPIRATORY SYSTEM

Issue	LOC	Source	Affil	Rationale/Comment
Upper respiratory tract infection	Avoid	Paris, 1979[7]	PT	

Issue	LOC	Source	Affil	Rationale/ Comment
Arthroses	RCI	Hertling and Kessler, 1996[6]	PT	
Autoimmune disease—advanced	CI	Cookson, 1979[8]	PT	In advanced autoimmune disease (i.e., ankylosing spondylitis), ligaments may become lax and spinal joints hypermobile. Vigorous manual techniques are CI.
Bone disease	ACI	Grieve, 1989[2,a,b]	PT	
	Caution	Cookson, 1979[8,b]	PT	
	Extreme caution	Kisner and Colby, 1996[1,c]	PT	
Connective tissue—weakened	Extreme caution	Kisner and Colby, 1996[1]	PT	Forceful mobilization, in the presence of weak connective tissue, such as from disuse, injury, surgery, or medications (corticosteroids), may destroy tissue.
Deformity—operative	Caution	Cookson, 1979[8]	PT	
Disc—herniation	RCI	Paris, 1979[7]	PT	Note: Disc herniation involves the partial expulsion of nuclear material from the annulus into the canal, with the majority of material remaining in the annulus.[1]
Disc—prolapse	RCI			This concern is dependent on skill level. Note: A disc prolapse results when the nuclear material frankly ruptures into the vertebral canal.[1]
Disc—prolapse, with neurological changes	ACI	Paris, 1979[7]	PT	This is a disc prolapse with serious neurological changes, including cord compression.
Hypermobility	RCI	Paris, 1979[7]	PT	Patients with hypermobility may have capsular or ligamentous necrosis. Anterior and posterior glides are contraindicated for anterior and posterior shoulder dislocations, respectively, during the rehabilitation phase (i.e., following reduction).[1]
	Caution	Cookson, 1979[8,d]	PT	
	Caution	Grieve, 1989[2]	PT	
	CI	Kisner and Colby, 1996[1]	PT	

Continued

Issue	LOC	Source	Affil	Rationale/Comment
Hypermobility in associated joints	Extreme caution	Kisner and Colby, 1996[1]	PT	These joints need to be stabilized so mobilization forces do not stress them.
Internal derangement	RCI	Hertling and Kessler, 1996[6]	PT	
Joint effusion	RCI	Hertling and Kessler, 1996[6]	PT	Do not stretch with joint mobilization because the joint capsule is already distended
	CI	Kisner and Colby, 1996[1]	PT	from the swelling and is limited by pain rather than fiber shortening.[1]
Joint inflammation	RCI	Hertling and Kessler, 1996[6]	PT	Do not stretch with joint mobilization as it will only increase pain, guarding, and
	CI	Kisner and Colby, 1996[1]	PT	tissue damage.[1]
Ligaments—laxity (generally)	Avoid	Paris, 1979[7]	PT	Note: Because a goal of joint mobilization is soft tissue stretching, using this technique on a lax joint is counterintuitive and may create further, unwanted instability.
Osteomyelitis	ACI	Paris, 1979[7]	PT	Osteomyelitis is characterized by inflammation of bone, usually due to bacterial infection, bone destruction, abscess formation, and reactive formation of new bone. Avoid any technique (e.g., such as massage) that may mechanically spread infection.[9]
Osteoporosis	Care	Grieve, 1989[2]	PT	Note: Osteoporosis (porous bone) is characterized by reduced bone mass, with
	ACI	Paris, 1979[7,d]	PT	susceptibility to fractures, particularly vertebral compression fractures that are not
	Caution	Cookson, 1979[8]	PT	usually associated with severe trauma.[9] Mobilize with care, especially over osteoporotic ribs.[2]
Rheumatica, polymyalgia	Care	Grieve, 1989[2]	PT	This condition is regarded as an inflammatory arthritis of axial and limb girdle joints.
Rheumatoid arthritis	CI	Cookson, 1979[8]	PT	This is an advanced autoimmune disease. Connective tissue is weakened and forceful
	Care	Grieve, 1989[2]	PT	peripheral mobilization may rupture tissue and lead to instability.[1] One source suggests
	Extreme caution	Kisner and Colby, 1996[1]	PT	gentle mobilization in RA, but patient must not be acutely inflamed, the cervical spine must be avoided, and depleted bone structure (especially rib) must be respected.[2]

Rheumatoid collagen necrosis—of the vertebral ligament	ACI	Grieve, 1989[2]	PT	The cervical spine is particularly vulnerable.
Scoliosis	RCI	Paris, 1979[7]	PT	
Spondylolisthesis	RCI	Paris, 1979[7]	PT	Note: Spondylolisthesis (*listhesis* means "slipping") is a defect in the isthmus that results in vertebral instability with a forward slipping of the spinal column from its base, common at the LS level. The ligament stability is relied upon.[9] Techniques involving a "degree of energy" are contraindicated for spondylolisthesis.[2]
	Care	Grieve, 1989[2]	PT	
Spondylolysis	RCI	Paris, 1979[7]	PT	Note: Spondylolysis may cause neurological signs if an osteophyte encroaches on the spinal canal or intravertebral foramina.[1]

a, More involved than "simple osteoporosis"; b, Of the spine; c, Concerns for the periphery; d, Active.

O00-O99 PREGNANCY, CHILDBIRTH, AND PUERPERIUM

Issue	LOC	Source	Affil	Rationale/Comment
First trimester of pregnancy	Avoid CI	Paris, 1979[7] Cookson, 1979[8]	PT	There is the danger of precipitating a miscarriage in the first trimester. Vigorous maneuvers are CI.[7]
Last stage of pregnancy	Avoid CI	Paris, 1979[7] Cookson, 1979[8]	PT PT	Ligament are lax during the last stage of pregnancy.[7] Vigorous maneuvers are CI.

Q00-Q99 CONGENITAL MALFORMATIONS, DEFORMITIES AND CHROMOSOMAL ABNORMALITIES

Issue	LOC	Source	Affil	Rationale/Comment
Deformity, congenital	Caution	Cookson, 1979[8]	PT	
Down syndrome	Strongly CI	Harris and Lundgren, 1991[4]	PT	Twenty-three percent of individuals with Down syndrome have patella instability, 10% have hip subluxations or dislocations, and 15% have atlantoaxial instability.
Prader-Willi syndrome	Strongly CI			This syndrome presents with generalized hypotonia.

R00-R99 SYMPTOMS, SIGNS, AND ABNORMAL CLINICAL AND LABORATORY FINDINGS (NOT ELSEWHERE CLASSIFIED)

Issue	LOC	Source	Affil	Rationale/Comment
Elderly persons with weakened connective tissue and reduced circulation	Extreme caution	Kisner and Colby, 1996[1]	PT	
Debilitation—general	RCI	Hertling and Kessler, 1996[6]	PT	E.g., poor general health.
	Avoid	Paris, 1979[7]	PT	
Inflammation	ACI	Grieve, 1989[2,a]	PT	
	CI	Cookson, 1979[8]	PT	
Pain, excessive	Extreme caution	Kisner and Colby, 1996[1]	PT	Determine cause of pain.

a, Active inflammatory.

S00-T98 INJURY, POISONING, AND CERTAIN OTHER CONSEQUENCES OF EXTERNAL CAUSES

Issue	LOC	Source	Affil	Rationale/Comment
Ligament, rupture	ACI	Paris, 1979[7]	PT	
Fracture—recent	ACI	Hertling and Kessler, 1996[6]	PT	
	ACI	Paris, 1979[7,a]	PT	
	Caution	Cookson, 1979[8]	PT	
	CI	Sprague, 1983[3]	PT	
	Extreme caution	Kisner and Colby, 1996[1,b]	PT	

a, Fracture; b, Use of joint mobilization (peripheral) depends on site of fracture and stabilization.

Y70-Y82 MEDICAL DEVICES

Issue	LOC	Source	Affil	Rationale/Comment
Total joint replacements	Extreme caution	Kisner and Colby, 1996[1]	PT	The replacement mechanism is "self-limiting."

PROCEDURAL CONCERN

Issue	LOC	Source	Affil	Rationale/Comment
Spasms that protect a joint	Advice	Grieve, 1989[2]	PT	Never push through spasms that are protecting a joint.
Temporary soreness after treatments	Advice			Patient instructions may relieve unnecessary anxiety between sessions. Warn patients of temporary aftereffects of treatments (i.e., soreness; other "after-effects").

ADVERSE EVENT

Source	Background	Therapy	Outcome	Follow-up/ Interpretation
Michaeli, 1993[5] **Mobility and complications** Descriptive (questionnaire) Aust Physiother	A survey was sent to 250 physiotherapists who completed a postgraduate course in South Africa between 1971 and 1989.	153 surveys were returned (61% response rate) with 228,050 manipulative procedures reported between 1971 and 1989. A total of 29 patients receiving spinal (cervical, thoracic, lumbar) manipulations experienced 52 mostly minor complications (most were from cervical manipulations). Another 58 patients receiving cervical mobilization had 129 complications, including the following case: A 75-year-old man suffered a minor CVA with aphasia (residual deficit 2 years later) a day	Dizziness, severe headaches, and nausea were the most common side effects for both cervical manipulation and mobilization. Complications after cervical manipulation included dizziness, nausea, severe headaches, nystagmus, blurred vision, brachialgia (also with neurological deficits), loss of consciousness, and acute wry neck. All patients recovered without sequelae with an average recovery of 6.3 days. Complications after cervical mobilization included dizziness, severe headaches,	The authors conclude that spinal manipulation is relatively safe (by physiotherapists in South Africa). Therapists should be aware of the potential risks with cervical mobilization.

or two following successive treatments for neck pain. (The mobilization was a grade 4 unilateral PA pressure to the occipito-atlantal and atlantoaxial joints and a rotatory mobilization described by patient as a "strong twisting movement." Note: Premanipulative procedures were not conducted and VBI symptoms were not reported by patient.)

nausea, brachialgia (also with neurological deficits), blurring vision, vomiting, nystagmus, increased pain >2 weeks, CVA, and skin clamminess. The majority had no sequelae. There was partial recovery noted in one person with a CVA and two patients with brachialgia with neurological deficits. No recovery was reported in another two patients with brachialgia with neurological deficits (loss of strength and reflexes).

REFERENCES

1. Kisner C, Colby LA: Therapeutic exercise: foundations and techniques, ed 3. Philadelphia: F.A. Davis; 1996.
2. Grieve GP: Contra-indications to spinal manipulation and allied treatments. Physiotherapy 75(8):445-453, 1989.
3. Sprague RB: The acute cervical joint lock. Phys Ther 63(9):1439-1444, 1983.
4. Harris SR, Lundgren BD: Joint mobilization for children with central nervous system disorders: indications and precautions. Phys Ther 71(12):890-896, 1991.
5. Michaeli A: Reported occurrence and nature of complications following manipulative physiotherapy in South Africa. Aust Physiother 39(4):309-315, 1993.
6. Hertling D, Kessler RM: Introduction to manual therapy. In Hertling D, Kessler RM, eds: Management of common musculoskeletal disorders: Physical therapy principles and methods, ed 3. Philadelphia: Lippincott-Raven; 1996.
7. Paris SV: Mobilization of the spine. Phys Ther 59(8):988-985, 1979.
8. Cookson JC: Orthopedic manual therapy: An overview. Phys Ther 59(3):259-267, 1979.
9. Brashear HR Jr, Raney RB Sr: Shand's handbook of orthopaedic surgery, ed 9. St. Louis: CV Mosby; 1978.

26 SPINAL MANIPULATION

OVERVIEW. Spinal manipulation (also called thrust, chiropractic adjustment) involves passive mechanical movement directed at a specific spinal joint or joint segment in order to restore movement or reduce pain. It is a high-velocity, low-amplitude maneuver performed at the end of the patient's spinal range, which the patient cannot stop or control. Theories for the pain relief following spinal adjustments include (1) mechanical/reflexive relaxation of soft tissue, (2) movement of a disc bulge away from pain-sensitive structure, or (3) proprioceptive input to the spinal cord to gate out pain.[1]

SUMMARY: CONTRAINDICATIONS AND PRECAUTIONS. Six sources cited a total of 47 concerns for spinal manipulation. Concerns ranged from eight to 31 per source, with a physical therapist citing the largest number. The largest proportion of concerns (about 40%) relate to musculoskeletal diseases. The most frequently cited concerns were vertebral artery disease and inflammatory joint disease (all six sources). Other frequently cited concerns included cauda equina syndrome, osteoporosis, metastatic cancer, and anticoagulation disorders. Two sources cited numerous ACIs.

Note: Although authorities suggest adverse events following manipulation are rare, numerous case reports of individuals sustaining vascular damage with subsequent neurologic impairment (particularly following cervical manipulation) have been published over the years in the medical literature.

The list of adverse events for spinal manipulation below is not exhaustive, nor should it suggest an incidence rate. Readers are also reminded that case reports are a weak form of evidence.

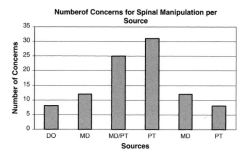

Number of Concerns for Spinal Manipulation per Source

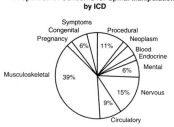

Proportion of Concerns for Spinal Manipulation by ICD

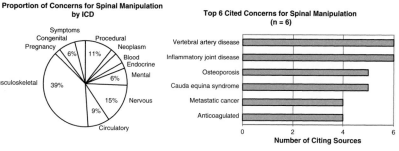

Top 6 Cited Concerns for Spinal Manipulation (n = 6)

CONTRAINDICATIONS AND PRECAUTIONS FOR MANIPULATION

C00-C97 NEOPLASMS

Issue	LOC	Source	Affil	Rationale/Comment
Carcinoma— metastatic	Special precautions	Greenman, 2003[2,c]	DO	Metabolic and systemic bone disease
	CI	Geiringer, 1990[3]	MD	**Of 172 patients who were manipulated over a 3-year period, Livingstone[5] described 12 patients who sustained injuries. In one case, he described a 70-year-old man with upper back pain, numb feet, and difficulty urinating who received a dorsal manipulation by a chiropractor. No x-rays were taken. After the third treatment, he developed paraplegia with anesthesia below T9 and leg weakness. Bone marrow results revealed multiple myeloma. Two months later, he developed bronchopneumonia and died.**
	CI	Tan, 1998[1,b]	MD/PT	
	ACI	Grieve, 1989[4,a]	PT	

a, Neoplastic, affecting bone or soft tissue of spine or other tissue, having an earlier history; b, Vertebral malignancy; c, Primary or metastatic. General note: Greenman's[2] guidelines apply to "manual medicine."

D50-D89 DISEASES OF BLOOD AND BLOOD FORMING ORGANS AND CERTAIN DISORDERS

Issue	LOC	Source	Affil	Rationale/Comment
Anticoagulation	CI	Geiringer, 1990[3]	MD	In 1976, Stewart-Wynne[7] described a 55-year-old man who was prescribed warfarin sodium (post-MI)
	CI	Tan, 1998[1]	MD/PT	and later sustained an iliopsoas hematoma and a femoral neuropathy following three spinal
	CI	Cyriax, 1982[6]	MD	manipulations for the treatment of acute left sciatica by an osteopath.
	ACI	Grieve, 1989[4,a]	PT	Cyriax[6] cites a case of a chiropractic manipulation in a person on warfarin with sciatic pain who subsequently developed an interspinal hematoma.
Hemophilia[b]	ACI	Grieve, 1989[4]	PT	The risk of hemarthrosis increases.
		Tan, 1998[1]		

a, Warfarin sodium; b, Blood disease.

E00-E90 ENDOCRINE, NUTRITIONAL AND METABOLIC DISEASES

Issue	LOC	Source	Affil	Rationale/Comment
Diabetes—severe	CI	Tan, 1998[1]	MD/PT	Tissue vitality may be low.[4]
	ACI	Grieve, 1989[4]	PT	

F00-F99 MENTAL AND BEHAVIORAL DISORDERS

Issue	LOC	Source	Affil	Rationale/Comment
Fixation—obsessive fixation (on pain)	CI	Tan, 1998[1]	MD/PT	
	ACI	Grieve, 1989[4]	PT	
Neurosis—nonorganic basis (for backache)	CI	Cyriax, 1982[6,a]	MD	Cyriax felt that if the patient's emotional status declined, the manipulation might be blamed.[6] Do not manipulate.
Neurosis—compensatory (litigation)	CI	Cyriax, 1982[6,a]	MD	The patient has no wish to get better. Treat after the suit is finished.

a, Lumbar.

G00-G99 DISEASES OF THE NERVOUS SYSTEM

Issue	LOC	Source	Affil	Rationale/Comment
Cauda equina syndrome	CI	Geiringer, 1990[3]	MD	Cauda equina syndrome presents with flaccid paralysis of bilateral LE, paralysis of the rectal and bladder
	CI	Tan, 1998[1]	MD/PT	sphincter, and aesthesis of the buttocks, perineum, and posterior legs and feet.[9]
	ACI	Maitland, 1986[8]	PT	Cyriax felt that spinal claudication would contraindicate manipulation because the cauda equina root
	CI	Cyriax, 1982[6,a]	MD	circulation is sufficiently compromised, thus suggesting a "considerable" bulge is present.
	ACI	Grieve, 1989[4]	PT	

Continued

Issue	LOC	Source	Affil	Rationale/Comment
CNS diseases—e.g., transverse myelitis	ACI	Grieve, 1989[4]	PT	A positive Lhermitte's sign may be present in disease of the cervical spinal cord and demyelinating conditions (e.g., sudden flexion of the neck leads to shooting limb paresthesia). Also positive cord pressure signs in the limb. **In 1959, Green and Jaynt[10] described a 31-year-old woman with possible multiple sclerosis who was vigorously manipulated by a chiropractor and was subsequently diagnosed with an acute brainstem vascular accident**.
Myelopathy	CI	Geiringer, 1990[3]	MD	Note: Myelopathy may suggest compression of the spinal cord (with cervical myelopathy, in the cervical region).[11] It may also refer to nonspecific pathological changes.[12]
	CI	Tan, 1998[1]	MD/PT	
	ACI	Maitland, 1986[8,b]	PT	Cyriax viewed UMN lesions as unsafe to manipulate as it could lead to tetraplegia.[6]
	CI	Cyriax, 1982[6,c]	MD	
	ACI	Grieve, 1989[4,d]	PT	
Neurological symptoms—in LE	ACI	Grieve, 1989[4]	PT	Neurological symptoms in LE that are caused by cervical or thoracic joint conditions. Symptoms in one or both lower limbs.
				Shvartzman and Abelson[13] describe a 49-year-old industrial worker with back pain and sensory loss over the right S1 dermatome (root signs) who received unspecified chiropractic that after 2 months led to severe leg pain, unsteady gait, and constipation. A laminectomy revealed an olive-sized cystic blood clot at the L1-L2, T11-T12 level.
Radiculopathy—multiple adjacent	CI	Geiringer, 1990[3]	MD	Manipulation with root pain complaints, but without objective signs, is controversial.
	CI	Tan, 1998[1,f]	MD/PT	
	ACI	Grieve, 1989[4,e]	PT	
Root pain—severe	ACI	Grieve, 1989[4]	PT	

| Root compression—4th sacral root | CI | Cyriax, 1982[6,g] | MD | The situation implies considerable posterior ligament bulging. Manipulation can lead to rupture and to protrusion and extrusion of the entire disc. **In 1943, Fisher[14] reported on a 32-year-old female baker who presented with chronic LBP with LE radiation and left leg weakness. She was adjusted by a chiropractor and subsequently developed cauda equina syndrome with a complete rupture of L5 disc. The surgeon believed the chiropractor made a small preexisting herniation complete**. |

a, Lumbar; b, Pressure on cord (e.g., mild bilateral foot paresthesia); c, Cervical; d, Cord (CNS) involvement; e, Involvement of >1 spinal nerve root on one side or >2 adjacent roots in only one lower limb; f, Objective radicular signs; g, Lumbar, absolute bar.

I00-I99 DISEASES OF THE CIRCULATORY SYSTEM

Issue	LOC	Source	Affil	Rationale/Comment
Aneurysm—local	CI	Tan, 1998[1]	MD/PT	Note: Aneurysms are abnormal dilations of vessels with a diameter greater or equal to 50% of normal. A permanent sac-like structure develops due to weakness. A thoracic aortic aneurysm can rupture under the force of elevated blood pressure.[15]
Atherosclerosis	CI	Tan, 1998[1]	MD/PT	Note: Atherosclerosis is the most common form of artery hardening (arteriosclerosis) and presents with fatty plaque deposits on the inner layer of arteries.[15] **Dozis[16] described a 39-year-old woman with neck and shoulder pain who sustained a cerebral infarct of the inferior right occipital lobe from an embolism following a chiropractic manipulation. The author proposed that endothelium was dislodged when the vertebrobasilar artery was stretched.**

Continued

Issue	LOC	Source	Affil	Rationale/Comment
Graft—aortic	CI	Cyriax, 1982[6,a]	MD	Concern of rupturing the graft.
Vertebral artery disease	Special precaution	Greenman, 2003[2,d]	DO	Maitland recommends screening first for symptoms suggesting vertebral artery. Evaluate vertigo and signs and symptoms of vertebrobasilar artery disease or vertebrobasilar insufficiency.[1] Greenman advocates
	CI	Geiringer, 1990[3]	MD	avoidance of extensive extension and rotation.[2] Cyriax was concerned about basilar ischemia and felt the correct technique involved strong traction with "little or no rotation."[6] Note: The vertebral-basilar
	CI	Tan, 1998[1,c]	MD/PT	circulation, which supplies the cerebellum, medulla, and caudal pons, can be affected by atherosclerosis
	Advice	Maitland, 1986[8]	PT	and embolic occlusion. Wallenberg syndrome or lateral medullary syndrome occurs with occlusion of the posterior inferior cerebellar artery (PICA). Locked-in syndrome is caused by complete occlusion of the basilar
	CI	Cyriax, 1982[6,b]	MD	artery at the pons/medulla.[17] **In 1974, Lyness and Wagman[18] reported on a 20-year-old woman**
	ACI	Grieve, 1989[4]	PT	**who received a cervical manipulation by an osteopath that lead to locked-in syndrome due to destruction of the ventral pons. The author speculated that congenital variation of her vertebral-basilar system resulted in insufficiency or spasm with compression of a larger vertebral artery during neck rotation.**
				In 1976, Mueller and Sahs[19] **described a 38-year-old man who had irregularities in the right and left vertebral arteries at the C2 level, received a spinal adjustment, and subsequently sustained brainstem dysfunction**.

a, Lumbar; b, Cervical; c, Vertebrobasilar artery disease; d, Vertebral artery conditions in cervical spine.

Issue	LOC	Source	Affil	Rationale/Comment
Adjacent segments are irritable or hypermobile	Precludes treatment	Grieve, 1989[4]	PT	Increased risk of aggravating other segments.
Anomalies—bony craniovertebral (most) and lumbosacral (some)	ACI	Grieve, 1989[4]	PT	An example is an unstable lumbosacral articulation.
Aseptic necrosis	CI	Tan, 1998[1]	MD/PT	Note: Osteochondrosis (also aseptic necrosis, epiphysitis) is a disorder of ossification centers in growing children. Epiphyses are most susceptible and covered with poorly vascularized articular cartilage.[9]
Bone diseases	ACI	Grieve, 1989[4]	PT	Note: Bone diseases are also highlighted under vertebral infections, osteoporosis,
	Special precautions	Tan, 1998[1]	MD/PT	and Paget's disease as they may occur from senility, extended steroid therapy,
		Greenman, 2003[2,n,o]	DO	endocrine disorders, gastrectomy, hormonal drugs.
Degenerative joint disease	CI	Geiringer, 1990[3,a]	MD	Note: In OA where the cartilage is affected, its ability to withstand stress declines.
	CI	Tan, 1998[1,b]	MD/PT	In the spine, the cervical and lumbar regions are most affected.[9]
	ACI	Grieve, 1989[4,c]	PT	
Deformity—spinal (frank deformity)	ACI	Grieve, 1989[4]	PT	Due to old pathology such as scoliosis or kyphosis from an adolescent
		Tan, 1998[1,d]	MD/PT	osteochondrosis.

Continued

Issue	LOC	Source	Affil	Rationale/Comment
Gout	ACI	Grieve, 1989[4]	PT	Note: In this disease, urate crystals deposits in synovium (sheaths membranes), articular cartilage and subcutaneous tissue causing irritation, and inflammation (hot, red, extreme pain). Gout seldom occurs in the spine.[9]
Hypermobility	Special precautions	Greenman, 2003[2,i]	DO	
	CI	Tan, 1998[1]	MD/PT	
	Prelude treatment	Grieve, 1989[4]	PT	
Inflammatory joint disease (inflammatory arthropathies), i.e., ankylosing spondylosis or RA, spondyloarthropathies	Special precautions	Greenman 2003[2,o]	DO	Neck manipulation is ACI for persons with ankylosing spondylitis or RA because the disease affects the spinal ligaments, which can subluxate in the cervical spine and result in sudden death. Forced movements in RA may also aggravate pain.[6]
	CI	Tan, 1998[1,p,q]	MD/PT	Note: In rheumatoid arthritis, the odontoid process erodes, the transverse ligament is disrupted, and C1 subluxates on C2, resulting in fatal cord compression from minor trauma.[9] **In 1952, Kunkle[20] reported a patient with Marie-Strumpell RA who was adjusted by a chiropractor and subsequently suffered a right brainstem infarct.**
	ACI	Maitland, 1986[8]	PT	
	CI	Cyriax, 1982[6,e]	MD	
	ACI	Grieve, 1989[4,f]	PT	
	CI	Geiringer, 1990[3,p]	MD	**In 1976, Rinsky[21] reported on a 44-year-old right-handed man with a history of ankylosing spondylitis and a fall (with a possible fracture at that time) who then received a cervical manipulation by a chiropractor that resulted in a complete C4 tetraplegia with a C3-C4 fracture.**
				In a 1978 review of 64 cases of ankylosing spondylitis with osteoporotic spines, Hunter and Dubo[22] reported 30 sustained spinal fractures due to

minor falls. The lower cervical area is a common site. In one recounted case report, a cervical fracture occurred in a patient while supine without head support. If minor trauma is suspected in this population, manage as a fracture initially.

Joint instability	Special precautions	Greenman 2005[2,j]	DO	See Instability.[2]
	CI	Geiringer, 1990[3]	MD	
	CI	Tan, 1998[1,g]	MD/PT	
	Precludes treatment	Grieve, 1989[4]	PT	
Joint irritability	Precludes treatment	Grieve, 1989[4]	PT	When movements are painful and joints are irritable.
Lumbago—hyperacute	CI	Cyriax, 1982[6,h]	MD	Note: Lumbago is pain in the lumbar (back) region.[12] The patient may be in so much lumbar pain as to not tolerate any movements of the spine.
Osteomalacia	CI	Tan, 1998[1,i]	MD/PT	
Osteoporosis	Special precautions	Greenman 2003[2,n]	DO	Note: Osteoporosis (porous bone) is characterized by reduced bone mass with susceptibility to fractures, particularly vertebral compression fractures that are not typically associated with severe trauma.[9] Most sources used the terms *bone disease* when expressing their concerns.
	CI	Geiringer, 1990[3]	MD	
	CI	Tan, 1998[1,j]	MD/PT	
	ACI	Maitland, 1986[8,k]	PT	
	ACI	Grieve, 1989[4]	PT	
Paget's disease	ACI	Grieve, 1989[4]	PT	Note: In the chronic bone disease Paget's (also osteotis deformans), resorption and proliferation of bone, bowing of the long bones, and thickening of the cranium occur. In the spine, collapses of 1 or more vertebral bodies leads to kyphosis.[9]

Continued

Issue	LOC	Source	Affil	Rationale/Comment
Rheumatologic disease—inactive	CI	Tan, 1998[l]	MD/PT	
Spondylosis	CI	Tan, 1998[l]	MD/PT	Spondylosis is characterized by ankylosing, destructive, or structural abnormality of the vertebral spine.[23] It may cause neurological signs if formed osteophytes encroach on the spinal canal or intravertebral foramina.[24]
	ACI	Grieve, 1989[4,r]	PT	
Vertebral infection	CI	Geiringer, 1990[3]	MD	Note: Osteomyelitis results in bone inflammation, usually due to bacterial infection, with bone destruction, abscess formation, and reactive formation of new bone. Avoid any technique such as massage that may mechanically spread infection.[9] **Livingston[25] described a 55-year-old woman with low back pain that was aggravated by PT treatment of "sonic waves" and "adjustments" of her spine. Years earlier, she experienced severe pain following a chiropractic adjustment that required 1 year of treatment and spinal surgery. Her x-ray, read as inflammation by the chiropractor, turned out to be a tuberculous abscess of the dorsal vertebrae. In 1925, Blaine[26] cited two additional cases, one (from a newspaper) of an 11-year-old girl with upper cervical vertebrae TB who received a spinal adjustment. The diseased bone collapsed, and death ensued.**
	CI	Tan, 1998[l]	MD/PT	
	ACI	Grieve, 1989[4,m]	PT	

a, DJD of the zygapophysis and uncovertebral joints of Luschka; b, DJD; c, Advanced changes; d, Fixed, also anomalies; e, Cervical; f, Also septic arthritis; g, Vertebral body dislocations, fractures; h, Lumbar; i, Hypermobility "clearly avoid"; j, Also osteopenia, osteomalacia, vertebral bone disease; k, Any conditions, such as steroids, that may lead to osteoporosis; l, Inactive; m, TB or osteomyelitis; n, Metabolic bone diseases; o, Primary joint diseases (e.g., RA, infectious arthritis); p, Spondyloarthropathies; q, Vertebral inflammation; rheumatic disease in cervical region; r, Calcified intervertebral disc (thoracic).

O00-O99 PREGNANCY, CHILDBIRTH, AND PUERPERIUM

Issue	LOC	Source	Affil	Rationale/Comment
Pregnancy	P	Maitland, 1986[8,a]	PT	The primary concern appears to be miscarriages. Cyriax felt that in the last months of pregnancy, manipulation was impractical.[6]
	CI	Cyriax, 1982[6,b]	MD	Grieve recommends no vigorous rotatory stress to the thoracolumbar spine after the fourth month of pregnancy and no manipulation
	CI/P	Grieve, 1989[4]	PT	at any time if there is a known risk of miscarriage.[4] Compression techniques are to be avoided in later stages of pregnancy.

a, Last months of pregnancy; b, Lumbar.

Q00-Q99 CONGENITAL MALFORMATIONS, DEFORMITIES, AND CHROMOSOMAL ABNORMALITIES

Issue	LOC	Source	Affil	Rationale/Comment
Genetic disorders, particularly in cervical spine	Special precautions	Greenman, 2003[2]	DO	E.g., Down syndrome
Laxity—genetic, developmental and congenital conditions	CI	Tan, 1998[1]	MD/PT	These conditions have an associated laxity or hypermobility:
	ACI	Grieve, 1989[4]	PT	• Down syndrome[2]
				• Ehlers-Danlos syndrome[1,4]
				• Marfan syndrome
				• Laxity syndromes[1]
				• Anomalies[1]
Odontoid process—deformation/ ligamentous laxity	CI	Cyriax, 1982[6,a]	MD	A deformed odontoid (or ligamentous laxity) can lead to vertebral instability and occlusion of the vertebral artery where the patient loses consciousness and falls to the floor. Cyriax suggests asking if there is any history of "drop attacks."[6]

a, Cervical.

R00-R99 SYMPTOMS, SIGNS

Issue	LOC	Source	Affil	Rationale/Comment
Protective spasms	Precludes treatment	Grieve, 1989[4]	PT	When the spasm serves to protect the area to be treated.
If no pain-free directions of vertebral motion	CI	Tan, 1998[1]	MD/PT	

PROCEDURAL CONCERNS

Issue	LOC	Source	Affil	Rationale/Comment
Relaxation—inability	Precludes treatment	Grieve, 1989[4]	PT	If the patient is unable to relax.
Forceful manipulations—if any evidence of nerve root involvement	Avoid	Maitland, 1986[8]	PT	Manipulation in presence of nerve root compression is controversial. A possible exception is if root symptoms are longstanding and patient then develops a mechanical derangement of the spine, unrelated to the chronic root pain.
Pain—undiagnosed	ACI	Grieve, 1989[4]	PT	
Skill—inadequate (of clinician)	CI	Geiringer, 1990[3]	MD	
Workup adequate	Advice	Maitland, 1986[8]	PT	Medical assessment and radiographs of spine are essential before manipulating person with vertebral disease.

Source	Background	Therapy	Outcome	Follow-up/Interpretation
Blaine, 1925[26] **Cervical manipulation, fracture/dislocation and death** Case report JAMA	An 18-year-old male presented with chest pain, numbness and weakness in his hands, and neck pain.	A violent manipulation to his neck by a chiropractor led to pain and limitation.	The patient sustained a fracture dislocation of atlas on axis, with an odontoid fracture. Over next 2 years progressive paralysis was followed by death.	Blaine also recounted two additional cases: (1) (from a newspaper) A 11-year-old girl with upper cervical vertebrae TB, who received a spinal adjustment. The diseased bone collapsed, and death ensued. (2) A 5-year-old child with bronchial pneumonia had the spine adjusted with great force in an unsupported, middle section of a table. The child cried out and died.
Davidson et al, 1975[27] **Cervical manipulation and vertebral artery pseudoaneurysm** Case report Radiology	A 42-year-old woman (no details)	Cervical manipulation was performed by a chiropractor for 4 weeks. On the fourth visit, the woman experienced rapid onset of dizziness, nausea, vertigo, diplopia, right ear tinnitus (a roaring sound), an inability to stand, paresis of the right 4th cranial nerve, right facial palsy, and rotatory nystagmus.	Her diagnosis was a right vertebral artery pseudoaneurysm.	At 3 months, she had neurosensory hearing loss and a residual upper facial paresis.

Continued

Source	Background	Therapy	Outcome	Follow-up/Interpretation
Dozis and Factor, 1997[16] **Cervical manipulation and embolic stroke** Case report Am J Ophthalmol	A 39-year-old female airline flight attendant presented with a complaint of shoulder and neck pain.	She underwent a chiropractic neck manipulation and experienced an immediate peripheral visual field loss, a small affected central area, and dizziness. (The dizziness later resolved.)	She was diagnosed with a left upper quadrant superior homonymous hemianopsia due to a cerebral infarct. MRI revealed an acute infarction of the ventromedial portion of the inferior right occipital lobe.	Her condition remained unchanged at 3 and 6 months. A follow-up MRI at 6 months revealed a $3.0 \times 1.5 \times 1.0$-cm area of encephalomalacia. The authors proposed that the deficits occurred when the vertebrobasilar artery was stretched and vascular endothelium was dislodged, leading to an embolic stroke. They recommend screening for stroke risk, hypertension, cervical spondylosis, and previous TIAs before manipulating.
Fisher, 1943[14] **Ruptured intervertebral disc and manipulation** Case report Ky Med J	A 32-year-old female baker presented with LBP for 15 years on and off, with radiation to the calf (left leg weaker).	She received a lower spine adjustment by a chiropractor. The next day, she experienced a saddle distribution of anesthesia and a loss of bowel and bladder function.	She was diagnosed with a complete rupture of the 5th intervertebral disc with pressure on the cauda equina.	She recovered following spinal surgery. The surgeon believed the chiropractor made a small preexisting herniation complete following manipulation.

Green and Jaynt, 1959[10] **Cervical manipulation and brainstem infarct** Case report JAMA	A 31-year-old woman with a tentative diagnosis of multiple sclerosis presented with a history of diplopia, blurred vision; also abdominal distension.	Vigorous manipulation by a chiropractor led to dizziness, vomiting, decreased power and sensation in the left arm and leg, slurred speech, diplopia, nystagmus, and a positive Babinski sign.	She was diagnosed with an acute brainstem vascular accident.	She recovered over the next few months.
Johnson et al, 1993[28] **Cervical self-manipulation and transient pontine ischemia** Case report Med J Aust	A healthy 26-year-old man presented with a 5-year history of chiropractic manipulation for intermittent neck aches. He was taught self-manipulation.	He performed abrupt, painful, rotation (self-manipulation) of his neck 60 degrees to each direction 2×/day. 10 minutes later, he experienced a "graying out" of vision in both eyes, visual illusions, nausea, vomiting, vertigo, left facial weakness, diplopia, and an unsteady gait.	The man was diagnosed with bilateral pontine ischemia.	The following week, symptoms resolved except for a mild left facial paralysis (x-rays and MRI were normal). Johnson suggested ischemia was precipitated by cervical manipulation which led to transient ischemia of the posterior cerebral artery and possibly a vertebral artery spasm.
Kanshepolsky et al, 1972[29] **Cervical manipulation and cerebellar infarct** Case report Bull Los Angeles Neurol	A 39-year-old woman presented with neck pain and a 2-year history of tension headaches.	She received a series of neck manipulations over a 2-week period by a chiropractor. Following one session, her legs gave out, and diplopia occurred but later resolved.	The diagnosis was cerebellar infarct. A suboccipital craniotomy revealed cerebellar necrosis.	Residual deficits included a right drift, hearing loss, and nystagmus.

Continued

Source	Background	Therapy	Outcome	Follow-up/Interpretation
Kunkle et al, 1952[20] **Traumatic brainstem thrombosis** Case report Ann Intern Med	A patient with joint pain, a diagnosis of Marie-Strumpell RA (ankylosing spondylitis) at age 14, and conversion hysteria with temporary left-arm paralysis at age 16 presented with frequent headaches (left occipital, frontal area).	After another session, she lost consciousness for a few minutes and then recovered. The next day, she was difficult to arouse and was hospitalized. She became comatose and developed decerebrate posturing. Adjustments were provided by a chiropractor. The sixth adjustment involved vigorous neck rotation and firm pressure over the right side of the neck. This led to sudden visual dimness, malaise, diplopia, moderate right limb weakness, left-sided numbness, dysphagia, and a dropped right upper lid.	The patient was hospitalized 10 days with a diagnosis of a right brainstem infarct.	Residual deficits remained.

Lyness and Wagman, 1974[18] **Cervical manipulation, congenital variation of vertebral-basilar system, and locked-in syndrome** Case report Surg Neurol	A 20-year-old woman complained of recurrent neck pain and headaches.	She underwent cervical manipulation by an osteopath that involved twisting her head to the left and then right. Later, she developed paralysis, extensor rigidity of all four limbs, an inability to speak or swallow, no neck mobility, and limited communication with eyes (yes/no code).	She was diagnosed with locked-in syndrome due to destruction of the ventral pons.	She had very limited voluntary recovery. Lyness et al. suggest that congenital variation of the vertebral-basilar system resulted in insufficiency or spasm with compression of a larger vertebral artery during neck rotation.
Miller and Burton, 1974[30] **Stroke and adjustment** Case series JAMA	A 52-year-old woman presented with a minor injury 10 years earlier and recurrent neck pain.	She underwent a series of manipulations by a chiropractor. Transient vertigo, nausea, vertigo, blurred vision, and scotomata occurred. This was followed by an inability to stand, increased numbness and left-sided weakness, diplopia, hoarseness, hiccups, spastic quadriplegia (> R side).	The diagnosis was stroke.	She improved over the next 5 months with physical therapy.
	A 35-year-old male aviator presented with chronic stiffness and a dull ache in the neck.	Forceful rotation and right neck manipulation was performed by a chiropractor. The patient lost consciousness for several seconds, awoke with blurred vision, vomited,	He was diagnosed as having a stroke due to an occluded posterior cerebral artery.	At 1 year (follow-up), the patient had intellectual deficits. The author recommendation is to stop treatment if the patient shows signs of vertebral-basilar ischemia.

Continued

Source	Background	Therapy	Outcome	Follow-up/Interpretation
		and developed diplopia and an occipital headache. He recovered after 30 minutes and then lost consciousness again after a second manipulation. Patient awoke with memory difficulties and an inability to stand.		
Mueller and Sahs, 1976[19] **Cervical manipulation and brainstem infarct or C2 dislocation** Case report Neurology	A 43-year-old right-handed woman complained of headaches for 10 years.	She had adjustments for 2 years. After a cervical manipulation, she experienced rapid onset of right-sided loss of control, vomiting, dysarthria, nausea, diplopia, trunk ataxia, and veering to right. The room appeared to tilt.	She was diagnosed with a brainstem dysfunction. Her odontoid process was initially noted to be displaced anteriorly and cephalically on radiographs.	She had residual diplopia and horizontal nystagmus. Note: Clinician type not reported.
	A 28-year-old right-handed woman presented with headaches for 2 weeks due to stress; she was taking birth control pills.	Mechanical manipulation of her neck led to vomiting and loss of consciousness. She awoke with left face numbness, dizziness, nausea, tinnitus, and a tendency to fall to her left.	She was diagnosed with a C2 anterior dislocation.	At 1 month, she displayed a mild unsteady gait and moderate dyssynergia on her left side. Note: Clinician type not reported.

	A 38-year-old right-handed man with a mild headache for 3 to 4 years, temporarily relieved with spinal adjustments.	A few hours following a mechanical adjustment, he experienced a headache, nausea, vomiting, dizziness, slurred speech, an inability to walk without assistance, and a right face droop. He was hospitalized with right limb ataxia.	His diagnosis was brainstem dysfunction. An arteriogram revealed an irregular right distal segment of the vertebral artery and a lateral "step off" of the left vertebral artery at the C2 level.	At 12 months, he had right headaches, mild dystaxia, right mild dysarthria. Note: Clinician type not reported.
Pratt-Thomas and Berger, 1947[31] **Manipulation, thrombus, and death** Case report JAMA	A 32-year-old male presented with persistent headache, nausea, and a giddy feeling.	He received an adjustment by a chiropractor that resulted in unconsciousness and death 24 hours later.	The diagnosis was contusion of the medulla oblongata with a complete block; a blood clot in the basilar, left anterior, inferior and right posterior inferior cerebellar arteries.	
	A 35-year-old female presented with hay fever.	She received an adjustment by a chiropractor that resulted in dizziness. She became unconscious and died in the evening.	The diagnosis was thrombosis of the posterior inferior cerebellar artery and basilar and right vertebral arteries; and edema and softening of cerebellum.	

Continued

Source	Background	Therapy	Outcome	Follow-up/Interpretation
Richard, 1967[32] **Lumbar manipulation, disc protrusion and L4-5 block** Case report NYS J Med	A 41-year-old female presented with a past medical history of transient back pain (2 years ago), occasional left leg radiating pain (1 year ago). She had chiropractic 6 months ago with some relief. Most recently, she experienced 3 weeks of increased back pain due to lifting.	She went to a chiropractor who applied pressure over her sacrum, thinking it was an unstable right sacroiliac joint. The patient felt a sharp sudden intense pain, weakness, and then needed assistance to walk. Over the next few days, she developed leg weakness, numbness in the perineum/buttocks/rectum, and voided less. The chiropractor told her she would "be all right" and instructed her to stretch her muscles by standing on her toes. She subsequently was in an MVA and experienced extreme lower limb weakness and burning pain of the rectum and perineum.	Her diagnosis was cauda equina compression due to disk prolapse. Myelogram revealed a complete block at the L4 to L5 lumbar vertebral level. A laminectomy revealed three larger disk fragments from L4 compressing on the cauda equina.	The patient regained bowel and bladder control and some LE strength in the following weeks; 18 months later, she could not feel bladder fullness. The author interviewed the chiropractor and noted that disk protrusion was not one of the chiropractor's diagnoses. Low back adjustments in patients with lumbar disk disease are dangerous.
Rinsky et al, 1976[21] **Cervical manipulation and ankylosing spondylitis and C4 tetraplegia** Case report Paraplegia	A 44-year-old right-handed man with a past medical history of ankylosing spondylitis (spine ankylosed in flexion and left	He received a cervical manipulation by a chiropractor and experienced immediate left-sided weakness and an inability to walk. He was hospitalized with progressive right-sided weakness and an inability to void.	He was diagnosed with a complete C4 tetraplegia. Radiographs suggested a fracture of C3-C4 (C3 posteriorly displaced on C4). Surgical decompression,	Injuries were permanent. The author felt the fracture was probably due to the original fall, but the spinal cord injury was due to the manipulation.

	hip fused); tingling left arm and neck pain (due to a fall).		laminectomy, and reduction were performed.	
Rivett and Milburn, 1997[33] **Cervical manipulation, complications, and underreporting** Descriptive (questionnaire) Physiotherapy	A questionnaire of complications in spinal manipulation occurring over the past 5 years ($N = 230$) was sent to all vascular surgeons, orthopedic surgeons, neurologists, and neurosurgeons in New Zealand.	The response rate was 63% ($n = 146$); 42 incidences were reported by 23 medical specialists. No deaths, but more than 40 cases experienced long-term adverse effects. Fourteen cases with CVA and two cases with undiagnosed multiple myeloma or metastatic prostate CA resulted in myelopathy (62% cervical, 24% lumbar, 14% thoracic) after manipulation.	Physiotherapists (New Zealand) were responsible for 14 (about 33%) of the complications. Chiropractors were responsible for 23 (over half). Physiotherapy complications included two CVAs, six radiculopathies, three disc prolapses, one pain exacerbation (complications were primarily located at the cervical level).	Rivett and Milburn suggested that complications are underreported and recommend a prospective study.
Schwarz et al, 1956[34] **Cervical manipulation and Wallenberg syndrome** Case report Arch Intern Med	A 28-year-old female complained of a head cold.	Cervical manipulation by a chiropractor led to immediate dizziness, numbness of the right face and left limbs, inability to swallow solid food, slurred nasal speech, and unsteady gait.	She was diagnosed with Wallenberg syndrome.	Three months later, she was less ataxic and almost completely recovered.

Continued

Source	Background	Therapy	Outcome	Follow-up/Interpretation
Smith and Estridge, 1962[35] **Cervical manipulation and brainstem infarct** Case series JAMA	A 33-year-old woman complained of pain and stiffness in her neck.	After a second cervical manipulation by a chiropractor, she experienced nausea, vomiting, vertigo, and limb incoordination. She went into a coma, was hospitalized, and placed on a respirator. Her pupils were fixed, tone was flaccid, and she died 3 days later.	The diagnosis was brainstem vascular accident.	
	A 48-year-old woman presented with a "crink" in her neck.	She was manipulated by an osteopath with a forceful rotation leading to severe headache, vertigo, sweating, nausea, and difficulty swallowing, speaking, and walking (she fell to right side). Her right upper eyelid drooped and she felt paresthesia (left limbs) but heaviness (right limbs).	Her diagnosis was occlusion of the posterior inferior cerebellar artery (Wallenberg syndrome).	Headaches persisted for 4 years.
	A 63-year-old man presented with a nervous stomach.	He received a neck adjustment by a chiropractor, which led to dizziness, an ataxic gait (unable to walk without support), numbness and weakness on his right side, hyperreflexia, and a right positive Babinski sign.	His diagnosis was a brainstem vascular accident due to compromised vertebral artery following neck manipulation.	One month later, there was no paresthesia, minimal L UE and RLE weakness, hyperreflexia, and a right positive Babinski sign. The author suggests the rarity of this complication may be due to abnormal vascular pattern in these patients (i.e., single vertebral artery).

Zauel and Carlow, 1977[36] **Cervical manipulation and ophthalmoplegia** Case report Ann Neurol	A 47-year-old woman presented with an occipital headache.	Forceful cervical manipulation was performed to her right side by a chiropractor. Immediate nausea, vomiting, diplopia, and right hemiparesis occurred. The patient had an adductor paralysis of the left eye and an abductor nystagmus of the right eye on right lateral gaze.	She was diagnosed with an acute internuclear ophthalmoplegia secondary to compromised vertebral-basilar circulation following cervical manipulation. Radiographs showed moderate hypertrophic degenerative changes, predominately at the C6 C7 level.	The author notes that if cervical spondylosis is present, do not undergo chiropractic manipulation.
Zimmerman et al, 1978[37] **Cervical manipulation and cerebellum infarct** Case report Neurology	A 7-year-old boy presented with a history of birth trauma (fractured clavicle) and headaches, especially following somersaults.	Repeated manipulation of the cervical spine by a chiropractor involved rotation with flexion or hyperextension. Several hours later, headaches, vomiting, left facial weakness, and transient cranial nerve deficits were experienced. The next day, no deficits remained and manipulations resumed after 2 weeks. At that time, the boy experienced headaches, diplopia, lethargy, decreased fine motor ability in the right hand, and gait ataxia.	He was diagnosed with a cerebellar infarct (from CT scan) with progressive cerebellar dysfunction and visual field deficit.	At 6 months, no visual deficit was evident and cerebral function was normal.

REFERENCES

1. Tan JC: Practical manual of physical medicine and rehabilitation: diagnostics, therapeutics, and basic problems. St. Louis: Mosby; 1998.

2. Greenman PE: Principles of manual medicine, ed 3. Philadelphia: Lippincott Wilkins & Williams; 2003.

3. Geiringer SR, deLateur BJ: Physiatric therapeutics 3. Traction, manipulation, and massage. Arch Phys Med Rehab 71(4-S):S264-S246, 1990.

4. Grieve GP: Contra-indications to spinal manipulation and allied treatments. Physiotherapy 75(8):443-453, 1989.

5. Livingston MC: Spinal manipulation causing injury. A three-year study. Clin Orthop Rel Res 81:82-86, 1971.

6. Cyriax J: Textbook of orthopaedic medicine, vol 1, Diagnosis of soft tissue lesions, ed 8. London: Bailliere Tindall; 1982.

7. Stewart-Wynne EG: Iatrogenic femoral neuropathy. BMJ 1:263, 1976.

8. Maitland GD: Vertebral manipulation, ed 5. London: Butterworths; 1986.

9. Brashear HR Jr, Raney RB Sr: Shands' handbook of orthopaedic surgery, ed 9. St. Louis: C.V. Mosby; 1978.

10. Green D, Jaynt RJ: Vascular accidents to the brain stem associated with neck manipulation. JAMA 170:522-524, 1959.

11. Walton JN: Essentials in neurology, ed 4. Philadelphia: J.B. Lippincott; 1975.

12. Dorland's illustrated medical dictionary, ed 24. Philadelphia: WB Saunders; 1965.

13. Shvartzman P, Abelson A: Complications of chiropractic treatment for back pain. Postgrad Med 83(7):57-58, 61, 1988.

14. Fisher ED: Report of a case of ruptured intervertebral disc following chiropractic manipulation. Ky Med J 41:14, 1943.

15. Goodman CC: The cardiovascular system. In: Goodman CC, Boissonnault WG, Fuller KS, eds: Pathology: implications for the physical therapist, ed 2. Philadelphia: W.B. Saunders; 2003.

16. Donzis PB, Factor JS: Visual field loss resulting from cervical chiropractic manipulation. Am J Ophthalmol 123(6):851-852, 1997.

17. Jensen FE: Cerebrovascular disease. In Loscalzo J, Creager MA, Dzau VJ, eds: Vascular medicine: A textbook of vascular biology and diseases, ed 2. Boston: Little, Brown; 1996.

18. Lyness S, Wagman AD: Neurological deficit following cervical manipulations. Surg Neurol 2:121-124, 1974.

19. Mueller S, Sahs AL: Brain stem dysfunction related to cervical manipulation: report of three cases. Neurology (Minneapolis) 26:547-550, 1976.

20. Kunkle EC, Muller JC, Odom GL: Traumatic brain-stem thrombosis: report of a case and analysis of the mechanism of injury. Ann Intern Med 36:1329-1335, 1952.

21. Rinsky LA, Reynolds GG, Jameson RM, et al: A cervical spinal cord injury following chiropractic manipulation. Paraplegia 13(4):223-227, 1976.

22. Hunter T, Dubo H: Spinal fractures complicating ankylosing spondylitis. Ann Intern Med 88(4):546-549, 1978.

23. Eisenberg MG: Dictionary of rehabilitation. New York: Springer; 1995.

24. Kisner C, Colby LA: Therapeutic exercise: foundations and techniques, ed 3. Philadelphia: F.A. Davis; 1996.

25. Livingston M: Paramedics, chiropractors and health planners [case reports, letter]. Can Med Assoc J 119(12):1391-1392, 1978.

26. Blaine ES: Manipulative (chiropractic) dislocations of the atlas. JAMA 85:1356, 1925.

27. Davidson KC, Weiford EC, Dixon GD: Traumatic vertebral artery pseudoaneurysm following chiropractic manipulation. Radiology 115:651-652, 1975.

28. Johnson DW, Whiting G, Pender MP: Cervical self manipulation and stroke. Med J Aust 158(4):290, 1993.

29. Kanshepolsky J, Danielson H, Flynn RE: Vertebral artery insufficiency and cerebellar infarct due to manipulation of the neck: report of a case. Bull Los Angeles Neurol Soc 37:62-66, 1972.

30. Miller RG, Burton R: Stroke following chiropractic manipulation of the spine. JAMA 229:189-190, 1974.

31. Pratt-Thomas HR, Berger KE: Cerebellar and spinal injuries after chiropractic manipulation. JAMA 133:600-603, 1947.

32. Richard J: Disk rupture with cauda equine syndrome after chiropractic adjustment. N Y State J Med 67(18):2496-2498, 1967.

33. Rivett DA, Milburn P: Complications arising from spinal manipulative therapy in New Zealand. Physiotherapy 83(12):626-632, 1997.

34. Schwarz GA, Geiger JK, Spano AV: Posterior inferior cerebellar artery syndrome of Wallenberg after chiropractic manipulation, Arch Intern Med 97:352-354, 1956.

35. Smith RA, Estridge MN: Neurologic complications of head and neck manipulations: report of two cases. JAMA 182:528-531, 1962.

36. Zauel D, Carlow TJ: Internuclear ophthalmoplegia following cervical manipulation. Ann Neurol 1(3):308, 1977.

37. Zimmerman AW, Kumar AJ, Gadoth N, Hodges FJ III: Traumatic vertebrobasilar occlusive disease in childhood. Neurology 28(2):185-188, 1978.

27 MUSCLE ENERGY TECHNIQUE

OVERVIEW. Muscle energy technique (MET) is a method that uses active isometric or isotonic contraction by the patient in a specific direction, and against a counterforce, in order to mobilize restricted joints, strengthen weak muscles, stretch tight muscles, and release hypertonicity. The technique has similar features to the *contract-relax* technique used in proprioceptive neuromuscular facilitation.[1]

SUMMARY: CONTRAINDICATIONS AND PRECAUTIONS. Two sources cited a total of 12 concerns for MET. Most concerns were either procedural (e.g., overly aggressive, particularly in inexperienced practitioners) or related to musculoskeletal problems that are also a concern for joint manipulation therapy (e.g., tissue fragility, hypermobility). Myositis is contraindicated because MET involves resisted movements that may further aggravate an inflamed condition. Note: If MET is viewed as a form of manipulation, other manipulative concerns may also apply (see Joint manipulation).[2]

SUMMARY: ADVERSE EVENTS. In a $119,000 settlement, a patient contended MET aggravated a lumbar disc condition that required surgery (see Adverse Events).[3]

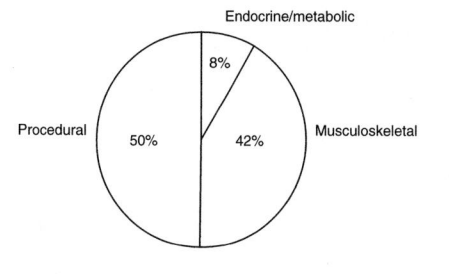

Proportion of Concerns for MET Based on ICD

Endocrine/metabolic 8%

Procedural 50%

Musculoskeletal 42%

CONTRAINDICATIONS AND PRECAUTIONS

E00-E90 ENDOCRINE, NUTRITIONAL, AND METABOLIC DISEASES

Issue	Level of Concern	Sources	Affil	Rationale/Comment
Diabetes	RCI	Tan, 1998[2]	MD/PT	

M00-M99 DISEASES OF THE MUSCULOSKELETAL SYSTEM AND CONNECTIVE TISSUE

Issue	Level of Concern	Sources	Affil	Rationale/Comment
Degenerative joint disease	RCI	Tan, 1998[2]	MD/PT	
Laxity—joint	RCI			
Myositis—concurrent	CI			The patient actively contracts during MET.
Osteoporosis	RCI			
Rheumatoid arthritis—noncervical	RCI			

PROCEDURAL CONCERNS

For Beginners of MET

Issue	Level of Concern	Sources	Affil	Rationale/Comment
Accurate diagnosis—working without Intensity (light)—use 20% of strength Pain—do not cause it	CI Advice	Chaitow, 2001[1]	DO	Inexperienced practitioners can overdose patient.

ADVERSE EVENTS

LITIGATION

Source	Background	Therapy	Outcome	Follow-up/Interpretation
2000, California[3] **Back surgery and MET** June 2002	In 2000, a California man presented with s/p L5-S1 diskectomy in 1998 due to a lifting injury and a subsequent decompressive hemilaminectomy in 2000 due to spinal stenosis.	He received a muscle energy technique by a physical therapist to address pelvic obliquity.	The patient contended he experienced immediate pain that required surgical repair of an L4-5 herniated disc following muscle energy technique. The plaintiff further contended the maneuver was unauthorized because the prescription required aquatic therapy, heat, and massage and specified "no flexion or extension exercise ever."	The defendants (physical therapist and company) contended therapy did not involve flexion or extension movements and that the patient previously had unremitting, chronic back pain. Mediation settlement: $119,000

REFERENCES

1. Chaitow L, Liebenson C, Murphy DR: Muscle energy techniques. Edinburgh, Scotland: Churchill Livingstone; 2001.
2. Tan JC: Practical manual of physical medicine and rehabilitation: diagnostics, therapeutics, and basic problems. St. Louis: Mosby; 1998.
3. Medical malpractice verdicts, settlements and experts, June 2002, p 50, loc 3.

Section E   PRESCRIPTION, APPLICATION, FABRICATION OF DEVICES AND EQUIPMENT

28   ADAPTIVE DEVICES

28.1 Bath Chair

OVERVIEW. A bath chair is an adaptive metal chair that is either stationary or designed with casters so it can be pushed by an attendant. It is used in the shower. Its name originates from Bath, England, where it functioned as an outdoor three-wheeled vehicle at the English spa.[1]

SUMMARY: CONTRAINDICATIONS AND PRECAUTIONS. One concern for bath chairs is body part entrapment (i.e., testicle; prolapsed rectum) from drainage holes located on the seats of some chair designs.[2-4]

CONTRAINDICATIONS AND PRECAUTIONS

VULNERABLE BIOLOGICAL TISSUE

Issue	LOC	Sources	Affil	Rationale/Comment
Body part entrapments	Safety notice Advice	MHPRA, 2003[2,3] Pain et al, 2003[4]	Gov (UK) OT	Drainage slot/holes on some shower and bath chairs can entrap body parts (see Adverse Events).

ADVERSE EVENTS

Source	Background	Event	Comments
MHPRA (Medicine and Healthcare Products Regulatory Agency), 2003[2,3] **Body entrapments and shower bath chairs** Safety notice Online	Safety notice: some shower and bath chairs have drainage slot/holes that can lead to body part entrapment.	Within a 3-month period, four cases of male genitalia entrapped in the drainage holes of seating equipment were reported, resulting in cuts, lacerations, and/or bruising. In one case an elderly woman with rectal prolapse was entrapped in holes of a bath hoist seat. In another two cases reported in May 1997, three males with entrapped testicles had to be cut free.	Consider using folded towel to minimize entrapment risk. Examine size, shape, and location of drainage hole to assess risk. Examine seats for cracks or distortions that may allow skin to be pinched. Note: The MDA is an executive agency of the Department of Health, UK.

REFERENCES

1. Eisenberg MG: Dictionary of rehabilitation. New York: Springer; 1995.
2. Safety notice MDA/2003/029 Medicines and Healthcare Products Regulatory Agency Bath and Shower seating equipment: Risk of injury Available at: http://www.mhra.gov.uk/. Accessed November 17, 2005.
3. MDA: 1997 Safety Notice: Bath and shower seating equipment: risk of injury, SN9709. London: Medical Devices Agency (MDA SN9709).
4. Pain H, McLellan L, Gore S: Choosing assistive devices. A guide for users and professionals. London: Jessica Kingsley; 2003.

28.2 Commode Chairs

OVERVIEW. A commode (also commode chair) is a stationary or wheeled, chair-like framework that holds a toilet utensil (i.e., a removable bedpan) under an open seat.[1,2] It can be used when individuals wish to empty their bladder (urinate) and/or evacuate their bowels (defecate).

SUMMARY: CONTRAINDICATIONS AND PRECAUTIONS. A 1993 British study of commode users identified two issues: privacy and follow-up/safety.[3]

CONTRAINDICATIONS AND PRECAUTIONS

F00–F99 MENTAL AND BEHAVIORAL DISORDERS

Issue	LOC	Sources	Affil	Rationale/Comment
Privacy—Consumers are concerned about privacy with regard to commode location	Advice	Naylor and Graham, 1993[3]	—	The concern is based on Naylor's 1993 study on the attitudes of 140 community-living commode users and their 105 caregivers in England who were randomly selected and interviewed with semistructured questionnaires (102 women, median age 75; 38 men, median age 71; median Barthel score for ADA was 15 [max 20]).

Issue	LOC	Sources	Affil	Rationale/Comment
Follow-ups	Advice	Naylor and Graham, 1993[3]	—	**See Naylor's 1993 study.** There is little monitoring of the commode after it is delivered to the home. Safety and comfort-related follow-ups about the commode are needed on a regular basis.
Inappropriate use—Standard commode use is inappropriate if the consumer is confined to one room	Advice			**See Naylor's 1993 study.** Consider providing a "chemical" seat, and air purifiers and ionizers to address odor if person confined to one room.

REFERENCES

1. Webster's third new international dictionary. Springfield (MA): Merriam-Webster; 1981.
2. Eisenberg MG: Dictionary of rehabilitation. New York: Springer; 1995.
3. Naylor JR, Graham P: Commodes: inconvenient conveniences. BMJ 307(6914):1258-1260, 1993.

28.3 Hospital Beds

OVERVIEW. A bed is a piece of furniture that one lies down and sleeps on and usually includes a frame, leg supports, springs, and a mattress.[1] Several types of beds are used to address different patient problems (i.e., trauma, pressure ulcers).

SUMMARY: CONTRAINDICATIONS AND PRECAUTIONS. Bed concerns generally center around safety issues (body entrapment fatalities; crushing injuries), proper patient selection (sizing, anthropometrics), and disadvantages of specific bed types (e.g., an inability to perform CPR). Both the FDA (US) and MDA (UK) have reported fatalities related to body entrapment involving poorly fitted or inappropriately selected bed rails.[2-4] (Also see Restraints.)

CONTRAINDICATIONS AND PRECAUTIONS

STANDARD ADJUSTABLE BEDS

Issue	LOC	Sources	Affil	Rationale/Comment
Bed adjustments—height, head, foot	Advice	Pierson and Fairchild, 2002[5]	PT	Improves access to patient and permits proper body mechanics.
Bed—replacement parts	P/Safety alert	FDA, 1995[2]	Gov	Not all bed parts are interchangeable. Variations in type may increase possibility for entrapment.
	Safety notice	MDA, 2001[3,a]	Gov	
				Check with manufacturer if parts (mattress, rail) are purchased separately.
				Replacement of bed parts should be of the dimension specified by the manufacturer.
Electric beds—crushing injuries	Hazard/ recommendation	Health Devices, 1989[6]	Org	**Four children died from crushing injuries sustained under a pedestal-style electric bed that was equipped with *walk-away down* features.**[6] That is, the bed keeps descending even after the control switch is released.
				Eliminate pedestal-style beds with walk-away down features. This hazard concern does not apply to four-poster beds or pedestal type beds with a "childproof" walk-away control.

Entrapment	P/Safety alert	FDA, 1995[2]	Gov	Entrapment has led to injuries and deaths. Inspect all hospital bed frames,
Identify high-risk individuals for bed entrapment:	Safety notice	MDA, 2001[3]	Gov	side rails, and mattresses for possible body entrapment.
• Confused				There should be no gaps wide enough to entrap a patient's head or body.
• Restless				Gaps can be created by the patient's weight compressing the mattress.
• Lacking motor control				**The FDA received 102 reports of head and body entrapment involving bed**
• Inappropriate patient size/				**side rails resulting in 68 deaths and 12 injuries (fractures, cuts, abrasions).**
weight for bed				**These incidences occurred in hospitals and in private homes.[2]**
				The MDA (UK) reports entrapments from poorly fitting bed rails and
				from U-shaped bed rails.[3]
Nurse call device	Advice	Pierson and Fairchild, 2002[5]	PT	Make sure the nurse call device is within reach of the patient.
Nursing schedules—for patient positioning	Advice			Adhere to nursing schedules for patient positioning. If the patient is not appropriately positioned for a treatment, reschedule when appropriate, temporarily position and then reposition, or treat in the position patient is found in.
Patient's selection	Advice			Standard beds (manual and electric) may not address the requirements of individuals who are acutely ill or traumatized.
Positioning—brain surgery patients	CI			Lowered-head position after brain surgery is contraindicated.
Safety rails—securing	Advice			Secure safety rails before leaving a patient (if rails are used).

Continued

Issue	LOC	Sources	Affil	Rationale/Comment
Side rails—not a substitute for protective restraints	P/Safety alert	FDA, 1995[2]	Gov	Bed side rails should not be used as a substitute for patient protective restraints. Follow your hospital protocol as well as government regulations with regard to vest or wrist protective restraints. **(Also see Restraints.)**
Tubing—IV lines or other	Advice	Pierson and Fairchild, 2002[5]	PT	Do not compress IV lines or other tubing with side rail **(also see Lines).**

a, Inspect rails.

TURNING FRAME (STRYKER WEDGE FRAME) (RARE USE TODAY)

Turning frames allows change in position from supine to prone and reverse in the horizontal plane while applying continuous cervical traction.

Issue	LOC	Sources	Affil	Rationale/Comment
Anthropometrics—tall or heavy patient **Contracture development** **Skin ulcerations—risk**	Disadvantages	Pierson and Fairchild, 2002[5]	PT	It may be difficult to position patient if tall (>6 feet) or heavy (>200 lb). Contractures may develop if patient is not exercised or positioned. Concern for skin shear and pressure due to limited positioning (assuming only prone and supine positions).

AIR-FLUIDIZED SUPPORT BED (CLINITRON)

Air-fluidized beds contain silicone-coated glass beads. Heated-pressured air flows through beads to support the patient. This type of bed may be indicated when the patient needs skin protection due to (1) an inability to easily change positions; (2) extensive pressure sores or risk; (3) extensive recent skin grafts; or (4) patient requirements of prolonged immobilization.

Issue	LOC	Sources	Affil	Rationale/Comment
Anthropometric	Disadvantages	Pierson and Fairchild, 2002[5]	PT	Tall and obese patients may not be comfortable in this bed.
CPR—poor surface rigidity				The bed may not be rigid enough to allow for effective chest compressions during CPR. A rigid wooden or plastic device may be needed under patient.
Fluid loss—increased				Evaporation of body fluids increases as air flows across the patient's skin. The patient may require extra fluids to compensate for any fluid loss.
Lung—pooling of fluids				The patient may require frequent position changes as there is a tendency for fluid to pool in lung lobes.
Sharp objects	P			Sharp objects can easily damage the bed cover.

POST-TRAUMA MOBILITY BEDS (KEANE, ROTO-REST)

Post-trauma beds are used to maintain seriously injured patients in stable position and in proper postural alignment. They use adjustable bolsters and allow side-to-side oscillations to reduce the amount of prolonged pressure over skin.

Issue	LOC	Sources	Affil	Rationale/Comment
Adverse responses	Disadvantages	Pierson and Fairchild, 2002[5]	PT	Patients may report motion sickness such as vertigo or nausea.
CPR—poor surface rigidity				The bed may not be rigid enough to allow for effective chest compressions during CPR. A rigid wooden or plastic device may be needed under patient.
Exercise may be restricted				Bolsters may interfere with movement and exercise.
Feelings of isolation				The patient may feel isolated because of a reduced visual orientation.

LOW AIR LOSS THERAPY BED

Low air loss therapy beds are designed with individually controlled pressure air bladders and may be indicated in patients with prolonged immobilization, at high risk of or with existing pressure ulcers.

Issue	LOC	Sources	Affil	Rationale/Comment
CPR—poor surface rigidit	Disadvantages	Pierson and Fairchild, 2002[5]	PT	The bed may not be rigid enough to allow for effective chest compressions during CPR. A rigid wooden or plastic device may be needed under patient.
Sharp objects				Sharp objects puncture air bladders.

Date	Device	Event	Outcome
MDA, 2001[3] **Bed entrapments with poorly fitting rails** Safety notice Online	Death risk from entrapment and asphyxiation of beds fitted with bed rails in poor condition.	Fatal incidences, especially in nursing/ residential homes, have been reported, due to lack of maintenance.	Advice: Bed rails should be compatible with the bed. Once fitted, bed rails should not permit gaps that will allow entrapment of a user's head or body. Rails should be inspected and maintained.
MDA, 2001[4] **Bed entrapments with inverted U-shaped rails** Safety notice Online	Inverted U-shaped bed grab handles, located on the sides of the bed, are used to help patients get in and out of bed or to pull themselves up	Reports of four cases of head entrapment in inverted U-shaped or similarly shaped bed grab handles.	Inverted U-shaped bed grab handles (which have enough space to fit a head through) should not be used to prevent individuals from falling out of bed.

REFERENCES

1. Webster's third new international dictionary. Springfield (MA): Merriam-Webster; 1981.

2. US Food and Drug Administration: FDA safety alert: entrapment hazard with hospital bed side rails. August 23, 1995, Center for Device and Radiological Health. Available at: http://www.fda.gov/cdrh/mdr/. Accessed November 7, 2005.

3. Safety notice SN 2001(35), Bed rails (cotsides) risk of entrapment and asphyxiation, supplement to HN2000(10). Available at: http://www.mhra.gov.uk/. Accessed November 17, 2005.

4. Medical Devices Agency: Bed grab handles: risk of head entrapment, SN 2001 (11). London: Medical Devices Agency; 2001. Available at: http://www.mhra.gov/uk/mda. Accessed November 17, 2005.

5. Pierson FM, Fairchild SL: Principles and techniques of patient care, ed 3. Philadelphia: W.B. Saunders; 2002.

6. Electric beds can kill children (update). Hazard update. Health Dev 18(9):323-325, 1989.

29   ASSISTIVE DEVICES

29.1 Canes

OVERVIEW. Canes are wooden or metal walking devices that are held in one hand and designed to aid in stability and to "take some of the weight off one foot."[1] Straight and quad canes offer one and four points of support, respectively. Hemi-walkers (walk-canes) offer four points of support with a wider base than that provided by a quad cane.[2]

SUMMARY: PRECAUTIONS. Some procedural concerns relate to proper fitting and appropriate use of canes. For example, canes are not designed to unweight a limb of a patient with a protected weight-bearing status. Twenty-six cane-related injuries were reported to the FDA from December 1990 to November 2002; the majority of injuries involved quad canes. Three quad cane-related deaths were reported to the FDA between 1997 and 2003.[3]

OTHER ISSUES. Mechanical failure: Two of the FDA-reported deaths have been associated indirectly with use of a quad cane that snapped **(also see Crutches)**. Note: Because users apply upper extremity force downward through the device, upper limb tissues and the device itself need to be sufficiently strong/healthy to withstand these compressive forces.

CONTRAINDICATIONS AND PRECAUTIONS

PROCEDURAL CONCERNS

Issue	LOC	Sources	Affil	Rationale/Comment
Cane measurement—too high	P	Tan, 1998[4]	MD/PT	Measurements: The cane top should be level with the patient's greater trochanter. Canes measured too high can lead to excessive elbow flexion and fatigue of the shoulder and elbow musculature.
Canes measurement—too low	P			Canes measured too low can result in less support.
Cane—placement	Advice	Pierson and Fairchild, 2002[5]	PT	If the cane is placed too far forward or to the side, it can result in lateral or forward leaning and reduced dynamic stability.
Ferrules—inspect regularly	P	Sainsbury, 1982[6]	OT	Inspect the feet of all products regularly for safety. Replace worn ones.
		Pain et al, 2003[7]	OT	
Quad canes lateral leg position	P	Tan, 1998[4]	MD/PT	Lateral legs of quad canes should projected away from the user during gait.
Weight-bearing precautions	P	Tan, 1998[4]	MD,PT	Do not use canes for patients with restricted weight-bearing gaits such as non–weight-bearing or partial weight-bearing gaits.[8]
	Advice	Schmitz, 2001[8]	PT	
		Pierson and Fairchild, 2002[5]	PT	

ADVERSE EVENTS

FOOD AND DRUG ADMINISTRATION REPORTS

FDA: Cane-Related Injuries[3]

Date	Device	Outcome	
12/12/90 to 11/6/02	26 cane-related injuries have been reported: 17 injuries involved quad canes 9 injuries involved straight canes	Body areas involved: 8 head, neck, nose, face 7 lower extremity (hip, knee thigh, shin, patella, ankle) 6 upper extremity (wrist, elbow, hand) 1 back; 3 ribs 6 unspecified	Injuries included: 9 fractures 8 unspecified 2 lacerations 1 concussion 1 nerve injury 1 sprain 1 laceration 1 bruise 1 seizure

Note: FDA reports do not necessarily establish cause-effect relationships between equipment and injury. Incidences may be due to equipment or user error. Also, some reports are alleged by attorneys.

FDA: Cane-Related Fatalities[3]

Date of Report	Brand	Fatal Event (death)
1/14/03	Quad cane large base	A dialysis patient's foot slipped under the base of the cane, resulting in a sprained ankle and fractured right patella. Following hospitalization, the patient was transferred to a skilled nursing facility for rehabilitation and died from complications due to an unrelated health condition.
2/12/01	Adjustable quad cane	Attorney alleged that while an individual used a quad cane, it snapped, and the individual fell, sustaining injury that subsequently led to death (no details).
2/04/97	Adjustable quad cane	Attorney reported that while an individual was using a quad cane to rise from a chair, the cane snapped and the individual fell, suffering a fractured spine. The individual subsequently died.

Note: Cane-related deaths. MDR and Maude[3] reported deaths.

REFERENCES

1. Eisenberg MG: Dictionary of rehabilitation. New York: Springer; 1995.
2. Miller-Keane encyclopedia and dictionary of medicine, nursing, and allied health, ed 7. Philadelphia: W.B. Saunders; 2003.
3. U.S. Food and Drug Administration: Center for Device and Radiological Health. Available at: http://www.fda.gov/cdrh/mdr/. Accessed November 7, 2005.
4. Tan JC: Practical manual of physical medicine and rehabilitation: diagnostics, therapeutics, and basic problems. St. Louis: Mosby; 1998.
5. Pierson FM, Fairchild SL: Principles and techniques of patient care, ed 3. Philadelphia: Saunders; 2002.
6. Sainsbury R, Mulley G: Walking sticks used by the elderly. BMJ 284:1751, 1982
7. Pain H, McLellan L, Gore S: Choosing assistive devices: A guide for users and professionals. London: Jessica Kingsley; 2003.
8. Schmitz TJ: Preambulation and gait training. In: O'Sullivan SB, Schmitz TJ, eds: Physical rehabilitation and treatment, ed 4. Philadelphia: F.A. Davis; 2001.

29.2 Crutches

OVERVIEW. Crutches are wooden or metal walking devices that extend from the floor to the vicinity of the elbow or the axilla. Axillary crutches terminate proximally with cross bars near the user's axilla, whereas forearm crutches (Loftstrand) end proximally with hinged open cuffs located just below the elbow.[1]

SUMMARY: CONTRAINDICATIONS AND PRECAUTIONS. Crutch concerns tend to be either musculoskeletal (arthritis, weakness), device-related (worn tips), or procedural (improper use of crutches). Cases report poor crutch usage, which has resulted in vascular (thrombosis) or neurological complications (neuropraxia).[2,3]

OTHER ISSUES. Note 1: Mechanical failure: While great emphasis has been placed on monitoring crutch tips for wear, the majority of crutch-related injuries reported to the FDA appear to have been mechanical failure-related (e.g., metal cracking, bolt failure). Only seven of 38 reported incidences involved the patient slipping.[4]

Note 2: Users apply downward force through the device in order to ambulate. Upper limb tissue (i.e., joints, bones, skin) and the device itself should be sufficiently strong/healthy to withstand these compression forces.

CONTRAINDICATIONS AND PRECAUTIONS

M00-M99 DISEASES OF THE MUSCULOSKELETAL SYSTEM AND CONNECTIVE TISSUE

Issue	LOC	Sources	Affil	Rationale/Comment
Arthritis—hand and wrist	CI	Schmitz, 2001[5a]	PT	Weight-bearing through arthritic hand and wrist is considered contraindicated. Use platform attachment on assistive device.
Weakness—upper limbs	P	Tan, 1998[6]	MD/PT	Adequate strength is needed to use crutches. A user should have sufficient strength to raise body 1 to 2 inches off floor.

a, In some arthritic patients.

Y70-Y82 MEDICAL DEVICES

Issue	LOC	Sources	Affil	Rationale/Comment
Crutch tips—worn	P	Tan, 1998[6] Pain et al, 2003[7]	MD OT	Monitor wear of tips and regularly inspect all products with feet for safety. Replace worn ones.

PROCEDURAL CONCERNS

Issue	LOC	Sources	Affil	Rationale/Comment
Crutches placement	Advice	Schmitz, 2001[5]	PT	Avoid parallel crutch and feet alignment because a parallel arrangement will decrease the base of support and affect the stability of the user. Keep crutches at least 4 inches in front and to the side of each foot, even at rest.[5]
Crowds/Small spaces	Disadvantage	Schmitz, 2001[5]	PT	For axillary crutch use, the base of the support (tripod configuration) may be awkward for the patient when ambulating in small spaces or in crowds.[5]
Posture/Leaning on pads	P	Tan, 1998[6]	MD/PT	Do not lean on axillary crutch pads for prolonged periods. Body weight should be borne through the hands rather than the bar or pads.[5] Leaning can lead to compressive forces in the axilla region with resultant neural and vascular damage.
	Advice/ Disadvantage	Schmitz, 2001[5]	PT	
		Pierson and Fairchild, 2002[8]	PT	
	P			**See crutch palsy case reports by Chevalier[2] in 2002 and by Poddar[3] in 1993, below.**
Training	P	Tan, 1998[6]	MD/PT	All patients should be properly trained in crutch use.[6]
Turning with crutches	Advice	Schmitz, 2001[5]	PT	Avoid pivoting on a single extremity because a small base of support can lead to a potential loss of balance. Instead, step in small circles.[5]

ADVERSE EVENTS

FDA REPORTS: CRUTCH-RELATED INJURIES

Source	Background	Incidence	Outcome	Interpretation/Comments
FDA[4] MDR and Maude Reports 5/07/93 to 7/02/96 5/03/88 to 4/16/93 5/7/87 to 4/25/88 **Crutches injuries**	38 reports of crutch-related injuries (involving both axillary and metal forearm devices).	Injury mechanism: General failure (broke, shattered) ($n = 17$) Connector, rivet, pin, bolt failure ($n = 9$) Slip ($n = 7$) Unknown ($n = 3$) Fit problem ($n = 1$) Chemical ($n = 1$)	Injury type: 41 reported injuries with crutches (more than one injury per event could occur) 22 nonspecific 8 fractures 4 bleeding, edema 2 lacerations 2 dislocations 1 tear 1 allergic rash 1 cast	Notes: Crutch type was not consistently reported (i.e., only three forearm and four laminated wood crutches were specified). It is difficult to determine from reports whether failure of the crutch resulted in falls or falls resulted in a broken crutch. Slips may be associated with worn crutch tips, but this was not specifically reported by FDA.

Note: FDA reports do not necessarily establish cause-effect relationships between equipment and injury. Incidences may be due to equipment or user error. Also, some reports are alleged by attorneys.

Source	Background	Incidence	Outcome	Interpretation/Comments
Chevalier et al, 2002[2] **Axillary crutch use and thrombosis** Case report from abstract (article in French) J Mal Vasc	A 65-year-old woman with childhood poliomyelitis and a 30-cm LLD used axillary crutches and presented with a subacute ischemia of right upper limb.	Dx: Axillary aneurysm with thrombosis due to chronic use of axillary crutches.	Treatment involved resection graft of aneurysm and thrombectomy to restore patency.	The authors state axillary crutches may result in arterial stenosis or aneurysms which can be further complicated by thrombosis, embolization, or axillary mass formation.
Poddar et al, 1993[3] **Axillary crutch use and radial palsy** Case report Clin Orthop Rel Res	A thin, 13-year-old boy with osteomyelitis of the left proximal tibial metaphysis (treated with IV antibiotics), with one leg casted and non–weight-bearing, was instructed on proper use of axillary crutches by physiotherapist.	After 5 weeks of crutch use, soreness in arms and forearms and inability to extend wrists bilaterally occurred. He could no longer use crutches. The neurological exam revealed a bilateral paresis of the radial, median, and ulnar nerves, with predominately radial involvement.	Dx: Bilateral (left worse) radial neuropraxia. EMG revealed denervation and recruitment of radial innervated muscles. A cast was reapplied and the crutches were discontinued. After 1 month, some recovery was noted; after 2-month follow-up, full recovery was observed.	The authors believe the radial nerve was affected due to its lateral location its closeness to the proximal humerus as compared with other nerves. Instruct patient not to bear excessive weight on the axillary bar. Consider forearm crutches (in pediatric patients). Caution user of axillary crutches of potential complication for detections.

REFERENCES

1. Eisenberg MG: Dictionary of rehabilitation. New York: Springer; 1995.
2. Chevalier J, Joly P, Dhoine P: Axillary aneurysm and crutches. J Mal Vasc 27(1):36-38, 2002.

3. Poddar SB, Gitelis S, Heydemann PT, et al: Bilateral predominant radial nerve crutch palsy. A case report. Clin Orthop Rel Res 297:245-246, 1993.
4. US Food and Drug Administration: Center for Device and Radiological Health. Available at: http://www.fda.gov/cdrh/mdr/. Accessed November 7, 2005.
5. Schmitz TJ: Preambulation and gait training. In: O'Sullivan SB, Schmitz TJ, eds: Physical rehabilitation and treatment, ed 4. Philadelphia: F.A. Davis; 2001.
6. Tan JC: Practical manual of physical medicine and rehabilitation: diagnostics, therapeutics, and basic problems. St. Louis: Mosby; 1998.
7. Pain H, McLellan L, Gore S: Choosing assistive devices: A guide for users and professionals. London: Jessica Kingsley; 2003.
8. Pierson FM, Fairchild SL: Principles and techniques of patient care, ed 3. Philadelphia: Saunders; 2002.

29.3 Lifts, Mechanical

OVERVIEW. A mechanical lift is a hydraulic-, battery-, or mechanically powered device used to lift and transfer or transport a patient in the horizontal or other required position from one place to another. The device includes straps and a sling to support the patient.[1]

SUMMARY: CONTRAINDICATIONS AND PRECAUTIONS. Mechanical lift concerns are either device-related (appropriate model for the task) or procedural-related (proper use of the device during transfers; proper maintenance).[2,3] Thirty-two lift-related deaths have been reported to the FDA from 1990 to 2002. In almost 80% of these cases, deaths were sling or strap related.[1]

CONTRAINDICATIONS AND PRECAUTIONS

Y70-Y82 MEDICAL DEVICES

Issue	LOC	Sources	Affil	Rationale/Comment
Load capacity	Advice	Health Devices, 1990[3,b]	Agency	Lifts should be designed to support at least 150% of its capacity rating to account for dynamic loading due to motion of the patient.
Type of activity	Recommendations	ECRI, 1997[2,a]		Ask if the lift is designed for transfers or for transportation, and use accordingly.
				Dynamic loading, which occurs during travel, may damage a lift if it is not intended for transportation of more than 1 to 2 feet.
				Most lifts are not designed to withstand dynamic loading (traveling with patient in the sling).
Type of residence	Advice	Health Devices, 1990[3]		Ask if the lift is designed for home or institutional use, and use accordingly. Some lifts cannot accommodate all patient sizes/weights for use in institutions. Some lifts are not designed to lift more than 200 lb and should be labeled accordingly.

a, The ECRI is a nonprofit, independent health services research agency that aims at improving the quality, cost-effectiveness, and safety of healthcare; b, *Health Devices* is the journal for the Emergency Care Research Institute (ECRI).

PROCEDURAL CONCERNS

Issue	LOC	Sources	Affil	Rationale/Comment
Environment—safety	Advice	Health Devices, 1990[3]	Agency	Clear floor of objects that should be avoided, such as throw rugs and cords.
Fabric slings—replacement	Advice			Fabric slings are not considered durable medical equipment and should be replaced every 1 to 3 years.
Inspection policy	Recommendations	ECRI, 1997[2]		Develop a policy for mechanical lift inspections and maintenance that includes:
				• Lifting mechanism
				• Hydraulic leaks (if hydraulic)
				• Frame/welds/cracks/signs of failure
				• Fasteners secured, i.e., chains, pins
				• Sling fabric wear
				• Hinges
				• Brakes
				• Casters
				Suggest inspections/maintenance every 6 months initially; less often later if warranted.
Leg position (of lift)	Advice	Health Devices, 1990[3]	Agency	The U bases on lifts can be unstable if the legs are closed. Spread U-shaped base open prior to using lift with patients.
Lift stability	Caution			All lifts may be unstable if moved abruptly.[3]
Service	Recommendations	ECRI, 1997[2]		Remove lifts with problems from service until corrected.
Valve position (of lift)	Caution			Valve on lifts must be closed. Prevent adjustable bar from descending and striking the patient's head when the patient has been lowered to the proper level.
Work space—sufficient	Advice			Have sufficient space to maneuver the lift.

ADVERSE EVENTS

Source	Background	Therapy	Outcome	Comment
Evaluation of patient lifts Descriptive Health Devices, 1990[3]	Fifteen patient lifts from eight manufacturers were evaluated for safety, human factors, and the design of the lifts and supports.	Healthy men and women ages 20 to 40 years with clinical experience but no disabilities participated in the testing.	Some lifts were better suited for home or for institutional use. Seven lifts (Arjo 218150; Handi-Move 1200; Hoyer C-CBL; Invacare 9901, 9916, 9917; and Porto-lift PL-1) were all rated acceptable for both home and institutional use. Hoyer C-HLA, Invacare 9902, Trans-Aid LAT-2 were Conditionally Acceptable—Not Recommended for institutional use because they should not be used with patients more than 200 lb. Century C-3 lift was Conditionally Acceptable—Not Recommended for home use because it was awkward to maneuver in narrow corridors with base fully extended.	Reported lift problems included: • Structural failure • Lift mechanism failure • Caster or brake failure • Overturning due to instability of lift Staff reported overturning as a frequent potential cause of patient injury.

FDA[1] MECHANICAL LIFT-RELATED DEATHS

Dates	Outcome	Possible Contributing Factors
MDR 7/26/96-8/31/90 and Maude 9/23/96-3/14/2002	34 deaths	• 14 strap not secured, slipped off, unhooked, knocked off, tangled • 7 patient fell from sling • 3 sling ripped • 2 incorrect sling size (from another company) • 1 poor positioning in sling • 1 leg not locked • 1 tripped on carpet • 1 foot support cracked • 1 broken lift in use • 1 worn hardware part • 1 wheel fell off • 1 unknown

REFERENCES

1. U.S. Food and Drug Administration: Center for Device and Radiological Health. Available at: http://www.fda.gov/cdrh/mdr/. Accessed November 7, 2005.
2. Emergency Care Research Institute Problem Reporting System: Proper use and inspection of patient lifts. Health Dev 26(6):254-255, 1997.
3. Anonymous: Patient lifts. Health Dev 19(3):67-96, 1990.

29.4 Vibratory Devices

OVERVIEW. A vibrator is a hand-held device that is powered by AC or battery and used to (1) stimulate muscle contraction in paralyzed muscles, (2) assist in postural drainage (used over the thorax), or (3) modulate pain (over acupuncture points).[1,2]

SUMMARY: CONTRAINDICATIONS AND PRECAUTIONS. Vibration-related concerns include (1) dosage settings (excessive amplitude or frequencies) that may irritate skin or (2) vibration use in some neurological populations where stimulation may facilitate unwanted responses (in the latter case, vibration has been used or suggested as an aid in diagnosis).

CONTRAINDICATIONS AND PRECAUTIONS

G00-G99 DISEASES OF THE NERVOUS SYSTEM

Issue	LOC	Sources	Affil	Rationale/Comment
Vibration with cerebellar dysfunction	Advice	Bishop, 1975[3]	PT	Vibration can reveal latent motor problems. In individuals with cerebellar disease, vibration may induced choreoathetotic movements.[3]

I00-I99 DISEASES OF THE CIRCULATORY SYSTEM

Issue	LOC	Sources	Affil	Rationale/Comment
Blood clots/immobilized areas	Caution	Umphred, 1995[2]	PT	There is an embolic concern of dislodging clots located in immobilized areas with vibration.

L00-L99 DISEASES OF THE SKIN & SUBCUTANEOUS TISSUE

Issue	LOC	Sources	Affil	Rationale/Comment
Skin—elasticity loss		Umphred, 1995[2]	PT	Friction of thin skin during vibration may cause tissue tears.

PROCEDURAL CONCERNS

Issue	LOC	Sources	Affil	Rationale/Comment
Amplitude—high	Advice	Umphred, 1995[2]	PT	Potentially, high-amplitude vibration can lead to skin ulceration.
Frequency—high, >200 Hz	Advice			Frequencies over 150 Hz can lead to discomfort and pain, whereas frequencies over 200 Hz can damage skin.
Infants	Caution			An unmyelinated nervous system may be overly stimulated from vibration.

REFERENCES

1. Eisenberg MG: Dictionary of rehabilitation. New York: Springer; 1995.
2. Umphred DA: Classification of treatment techniques based on primary input systems: Inherent and contrived feedback/loops systems and their potential influence on altering a feedforward motor system. In: Umphred DA, editor: Neurological rehabilitation. St. Louis: Mosby; 1995.
3. Bishop B: Vibration stimulation II. Vibratory stimulation as an evaluation tool. Phys Ther 55:29-33, 1975.

29.5 Walkers

OVERVIEW. A walker is a mechanical device with four legs and a metal frame used to provide moderate weight support while ambulating.[1]

SUMMARY: CONTRAINDICATIONS AND PRECAUTIONS. Adult walker concerns tend to be procedural[2-4] (e.g., using the device properly, monitoring it for wear). Other concerns are device-related (i.e., difficulty in managing a component part).[2] Three deaths and about 133 injuries have been reported to the FDA over a 14-year period (from 11/11/91 to 8/06/04).[1] In a separate matter, both the American Academy of Pediatrics[5,6] and the Consumer Product Safety Commission[7] have voiced grave safety concerns over use of infant (baby) walkers, where 34 related deaths have occurred from 1973 to 2001.

CONTRAINDICATIONS AND PRECAUTIONS

M00-M99 DISEASES OF THE MUSCULOSKELETAL SYSTEM AND CONNECTIVE TISSUE

Issue	LOC	Sources	Affil	Rationale/Comment
Arthritis—hand and wrist	CI	Schmitz, 2001[4,5,a]	PT	Weight-bearing through an arthritic hand and wrist is considered contraindicated. Use a platform attachment on the assistive device.

a, In some arthritic patients.

Issue	LOC	Sources	Affil	Rationale/Comment
Brakes—pressure activated **Brakes—cable**	Advice	Pain et al, 2003[2]	OT	Pressure brakes (where one presses down on wheeled walkers to engage brakes) may not be appropriate for people with painful wrists or who have a "slight" body type. Cable brakes (where users curl their fingers around the device and then squeeze to engage brakes) may be difficult to operate for a person with painful arthritic hands.

PROCEDURAL CONCERNS

Issue	LOC	Sources	Affil	Rationale/Comment
Rubber ferrules—inspect	Advice	Pain et al, 2003[2]	OT	Regularly inspect for safety on all products with feet. Replace worn feet.
Walker—folding-locking mechanism				Folding models are less stable when one places weight on them (they "give way a little").
Walker—folding—stability				Monitor the locking mechanism on folding wheeled walking frames regularly.
Walker—levelness	Advice	McConnell, 2001[3]	Nurs	Confirm that walker is level before patient uses it (i.e., after adjusting its height).
Walker—reciprocal	Advice	Schmitz, 2001[4]	PT	Some stability is lost with this type of walker.
Walker—seats surfaces				Assess the stability of the seat surface.
Walker—stair-climbing	Avoid			These walkers are extremely unsafe on stairs and should be avoided.
Walker—stepping too close to crossbar	Caution			Stepping too close to walker's crossbar can decrease the user's base of support and may increase risk of falls.
Wheel—rolling, attachments				Stability of the walker is reduced.

ADVERSE EVENTS

INFANT WALKERS

Issue	LOC	Sources	Affil	Rationale/Comment
Pediatrics, 2001[5] **Infant walker** The AAP recommends a ban on sale and manufacturer of infant walkers.	Position statement	AAP, 2001[5]	Academy	There is considerable risk for major and minor injuries (with unclear benefits) using infant walkers.[5,6] The Academy suggests a stationary activity center as a safer alternative to mobile walkers for infants. Those parents who insist on using an infant walker should use walkers that meet ASTM F977-96 standards (i.e., wider than 36-inch doorway, and braking system) to prevent rolling down steps.

CPSC REPORTS

Date	Device	Event		Comment
CPSC, 2001[7] **Infant walkers and deaths** Announcement Online	US CPSC indicates children sustain injuries from baby walkers more than any other nursery product.	Most injuries are related to falls down stairs. Since 1973, 34 walker-related deaths have been reported.	New standards certified by the Juvenile Products manufacturers Association. Two requirements: The walker must be too wide to fit through standard doorway	Other alternative: stationary activity center (no wheels). Safety tips: • Gate on top of stairs; close the door • Visually monitor children • Keep child away from hot surfaces • Keep child away from water (toilet, pools) • Caution with regard to dangling appliance cords

or The walker must have gripping mechanism to stop at edge of a step.	• Avoid areas of uneven floors such as carpet edges that may lead to tip-overs (From: Consumer Product Safety Alert: Stair Steps and Baby Walkers Don't Mix)

FDA REPORTS[1]

Date	Device	Event	Outcome
Walker use and death[1] 10/22/93	Guardian walker	The user was sitting at the edge of the bed and tried to use the walker to stand. The user fell, hit head, and was admitted to an ICU.	The user died a few days later.

Note: FDA reports do not necessarily establish cause-effect relationships between equipment and injury. Incidences may be due to equipment or user error. Also, some reports are alleged by attorneys.

MDA

Date	Device	Event	Comment
MDA, June 2001[8] **Tri-wheel walkers and collapsing** Safety notice On line	Three-wheeled walkers (i.e., one wheel in front), also called rollators, delta walkers, or tri-wheel walkers	There are reports of tri-wheel walkers in the UK collapsing during use and causing serious injury because of loose central-locking mechanisms. Other safety concerns include brake adjustment, locking handles (for height adjustments), front wheel movement, and inadequate maintenance instructions.	Inspect the central locking mechanism (Is it loose or missing?). Tighten all fasteners (screws, nuts, bolts) and locking handles. Check that front wheel (caster) freely swivels.

REFERENCES

1. U.S. Food and Drug Administration: Center for Device and Radiological Health. Available at: http://www.fda.gov/cdrh/mdr/. Accessed November 7, 2005

2. Pain H, McLellan L, Gore S: Choosing assistive devices: A guide for users and professionals. London: Jessica Kingsley; 2003.

3. McConnell EA: Clinical do's and don'ts: teaching your patient to use a stationary walker. Nursing 31(10):17, 2001.

4. Schmitz TJ: Preambulation and gait training. In: O'Sullivan SB, Schmitz TJ, eds: Physical rehabilitation and treatment, ed 4. Philadelphia: F.A. Davis; 2001.

5. American Academy of Pediatrics Committee on Injury and Poison Prevention: Injuries associated with infant walkers. Pediatrics 108(3): 790-792, 2001.

6. Siegel AC, Burton RV: Effects of baby walkers on motor and mental development in human infants. J Dev Behav Pediatr 20(5):355-361, 1999.

7. Consumer Product Safety Commission: CPSC gets new, safer baby walkers on the market, CPSC Document # 5086. Available at: http://www.cpsc.gov/CPSCPUB/PUBS/5086.pdf. Accessed November 17, 2005.

8. Medical Devices Agency: Rollators: risk of collapse and other issues, SN 2001 (16). London: Medical Devices Agency; 2001. Available at: http://www.medical-devices.gov.uk. Accessed November 7, 2005.

29.6 Manual Wheelchairs

OVERVIEW. A manual wheelchair is a locomotor device consisting of a seat and wheels which can be self-propelled or pushed by an attendant.[1]

SUMMARY: CONTRAINDICATIONS AND PRECAUTIONS. Few authorities have published contraindication guidelines for wheelchairs. Tan[2] mentions nine concerns, three of which are absolute: poor judgment, blindness, and ischial ulcers. The largest proportion of concerns are musculoskeletal related. Three concerns appear directed toward individuals who either self-propel (i.e., visual concerns) or only have access to standard wheelchairs (i.e., devices that may not address postural defects or trunk weakness).

Adverse events (injuries and deaths) reported to the FDA include tipping (falling out of wheelchair), burns while in the chair, and asphyxiation (from the device or straps).

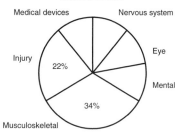

Proportion of Concerns for Manual Wheelchairs Based in ICD

Medical devices
Nervous system
Injury
22%
Eye
Mental
34%
Musculoskeletal

CONTRAINDICATIONS AND PRECAUTIONS

F00-F99 MENTAL AND BEHAVIORAL DISORDERS

Issue	LOC	Sources	Affil	Rationale/Comment
Judgment—poor	ACI	Tan, 1998[2]	MD/PT	

G00-G99 DISEASES OF THE NERVOUS SYSTEM

Issue	LOC	Sources	Affil	Rationale/Comment
Nerve compression—disc	RCI	Tan, 1998[2]	MD/PT	

H00-H59 DISEASES OF THE EYE

Issue	LOC	Sources	Affil	Rationale/Comment
Blindness	ACI	Tan, 1998[2]	MD/PT	

M00-M99 DISEASES OF THE MUSCULOSKELETAL SYSTEM AND CONNECTIVE TISSUE

Issue	LOC	Sources	Affil	Rationale/Comment
Orthopedic condition—postop	RCI	Tan, 1998[2]	MD/PT	Pelvic or proximal femur surgical postop condition.
Postural defects	RCI			
Trunk weakness	RCI			

S00-T98 INJURY, POISONING, AND CERTAIN OTHER CONSEQUENCES OF EXTERNAL CAUSES

Issue	LOC	Sources	Affil	Rationale/Comment
Fracture—vertebral	RCI	Tan, 1998[2]	MD/PT	
Pressure ulcer—ischial	ACI			Consider prone positioning on a gurney.

Y70-Y82 MEDICAL DEVICES

Issue	LOC	Sources	Affil	Rationale/Comment
Latex equipment—related allergies Positional devices containing latex: • Wheelchair wheels • Wheelchair cushions • Wheelchair seat backs	Avoid	Scoggin and Parks, 1997[3]	OT	Protein in the rubber has a cumulative effect from exposure early in life and from multiple surgical interventions. Responses include watery eyes, hives, sneezing, nasal congestion, wheezing, local rashes, and coughing. Life-threatening anaphylactic shock associated with latex gloves and materials during medical procedures is also noted. Consider fabric covers or blanket rolls over positioning devices if a user is allergic to latex. **Individuals with spina bifida are particularly susceptible.**

WHEELCHAIR TRANSPORTATION IN MOTOR VEHICLES: ISSUES

Issue	LOC	Sources	Affil	Rationale/Comment
Unoccupied wheelchairs—securing The unoccupied wheelchair should be secured if the individual is removed from the wheelchair (i.e., into appropriate, approved, safe seating), during transportation. **Fastening device—to floor** Secure wheelchairs with a fastening device that is attached to the floor.	Recommend	AAP, 2001[4]	MD/Academy	The procedure helps to prevent the device from becoming a dangerous projectile in the event of a crash or sudden vehicle stop. As of August 2001, most wheelchairs have not been manufactured as certified transit devices and are not subjected to crash-testing requirements. If occupied, it should have a four-point tie-down device (tested) capable of restraining the wheelchair during frontal impact at 30 mph and 20 g.

Restraint system—to wheelchair frame	The restraint system should be attached to the frame of the wheelchair, not to the occupant, and not to the wheels of the wheelchair.
Orientation of person—forward facing	For persons occupying wheelchairs: they should be secured in a forward-facing position.

ADVERSE EVENTS

WHEELCHAIR-RELATED INJURIES

Source	Background	Event	Outcome	Comment
Dudley et al, 1992[5] **Wheelchair accidents** Descriptive (random questionnaire) Clin Rehab	A random sample of wheelchair users (250 of 4334) in Leeds Eastern Health District (UK) was surveyed with a 91% response rate.	Reports of wheelchair accidents	A total of 174 questionnaires were completed; 48 respondents reported wheelchair accidents to self or another. 97% of accidents reported by wheelchair user involved falls.	Author recommendations: 1. Regular wheelchair maintenance, 2. Educate attendant on folding wheelchair 3. Environment-friendly curbs

Continued

Source	Background	Event	Outcome	Comment
Gray, 1992[6] **Falls** Descriptive Dev Med Child Neurol	Muscle disease clinic and hospital describe wheelchair-dependent children (at least 1 year) with neuromuscular disease falling out of wheelchairs with resulting fractures.	Diagnoses of those who fell: 11 Duchenne muscular dystrophy 1 Becker muscular dystrophy 1 spinal muscular atrophy	Falls (8) Slips out of wheelchair (3) [worn seat belt (1)] Tips during transfers (2) Falls off wheelchair ramp (1)	Author stresses importance of (1) proper fit, (2) operation on all surfaces, (3) proper positioning and use of seat belt (not positioned high around waist area)
James, 1970[7] **Fall** Case report (potential litigation) Phys Ther	15-year-old wheelchair-dependent girl with cerebral palsy attended PT at a hospital.	As PT stepped from front to rear of wheelchair to move patient into the treatment area, the patient fell face forward out of the wheelchair.	The girl dislodged upper front tooth, broke adjoining capped tooth, bruised nose severely, and blackened both eyes. The parents initiated legal action against the hospital but dropped the case later because of the excellent rapport between the parents, patient, and PT.	The PT's insurance company paid $424.43 in dental and other expenses. (Note: No information provided about seatbelt use.)
Kirby and Ackroyd-Stolarz, 1995[8] **Wheelchair injuries** Database review Am J Phys Med Rehab	Wheelchair injury reports received by the FDA from 1975 to 1993 were reviewed.	651 adverse reports identified Injury type • 45.5%: fracture • 22.3%: contusion/abrasion • 20.1%: other Device involved • 52.8%: scooters • 24.6%: power wheelchair • 22.6%: manual wheelchair	Contributing factors • 60.5%: engineering • 25.4%: environmental • 9.6%: occupant • 4.6%: system Tip direction: most common • Forward—manual and power • Sideways—scooters	Authors state: "Use of these devices is not without risk" Three most common environmental factors: • 26.3% inclined, ramp, curb cuts • 21.9% change in surface • 21.5% driveway, street, sidewalk

Ummat and Kirby, 1994[9] **Wheelchair accidents** Database review Am J Phys Med Rehab	The National Electronic Injury Surveillance System (NEISS) databases (representative of US emergency rooms) from 1986 to 1990, 1991, and 1992 of nonfatal wheelchair-related accidents.	Reviewed data from 127 ERs; 2066 accidents were identified. An average national estimate of 36,559 accidents per year were serious enough to require ER visits ($P = .007$) with an upward trend over time.	Causes • 73.2% falls and tips • 41.4% ramps • 16.9% transfers Locations • 50.8% at home Types of injuries • 32.8% contusions/abrasions • 28% lacerations • 20.2% fractures • 10.3% sprains and strains	NEISS uses a national probability sample of all hospital ERs in the US and territories. Note: Data do not include accidents not resulting in ER visits (i.e., less serious injuries).

STAIR-CLIMBING WHEELCHAIR-RELATED INJURIES

FDA Reports[1]

Date of Report	Brand	Event
8/08/88	Quadra stair-climbing wheelchair	The user fell and fractured the hip when a wheel came off the unit while on the stairs.
12/30/86	Model 40 stair	A rivet that holds the handles on came loose and resulted in a fall but no injuries.

FDA Reports: Stair-climbing wheelchair (IMK)

WHEELCHAIR-RELATED FATALITIES

Source	Background	Therapy	Outcome	Follow-up/Interpretation
Calder and Kirby, 1990[10] Database review Am J Phys Med Rehab	Death certificates from a complete database from 1973 to 1987 from the National Information Clearinghouse, Consumer Product Safety Commission were reviewed.	770 wheelchair-related deaths were identified: • 77.4% falls and tips • 11% environmental (stairs in 60%) • 6.2% fatal burns (57% smoking-related) • 5.7% asphyxia from restraints	Location • 52.9% institutions • 27.5% home • 7.9% hospitals	Authors indicate some fatalities are preventable: • Transfer-related—viewed as high risk activity ($n = 70$): consider (1) training, (2) turning casters in forward position to increase device stability • Smoking-related—presumably in weak, immobile, decreased mental facility: (1) fire-retardant clothes, (2) use smoke detectors • Restraint-related: (1) monitor and (2) proper design • Environment (e.g., stairs): take into consideration

FDA Reports[1]: Fatalities

Date of Report	Brand	Fatal Event
11/21/2002	Breezy	User did not engage wheel locks, rolled down a slope, could not stop, and ran into a metal fence. The user sustained multiple fractures and, after 2 months, developed a lung infection.
11/20/02	Activx	User fell rearward from wheelchair in exercise room of a nursing home. Push canes were broken. Anti-tippers had been cut down to increase clearance for attendant.
10/17/02	Wheelchair, transport	User fell backward and hit head.

11/19/2001	Quickie	User was transported from school to home, did not recline wheelchair or secure with pin, and fell off lift. The wheelchair tipped forward and user hit head, developed a hematoma, and died 5 days later.
09/11/01	Invacare manual wheelchair	User fell out of wheelchair and hit head.
02/22/01	Tracer	User tipped out of wheelchair while traveling in a van, fractured leg and subsequently died. The wheelchair was not properly secured in the van and tipped over when the van took a sharp turn.
07/10/00	Mechanical wheelchair	An attendant transported wheelchair backwards up a ramp. The left handgrip came off the wheelchair and wheelchair rolled down a ramp and tipped. The user hit head.
02/24/99	Quickie P210	Wheelchair overturned on patient, pinning patient and crushing throat, resulting in traumatic asphyxia.
11/05/98	Ride-Lite 9000	User dropped lighter on lap and was engulfed in flames.
10/31/98	Rolls 1000	User dropped a burning sponge curler on lap.
12/22/97	Ride-Lite 9000	Short sleeve caught on fire when user was in contact with burning stove. User sustained second- and third-degree burns and later died.
08/15/97	Tracer	Patient found out of chair on floor, wheelchair tipped forward, and seat belt around neck, allegedly resulting in death.
07/31/96	Rolls 1000E	User was transported in a van using a "tie down" system (manual warned against this manner of transportation). The rear wheel bent and the user struck her head on side of the van. A head injury and death ensued.
10/25/95	Quickie manual wheelchair	A child pulled own feet out of restraint, slid down the chair, and was caught on the position belt; child suffered positioning asphyxia.
09/21/94	Quickie	While crossing a threshold from room to room, a wheelchair flipped backwards and the user fractured a rib.
08/26/93	Rolls 4000	User was sitting at the front edge of the seat, leaned forward to pick up something, tipped the wheelchair and struck head on floor. The user developed cerebral edema and expired 3 days later. The chair was equipped with front anti-tippers.
04/26/91	Quickie wheelchair	Attorney alleged user slid down chair and strangled by chest brace on wheelchair.
09/18/86	E & J	Attorney alleges wrongful death in rehab center involving a wheelchair. No details.

Note: FDA reports do not necessarily establish cause-effect relationships between equipment and injury. Incidents may be due to equipment or user error. Also, some reports are alleged by attorneys.

REFERENCES

1. U.S. Food and Drug Administration: Center for Device and Radiological Health. Available at: http://www.fda.gov/cdrh/mdr/. Accessed November 7, 2005
2. Tan JC: Practical manual of physical medicine and rehabilitation: diagnostics, therapeutics, and basic problems. St. Louis: Mosby; 1998.
3. Scoggin AE, Parks KM: Latex sensitivity in children with spina bifida: implications for occupational therapy practitioners. Am J Occup Ther 51(7):608-611, 1997.
4. American Academy of Pediatrics, Committee on Injury and Poison Prevention: School bus transportation of children with special health care needs. Pediatrics 108(2):516-518, 2001.
5. Dudley NJ, Cotter DHG, Mulley GP: Wheelchair-related accidents. Clin Rehab 6(3):189-194, 1992.
6. Gray B, Hsu JD, Furumasu J: Fractures caused by falling from a wheelchair in patients with neuromuscular disease. Dev Med Child Neurol 34(7):589-592, 1992.
7. James CA Jr: Medico-legal considerations in the practice of physical therapy. Phys Ther 50(8):1203-1207, 1970.
8. Kirby RL, Ackroyd-Stolarz SA: Wheelchair safety—adverse reports to the United States Food and Drug Administration. Am J Phys Med Rehab 74(4):308-312, 1995.
9. Ummat S, Kirby RL: Nonfatal wheelchair related accidents reported to the National Electronic Injury Surveillance System. Am J Phys Med Rehab 73(3):163-167, 1994.
10. Calder CJ, Kirby RL: Fatal wheelchair-related accidents in the United States. Am J Phys Med Rehab 69(4):184-190, 1990.

29.7 Power Mobility (Power Wheelchairs and Scooters)

OVERVIEW. A powered wheelchair is a battery-operated device with a frame and wheels that is used to provide locomotion to persons restricted to a sitting position.[1] Power scooters (i.e., golf cart–like devices), which generally require better manipulative, transfer, and sitting skills than power wheelchairs, are also included under Adverse Events.

SUMMARY: CONTRAINDICATIONS AND PRECAUTIONS. Few sources have published formal guidelines for power wheelchairs. Four sources, who offer nine nonoverlapping concerns, are included below. Three Medical Devices concerns center around electromagnetic interference (erratic power performance), latex allergies (from wheelchair components), and O_2 cylinder placement near power wheelchairs (i.e., sparks, flash fires, explosions).

Note: Other concerns such as ischial pressure ulcers, mentioned under manual wheelchairs, may also be applicable for power mobility (**also see Manual wheelchairs**).

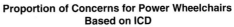

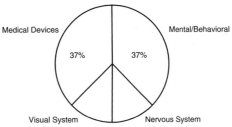

CONTRAINDICATIONS AND PRECAUTIONS

POWER WHEELCHAIR

F00-F99 MENTAL AND BEHAVIORAL DISORDERS

Issue	LOC	Sources	Affil	Rationale/Comment
Inattention	CI	Tan, 1998[2]	MD/PT	
Irresponsibility	CI			
Poor judgment	CI			

G00-G99 DISEASES OF THE NERVOUS SYSTEM

Issue	LOC	Sources	Affil	Rationale/Comment
Inability to control switches	CI	Tan, 1998[2]	MD/PT	
Involuntary motions	CI			

Issue	LOC	Sources	Affil	Rationale/Comment
Blindness	CI	Tan, 1998[2]	MD/PT	**Note: In 1998, Greenbaum argued that visual limitations were not an absolute CI for power mobility. The author described a case of an individual who was legally blind but was able to operate a power wheelchair with the aid of a guide dog.**

Medical Devices

Issue	LOC	Sources	Affil	Rationale/Comment
Electromagnetic interference (EMI) Signals in the environment (electromagnetic energy) may be a potential hazard to users of power wheelchairs and power scooters, causing erratic unintentional movements with instances of serious injury.	Advice	FDA, 1994[3]	Gov	**In 1994, Witters and Ruggera[5] demonstrated EMI susceptibility in both power wheelchairs and scooters when examining the performance of brake release and wheel movements in these devices.** Electromagnetic interference (and steps to protect from EMI hazards): Power wheelchairs/scooters should have a minimal immunity level of 20 volts per meter (a reasonable protection from common EMI sources). The higher the value, the better the protection. Warn that additional components or modification of the chair may make it more susceptible to EMI. Inform user of EMI problems (i.e., radio-wave sources). Do not turn on hand-held communication devices such as CB radios, walkie-talkies, or cellular phones while the wheelchair is turned on.

Continued

Issue	LOC	Sources	Affil	Rationale/Comment
				Avoid coming close to nearby transmitters such as radio/TV stations. Mobile transceivers include police, fire, ambulance, and taxi vehicles. (Cordless telephones, laptop computers, AM/FM radios, TV sets, CD players, electric shavers, and hair dryers are less likely to cause EMI problems, according to an FDA letter of 1994.[4])
				If unintentional movement occurs, turn off power chair as soon as it is safe to do so. Report incidents to the manufacturer.
Latex equipment—related allergies Positional devices containing latex: • Wheelchair wheels, • Wheelchair cushions, • Wheelchair seat backs	Avoid	Scoggin and Parks, 1997[6]	OT	Protein in the rubber has a cumulative effect from exposure early in life and from multiple surgical interventions. Responses include watery eyes, hives, sneezing, nasal congestion, wheezing, local rashes, coughing; also life-threatening anaphylactic shock associated with latex gloves and materials during medical procedures. Consider fabric covers or blanket rolls over positioning devices if allergic to latex. **Individuals with spina bifida are particularly susceptible.[6]**
Oxygen use and power wheelchairs	Advice on pressured oxygen cylinders near power wheelchair	Health Devices, 1992[7]	Org	The situation is reasonably safe if the O_2 cylinder is secured and protected (immobilized; protect stem and regulator from being broken off or bumped, leading to O_2 leakage and accumulation). Oxygen should not be allowed to accumulate under patient's clothing or near upholstery or electric controls, motor, or battery. • Never smoke, as O_2 increases ignitability and flammability. • Secure the O_2 cylinder. • Never charge or replace the batteries in an O_2-enriched atmosphere—it can lead to sparks and flash fires or explosions.

- Ensure that O_2 line is not draped near moving components (e.g., power recliner), leading to entanglement, patient injury, leaks in the O_2 line, and wheelchair damage.
- Monitor entire tubing daily for leaks.
- Turn off O_2 source if not in use.

ADVERSE EVENTS

PEER-REVIEWED ARTICLES

Source	Background	Therapy	Outcome	Follow-up/Interpretation
Becker et al, 1991[8] **Injury and scooter malfunction** Case report J Emerg Med	A 50-year-old male with a 3-year history of MS and progressive spastic paraplegia used a three-wheeled platform mobility aid (scooter).	The patient fell, sustaining a 3-cm laceration on his left thenar eminence (required sutures) when scooter uncontrollably accelerated.	Examination of the device revealed detachment of the mechanism that returns an accelerating handle to a neutral position (a defect in the speed control regulator).	The defect was due to a resistance arm that had been inappropriately welded to its base, which was subsequently corrected (reported to manufacturer).

Continued

Source	Background	Therapy	Outcome	Follow-up/Interpretation
User Experience Network, 1992[7] **Oxygen use and power wheelchairs** Health Devices, 1992[7]	ECRI on D or E cylinder of pressured oxygen near power wheelchair.	Reasonably safe if cylinder is secured and protected (immobilized; protect stem and regulator from being broken off or bumped, leading to O_2 leakage and accumulation). Oxygen not allowed to accumulate under patient's clothing or near upholstery or electric controls, motor, battery.	Never smoke, as O_2 increases ignitability and flammability. Secure the O_2 cylinder. Never charge or replace the batteries in an O_2-enriched atmosphere— can lead to sparks and flash fires or explosions. O_2 line is not draped near moving components, such as a power recliner, leading to entanglement, patient injury, leaks in the O_2 line, and wheelchair damage. Check entire tubing daily for leaks. Turn off O_2 source if not in use.	
Witters and Ruggera, 1994[5] **Power wheelchairs and EMI** Laboratory (device) testing Proc RESNA	EMC testing of chairs to various electric field intensities over a 1 MHz to 1 GHz frequency range and field strength from 3 V/m to 40 V/m using a gigahertz transverse electromagnetic cell in an anechoic chamber.	During exposure, chairs (power scooter) were monitored for brake release and wheel movements during (1) stationary (with power on) and (2) moving (wheels rotating at 25-50% maximum) conditions.	Results: All chairs exhibited their own degree of susceptibility with newer models affected by low field strengths (5 V/m—similar to that of a 4-watt handheld radio at 7 feet).	Medical devices are another source of EM interference. Most EMI can be eliminated by good design and shielding techniques. Note: Frequency range tested included sources such as radio, TV, microwave, cellular phones. Type and number of chairs tested not reported. Statistics not reported.

FDA REPORTS[1]

Power Wheelchair–Related Fatalities

Date Reported	Brand Name	Fatal Event
3/17/2003	Invacare power wheelchair	The user tipped backwards in the wheelchair with the head pinned into the chest area (not breathing); died of suffocation.
2/11/2003	Invacare power wheelchair	User was severely burned and died in wheelchair, possibly due to external ignition (cigarette or candle).
1/28/2003	Pride Jazzy	Apartment fire.
1/21/2003	Invacare power wheelchair	User was traveling down a highway and was struck by an automobile.
10/18/2002	Pride Jazzy	User was in an assisted living center, smoking. A small fire resulted in thermal injuries and death.
9/27/2002	Quickie	User fell out of chair, hit head, required surgery, and died about 6 weeks later.
6/5/2002	Invacare power wheelchair	User popped a wheelie while on a van lift, fell 3 feet off ramp with wheelchair on top of user.
4/29/2002	Pride	User drove full speed onto a van lift, hit head on the van's door opening, fracturing neck.
4/29/2002	Pride	User drove too close to creek, traveled down bank into water, fell face first in 18-inch water depth and drowned.
3/01/2001	Action Storm	Wheelchair caught fire when a candle ignited clothes.
6/05/2000	Ranger II	Attorney reports a wheelchair cord entangled as user tried to enter a room.
5/11/2000	Rascal	User was on street and was thrown off wheelchair when it rocked side to side and tipped over.
7/26/99	Power 9000	Wheelchair caught fire in apartment.
1/05/99	Ranger II	Accidental short in wire (battery) led to a fire.
12/18/1998	Ranger X	Attorney reported wheelchair acting erratically. User fell and died.
10/10/1998	Bounder Plus	User fell backwards off a van lift while in a power wheelchair.
11/06/1997	Power 9000	User fell out of wheelchair, sustained abrasions, and died 2 weeks later.

Continued

Date Reported	Brand Name	Fatal Event
8/25/1997	Arrow	User was struck by a truck while on a dark street (owner's manual warns against driving on streets or highways).
2/11/1997	P100 Power Wheelchair	User was on wheelchair while charging battery exploded, severely injuring user.
10/11/1996	Arrow XT	Attorney reported fire, smoke inhalation, and death. Also noted: unauthorized components used.
8/17/95	Max 30/Permobil	Charger/cable caused fire on wheelchair, fire in room, and death.
10/5/94	Rascal convertible	A female user with multiple sclerosis misjudged position of step, ran front wheels off steps, and fell down steps (reported by husband).
4/9/90	Everest & Jennings	Wife found husband in back yard, possibly dead from positional asphyxia. Wheelchair reported broken.

Note: FDA reports do not necessarily establish cause-effect relationship between equipment and injury. Incidences may be due to equipment or user error. Also, some reports are alleged by attorneys.

Scooter-Related Fatalities[1]

Date Reported	Brand Name	Fatal Event
1/28/03	Pride Scooter	Fire in the garage.
7/31/02	Rascal 3W	Tipped over in yard.
3/20/02	Rascal	The user was struck from behind and was thrown from the unit.
1/03/02	Chauffeur 3W	No details.
10/15/01	Rascal	The user was hit by a vehicle while crossing an intersection.
4/06/01	Golden companion	Lift contributed to accident.
12/21/00	Vehicle (4-wheel)	Unit traveling too fast down hill and turned sharply, falling on top of user. Hospitalized 2 weeks and died.
10/24/00	Pride	No details.
10/27/99	Pacesaver	Struck by car while crossing a highway at night. Manual warns against driving on busy streets.
6/4/99	Pacesaver	Run over by a large truck situated 6 inches in front of scooter. Location: construction site. Driver did not see user.

4/19/99	Tri-rolls	Attorney reports brakes failed.
3/4/99	Ranger "Solo"	Attorney reports user fell off unit, developed pneumonia.
12/02/98	Pride Shuttle	User unable to travel up hill due to low battery. Then backed down hill backwards by placing unit in neutral without brakes, hit curb backwards, fell on curb and sidewalk.
10/29/98	Pride	No details.
10/29/98	Brand unknown	Husband allegedly wired unit to accommodate a second battery in order to secure a quicker charge.
10/09/98	Rascal	Unit on lawn near sloped area, flipped over on patient, puncturing lung.
9/23/98	Rascal	User fell and hit head. The device's tiller arm was loose and unstable. A new one was on order. Cautioned not to use.
12/23/97	Sterling	While user was crossing railroad tracks, a wheel became stuck in gap and the user was struck by train.
8/30/96	Pacesaver	A street sweeper traveling on northbound lane but going in reverse did not see scooter and hit it.
3/21/96	Scout	An 81-year-old person with COPD found next to scooter with O_2 line entangled and cut under unit.
7/29/94	Bravo	An 81-year-old tipped unit, fell, and fractured hip; the patient developed a blood clot 3 months s/p repair.
2/28/94	Amigo RWD	User sitting in unit; unit caught fire.
2/8/94	Lark	User purchased a refurbished unit. On the way home, it tipped in street and user hit head.
9/22/92	Pace Saver Excel	User drove backwards off subway platform and into a high-voltage line.
3/24/92	Amigo FWD	User negotiated a steep, narrow ramp covered with artificial turf. The unit overturned. The user struck head, was hospitalized, and developed pneumonia.
7/12/90	Bravo	An 86-year-old female with emphysema fell, fractured a hip, and died 5 days later. A wheel had detached due to a broken weld.
8/19/88	Rascal	A traffic light changed while user was crossing street; user was struck by car.
12/23/86	Rascal	An attorney reported seat post ripped out of engine housing. It had been previously repaired by an unauthorized company.
12/16/86	Rascal	User tipped backwards at home.
11/06/86	Rascal 3W	While ascending a ramp at a grocery store, user fell sideways off ramp.

Note: FDA reports do not necessarily establish cause-effect relationships between equipment and injury. Incidences may be due to equipment or user error. Also, some reports are alleged by attorneys.

REFERENCES

1. U.S. Food and Drug Administration: Center for Device and Radiological Health. Available at: http://www.fda.gov/cdrh/mdr/. Accessed November 7, 2005.

2. Tan JC: Practical manual of physical medicine and rehabilitation: diagnostics, therapeutics, and basic problems. St. Louis: Mosby; 1998.

3. Greenbaum MG, Fernandes S, Wainapel SF: Use of a motorized wheelchair in conjunction with a guide dog for the legally blind and physically disabled. Arch Phys Med Rehab 79(2):216-217, 1998.

4. Alpert S. Dear Powered Wheelchair/Scooter or Accessory/Component Manufacturer [letter]. Center for Devices and Radiological Health. Department of Health and Human Services. Public Health Services, FDA, May 26, 1994.

5. Witters DM, Ruggera PS: Electromagnetic compatibility (EMC) of powered wheelchairs and scooters. Proceedings of the RESNA 1994 Annual Conference, June 17-22, 14:359-360, 1994.

6. Scoggin AE, Parks KM: Latex sensitivity in children with spina bifida: implications for occupational therapy practitioners. Am J Occup Ther 51(7):608-611, 1997.

7. User Experience Network: safe use of supplemental oxygen with powered wheelchairs. Health Devices 21(8):291, 1992.

8. Becker DG, Washington BV, Devlin PM, et al: Injury due to uncontrolled acceleration of an electric wheelchair. J Emerg Med 9(3): 115-117, 1991.

30   EXERCISE EQUIPMENT

This section includes advice/concerns for therapeutic or exercise equipment commonly found in the gym of a physical rehabilitation facility and include finger ladders, free and machine weights, hand blocks, overhead pulleys, skate board, Swiss balls, supported treadmills, Theraband, and toys. Adverse events associated with equipment such as isokinetic machinery, treadmills, stationary bicycles, and latex materials are also reported.

FINGER LADDER (WALL CLIMBING)

Issue	LOC	Sources	Affil	Rationale/Comment
Teach proper motion	P	Kisner and Colby, 1996[1]	PT	The concern is substitution (i.e., improper technique). Avoid trunk substitution (side bending), toe-raising, or shoulder shrugging.
	Advice	Tan, 1998[2]	MD/TP	

FREE WEIGHTS (BARBELLS)

Issue	LOC	Sources	Affil	Rationale/Comment
Backing into others—avoid	P	Baechle and Groves, 1992[3]	—	
Coordination requirements	Advice			Greater coordination is required with free weights (i.e., no guides) than with machines.
Dropping risk	Advice	Joynt, 1988[4]	MD	The concern is probably injury (from falling weights) during isotonic barbell exercises.
Loading bars—evenly	P	Baechle and Groves, 1992[3]	—	When bar is evenly loaded, it is balanced (i.e., less inclined to tip to one side).
Locking barbells (secure)	P			Secure weights to prevent weight from sliding off bar and injuring a body part.
Protruding bars	P			Be aware of extended (protruding) bars at the gym. Avoid "walking into one."

Continued

Issue	LOC	Sources	Affil	Rationale/Comment
Storing equipment	P			Avoid tripping over equipment or making equipment accessible to unsupervised children. The weights may be too heavy for the child to safely manage alone.

HAND BLOCKS

Issue	LOC	Sources	Affil	Rationale/Comment
Blocks should have stable base	Advice	Moy, 1987[5]	—	

MACHINE WEIGHTS

Issue	LOC	Sources	Affil	Rationale/Comment
Hands—between weight stacks	Advice	Baechle and Groves, 1992[3]	—	Do not place hands between weight stacks when adjusting the load.
Hands—near mechanical parts	Advice			Do not place hands near chains, belts pulleys, or cams.
Keys—inserting	Advice			Insert key all the way into weight stack.
Lifts—speed of	Advice			Lifts should be slow and controlled. Uncontrolled momentum of fixed or variable resistance machines can result in muscle, tendon, and joint injuries.

Positioning—assuming	Advice	Assume stable, properly adjusted, secured (belts) position.
Wear—monitor	Advice	Monitor the following:
		• Frayed cables and belts
		• Worn pulleys and chains
		• Broken welds
		• Loose pads
		• Rough or uneven machine movements

OVERHEAD PULLEYS

Issue	LOC	Sources	Affil	Rationale/Comment
Teach proper motion for shoulder abduction/flexion	P	Kisner and Colby, 1996[1]	PT	Increased pain and reduced mobility may occur due to compression of the humerus against acromion process during shoulder flexion or abduction. Discontinue shoulder exercise if this occurs. **In a 1990 experiment, Kumar et al.[6] reported that 62% of stroke patients assigned to an overhead pulley exercise group experienced shoulder pain.**

SKATE BOARD/POWDER BOARD

Issue	LOC	Sources	Affil	Rationale/Comment
Hip surgery	P	Kisner and Colby, 1996[1]	PT	If hip surgery, position hip properly while side-lying. Avoid hip adduction for patients with THR.

SWISS BALL

A00-B99 CERTAIN INFECTIONS AND PARASITIC DISEASES

Issue	LOC	Sources	Affil	Rationale/Comment
Cross-contamination—avoid	CI/P	Carriere, 1998[7]	PT	Use with same patient; wash before use.

F00-F99 MENTAL AND BEHAVIORAL DISORDERS

Issue	LOC	Sources	Affil	Rationale/Comment
Fear of falling off ball	CI	Houglum, 2001[8]	PT/ATC	Don't use Swiss ball.

G00-G99 DISEASES OF THE NERVOUS SYSTEM

Issue	LOC	Sources	Affil	Rationale/Comment
Ventricular peritoneal shunt	CI/P	Carriere, 1998[7]	PT	Check with surgeon if patient has a ventricular peritoneal shunt. Note: No explanation provided—perhaps pressure or drainage/positional-related concern for the shunt.

M00-M99 DISEASES OF THE MUSCULOSKELETAL SYSTEM AND CONNECTIVE TISSUE

Issue	LOC	Sources	Affil	Rationale/Comment
Pain with exercise	CI/P	Carriere, 1998[7]	PT	
Amputation—lower limb	CI/P			Balance (center of gravity) is affected without prosthesis.
Osteoporosis	CI/P			Avoid falls (e.g., off ball).
NWB status—sitting exercises	CI/P			

PROCEDURAL CONCERNS

Issue	LOC	Sources	Affil	Rationale/Comment
Clothes—belt buckles	Safety	Houglum, 2001[8]	PT/ATC	May puncture ball.
Clothes—oversized	CI/P	Carriere, 1998[7]	PT	Clothes may become entangled.

Continued

Issue	LOC	Sources	Affil	Rationale/Comment
Clothes—slippery	CI/P	Carriere, 1998[7]	PT	Avoid slippery clothing. The patient may slip off ball. Use rubber soles.
	Safety	Houglum, 2001[8]	PT/ATC	
Combined activities	Safety	Houglum, 2001[8]	PT/ATC	Avoid bouncing while bending, twisting, rotating spine. Combining activities may injure spine.
Environments—hot, sunny	CI/P	Carriere, 1998[7]	PT	Do not fully inflate ball in hot, sunny environment. Air expands and ball may burst.
Hair—loose	CI/P	Carriere, 1998[7]	PT	Hair may become entangled.
	Safety	Houglum, 2001[8]	PT/ATC	Restrain hair if necessary.
Injury—related contraindications	CI	Houglum, 2001[8]	PT/ATC	If any injury contraindicates the exercise on the Swiss ball (e.g., weight sitting on ball with foot support when patient has a non–weight-bearing status). (Also see Musculoskeletal concerns.)
Lines (i.e., IV lines)—monitor	CI/P	Carriere, 1998[7]	PT	Lines may constrain position.
Mat—nonslippery	CI/P	Carriere, 1998[7]		Use ball on firm, nonslippery mat. Soft mats decrease rolling. Avoid carpet skin burns. Concrete is dangerous.
Overinflating ball	CI/P	Carriere, 1998[7]	PT	Avoid overinflating as ball may burst.
Pediatric patients—supervise	CI/P	Carriere, 1998[7]		Avoid falls from large balls.
Skin protection from abrasions	Safety	Houglum, 2001[8]	PT/ATC	If weight-bearing on knees, wear sweatpants to protect skin.
Symptom exacerbated	CI	Houglum, 2001[8]	PT/ATC	If symptoms exacerbated with Swiss ball exercise (e.g., increased dizziness, pain). (Also see Musculoskeletal concerns.)

SUPPORTED TREADMILL AMBULATION TRAINING[a,b]

Issue	LOC	Sources	Affil	Rationale/Comment
Treadmill	Required	Wilson et al, 2000[9]	MS	Requirements: • 140×60 cm minimal walking surface. • 75 cm maximal walking surface width (to allow access to midline of the treadmill). • 0.3 km/hr minimal speed. • 140 kg at 0.3 km/hr power to move (so that treadmill does not stall at slow speed). • Handrails (for balance). • Safety-stop apparatus (for emergencies).
Unloading system (the mechanism that lifts and unweights the patient)	Required			Requirements: • Unload up to 40% body weight with reliable reporting. • Two-point suspension (50 cm apart—shoulder width) to permit weight-shifting activities. • Allows 5 cm of vertical displacement. • Fall prevention system (if maximal load is a 250-lb person, the authors recommend a system able to unload 100 lb for training and offer a 300% safety factor, i.e., 750 lb, to prevent falls). • Accessible controls for adjustments. • Spring support system.

Continued

Issue	LOC	Sources	Affil	Rationale/Comment
Harness	Required			Requirements: • The unloading system as two points of attachment. • Comfort provided (during unloading) by using support across buttocks, around thighs and ribs (without impinging on brachial plexus or pectoral area [for females]). • Easy to doff and don. • Harness promotes upright posture.
Therapist area	Required			Requirements: • 25 cm width seating space (adequate) with back support (i.e., firm molded cushion). • Access to patient's legs.

a, These authors' recommendations were based on clinical experience, anthropometric data, engineering principles, and experience using three patients with chronic spinal cord injuries who met the criteria of adequate LE ROM, grade 3 or more bilateral triceps strength, ASIA scale of C or D, DTR intact at quads and Achilles tendons, and no spasticity that would interfere with standing. b, Additional recommendations (beyond required) include a ramp for wheelchair access, small speed increments (0.15 km/hr), and an ergonomically designed lift system to elevate the walking surface.

THERABAND (CONTAINS LATEX)

Q00-Q99 CONGENITAL MALFORMATIONS, DEFORMITIES, AND CHROMOSOMAL ABNORMALITIES (SPINA BIFIDA)

Issue	LOC	Sources	Affil	Rationale/Comment
Spina bifida	Avoid	Scoggin and Parks, 1997[10]	OT	Protein in the rubber has a cumulative effect from exposure early in life and from multiple surgical interventions. Responses include watery eyes, hives, sneezing, nasal congestion, wheezing, local rashes, coughing; also life-threatening anaphylactic shock associated with latex gloves and materials used during medical procedures. Consider naturally weighted toys instead of latex-containing Theraband in this population.

TOYS

Issue	LOC	Sources	Affil	Rationale/Comment
Contamination—soft toys	FYI	Merriman et al, 2002[11]	—	**In a study of six general practitioner waiting rooms, Merriman[11] found that 90% of soft toys and 13% of hard toys showed high total bacterial and coliform counts of contamination.**

ADVERSE EVENTS

Source	Background	Therapy	Outcome	Follow-up/Interpretation
Carman and Chang, 2001[12] **Treadmills and pediatric hand injuries** Chart review Ann Plast Surg	The author reported 12 children with treadmill-related UE injuries between September 1996 and March 2000 at the Children's Hospital in Philadelphia.	Child ages ranged from 14 month to 7 years. Injuries occurred at home with a motorized treadmill. Six occurred while an adult supervised the unit; four occurred while unsupervised.	Injury types included abrasions and lacerations. Ten children sustained partial or full-thickness burns on volar hand and digits. Six children required surgery.	Mechanism: The child's hand caught under back end of the treadmill where the belt wraps around the rear roller.
Fraser-Moodie and Cox, 1974[13] **Exercise (slim) wheel and rectus abdominis hematoma** Case series Br J Surgery	A 63-year-old housewife.	She used an exercise wheel for the first time and experienced severe central abdominal pain, worse with coughing. She vomited twice.	At first, a 10 cm × 6 cm right lower quadrant tender mass was noted. Later periumbilical bruising was observed and then lumbar, buttocks, and suprapubic bruising were observed.	The exercise wheel (also called slimming wheel) is a device you roll on the floor while moving from a kneeling toward a more prone position. It was a popular method of losing weight and keeping fit in 1974. All three patients who used the slimming wheel were obese, middle-aged, unfit patients and sustained rectus abdominis hematoma.

	A 61-year-old female laundress lost 10 kg of weight using the exercise wheel for several months.	She complained of acute abdominal pain, worse near her right iliac fossa with round tender mass (10-cm diameter) noted.	She underwent laparotomy with a diagnosis of torsion of an ovarian cyst. A 300-ml blood clot cleared, and fresh bleeding from the ruptured inferior epigastric artery was noted when the abdominal muscles were retracted.
	A 49-year-old man used an exercise wheel twice a day for 6 months and lost 8 kg of weight.	He complained of a lump and soreness in the abdomen for several weeks, located to the right of his midline above the umbilicus.	A hard, nontender, 2-cm (diameter) fibrous nodule was surgically excised.
Kumar et al, 1990[6] **Pulleys, pain, and stroke patients** Experiment Am J Phys Med Rehab	28 patients with a diagnosis of stroke.	Patients were assigned to (1) therapist ROM, (2) skateboard, or (3) overhead pulley groups. Groups did not differ on side or extent of involvement or presence of subluxation.	Shoulder pain from ROM, skateboard, and overhead pulley groups were 8%, 12%, and 62%, respectively ($P = .014$). The authors recommend avoiding overhead pulley exercises in the rehabilitation of stroke patients.

CPSC[14]

Source	Background	Therapy	Outcome	Follow-up/Interpretation
Exercise bicycle, treadmill, and stair climbers— related pediatric injuries	An estimated 8700 children under 5 years of age and 16,500 children between the ages of 5 to 14 injure themselves on exercise equipment per year.	Injuries are related to stationary bicycle, treadmill, and stair climber equipment use.	Injuries include fractures and amputations (20% of injuries).	Warning: Keep children away from exercise equipment. Use a chain guard with bicycles. Store or lock equipment when not in use.

FOOD AND DRUG ADMINISTRATION REPORTS

FDA[15] (also see Testing: Isokinetic testing)

Date	Equipment	Event
6/25/99	Kincom 125 E	A patient s/p hip fracture repair was exercising (150/75) and felt a sharp pain. A hairline fracture was reported; no malfunction was found.
4/19/99	Kincom 125 A/P	The PTA heard a "pop" on the second set of 10 repetitions of very strenuous quad exercises; patient sustained a patella fracture. No unit malfunction found.
5/28/97	Cybex	During passive mode exercise of the left knee (flexion and extension), the knee bent further than anticipated. The mechanical stop was not set.
5/03/95	Cybex	A patient with a surgical repair (no details) felt pain while on the unit but was told to continue, resulting in reinjury and requiring surgery.

12/09/94	Lido Active Multijoint	A therapist with carpal tunnel syndrome aggravated the condition while adjusting the unit's position.
3/02/94	Kincom 500 H	A patient sustained a hyperextension injury (no details) during a knee exercise. Note: No unit malfunction was found.
2/14/94	Kincom 125 E	A user sustained a femoral fracture during a prone knee flexion exercise for the hamstrings when the unit's lever arm loosened, detached from the actuator, and hyperextended the user's leg.
10/29/93	Kincom II	An employee's hand was pinned against a computer when the unit's actuator arm moved.
7/14/93	Kincom 125 E+	A girl sustained an open distal phalanx fracture of the left ring finger (no details).
5/10/93	Kincom I	A man sustained a laceration to the lower leg during quadriceps testing at 80 degrees/sec in concentric/eccentric mode when the unit's head tilted unexpectedly.
3/23/93	Kincom 500 H	A female s/p knee arthroscopic surgery was exercising and fractured the patella on her involved side (no details of protocol).
11/06/92	Kincom II	During knee testing (comparison) at 180 degrees/sec eccentric mode, the user felt knee pain (no details).
7/28/92	Kincom 125 E Plus	Patient with ACL exercising quadriceps test at 130 degrees/sec (80 to 90 degrees) started isokinetic before machine was ready and tore left ACL while it was in an isometric mode.
6/26/92	Kincom 125 E	The user fractured a patella (no details).
4/01/92	Kincom III	A patient with an autograph ACL reconstruction sustained a ruptured autograph during a 45 degrees/sec leg press when the table top slipped backward, resulting in full extension of the patient's knee.
3/11/92	Kincom 125 E+	During a demonstration of the unit in the passive mode, a child's finger was caught in the actuator, resulting in 70-80% finger severance. The finger was reattached.
11/19/90	Kc 125 Muscle Testing	A patient sustained an upper chest and rib pain/laceration during left shoulder exercise when an aide unstrapped the patient from the unit while it was still in operation (programmed).
11/26/86	Kincom	The individual's wrist broke; the cause was not determined.

Note: FDA reports do not necessarily establish cause-effect relationships between equipment and injury. Incidences may be due to equipment or user error. Also, some reports are alleged by attorneys.

FDA—LATEX SENSITIVITY

Latex, a natural rubber product from a rubber tree, contains proteins. The protein can become airborne and inhaled. Avoid areas where one may inhale powder from latex gloves; tell employer and health care providers of latex allergy; wear a medical alert bracelet.

Source	Background	Outcome	Affil	Comments
Snider, 1997[16] FDA and Latex	FDA received more than 1700 reports of severe allergic reactions related to latex-made medical devices. **In 1989, six deaths occurred in children with spina bifida due to reactions from latex cuffs located on the tip of barium enema catheters.**	Two groups at risk are health care workers and children with spina bifida, persons with conditions that involve multiple surgical procedures. Medical devices containing latex include surgical gloves, anesthesia equipment, adhesive bandages, and intravenous catheters.	Gov	Items with hypoallergenic labeling may not be safe for people with latex sensitivity because although levels of latex protein are reduced, they can still cause allergic reactions in sensitive individuals.
Scoggin and Parks, 1997[10] Review article Latex exposure in persons with spina bifida AJOT	Avoid	Medical devices with latex	OT	Protein in the rubber has a cumulative effect from exposure early in life and from multiple surgical interventions. Responses include watery eyes, hives, sneezing, nasal congestion, wheezing, local rashes, coughing; also life-threatening anaphylactic shock associated with latex gloves and materials used during medical procedures. If in doubt, contact the manufacturer.

Devices containing latex:
    Latex gloves
    Theraband
    Wheelchair parts (wheels, cushions, seat
        backs)
    Balloons
    Rubber catheters
    Adhesive tape and bandages
    Elastic in diapers
    Foam padding
    Rubber squeeze toys
    Pacifiers with latex
Alternatives:
    Latex-free gloves
    Nonrubber balls and balloons
    Pacifiers with silicone nipples
    Naturally weighted toys instead of
        Theraband

a, Latex Allergy: A prevention guide, available at: http://www.cdc.gov/niosh/98-113.html.

LITIGATION

Year State	History	Therapy	Device	Complication	Comments Award
2001, California[17] **Rowing machine and reinjured back**	A man tripped, fell, and injured his back working as a warehouse laborer. He had a lumbar laminectomy and a L4-L5 disc resection (1998).	Physical therapy	He went to physical therapy for reconditioning. An unlicensed PT aide instructed him on an "upright row" maneuver on a rowing machine. A nylon lock nut separated from a bolt, causing the weight stack to fall. Patient stumbled backward.	He reinjured his back.	The physical therapy service was not sued. (Assembly company pursued a cross-complaint against PT service claiming failure of PT to inspect equipment as per owner's manual and adequately supervise/instruct patient.) $180,000 settlement; suit involving indemnity.
1999, Illinois[18] **Stool with wheels and shoulder injury**	A 55-year-old woman received quadriceps strengthening exercises.	Hospital; outpatient PT	The physical therapist instructed the patient to sit on a four-legged stool with wheels and push the stool backwards using her feet. The stool tipped over and the patient fell to floor.	She sustained a rotator cuff impingement injury (syndrome).	The defendants claimed the patient performed exercise safely three times and was properly instructed, assessed, and observed. Verdict for the plaintiff: $188,500.
1999, Massachusetts[19] **Stairmaster and fall**	A 63-year-old male presented with weak arms and a weak leg due to polio; s/p leg fracture.	Hospital	He received physical therapy 3x/wk using a stair-climbing apparatus (five steps). The therapist allegedly left patient alone on fourth step for 1½ minutes (to talk to a friend).	The patient's leg collapsed and he fell and refractured his weak leg. The patient required an air cast for 2 weeks and claimed emotional distress.	$222,811 post verdict settlement.

| 1997, Texas[20] **Styrofoam log and back injury** | Male plaintiff (no details). | Rehabilitation facility; physical therapy | The patient was standing on a Styrofoam log when it rolled out from under him and he fell. | He sustained nerve injury to his back. | He claimed the standard of care was breached. $127,500 verdict (the defendant was found 51% negligent). |
| 1997, Texas[21] **Roman chair and back injury** | A woman presented with back pain. | Physician and PT facility | She received physical therapy for her back injury using a Roman chair (no details on equipment or exercise performed). | Allegedly, the "Roman chair" aggravated her old back injuries and she subsequently sustained a new injury. | $1 million verdict. |

Note: Awards and settlements do not necessarily prove a cause-effect relationship between equipment or therapy and injury.

REFERENCES

1. Kisner C, Colby LA: Therapeutic exercise: foundations and techniques, ed 3. Philadelphia: FA Davis; 1996.
2. Tan JC: Practical manual of physical medicine and rehabilitation: diagnostics, therapeutics, and basic problems. St. Louis: Mosby; 1998.
3. Baechle TR, Groves BR: Weight training: steps to success. Champaign (IL): Human Kinetics; 1992.
4. Joynt RL: Therapeutic exercise. In Delisa JA, editor: Rehabilitation medicine: principles and practice. Philadelphia: J.B. Lippincott; 1988.
5. Moy A: Assessment of manual bed aids. DHSS Disability Equipment Assessment Programme. London: HMSO; 1987.
6. Kumar R, Metter EJ, Mehta AJ, et al: Shoulder pain in hemiplegia. The role of exercise. Am J Phys Med Rehab 69(4):205-208, 1990.
7. Carriere B: The Swiss ball: theory, basic exercise, and clinical application. Berlin: Springer; 1998.
8. Houglum PA: Therapeutic exercise for athletic injuries. Champaign (IL): Human Kinetics; 2001.

9. Wilson MS, Qureshy H, Protas EJ, et al.: Equipment specifications for supported treadmill ambulation training. J Rehab Res Dev 37(4): 415-422, 2000.

10. Scoggin AE, Parks KM: Latex sensitivity in children with spina bifida: implications for occupational therapy practitioners. Am J Occup Ther 51(7):608-611, 1997.

11. Merriman E, Corwin P, Ikram R: Toys are a potential source of cross-infection in general practitioners' waiting rooms. Br J Gen Pract 52(475):138-140, 2002.

12. Carman C, Chang B: Treadmill injuries to the upper extremity in pediatric patients. Ann Plast Surg 47(1):15-19, 2001.

13. Fraser-Moodie A, Cox S: Haematoma of rectus abdominis from the use of an exercise wheel: a report of 3 cases. Br J Surg 61(7): 577, 1974.

14. Consumer Product Safety Commission: Prevent Injuries to children from exercise equipment, CPSC Document No 5028. Available at: http://www.cpsc.gov/cpscpub/pubs/5028.html. Accessed November 7, 2005.

15. U.S. Food and Drug Administration: Center for Device and Radiological Health. Available at: http://www.fda.gov/cdrh/mdr/. Accessed November 7, 2005.

16. Snider S: FDA talk paper: Latex labeling required for medical devices 1997. Available at: http://www.fda.gov/bbs/topics/ANSWERS/ANS00826.html. Accessed November 8, 2005.

17. Medical malpractice verdicts, settlements and experts, September 2001, p 45, loc 2.

18. Medical malpractice verdicts, settlements and experts, September 1999, p 37, loc 3.

19. Medical malpractice verdicts, settlements and experts, April 1999 p 38, loc 1.

20. Medical malpractice verdicts, settlements and experts, July 1997, p 41, loc 3.

21. Medical malpractice verdicts, settlements and experts, July 1997, p 41, loc 2.

31.1 Casting (Includes serial casting; casting for burns)

OVERVIEW. A cast is a rigid casing applied around a body part.[1] Serial casting involves recasting over time and is used to treat contractures by affecting muscle length, soft tissue extensibility, and possibly affecting muscle spindle excitability. The applied load on soft tissue is low and duration is long (i.e., not a quick stretch). Casting of burns offers plastic deformation of connective tissue, biomechanical realignment of joint structures, and protection of exposed tendons, fragile skin, or wounds.

SUMMARY: CONTRAINDICATIONS AND PRECAUTIONS. Four sources (one burn- and three neurologically related) cited a total of 25 concerns for casting. Concerns ranged from 4 to 13 per source with the burn source citing the largest number. The largest proportion of concerns was procedural (about 45%). Six shared concerns (by two sources) were agitation, allergies, fragility, heterotopic ossification, excessive edema, and open wounds.

In a 2002 retrospective study, Pohl et al found fewer complications (i.e., ulcers, pain, swelling) in patients with cerebral spasticity when short intervals between serial casting were used.[2]

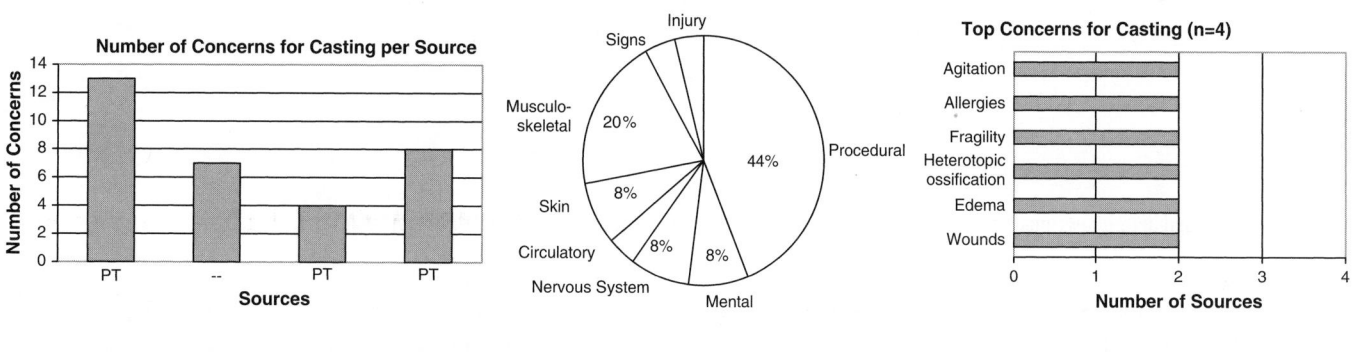

Number of Concerns for Casting per Source

Proportion of Concerns for Casting Based on ICD

Top Concerns for Casting (n=4)

CONTRAINDICATIONS AND PRECAUTIONS

Serial Casting/Casting

F00-F99 MENTAL AND BEHAVIORAL DISORDERS

Issue	LOC	Sources	Affil	Rationale/Comment
Agitation	CI	Staley and Serghiou, 1998[3,a]	PT	There is an increase risk of injury in agitated or self-abusive
	P	Goga-Eppenstein, 1999[4]	PT	patients.
	Advice	Booth, 1983[5,b]	PT	Assess tolerance for procedure and joint immobilization. Do not give a fiberglass cast to an agitated patient because splintered ends that may develop on the case are sharp.

| Cognitive/emotional state | P | Staley and Serghiou, 1998[3,a] | PT | Patients with a related cognitive or emotional state may hinder true range of motion. |

a, Guidelines written for burn patients; b, Guidelines written for head-injured patients with spasticity.

G00-G99 DISEASES OF THE NERVOUS SYSTEM

Issue	LOC	Sources	Affil	Rationale/Comment
Decerebrate/decorticate extensor spasticity—severe	CI	Cusick, 1990[6,a]	PT	
Insensate—legs	P	Staley and Serghiou, 1998[3]	PT	

a, Guideline written for patients with neuromuscular deficits.

I00-I99 DISEASES OF THE CIRCULATORY SYSTEM

Issue	LOC	Sources	Affil	Rationale/Comment
Hypertension	P	Staley and Serghiou, 1998[3]	PT	Do not cast bilateral extremity if hypertension is present.

L00-L99 DISEASES OF THE SKIN AND SUBCUTANEOUS TISSUE

Issue	LOC	Sources	Affil	Rationale/Comment
Allergy—to materials	P	Staley and Serghiou, 1998[3]	PT	Patient may be sensitive to plaster or to cotton/synthetic stockinette material.
	P	Goga-Eppenstein, 1999[4]	PT	For plaster, test with a small wet strip on skin and observe for reaction.
Fragile skin	P	Staley and Serghiou, 1998[3]	PT	Exercise extreme care using padding to avoid pressure if there is a minor
	P	Goga-Eppenstein, 1999[4]	PT	abrasion or potential for breakdown.

M00-M99 DISEASES OF THE MUSCULOSKELETAL SYSTEM AND CONNECTIVE TISSUE

Issue	LOC	Sources	Affil	Rationale/Comment
Bony abnormality or obstruction	CI	Cusick, 1990[6]	PT	
Contractures >3 years (long-standing, static) following brain injury	CI			May try, but few gains are expected.
Contractures—plantar flexion (severe)	CI			
Heterotopic ossification	CI	Staley and Serghiou, 1998[3]	PT	Stretching inflamed tissue can aggravate condition.[6]
	CI	Cusick, 1990[6]	PT	
Hypoextensibility (static) in persons with cerebral palsy	CI	Cusick, 1990[6]	PT	The problem may be trophic in nature if there is no persistent hypertonicity.

R00-R99 SYMPTOMS, SIGNS

Issue	LOC	Sources	Affil	Rationale/Comment
Edema—excessive	CI	Staley and Serghiou, 1998[3]	PT	Wait until swelling subsides.[6]
	CI	Cusick, 1990[6]	PT	

S00-T98 INJURY, POISONING, AND CERTAIN OTHER CONSEQUENCES OF EXTERNAL CAUSES

Issue	LOC	Sources	Affil	Rationale/Comment
Wounds—open	P	Staley and Serghiou, 1998[3]	PT	
	CI	Cusick, 1990[6]	PT	

PROCEDURAL CONCERNS

Issue	LOC	Sources	Affil	Rationale/Comment
Bony prominences—pad well **Dry cast**	Advice	Booth, 1983[5]	PT	Let lower extremity cast dry 24 hours before weight bearing to prevent deformation of cast.
Instructions—Provide instructions for monitoring and warning signs	P			Remove cast if warning signs are noted to avoid skin breakdowns and DVTs. Provide patient with a letter informing the purpose of cast in the event a casted outpatient notes warning signs and must have cast removed in an emergency room. Warning signs: • Swollen fingers/toes • Poor or absent distal pulses • Dusky veins • Pain • Paresthesia • Poor nail-bed refill • After pressure skin blanching
Noncompliance—with follow-up appointment **Noncompliance—with cast maintenance**	CI	Staley and Serghiou, 1998[3]	PT	

Noncompliance—with circulatory/ulceration monitoring				
Positioning of joint—during casting	P	Goga-Eppenstein, 1999[4]	PT	Position the joint in submaximal range for casting. If muscle-related throbbing lasting 4 hours after casting, the joint may have been overstretched and should be recast.
Reliability	P	Staley and Serghiou, 1998[4]	PT	Consider if there may be questionable return of the patient for a timely removal of the cast.
Scratching—inside cast	P	Goga-Eppenstein, 1999[4]	PT	Avoid scratching inside cast with a stick as it may lead to skin breakdown.
Upper limb casting—bilateral	P			Make sure medical staff does not require access to the casted upper limbs (i.e., for blood pressures or to draw blood).
Wet cast	P			Avoid getting cast wet as it may lose shape. Inner padding may irritate skin and lead to breakdown. When taking baths or showers, protect cast with plastic bag secured proximally.

EVIDENCE

Source	Background	Therapy	Outcome	Follow-up/Interpretation
Pohl et al, 2002[2] **Serial casting frequency and complications** Retrospective	Review from 1997 to 2001 of 105 adults with cerebral spasticity (severe to moderate) with fixed contractures due to muscle tone in a German rehabilitation center.	172 serial casted joints (fiberglass) of elbows (42), knees (21), ankles (68) and wrist (41). Casts were changed (1) every 5-7 days (median 6.9) ($P = 56$, 39.2 years median age; from 1997 to 1998) or (2) every 1-4 days (2.7 median)	Complications were noted in 29.3% of the long cast changing interval group and in 8.8% of the short cast changing interval group ($p = .001$). Complications included: • Pressure ulcers, grade 1 and 2 (23 from the long; 6 from the short interval group)	Authors believe short changing intervals during serial casting result in fewer complications.
Arch Phys Med Rehab	Dx included ischemic stroke, hemorrhage, TBI, hypoxia, subarachnoid hemorrhage.	($n = 49$; 44.6 years median age; from 1997 to 2001).	• Pain (1 in each group) • Swelling (3 from the long interval group)	

REFERENCES

1. Eisenberg MG: Dictionary of rehabilitation. New York: Springer; 1995.

2. Pohl M, Ruckriem S, Mehrholz J, et al: Effectiveness of serial casting in patients with severe cerebral spasticity: a comparison study. Arch Phys Med Rehab 83(6), 784-790, 2002.

3. Staley M, Serghiou M: Casting guidelines, tips, and techniques: Proceedings from the 1997 American Burn Association PT/OT Casting workshop. J Burn Care Rehab 19(3):254-260, 1998.

4. Goga-Eppenstein P, Hill JP, Seifert TM, Yasukawa AM: Precautions and competency in cast application. Casting protocols for the upper and lower extremities. The Rehabilitation Institute of Chicago Publication Series. Gaithersburg (MD): Aspen Publications; 1999.

5. Booth BJ, Doyle M, Montgamery J: Serial casting for the management of spasticity in the head-injured adult. Phys Ther 63(12):1960-1965, 1983.

6. Cusick BD: Progressive casting and splinting for lower extremity deformities in children with neuromotor dysfunction. Tucson (AZ): Therapy Skill Builders; 1990.

31.2 Orthotics

OVERVIEW. An orthosis is an external device that is worn on a body part to support, correct, or prevent deformities or to align body structures for improved function.[1] Webster's dictionary[2] defines it as a straightening treatment for the maladjusted. The term splint varies in meaning and may refer to either a hand orthosis[3] or a temporary external device.[1] Some examples of orthoses include body jackets, hand splints, ankle foot orthoses, knee cages, elastic stockings, and corrective shoes.

SUMMARY. Concerns for spinal and lower and upper limb (including hand splints) orthotics are varied and depend in large part on the patient's clinical presentation and involved body region. Skin monitoring is recommended in most, if not all, orthotic applications. In general, orthotic concerns include skin ulceration in insensate or poorly vascularized skin, skin allergies from splint materials, contracture promotion (e.g., using UE slings in persons with UMN lesions), worsened spasticity (e.g., using dynamic splints in persons with UMN lesions), and orthotics that either fail to adequately stabilize critical body segment (e.g., high cervical fracture) or fail to control a crucial movement component (e.g., deleterious rotational forces). In addition to pressure ulcer complications, pressure-related neuropathies[4,5] and compartmental syndromes[6] have been reported with orthotic use.

CONTRAINDICATIONS AND PRECAUTIONS

LOWER LIMB ORTHOTICS: GENERAL CONCERNS (INCLUDES SHOE ORTHOSES)

G00-G99 DISEASES OF THE NERVOUS SYSTEM

Issue	LOC	Sources	Affil	Rationale/Comment
Sensation—impaired	Advice	Tan, 1998[1]	MD/PT	Monitor skin regularly for redness, trophic changes, abrasions, dermatitis.

I00-I99 DISEASES OF THE CIRCULATORY SYSTEM

Issue	LOC	Sources	Affil	Rationale/Comment
Circulation—impaired	Advice	Tan, 1998[1]	MD/PT	Monitor skin regularly for redness, trophic changes, abrasions, dermatitis.

Issue	LOC	Sources	Affil	Rationale/Comment
Discomfort—investigate any	Advice	Tan, 1998[1]	MD/PT	Discomfort may lead to decreased use. **In 1969, Weitz[6] described a 20-month-old boy with tibia varus deformity LLE who was fitted for LLB using a lateral strap applied to the middle half of his leg to correct deformity. He cried a few hours after wearing the brace, and subsequently developed a compartment syndrome.**

ANKLE–FOOT ORTHOSES: GENERAL (THERMOPLASTIC)

(Off-the-Shelf or Custom-Made)

Issue	LOC	Sources	Affil	Rationale/Comment
Edema—fluctuating	CI	Tan, 1998[1]	MD/PT	Especially for solid AFO, spiral AFO, hemispiral AFO.
Strength of hip and knee—inadequate	CI			

ANKLE–FOOT ORTHOSES: SPIRAL

Issue	LOC	Sources	Affil	Rationale/Comment
Deformity fixed—ankle with <90 degrees of dorsiflexion	CI	Tan, 1998[1]	MD/PT	

Continued

Issue	LOC	Sources	Affil	Rationale/Comment
Imbalanced forces—acting on ankle foot complex	CI			
Instability—medial lateral ankle (severe)	CI			
Spasticity (moderate to severe)	CI			

ANKLE–FOOT ORTHOSES: HEMI-SPIRAL

Issue	LOC	Sources	Affil	Rationale/Comment
Deformity—fixed—ankle with <90 degrees of dorsiflexion	CI	Tan, 1998[1]	MD/PT	
Deformity valgus—ankle	CI			
Spasticity (severe) with sustained clonus	CI			

WEIGHT-BEARING ORTHOSES

Used to reduce or eliminate lower limb weight bearing

Issue	LOC	Sources	Affil	Rationale/Comment
Circulation—peripheral (in weight-bearing area)	Advice	Tan, 1998[1]	MD/PT	Peripheral circulation must tolerate pressure from the orthosis.
Skin—in weight-bearing area	Advice			Skin must tolerate pressures from orthosis.

FEMORAL FRACTURE ORTHOSES

Used for middle and distal third femur fractures following a period of immobilization and once callus formation is noted

Issue	LOC	Sources	Affil	Rationale/Comment
Fractures—proximal femoral	CI	Tan, 1998[1]	MD/PT	Varus angulation cannot be controlled well using this orthotic.

UPPER LIMB ORTHOTICS

Hand Splints

F00-F99 MENTAL AND BEHAVIORAL DISORDERS

Issue	LOC	Sources	Affil	Rationale/Comment
Limited communication in children—splinting burns	Extreme caution	Helm, 1982[7]	MD	The child may have limited verbal ability to communicate discomfort if splint is mal-fitting, leading to unnecessary pain and necrosis.

Vulnerable Biological Tissue: Skin Areas

Vulnerable to pressure injuries from their respective splints

Issue	LOC	Sources	Affil	Rationale/Comment
For C-bar of opponens cuff • Palmar surface of metacarpal joint of thumb and index finger	P	Malick, 1980[8]	OT	Precaution: The forces used to align the body part correctly may result in pressure areas.

Continued

Issue	LOC	Sources	Affil	Rationale/Comment
For dorsal splints				
• Dorsal metacarpal phalange joint				
• Head of ulna with wrist strap				
• Head of ulna with forearm section				
For lumbrical bar				
• Dorsal surface of first phalange of each finger				
For opponens bar				
• Metacarpal of thumb distal to the ulna head				
For palmar splint				
• Head of ulnar with wrist strap				
• Head of ulna with forearm section				
For palmar resting-pan splints				
• Palmar surface of distal finger joints, especially with flexion contractures or spasticity				
For wrist cock-up splint				Particularly when a wrist flex contracture is present.
• Center of the palm				
Thenar eminence—base				
Proximal end—splint				

PROCEDURAL CONCERNS

Issue	LOC	Sources	Affil	Rationale/Comment
Encircling the hand tightly	P/Avoid	Malick, 1980[8]	OT	
Exercise	Advice			Exercise in conjunction with splint use, as indicated.
Flame (open)—near splint (Aquaplast or Orfit materials)	P	Cusick, 1990[9]	PT	Avoid flames in splints fabricated with Aquaplast or Orfit materials. The splint may burn.
Forearm piece—too short	P/Avoid	Malick, 1980[8]	OT	
Forearm piece—too long	P/Avoid			Fabricating the forearm piece too long may impede elbow flexion and impinges the elbow area.
Heat source (near) >100 °F (Aquaplast or Orfit materials) • Radiator • Hot bath • Hot shower • Dashboard of car • Windowsill on sunny day	P	Cusick, 1990[9]	PT	Avoid heat sources in splints fabricated with Aquaplast or Orfit Materials; the splint may lose its shape.
Monitoring—skin	Advice	Tan, 1998[1]	MD/PT	The skin areas under the orthotic should be free of blemishes once the orthotic has been removed for 10 minutes.
Positioning—in finger joint hyperextension	P/Avoid	Malick, 1980[8]	OT	

Continued

Issue	LOC	Sources	Affil	Rationale/Comment
Pressure areas—over bony prominences	P/Avoid			
Schedule—static splints	Advice			All static splint should be worn intermittently unless otherwise specified.

Shoulder Sling (Arm Sling)

Shoulder slings (i.e., figure-8 style) position the shoulder joint in elbow flexion and shoulder abduction, internal rotation

G00-G99 DISEASES OF THE NERVOUS SYSTEM

Issue	LOC	Sources	Affil	Rationale/Comment
Hemiplegia with flexion synergy	Controversial CI	Tan, 1998[1] Miner and Nelson, 1995[10,a]	MD/PT OT	This sling practice is discouraged by NDT therapists. It is believed to encourage flexion synergy, flexion tone, and contracture development.

a, For UMN lesions. The Royal hemi-sling (i.e., with cuff encircling upper arm), or Hook hemi-harness arm slings may not approximate the glenohumeral joint in large patients.

Arm Abduction Orthoses (Airplane Splint)

G00-G99 DISEASES OF THE NERVOUS SYSTEM

Issue	LOC	Sources	Affil	Rationale/Comment
Thoracic outlet syndrome—shoulder should be less than 90 degrees abduction	CI	Miner and Nelson, 1995[10]	OT	Avoid overstretching nerve, vascular, or skin structures with this orthosis.

Balanced Forearm Orthosis

G00-G99 DISEASES OF THE NERVOUS SYSTEM/M00-M99 MUSCULOSKELETAL/SIGNS AND SYMPTOMS

Issue	LOC	Sources	Affil	Rationale/Comment
Contractures	CI	Miner and Nelson, 1995[10]	OT	
Sitting tolerance, lack	CI			
Spasticity, extreme	CI			

Dynamic Elbow Splints (Dynasplints; Turnbuckle Splints)

Dynamic elbow splints increase range by exerting a load on soft tissue over an extended period of time

G00-G99 DISEASES OF THE NERVOUS SYSTEM

Issue	LOC	Sources	Affil	Rationale/Comment
Spastic muscle	Do not use	Tan, 1998[1]	MD/PT	The dynamic nature of the splint may lead to further increased
	CI	Miner and Nelson, 1995[10]	OT	tone if muscle tone is high.

Air Splint (Elbow)

G00-G99 DISEASES OF THE SKIN

Issue	LOC	Sources	Affil	Rationale/Comment
Allergies	CI	Miner and Nelson, 1995[10]	OT	These plastic splints are inflatable to maintain elbow extension or for weight-bearing activities. Note: The plastic material contacts/covers the skin surfaces.
Heat intolerance	CI			

Tone-Reduction Orthoses

INJURIES/M00-M99 DISEASES OF THE MUSCULOSKELETAL SYSTEM

Issue	LOC	Sources	Affil	Rationale/Comment
Fractures	CI	Miner and Nelson, 1995[10]	OT	These orthoses (e.g., cone splints, finger abduction splint; also see air splint) use firm palm pressure, reflex inhibiting positions (digital extension with abduction), or surface contact to affect underlying muscle activity.
Open skin lesions	CI			

Tenodesis orthoses

M00-M99 DISEASES OF THE MUSCULOSKELETAL SYSTEM

Issue	LOC	Sources	Affil	Rationale/Comment
Range of motion, inadequate	CI	Miner and Nelson, 1995[10]	OT	The wrist must be capable of first extending to pull the thumb into opposition with the index and middle digits.

Gloves

Issue	LOC	Sources	Affil	Rationale/Comment
Circulation—compromised	CI	Miner and Nelson, 1995[10]	OT	
Open wounds	CI			
Scars—sensitive to shear forces	CI			

SPINAL ORTHOTICS

Spinal Orthoses: General Concerns

PROCEDURAL CONCERNS

Issue	LOC	Sources	Affil	Rationale/Comment
Check out—breathing	Advice	Tan, 1998[1]	MD/PT	Orthoses should permit unrestricted breathing and digestion. In 1978, Gryboski et al[11] described four cases of patients who developed esophagitis after TLSO application. In 1981, Kling et al[12] described a girl with scoliosis who developed esophagitis after Boston TLSO use.
Check out—digestion and chewing	Advice			

Continued

Issue	LOC	Sources	Affil	Rationale/Comment
Check out—sitting	Advice			Orthoses should permit comfortable sitting.
Monitoring—skin	Advice			10 minutes after an orthotic is removed, skin areas should be free of blemishes.[1] **In 1994, Liew and Hill reported two multiple trauma patients who developed occipital ulcers that required surgical interventions after wearing a hard (polyethylene) cervical collar for 8 to 10 days.[13]**

Helmet (Cranial Orthosis)

F00-F99 MENTAL AND BEHAVIORAL DISORDERS

Issue	LOC	Sources	Affil	Rationale/Comment
Psychosocial issues	CI	Bussel et al, 1995[14]	MD	This concern is related to long-term use of helmets.

L00-L99 DISEASES OF THE SKIN AND SUBCUTANEOUS TISSUE

Issue	LOC	Sources	Affil	Rationale/Comment
Dermatological conditions	CI	Bussel et al, 1995[14]	MD	There may be heat-related irritation from helmet use.

Soft Foam Cervical Collar[a]

Plastic Collar[b]

Semirigid Plastic Collar with Chin and Occipital Piece[c]

S00-T98 INJURY, POISONING, AND CERTAIN OTHER CONSEQUENCES OF EXTERNAL CAUSES

Issue	LOC	Sources	Affil	Rationale/Comment
Ligamentous or bony injury	CI	Bussel et al, 1995[14]	MD	These collars offer either little or no control of motion.

a, No control offered; b, Inadequate extension, rotation or lateral flexion control; c, Offers only minimal rotation and lateral flexion control.
Note: Hard cervical collars used for prolonged durations may result in occipital pressure ulcers.[12]

Custom Cervical Bivalve

S00-T98 INJURY, POISONING, AND CERTAIN OTHER CONSEQUENCES OF EXTERNAL CAUSES

Issue	LOC	Sources	Affil	Rationale/Comment
Occipital or chin injuries	CI	Bussel et al, 1995[14]	MD	This total contact collar may be poorly tolerated.
Open wounds	CI			

Philadelphia Collar (CO)

Philadelphia Collar with Thoracic Extensions (CTO)

M00-M99 DISEASES OF THE MUSCULOSKELETAL SYSTEM AND CONNECTIVE TISSUE
R00-R99 SYMPTOMS AND SIGNS

Issue	LOC	Sources	Affil	Rationale/Comment
Cervical spine instability	CI	Bussel et al, 1995[14]	MD	This collar is designed for stable midcervical injuries. This total
Poor tolerance of pressure on thorax, chin, occiput, or sternum	CI			contact collar may be poorly tolerated.

Two or Four Poster (CO)

Two or Four Poster with Thoracic Extensions (CTO)

S00-T98 INJURY, POISONING, AND CERTAIN OTHER CONSEQUENCES OF EXTERNAL CAUSES
R00-R99 SYMPTOMS AND SIGNS

Issue	LOC	Sources	Affil	Rationale/Comment
Poor tolerance of pressure	CI	Bussel et al, 1995[14]	MD	These orthoses are designed for stable cervical fractures.
Unstable cervical fracture	CI			

Sternal Occipital Mandibular Immobilizer (SOMI) (CTO)

S00-T98 INJURY, POISONING, AND CERTAIN OTHER CONSEQUENCES OF EXTERNAL R00-R99 SYMPTOMS, SIGNS

Issue	LOC	Sources	Affil	Rationale/Comment
Poor tolerance of pressure	CI	Bussel et al, 1995[14]	MD	The SOMI controls extension poorly.
Unstable injuries, particularly in extension	CI			

Halo

S00-T98 INJURY, POISONING, AND CERTAIN OTHER CONSEQUENCES OF EXTERNAL CAUSES

Issue	LOC	Sources	Affil	Rationale/Comment
Cranial fractures	CI	Bussel et al, 1995[14]	MD	The ring of the halo must be fixed to the skull.

PROCEDURAL CONCERNS

Issue	LOC	Sources	Affil	Rationale/Comment
Shoulder abduction > 90 degrees	P	Pomerantz and Durand, 2005[15]	MD	There is a danger of exerting large distractive forces at the
Shoulder shrugging	Avoid			vertebral segment with these motions.

Note: Halo orthotics, used to control high cervical fractures, have several potential complications: loose pins, pin infections, pressure ulcers, reduced vital capacity, brain abscesses, neck pain, and psychological trauma.[1]

Corsets (Flexible Spinal Orthosis)

J00-J99 DISEASES OF THE RESPIRATORY SYSTEM

Issue	LOC	Sources	Affil	Rationale/Comment
Respiratory distress—severe	CI	Bussel et al, 1995[14]	MD	For LSO and TLSOs due to total contact and circumferential pressure exerted.

L00-L99 DISEASES OF THE SKIN AND SUBCUTANEOUS TISSUE

Issue	LOC	Sources	Affil	Rationale/Comment
Skin irritation	CI	Tan, 1998[1,a]	MD/PT	This is a general concern regarding corsets (i.e., prescribing a corset if irritation exists).

M00-M99 DISEASES OF THE MUSCULOSKELETAL SYSTEM AND CONNECTIVE TISSUE

Issue	LOC	Sources	Affil	Rationale/Comment
Spinal asymmetry—scoliosis	CI	Bussel et al, 1995[14]	MD	For TLSOs: Prefabricated TLSO corsets are difficult to fit over a scoliosis.

S00-T98 INJURY, POISONING, AND CERTAIN OTHER CONSEQUENCES OF EXTERNAL CAUSES

Issue	LOC	Sources	Affil	Rationale/Comment
Multiple rib fractures	CI	Bussel et al, 1995[14]	MD	For prefabricated thoracic rib belt: if thoracic mechanical stability is compromised.

Williams Flexion LSO

Extension Control

Issue	LOC	Sources	Affil	Rationale/Comment
Traumatic compression fractures (or pathologies where flexion is not to be performed)	CI	Bussel et al, 1995[14]	MD	This orthosis is designed for spondylolysis and spondylolisthesis; it permits flexion but stops lumbar spine extension.

CASH or Jewett TLSO

Flexion Control

S00-T98 INJURY, POISONING, AND CERTAIN OTHER CONSEQUENCES OF EXTERNAL CAUSES

Issue	LOC	Sources	Affil	Rationale/Comment
Unstable fractures (or pathology that should not permit extension (e.g., spondylolisthesis)	CI	Bussel et al, 1995[14]	MD	This orthosis is designed for thoracolumbar traumatic compression fractures; it permits free extension but stops flexion. It does not control rotation.

Body Jackets

G00-G99 DISEASES OF THE NERVOUS SYSTEM

Issue	LOC	Sources	Affil	Rationale/Comment
Insensate	Extra precaution	Pomerantz and Durand, 2005[15]	MD	Use care when fitting a person without sensation to a custom-molded total-contact TLSO.

L00-L99 DISEASES OF THE SKIN AND SUBCUTANEOUS TISSUE

Issue	LOC	Sources	Affil	Rationale/Comment
Skin/heat sensitivity	CI	Bussel et al, 1995[14]	MD	Body jackets are designed for the management of traumatic or postsurgical fractures and fusions. They provide total contact.

Custom Body Jacket for Scoliosis

G00-G99 DISEASES OF THE NERVOUS SYSTEM

Issue	LOC	Sources	Affil	Rationale/Comment
Nonprogressive paralytic curves	CI	Bussel et al, 1995[14]	MD	The custom TLSO is designed for flexible scoliotic curves in growing spines.

M00-M99 DISEASES OF THE MUSCULOSKELETAL SYSTEM

Issue	LOC	Sources	Affil	Rationale/Comment
Adult curves	CI	Bussel et al, 1995[14]	MD	The custom TLSO is designed for flexible scoliotic curves in growing spines.
T8 curves, above	CI			

Milwaukee CTLSO

G00-G99 DISEASES OF THE NERVOUS SYSTEM

Issue	LOC	Sources	Affil	Rationale/Comment
Neuromuscular scoliosis	CI	Bussel et al, 1995[14]	MD	Patients with paralysis will not be able to withdraw from the orthotic pads.

ADVERSE EVENTS

Source	Background	Therapy	Outcome	Follow-up/Interpretation
Gryboski et al, 1978[11] **Esophagitis and TLSO** Case series (2 of 4 reported here)	A 5 1/2-year-old girl with scoliosis was placed in a TLSO.	Epigastric pain developed 4 weeks later.	Dx: Esophagitis. Removal of brace and instituting antireflux measures led to relief of symptoms in 1 week. Later she resumed use.	TLSOs produce abdominal compression, causing symptoms within 1-2 months.

Continued

Source	Background	Therapy	Outcome	Follow-up/Interpretation
Lancet	A child 3 years 4 months old with scoliosis was placed in a scoliotic brace at 2 years of age.	The child vomited after feeding.	Dx: Esophagitis.	Mechanism (in two patients): Intragastric pressure was greater than esophageal pressure only when brace was worn.
Johnson et al, 1977[16] **Airplane splint, Erb's palsy, and contractures**	32 infants diagnosed with Erb's palsy (11 followed for 18 years).	Shoulder external rotation deformity noted in infants who wore an airplane splint for a few weeks to a few months.		
Retrospective and case series Arch Phys Med Rehab	An infant boy with right Erb's palsy was placed in an airplane splint (in abduction and external rotation) from age 2 months to 7 months.	At 13 months, his shoulder was fixed in external rotation and 50-degree abduction.	At 6 years, the attitude of the shoulder remained and the mother was unable to put the child's hand to his mouth.	
Kling et al, 1981[12] **TLSO and esophagitis** Case report Clin Orthop Rel Res	A tall, slender 14-year-old girl presented with idiopathic adolescent scoliosis (right thoracic 25 degree; left thoracolumbar 20 degree). Her curve progressed despite being cast for 4 weeks and wearing a Milwaukee brace for 8 months (23 hours/day).	She was prescribed a Boston TLSO to control increasing rotation of her lower curve. After 4 months of full-time use, the patient experienced mid-epigastric pain radiating to her back, eructation, and a sour taste in her mouth, which was worse when supine/sitting and before breakfast.	Dx: Chronic esophagitis. Gastroesophageal manometry revealed intragastric pressure 2 mm higher than lower esophageal sphincter pressure only with the brace on. Esophageal biopsy: nutrient papillae to 70-80% of mucosal thickness. Symptoms resolved after 3 weeks with removal of the brace, elevation of the head of bed,	The authors postulated that the orthosis increased intragastric pressure, allowing reflux and esophagitis.

Ryan et al, 2003[4] **AFO and peroneal palsy** Case report Pediatr Neurol	A 13-year-old boy presented with mild hemophilia and cardiomyopathy. He was supine, confused, and immobile and received factor replacement, transfusions, and extracorporeal membrane oxygenation while awaiting a donor heart.	He received bilateral prefabricated soft-foam AFOs to prevent contractures for 5 days (schedule: 2 hours on/ 2 hours off)	antacids, anticholinergics, and frequent feedings. Symptoms returned with orthotic use and led to a modified schedule of reduced wearing time of brace. He developed bilateral peroneal palsies with 0/5 dorsiflexion 2/5 eversion, 3/5 g toe extension and light touch loss on lateral legs and feet 1 week s/p cardiac transplantation. Electrodiagnoses confirmed peroneal neuropathies.	Paresthesia resolved in several weeks. He required ankle bracing for 4 months due to foot drop. At 6 months, lateral leg muscle wasting and dorsiflexion improved to 4/5. The authors believe local pressure over the fibular head due to a poorly fitted orthosis in conjunction with immobility and positioning (supine with externally rotated hips) contributed.
Weitz and Carson, 1969[6] **Compartment syndrome and LLB** Case report Bull Hosp Joint Dis	A 20-month-old boy with tibia varus deformity LLE was fitted for LLB using a lateral strap applied to the middle half of his leg to correct deformity.	The infant cried after a few hours after wearing brace and refused ambulation. A swollen left leg was noted. X-rays at the ER were negative.	Dx: Tibial compartment syndrome. Decompression fasciotomy of anterior tibial compartment. Muscles were grayish brown and ischemic.	The authors postulate pressure was applied on the anterior lateral calf while weight bearing, leading to compression and increased capillary permeability to fluid and plasma.

Continued

Source	Background	Therapy	Outcome	Follow-up/Interpretation
		Two days later, the infant exhibited decreased appetite and increased agitation. He was hospitalized the next day. Later, he was unable to dorsiflex the ankle and pulse was noted absent.	Two months post surgery, he was able to dorsiflex ankle; 6 months later, he regained full return of power to ankles and toes.	

REFERENCES

1. Tan JC: Practical manual of physical medicine and rehabilitation: diagnostics, therapeutics, and basic problems. St. Louis: Mosby; 1998.
2. Webster's third new international dictionary. Springfield (MA): Merriam-Webster; 1981.
3. Linden CA, Trombly CA: Orthoses: kinds and purposes. In Trombly CA, editor: Occupational therapy for physical dysfunction, ed 4. Baltimore (MD): Williams & Wilkins; 1995.
4. Ryan MM, Darras BT, Soul JS: Peroneal neuropathy from ankle-foot orthosis. Pediatr Neurol 29(1):72-74, 2003.
5. Fischer AQ, Strasburger J: Footdrop in the neonate secondary to use of footboards. J Pediatr 101:1003-1004, 1982.
6. Weitz EM, Carson G: The anterior tibial compartment syndrome in a twenty month old infant. Bull Hosp Joint Dis 30(1):16-20, 1969.
7. Helm PA, Kevorkian CG, Lushbaugh M, et al: Burn injury: rehabilitation management in 1982. Arch Phys Med Rehab 63:6-16, 1982.
8. Malick MH: Manual on static hand splinting. Pittsburgh (PA): Harmarville Rehabilitation; 1980.

9. Cusick BD: Progressive casting and splinting for lower extremity deformities in children with neuromuscular dysfunction. Tucson (AZ): Therapy Skill Builders; 1990.

10. Miner LJ, Nelson VS: Upper limb orthoses. In: Redford JB, Basmajian JV, Trautman P, eds: Orthotics: clinical practice and rehabilitation technology. New York: Churchill-Livingstone; 1995.

11. Gryboski JD, Kocoshis SA, Seashore JH, et al: "Body-brace" oesophagitis, a complication of kyphoscoliosis therapy. Lancet 2(8087):449-451, 1978.

12. Kling TF, Drennan JC, Gryboski JD: Esophagitis complicating scoliosis management with the Boston thoracolumbosacral orthosis. Clin Orthop Rel Res 159:208-210, 1981.

13. Liew SC, Hill DA: Complication of hard cervical collars in multi-trauma patient. Aust N Z J Surg 64(2):139-140, 1994.

14. Bussell M, Merritt J, Fenwick L: Spinal orthoses. In: Redford JB, Basmajian JV, Trautman P, eds: Orthotics: Clinical practice and rehabilitation technology. New York: Churchill-Livingstone; 1995.

15. Pomerantz F, Durand E: Spinal orthosis. In: Delisa JA, editor: Physical medicine and rehabilitation: principles and practice, ed 4, vol 2. Philadelphia: Lippincott Williams & Wilkins; 2005.

16. Johnson EW, Alexander MA, Koenig WC: Infantile Erb's palsy (Smellie's palsy). Arch Phys Med Rehab 58(4):175-178, 1977.

32 PROSTHETICS

OVERVIEW. A prosthesis is an artificial mechanical or electrical body part used to replace a missing one; the word literally means "placed instead."[1]

SUMMARY: CONTRAINDICATIONS AND PRECAUTIONS. Overall, prosthetic sources will often indicate whether patients are poor candidates for prosthetic training; contraindications are not frequently listed. Gitter and Bosker[2] indicate that a prosthetic candidate should have a reasonable cardiovascular reserve, adequate wound healing, good soft tissue coverage, sufficient range of motion and strength, motor control, and learning ability to use the prosthesis. With borderline cases, less costly trials (e.g., rigid dressing [removable] with pylon and foot) can be considered. Based on an older, 1977 retrospective review, Couch[3] identified dementia and debility as two contraindications for a prosthesis. Depending on the type of prosthesis, other concerns include skin grafts, skin hypersensitivity, short stump length,[3] blindness,[3] and commitment to the rehabilitation process. General prosthetic concerns as well as guidelines for ICEROSS Socket Systems and Patella Tendon Bearing Socket are noted below.

CONTRAINDICATIONS AND PRECAUTIONS

PROSTHESES: GENERAL

E00-E90 ENDOCRINE NUTRITIONAL AND METABOLIC DISEASES

Issue	LOC	Sources	Affil	Rationale/Comment
Body weight fluctuations	Poor candidate	Gitter and Bosker, 2005[2]	MD	

F00-F99 MENTAL AND BEHAVIORAL DISORDERS

Issue	LOC	Sources	Affil	Rationale/Comment
Dementia	CI	Couch et al, 1977[3]	MD	**In 1977, Couch et al[3] conducted a retrospective chart review of 150 patients who survived amputation; 37 (25%) failed rehabilitation attempts were attributed to patient dementia.**

G00-G99 DISEASES OF THE NERVOUS SYSTEM

Issue	LOC	Sources	Affil	Rationale/Comment
Flail shoulder and elbow for transradial amputations	Poor candidate	Gitter and Bosker, 2005[2]	MD	
Polyneuropathy, severe	Poor candidate			
Sensation-impaired	Advice	Tan, 1998[4]	MD/PT	Residual stump skin must be checked regularly for redness and abrasions.

H00-H59 DISEASES OF THE EYE

Issue	LOC	Sources	Affil	Rationale/Comment
Blindness	Rehab failure	Couch et al, 1977[3]	MD	**See Couch, 1977, below.**

I00-I99 DISEASES OF THE CIRCULATORY SYSTEM

Issue	LOC	Sources	Affil	Rationale/Comment
Coronary artery disease—severe	Poor candidate	Gitter and Bosker, 2005[2]	MD	
Circulation—impaired	Advice	Tan, 1998[4]	MD/PT	Residual stump skin must be checked regularly for redness, trophic changes, and abrasions.
	Poor candidate	Gitter and Bosker, 2005[2,a]	MD	

a, Dysvascular LE amputation.

J00-J99 DISEASES OF THE RESPIRATORY SYSTEM

Issue	LOC	Sources	Affil	Rationale/Comment
Pulmonary disease	Poor candidate	Gitter and Bosker, 2005[2]	MD	

M00-M99 DISEASES OF THE MUSCULOSKELETAL SYSTEM AND CONNECTIVE TISSUE

Issue	LOC	Sources	Affil	Rationale/Comment
Arthritis—multiple joint	Poor candidate	Gitter and Bosker, 2005[2]	MD	
Contracture, 30-degree flexion contracture in transfemoral amputation	Poor candidate			
Short transfemoral amputation, bilateral—in persons over 45 years of age	Poor candidate			

S00-T98 INJURY, POISONING, AND CERTAIN OTHER CONSEQUENCES OF EXTERNAL CAUSES

Issue	LOC	Sources	Affil	Rationale/Comment
Open wound	Poor candidate	Gitter and Bosker, 2005[2]	MD	Incisions that are healing poorly.

R00-R99 SYMPTOMS, SIGNS

Issue	LOC	Sources	Affil	Rationale/Comment
Debility	CI	Couch et al, 1977[3]	MD	**Based on Couch's 1977 retrospective chart review of 150 patients who survived amputation, 24 (16%) failed rehabilitation attempts were attributed to debility.**
Prognosis—poor	Poor candidate	Gitter and Bosker, 2005[2,a]	MD	

a, Or short life expectancy.

Note: In Couch et al (1977), other reasons for prosthetic training failure were attributed to: stroke 14 (9%), stump pain 5 (3%), blindness 3 (2%), and joint contractures 3 (2%); 6 (4%) were indeterminate.

ICELANDIC ROLL-ON SILICONE SOCKET (ICEROSS) SOCKET SYSTEM

F00-F99 MENTAL AND BEHAVIORAL DISORDERS

Issue	LOC	Sources	Affil	Rationale/Comment
Commitment—poor	ACI	McCurdie et al, 1997[5]	Royal Hospitals	Poor commitment to prosthetic rehabilitation.
Hygiene—poor	ACI			

L00-L99 DISEASES OF THE SKIN AND SUBCUTANEOUS TISSUE

Issue	LOC	Sources	Affil	Rationale/Comment
Scars—unhealed	ACI	McCurdie et al, 1997[5]	Royal Hospitals	

S00-T98 INJURY, POISONING, AND CERTAIN OTHER CONSEQUENCES OF EXTERNAL CAUSES

Issue	LOC	Sources	Affil	Rationale/Comment
Ulceration	ACI	McCurdie et al, 1997[5]	Royal Hospitals	

PATELLA TENDON BEARING SOCKET

G00-G99 DISEASES OF THE NERVOUS SYSTEM

Issue	LOC	Sources	Affil	Rationale/Comment
Hypersensitive stump	CI/ not indicated	Engstrom and Van de Ven, 1993[6]	PT	(Or with adherent scarring, possibly anesthetic.)
Hyposensitive stump	CI/ not indicated			

L00-L99 DISEASES OF THE SKIN AND SUBCUTANEOUS TISSUE

Issue	LOC	Sources	Affil	Rationale/Comment
Skin graft	CI/ not indicated	Engstrom and Van de Ven, 1993[6]	PT	Stumps not tough enough for PTB.

M00-M99 DISEASES OF THE MUSCULOSKELETAL SYSTEM AND CONNECTIVE TISSUE

Issue	LOC	Sources	Affil	Rationale/Comment
Contracture—knee flexion Instability—knee joint Stump—very short	CI/not indicated	Engstrom and Van de Ven, 1993[6]	PT	Greater than 25-degree knee flexion contracture.

Q00-Q99 CONGENITAL MALFORMATIONS, DEFORMITIES, AND CHROMOSOMAL ABNORMALITIES

Issue	LOC	Sources	Affil	Rationale/Comment
Malformation—of patella or knee joint region	CI/not indicated	Engstrom and Van de Ven, 1993[6]	PT	(I.e., congenital; fractures.)

PROCEDURAL CONCERNS/MISCELLANEOUS

Issue	LOC	Sources	Affil	Rationale/Comment
Occupation—heavy work	CI/not indicated	Engstrom and Van de Ven, 1993[6]	PT	(Heavy work, i.e., farming, oil rig work.)

ADVERSE EVENTS

Source	Background	Therapy	Outcome	Follow-up/Interpretation
Couch et al, 1977[3] **Prosthesis and rehabilitation failure** Chart review Am J Surg	150 patients who survived major leg amputation were followed for rehabilitation success using a prosthesis.	93 patients were given prostheses. Of these, 76% of unilateral AK and 90% of unilateral BK amputees had successful prosthetic rehabilitation.	Reasons for rehabilitation failure in this sample: • 25% debility • 16% dementia • 9% stroke • 3% stump pain • 2% blindness • 2% joint contracture • 4% indeterminate	The authors state most common reason CI for a prosthesis were debility and dementia.

REFERENCES

1. Eisenberg MG: Dictionary of rehabilitation. New York: Springer; 1995.
2. Gitter A, Bosker G: Upper and lower extremity prosthetics. In Delisa JA, editor: Physical medicine and rehabilitation: principles and practice, ed 4, vol 1. Philadelphia: Lippincott Williams & Wilkins; 2005.
3. Couch NP, David JK, Tilney NL, et al: Natural history of the leg amputee. Am J Surg 133(4):469-473, 1977.
4. Tan JC: Practical manual of physical medicine and rehabilitation: diagnostics, therapeutics, and basic problems. St. Louis: Mosby; 1998.
5. McCurdie I, Hanspal R, Nieveen R: ICEROSS—a consensus view: a questionnaire survey of the use of ICEROSS in the United Kingdom. Prosthet Orthot Int 21(2):124-128, 1997.
6. Engstrom B, Van de Ven C: Physiotherapy for amputees: the Roehampton approach, ed 2. Edinburgh, Scotland: Churchill Livingstone; 1993.

33 | PROTECTIVE DEVICES

33.1 Cushions

OVERVIEW. A cushion is a case filled with soft or resilient material that can be used during sitting, reclining, or kneeling activities.[1] Examples include use of wheelchair cushions for sitting and use of a bed pillow for head support.

CONTRAINDICATIONS AND PRECAUTIONS

Issue	LOC	Sources	Affil	Rationale/LOE/Comment
Boomerang pillow—reduced lung capacity due to age	CI	Roberts, 1995[2]	Nurs	**Based on an exploratory, repeated-measures study in 1995, Roberts et al[2] found a 20% reduction in mean minute volume in elderly nursing home patients without obvious lung disease while using the V-shaped pillow in supine.** (See proposed mechanism below.)
Gel cushions—long-term use	Advice	Garber, 1985[3]	OT	Long-term wheelchair users of gel cushions may lose tolerance for other cushion types. Note: Mechanism/evidence unclear.

ADVERSE EVENTS

Source	Background	Therapy	Outcome	Follow-up/Interpretation
Roberts et al, 1995[2] **Boomerang pillow and reduced breathing volume** Repeated measures (exploratory) Clin Nurs Res	A convenience sample of 18 frail women ages 65 to 80 from an Australian nursing home population who were cognitively intact, ambulatory with assist, and with no "overt" respiratory disease were studied.	Subjects were measured for mean minute volume at baseline, and at 5 and 10 minutes while using the boomerang pillow in supine.	There was a significant reduction in mean minute volume ($p = .02$) with a 20% reduction (0.7 liter change) noted with boomerang pillow.	The authors suggest that the boomerang pillow may be contraindicated in those with reduced lung capacity due to age and a need for further research with a larger sample. Mechanism: Because of its "V" shape, it causes slumping posture (posterior convexity of lumbar spine and flexed shoulders), thus restricting chest expansion during inspiration. Note: This population had no obvious respiratory disease.

REFERENCES

1. Webster's third new international dictionary. Springfield (MA): Merriam-Webster; 1981.
2. Roberts KL, Brittin M, deClifford J: Boomerang pillows and respiratory capacity in frail elderly women. Clin Nurs Res 4(4):465-471, 1995.
3. Garber SL: Wheelchair cushions: a historical review. Am J Occup Ther 39(7):453-459, 1985.

33.2 Restraints

OVERVIEW. A restraint is a device used to help immobilize a patient. A physical restraint is a manual, physical, or mechanical device that the patient cannot easily remove and that restricts freedom to move. Drug restraints are nonstandard medication treatments, used to control patient behavior and restrict freedom of movement.[1] The purpose/rationale of using restraints has been to reduce fall-related injuries from chairs, beds, and during ambulation, to reduce wandering-related injuries, and to implement invasive medical care such as IV lines. Despite these reasons, physical restraint use has led to instances of strangulation, chest compression asphyxiation, escape-related trauma, and skin and nerve injuries.[2]

SUMMARY: CONTRAINDICATIONS AND PRECAUTIONS. Patient injuries and fatalities are major concerns with restraint use. Recommendations and Position Statements for restraint use on patients are listed from the Food and Drug Administration[3] and American Geriatric Society,[4] respectively. Thirteen issues are listed; six (about 45%) are shared concerns. Issues include (1) use of alternatives, (2) discontinuation, (3) regulation, (4) removal, (5) staff training, and (6) proper use. Rubin et al,[5] in a 1993 descriptive study (case series), noted that restraints used in chairs, wheelchairs, and beds can be lethal, even if applied correctly.

PROCEDURAL CONCERNS

Issue	LOC	Sources	Affil	Rationale/Comment
Alternatives to restraints	Position statement	AGS, 1991[4,a]	Org	Encourage research into alternatives to restraint use.
	Recommendation	FDA, 1992[3]	Gov	Seek alternatives when possible.
Comfortable application	Recommendation	FDA, 1992[3]	Gov	
Consent—obtaining	Recommendation			Obtain consent from patient or family.
Discontinuation issues				
Remove or discontinue at reasonable intervals.	Position statement	AGS, 1991[4,a]	Org	Remove to evaluate need and effectiveness of the device.
Discontinue use as soon as feasible.	Recommendation	FDA, 1992[3]	Gov	Discontinue to allow normal body functions.
Restraints applied above IV site	Avoid	Pierson and Fairchild, 2002[1]	PT	Avoid restraints above an infusion site.
Policies—for institutions	Recommendation	FDA, 1992[3]	Gov	Have and display clear policies; train staff.
Regulations				
Follow local and state laws regarding restraints.	Recommendation	FDA, 1992[3]	Org	Short-term use may be indicated for emergent treatment that
Requires an order and renewed in compliance with state and federal regulations.	Position statement	AGS, 1991[4,a]	Gov	results in a less confused patient, or if patient poses significant harm to self or others.
Removal issues				
The device must be checked and removed from patient periodically.	Position statement	AGS, 1991[4,a]	Org	Removal allows exercise of the restrained limb, walking,
Remove as often as possible.	Recommendation	FDA, 1992[3]	Gov	hydration, social interaction, and bathroom activities.

Staff training	Position statement	AGS, 1991[4,a]	Org	Train for proper use and safety. Complications can be reduced with patient education, staff training, and better product labeling.[2]
	Recommendation	FDA, 1992[3]	Gov	
Understand behavior	Position statement	AGS, 1991[4,a]	Org	Understand the behavior that precipitates a decision to use restraints in the first place. Look at both patient and staff behavior.
Use as directed	Position statement	AGS, 1991[4,a]	Org	Use as directed by the manufacturer to prevent pressure-related injuries.
	Recommendation	FDA, 1992[3]	Gov	Misuses include choosing the wrong patients (i.e., the chronically agitated may become more agitated), the wrong sizing, and the wrong application (note the front and back of the device).
Use least restrictive device	Position statement	AGS, 1991[4,a]	Org	
Use sparingly—restraints	Position statement			Use restraints very sparingly in nonemergency situations. Reassess regularly for safer alternatives.
				The FDA estimates 100 deaths from improper use of restraints annually. Most occur when patient tries to get out of the restraint.[3]

a, The AGS Clinical Practice Committee Position Statement was developed and approved in May 1991 and reviewed in May 1997 and 2002.

ADVERSE EVENTS

Source	Background	Therapy	Outcome	Follow-up/Interpretation
Bunai et al, 2001[6] **Restraint, MVA, and death** Case report J Forens Sci	A 59-year-old man sat in a wheelchair while traveling in a van and was involved in an MVA.	Initially, only bruising was noted; 8 hours later, severe abdominal pain was reported. He died 20 hours after the accident.	Dx: Blunt pancreatic trauma caused by a wheelchair restraint system during the accident.	
Rubin et al, 1993[5] **Restraints and deaths** Descriptive/Case series Arch Fam Med	Questionnaires regarding restraint-related deaths were distributed to chief death investigators from 37 jurisdictions.	A total of 63 cases of asphyxial deaths due to restraints were reported from 23 jurisdictions. Ages ranged from 26 weeks to 98 years; 61% in nursing homes. Most restraints (57 of 63) were properly applied. Incidences were bed- or chair-related and most involved a vest restraint.	Type of restraint involved: 1. Chair (wheelchair or geriatric recliner) Vest (16) Waist (3) 2. Bed Vest (19) Waist (8) Rail (13) Wrist (2)	Restraints are potentially lethal, even when applied correctly.

REFERENCES

1. Pierson FM, Fairchild SL: Principles and techniques of patient care, ed 3. Philadelphia: Saunders; 2002.
2. Miles SH, Meyers R: Untying the elderly: 1989 to 1993 update. Clin Geriatr Med 10(3):513-525, 1994.

3. Food and Drug Administration: Safe use of physical restraint devices. Rockville (MD): FDA Backgrounder; 1992.

4. American Geriatric Society: Position statement. Restraint use. Available at: http://www.americangeriatrics.org/products/positionpapers/restraintsupdatePF.shtml. Accessed November 9, 2005.

5. Rubin BS, Dube AH, Mitchell EK: Asphyxial deaths due to physical restraint. A case series. Arch Fam Med 2(4):405-408, 1993.

6. Bunai Y, Nagai A, Nakamura I, et al: Blunt pancreatic trauma by a wheelchair user restraint system during a traffic accident. J Forens Sci 46(4):965-967, 2001.

34 SUPPORTIVE DEVICES

34.1 Elastic Supports (Compression Supports)

OVERVIEW. An elastic support is an article of clothing that offers some degree of compression around a body part in order to help prevent DVT (16-18 mm Hg—antiembolism stocking), control scar formation (20-30 mm Hg), control edema in ambulators (30-40 mm Hg),[1] or assist in venous circulation return.[2] An example of an elastic support is a compression garment.

SUMMARY: CONTRAINDICATIONS AND PRECAUTIONS. Two sources list seven concerns for compression supports. Concerns ranged from four to six per source; three shared issues included (1) treating edema, (2) peripheral artery disease, and (3) donning difficulties. The concerns of Scholten et al[3] are targeted to a stroke population. The FDA[4] has received reports of neuropathy and skin blistering as a possible complication of compression support therapy.

CONTRAINDICATIONS AND PRECAUTIONS

COMPRESSION SUPPORTS

I00-I99 DISEASES OF THE CIRCULATORY SYSTEM

Issue	LOC	Sources	Affil	Rationale/Comment
Edema—treating	P	Redford, 1986[5]	MD	Compression support is designed to maintain edema reduction, not treat it.
Gross edema of legs (beyond the knee)	CI	Scholten et al, 2000[3,a]	Dept Med	Compression level may be insufficient for treatment of edema. **Based on Scholten et al (2000) descriptive study in persons with stroke.[3]**
Peripheral artery disease	CI	Redford, 1986[5]	MD	Excessive compression support in persons with peripheral arterial disease may
	CI	Scholten et al, 2000[3,b]	Dept Med	increase danger of gangrene. **Based on Scholten et al (2000) descriptive study in persons with stroke.[3]**
Venous ulceration causing skin breakdown	CI	Scholten et al, 2000[3]	Dept Med	**Based on Scholten et al (2000) descriptive study in persons with stroke.[3]**

a, Marked dependent edema; b, <0.8 ABI.

L00-L99 DISEASES OF THE SKIN AND SUBCUTANEOUS TISSUE

Issue	LOC	Sources	Affil	Rationale/Comment
Cellulitis	CI	Scholten et al, 2000[3]	Dept Med	**Based on Scholten et al (2000) descriptive study in persons with stroke.[3]**
Skin disorders	CI	Redford, 1986[5]	MD	(I.e., moist dermatoses and cutaneous infections.)

PROCEDURAL CONCERNS

Issue	LOC	Sources	Affil	Rationale/Comment
Donning—difficulty	P	Redford, 1986[5]	MD	Persons with hemiplegia, paraplegia, organic brain syndrome or others who cannot independently
	CI	Scholten et al, 2000[3]	Dept	don supports will need assistance from others. Leg deformity may also make donning difficult.[3]
			Med	Consider this factor before prescribing. **Based on Scholten et al (2000) descriptive study in persons with stroke who presented with leg deformities.[3]**
Tolerability—poor	CI	Scholten et al, 2000[3]	Dept	Intolerance was often due to skin irritation.
			Med	**Based on Scholten et al (2000) descriptive study in persons with stroke.[3]**

ADVERSE EVENTS

Source	Background	Therapy	Outcome	Follow-up/Interpretation
Scholten et al, 2000[3] **Screening, CVA, and compression stockings** Descriptive Age Aging	112 consecutive stroke patients were assessed for tolerance and contraindications for graduated compression stockings.	Of 112 patients, 94 (84%) had no contraindications for stocking use. Noted contraindications were ankle-brachial index <0.8, marked dependent leg edema, and severe venous ulceration; 95% tolerated the stockings during hospital stay.	Based on the data, graduated elastic compression stockings were well tolerated if patients were screened for contraindications.	**Contraindications listed included:** • Incipient ischemia due to peripheral vascular insufficiency (Doppler measures <0.8 ABI) • Poor tolerability • Gross edema of legs (beyond the knee) • Venous ulceration causing skin breakdown • Cellulitis • Leg deformity making donning of stocking difficult

FDA REPORTS[4]

Stocking, elastic

Date	Device	Event	Outcome
8/01/88	Anti-embolism stocking (Pulsatile, Pharmaseal)	The stocking was prescribed for 4 days following a surgery.	The patient sustained a peroneal nerve compression with a resultant foot drop.
11/23/88	TED sequential compression device	A 76-year-old woman with arteriosclerotic disease and carotid endarterectomy was placed in the device prior to surgery. In the recovery room, the patient complained of "tightness." The following evening, she complained of severe leg pain.	When the device was removed, 1 × 2 inch bilateral blisters were noted below her knees on the lower legs.

Note: FDA reports do not necessarily establish cause-effect relationships between equipment and injury. Incidences may be due to equipment or user error. Also, some reports are alleged by attorneys.

REFERENCES

1. Cameron MH: Physical agents in rehabilitation: from research to practice. St. Louis: Saunders; 2003.
2. Pierson FM, Fairchild SL: Principles and techniques of patient care, ed 3. Philadelphia: Saunders; 2002.
3. Scholten P, Bever A, Turner K, et al: Graduated elastic compression stockings on a stroke unit: a feasibility study. Age Aging 29(4):357-359, 2000.
4. U.S. Food and Drug Administration: Center for Device and Radiological Health. Available at: http://www.fda.gov/cdrh/mdr/. Accessed on November 7, 2005.
5. Redford JB: Orthotics etcetera. Baltimore (MD): Williams & Wilkins; 1986.

34.2 Lines

Lines are medical devices that use tubing to infuse fluid, infuse or obtain blood, or monitor hemodynamics. Whereas central lines access a patient's heart from a peripheral vessel, peripheral lines access the patient's circulation from a peripheral vessel. Intracranial pressure (ICP) monitors measure the pressure of brain tissue against the skull.[1,2] Concerns when treating patients who have these lines are listed below.

A critical concern when treating patients is the dislodgment of IV lines or catheters because it can lead to a fatal air embolism. See Philips and Lee (1990),[3] Zafonte et al (1996),[4] and an Ohio lawsuit[5] below.

PERIPHERAL LINES

Arterial Lines (A Line)

Arterial lines are peripheral lines, inserted into the artery (e.g., radial, dorsal, pedal, axillary, brachial, or femoral) to continuously measure blood pressure or obtain blood samples.[2]

Issue	LOC	Sources	Affil	Rationale/Comment
Ask for assistance—moving patients	Advice	Collins, 1997[2]	PT	Avoid dislodging lines when moving a patient.
Exercising	P	Pierson and Fairchild, 2002[1]	PT	Exercise with A lines is possible, but avoid disturbing the inserted needle, occluding, or disconnecting the line, or disrupting the catheter.

Intravenous (IV) Infusion Lines

Intravenous (IV) infusion lines are peripheral lines used to obtain venous blood samples, to infuse fluids, nutrients, electrolytes, or medication, or to insert catheters into the central circulatory system to monitor physiologic conditions.[1] IV line precautions also apply to patient-controlled analgesia (PCA).[1a]

Issue	LOC	Sources	Affil	Rationale/Comment
Ask for assistance—moving patients	Advice	Collins, 1997[2]	PT	Avoid dislodging lines when moving a patient.
Blood pressure measures—taken above IV site	Advice	Pierson and Fairchild, 2002[1]	PT	Avoid applying a blood pressure cuff above the infusion site.
Elbow position				If infusion site is located in the antecubital area, do not flex the elbow.
Infusion site placement—at heart level				Ambulators are instructed to grasp the IV line support pole so the infusion site will be at heart level. If the infusion site remains in a dependent position, a retrograde flow of blood may occur into the IV line tubing. Similar procedures are observed when patients are treated in bed or on a treatment mat.
Infusion site problems, monitor for				Observe for edema, discomfort, reduced fluid flow, or infections before and after treatments.
Prolonged positioning with infusion site above the level of the heart				Avoid activities that require the infusion site to be elevated above the level of the heart for a prolonged period of time so the proper direction of fluid flow can be maintained.
				Report problems to nursing.
Restraints applied—above IV site				Avoid restraints located above the infusion site.
Tube—occlusions, disruptions, stretching				Avoid disrupting connections, occluding tubes, stressing infusion sites, or interrupting circulatory flow. Do not overstretch tubing during exercise.

a, Patient-controlled analgesia (PCA) is used to self-administer a small predetermined dose of pain medication intravenously on demand. The device is connected to the patient via an IV line.[1]

CENTRAL LINES

Swan-Ganz Catheter (Pulmonary Artery Catheter)

A Swan-Ganz catheter is an IV tube that is inserted into the internal jugular or femoral vein and is passed into the pulmonary artery to provide accurate continuous measurement of pulmonary artery (PA) pressure.[1] Swan-Ganz catheter precautions also apply to central venous pressure catheters (CVPs)[a] and indwelling right atrial catheters (e.g., Hickman).[1,b]

Issue	LOC	Sources	Affil	Rationale/Comment
Ask for assistance—moving patients	Advice	Collins, 1997[2]	PT	Avoid dislodging lines when moving a patient.
Exercising	P	Pierson and Fairchild, 2002[1]	PT	Exercise is possible, but mobility may need to be restricted near the catheter insertion (i.e., for the subclavian vein, avoid shoulder flexion; for the femoral vein, avoid hip flexion and abduction).

a, CVPs measure pressure in the right atrium or superior vena cava.[1] b, The indwelling right atrial catheters (e.g., Hickman) are inserted through the cephalic or internal jugular vein, through the superior vena cava, and to the right atrium (near tip). It allows the administration of medications, the withdrawal of blood for testing, the measurement of CVP, and hyperalimentation (into superior vena cava).[1]

Total Parenteral Nutrition (TPN) or Hyperalimentation Devices (Intravenous Feeding)

A catheter is inserted into the subclavian vein (or jugular or other vein and passed into the subclavian vein) and used to provide nutrients when the patient does not eat.[1]

Issue	LOC	Sources	Affil	Rationale/Comment
Alarm	Advice	Pierson and Fairchild, 2002[2]	PT	An infusion pump administers fluid and nutrients at a preselected flow rate. An alarm sounds if the fluid source is empty or the system becomes unbalanced.

Continued

Issue	LOC	Sources	Affil	Rationale/Comment
Connections—secure	Advice			Ensure that connections are secure before and after exercise. A disrupted or lost connection may result in development of an air embolus, which is a life-threatening event.
Shoulder motion restrictions	Advice			Shoulder motion on the side of the infusion site may be restricted, especially abduction and flexion. Exercise but do not disrupt, disconnect, or occlude tubing or stress the infusion site.

INTRACRANIAL MONITORING

Intracranial pressure (ICP) monitors measure pressure against the skull by brain tissue blood or cerebral spinal fluid (CSF); some monitors can also be used to withdraw CSF fluid. Individuals with closed head injuries, cerebral hemorrhages, brain tumors, and overproduction of CSF are monitored (normal pressure is 4-15 mm Hg). Fluctuations up to 20 mm occur during a variety of routine activities.[1]

Issue	LOC	Sources	Affil	Rationale/Comment
Activities causing rapid increase in ICP	Advice	Pierson and Fairchild, 2002[1] Collins, 1997[2,a]	PT PT	Isometric exercise and the Valsalva maneuver should be avoided as they can increase ICP.[1] Also avoid extreme hip flexion, lateral neck flexion, and coughing.
Body positioning	Advice	Pierson and Fairchild, 2002[1]	PT	Avoid neck flexion, hip flexion greater than 90 degrees, and lying in prone position.

Head position from horizontal	Advice	Pierson and Fairchild, 2002[1]	PT	Head should not be lowered more than 15 degrees below the horizontal.[1]
		Collins, 1997[2]	PT	Venous drainage is maximal with head of bed elevated 30 degrees. Lowering the angle may increase ICP.[2]
Tube occlusion	Advice	Pierson and Fairchild, 2002[1]	PT	Avoid disrupting disconnection or occlusion of the tube.
Sustained elevation of ICP	Advice	Collins, 1997[2]	PT	Momentary elevation of ICP occur normally but sustained increased are a concern and should be reported.

a, In addition to head angle (lower), pain can increase ICP.

ADVERSE EVENTS

Source	Background	Therapy	Outcome	Follow-up/Interpretation
Phillips and Lee, 1990[3] **IV catheter, prematurity, and fracture** Case Series BMJ	A girl (690 g, 25 weeks' gestation) presented with a diagnosis of severe hyaline membrane disease (on prolonged ventilation), septicemia, patent ductus arteriosus, hydrocephalus with IVH, on parenteral and nasojejunal feeding.	At 10 weeks, an intravenous catheter was inserted into her vein on the left dorsal wrist. Soft tissue swelling was later noted and x-rays revealed a distal fracture of the radial metaphyses and ulna (with no loss of bone density or cortical thinning; serum phosphate was mildly high at 1.69 mmol/L).	The premature infant was treated with immobilization and calcium, phosphate, vitamin D supplements. Healing occurred (time for healing not noted).	Premature infants <28 weeks, even without definitive evidence of bone disease, are at risk of fractures. Handle premature infants with care during minimally invasive procedures (e.g., starting an intravenous infusion), to avoid trauma-related long bone fractures.

Continued

Source	Background	Therapy	Outcome	Follow-up/Interpretation
Zafonte et al, 1996[4] **Air embolism and agitated patient with central venous catheter** Brain Inj	A 38-year-old, extremely agitated, male patient with a left frontal intracerebral hematoma due to a traumatic head injury had a central venous catheter in place for chest/abdominal injuries.	The patient, while agitated, twisted off one of the ports of the central venous catheter with his teeth. O_2 saturations declined to 70%. His course improved following several days of ventilatory support.	Dx: Air embolism.	Air embolisms are a potential complication anytime a needle is inserted in the venous system. The author recommended taping and padding all venous access ports. Other strategies include using a tee shirt to cover the site or adding a "fake" catheter on opposite side to distract patients.

LITIGATION

State, Date	History Location	Device	Complication	Comments/Award
2000, Ohio[5] **Dislodged central line and death**	A 58-year-old retired male with a history of brain cancer was hospitalized for complications.	In the hospital, a physical therapist dislodged a central intravenous line (that provided nutrition) as it became caught on the hospital bed during an attempt to move patient to an upright position.	Air was allowed to enter the patient's arteries. The patient died suddenly from an air embolism.	The plaintiff's therapist should not have allowed line to become dislodged. $750,000 settlement.

Note: Awards and settlements do not necessarily prove a cause-effect relationship between equipment and injury.

REFERENCES

1. Pierson FM, Fairchild SL: Principles and techniques of patient care, ed 3. Philadelphia: Saunders; 2002.
2. Collins SM: Peripheral and central lines and intracranial pressure monitoring IV-A. In Paz JC, Panik M, eds: Acute care handbook for physical therapists. Boston: Butterworth-Heinemann; 1997.
3. Phillips RR, Lee, SH: Fractures of long bones occurring in neonatal intensive therapy units. BMJ 301(6745):225-226, 1990.
4. Zafonte RD, Hammond FD, Rahimi R: Air embolism in the agitated brain injury patient: an unusual complication. Brain Inj 10(10):759-762, 1996.
5. Medical malpractice verdict settlement, and experts, November 2000, p 51, loc 1.

34.3 Mechanical Ventilation

Mechanical ventilation uses positive pressure to move air into and inflate the patient's lungs. Concerns center around familiarity with the equipment, communicating with patients, and anticipating patient complications associated with long-term support.[1,2]

Issue	LOC	Sources	Affil	Rationale/Comment
Alarms	Advice	Pierson and Fairchild, 2002[1]	PT	Auditory or visual alarms are activated by stimuli (disconnected tube, coughing, movement of tubing, change in respiration pattern). Determine cause of the alarm and how to return system to normal function.
Communicating with patient				Must use nonverbal means of communicating—head nods.

Continued

Issue	LOC	Sources	Affil	Rationale/Comment
Complication with prolonged ventilatory support	Advice	Collins, 1997[2]	PT	The patient is at risk for developing contractures, skin ulcers, pulmonary complications, and deconditioning.
Disconnecting or obstructing tubes/connectors	Advice	Pierson and Fairchild, 2002[1]	PT	Avoid disconnecting the tube of the ventilator from the ETT and bending, kinking, or occluding the connector tubing or obstructing it by the weight of the patient's extremities or trapping it under the bed rail.
Exercise tolerance—monitor closely				These patients may not tolerate exercise as well as others not on ventilators, so monitor closely (i.e., vitals, change in respiration pattern, syncope, or cyanosis).
Tube lengths				Tubing must be sufficiently long to allow physical activities such as exercise, bedside activities, sitting, and ambulation.

REFERENCES

1. Pierson FM, Fairchild SL: Principles and techniques of patient care, ed 3. Philadelphia: Saunders; 2002.
2. Collins SM: Mechanical ventilation III-B. In Paz JC, Panik M, eds: Acute care handbook for physical therapists. Boston (MA): Butterworth-Heinemann; 1997.

34.4 Supplemental Oxygen Delivery Systems

Supplemental oxygen is provided to patients who experience tissue hypoxia (i.e., Pao_2 [partial pressure of arterial oxygen] is <60 mm Hg) or when arterial saturation (Sao_2) is less than 90%.[1] (**Also see O_2 tanks in power wheelchairs mobility.**)

Issue	LOC	Sources	Affil	Rationale/Comment
Humidification	Advice	Pierson and Fairchild, 2002[2]	PT	Oxygen should be humidified to reduce its drying effects on respiratory mucous membrane.
Respiratory distress—monitor	Advice / Advice	Pierson and Fairchild, 2002[2] / Collins, 1997[1]	PT / PT	Be alert to signs of respiratory distress (i.e., dyspnea, shortness of breath, cramping in calf muscles, cyanosis of nail beds or lips, distress). Exercise or activity should cease and oxygen delivery evaluated for improper function. Do not place supine. Allow patient to lean forward slightly if seated; rest forearms on thighs or armrest to relieve symptoms. Monitor Sao_2, Pao_2, and hemodynamics prior to, during, and after (PT) intervention.[1]
Respiratory drive	Advice	Collins, 1997[1]	PT	Respiratory drive can be depressed by supplemental O_2 in persons with chronic lung disease.
Tube—disruptions	Advice	Pierson and Fairchild, 2002[2]	PT	Avoid disrupting, disconnecting, or occluding the tubing.
Full tank	Advice	Collins, 1997[1]	PT	Make sure tank is full before performing activities that require O_2.

REFERENCES

1. Collins SM: Supplemental oxygen delivery systems III-A. In Paz JC, Panik M, eds: Acute care handbook for physical therapists. Boston (MA): Butterworth-Heinemann; 1997.
2. Pierson FM, Fairchild SL: Principles and techniques of patient care, ed 3. Philadelphia: Saunders; 2002.

34.5 Tubes

Tubes are medical devices with hollow elongated channels used in feeding systems, to drain a body system (genitourinary or gastrointestinal), or to drain a body space (i.e., edema after surgery).[1] Examples include nasogastric, gastrostomy, and jejunostomy tubes.[2] Concerns for treating patients who have feeding tubes, drainage tubes, ostomy devices, and chest drainage tubes are listed below.

FEEDING TUBES

Nasogastric tube (NGT)

Nasogastric tubes are hollow elongated channels inserted through a nostril and terminating in patient's stomach. They can be used for enteral feeding (and medications) and gastric drainage (e.g., to obtain gas specimens).[1,2]

Issue	LOC	Sources	Affil	Rationale/Comment
Bronchial pulmonary hygiene treatments	Advice	Collins, 1997[2]	PT	Enteral feeding should be turned off temporarily prior to and during treatment.
Eating and drinking—restrictions	Advice	Pierson and Fairchild, 2002[3]	PT	The patient will not be able to eat food or drink fluids by mouth while NG tube is in place.
Head and neck movement—restrictions	Advice			Exercise movements involving the head and neck should be avoided, especially flexion or forward bending.
Mobility treatments	Advice	Collins, 1997[2]	PT	Enteral feedings can be disconnected temporarily for mobility. Confirm with nursing.

Gastrostomy Tube (G tube)

Gastrostomy tubes are hollow elongated channels inserted directly into the stomach through an incision in the patient's abdomen and can be used for enteral feeding and gastric drainage.[1,3]

Issue	LOC	Sources	Affil	Rationale/Comment
Accidental removal—G Tube	Advice	Pierson and Fairchild, 2002[3,a]	PT	Be aware of tube placement and avoid removing it during exercise. Note: The distal tubing may inadvertently become caught (e.g., on furniture, wheelchair) and pulled out.
Bronchial pulmonary hygiene treatments	Advice	Collins, 1997[2,b]	PT	Enteral feeding should be turned off temporarily prior to and during treatment.
Mobility treatments	Advice			Enteral feedings can be disconnected temporarily for mobility. Confirm with nursing.

a, Referred to as gastric tube; b, Also applies to jejunostomy (J tube) enteric feedings (placed in jejunum).

DRAINAGE TUBES

Urinary Catheters

Urinary catheters are tubular medical devices that drain the bladder. Types include Foley, external, and suprapubic catheters.[2]

Issue	LOC	Sources	Affil	Rationale/Comment
Collection bag location	Advice	Pierson and Fairchild, 2002[3]	PT	Drainage tubes should be located below the region drained as it relies on gravity.[2] The collection bag should not be positioned
	Advice	Collins, 1997[2,a]	PT	above the level of the bladder for more than a few minutes. Do not place bag on the patient's lap while sitting in a wheelchair or on the abdomen when on a stretcher. During gait, position bag below the level of the bladder.[3]
Straps and tape—tightness	Advice	Pierson and Fairchild, 2002[3]	PT	To avoid occlusion of the urethra or the blood supply of the penis, tape or strap must not be applied too tightly.
Tube slack—lower extremity exercise	Advice			Avoid disruption, disconnecting, stretching, or occluding the drainage tube during lower extremity exercise. Determine how much free tubing is available before initiating exercise to avoid excessive tension on tubing.

a, Also apply to other drainage tubes: e.g., rectal catheter, suprapubic tube, Jackson-Pratt drain, Hemovac.

OSTOMY DEVICES

An ostomy is a surgically created body opening used to discharge body wastes. The device or pouch collects the body waste.[4]

Issue	LOC	Sources	Affil	Rationale/Comment
Gas or waste leakage—activity-induced	Advice	Pierson and Fairchild, 2002[3]	PT	Avoid activities that may cause the patient to experience social embarrassment (leakage of waste or intestinal gas). A patient with a recent ostomy may be concerned about whether the system will function properly.
Pouch—stresses on	Advice			Avoid excessive stress to the attachment of the pouch during treatment.
Scheduling visits	Advice			Schedule treatments after the pouch has been emptied.

CHEST DRAINAGE SYSTEMS

Chest Tubes

A chest tube consists of a hollow elongated channel connecting the pleural cavity to a drainage container and serves to drain air or fluid from a pleural space in order to promote normal intrapleural pressures and mechanics.[3,4]

Issue	LOC	Sources	Affil	Rationale/Comment
Collection bottle—placement	Advice	Pierson and Fairchild, 2002[3]	PT	If ambulating, collection bottles should be kept below the level of the inserted tube location.
Tube disruption	Advice			Avoid pulling, disrupting, disconnecting, or occluding tubing.
Modify hand placement	Advice	Panik, 1997[5]	PT	Avoid pressing directly on the chest tube during bronchopulmonary or mobility treatments.
Monitor breath sounds	Advice			Monitor for changes in breath sounds before and following activity.

REFERENCES

1. Webster's third new international dictionary. Springfield (MA): Merriam-Webster; 1981.
2. Collins SM Supplemental Oxygen Delivery Systems III-A. In Paz JC, Panik M, eds: Acute care handbook for physical therapists. Boston (MA): Butterworth-Heinemann; 1997.
3. Pierson FM, Fairchild SL: Principles and techniques of patient care, ed 3. Philadelphia: Saunders; 2002.
4. United Ostomy Association, Inc: Home page. Available at: http://www.uoa.org/ostomy_main.htm. Accessed November 9, 2005.
5. Panik M: Chest tubes. In Paz JC, Panik M, eds: Acute care handbook for physical therapists. Boston (MA): Butterworth-Heinemann; 1997.

35   BREATHING

35.1 Breathing Strategies

INCENTIVE RESPIRATORY SPIROMETRY

OVERVIEW. Incentive respiratory spirometry involves a technique of taking slow deep breaths for a sustained maximal inspiration (fully inflate lungs) using a medical device that provides visual feedback. It is used to prevent or treat atelectasis after surgery and to treat restrictive lung defects associated with dysfunctional diaphragm or quadriplegia.[1]

SUMMARY: CONTRAINDICATIONS AND PRECAUTIONS. Four sources cited a total of nine concerns for incentive spirometry. Concerns ranged from one to four per source, with the American Association of Respiratory Care (AARC)[1] and a physician citing the largest number and a physical therapist citing the fewest. The largest proportion of concerns were device-related, such as how the device is used. The most frequently cited concerns were patients who either had a limited vital capacity or were uncooperative.

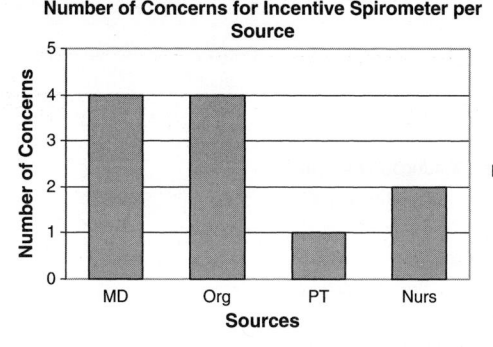

Number of Concerns for Incentive Spirometer per Source

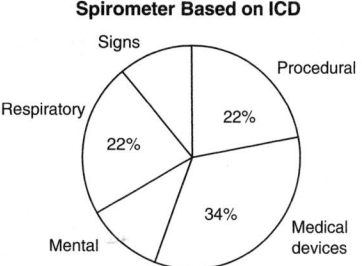

Proportion of Concerns for Incentive Spirometer Based on ICD

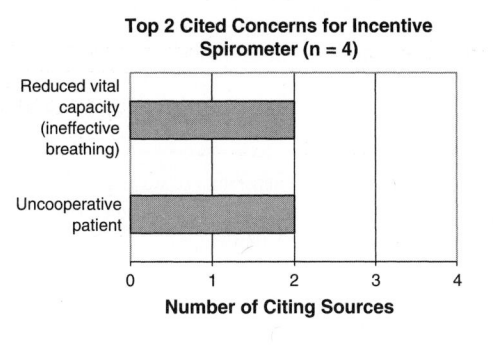

Top 2 Cited Concerns for Incentive Spirometer (n = 4)

F00-F99 MENTAL AND BEHAVIORAL DISORDERS

Issue	LOC	Sources	Affil	Rationale/Comment
Uncooperative patient	Advice	Peruzzi and Smith, 1995[2]	MD	Patient must be cooperative and motivated.
	CI	AARC, 1991[1]	Org	

J00-J99 DISEASES OF THE RESPIRATORY SYSTEM

Issue	LOC	Sources	Affil	Rationale/Comment
Tachypneic	Advice	Peruzzi and Smith, 1995[2]	MD	Patient should not be tachypneic.
Vital capacity limited	Advice	Peruzzi and Smith, 1995[2]	MD	Patient must be able to deep-breathe effectively. The AARC considers
	CI	AARC, 1991[1]	Org	inspirometry CI if vital capacity is <10 mL/kg or inspiratory capacity < $\frac{1}{3}$ of predicted. Peruzzi and Smith advise that vital capacity be >14 mL/kg or inspiratory capacity should be >12 mL/kg.

R00-R99 SYMPTOMS, SIGNS INVOLVING

Issue	LOC	Sources	Affil	Rationale/Comment
Fever	Advice	Peruzzi and Smith, 1995[2]	MD	Patient should not have high fever (102° F).

Medical Device

Issue	LOC	Sources	Affil	Rationale/Comment
Device—inaccessibility	Advice	Pullen, 2003[3]	Nurs	Do not place device out of the patient's reach.
Device—hygiene	Advice			Do not let patient use disposable mouthpiece for more than 24 hours. Clean mouth piece with water and shake dry after use.
Device—operation	CI	AARC, 1991[1]	Org	Understand how to use the device and demonstrate its proper use.

PROCEDURAL CONCERNS

Issue	LOC	Sources	Affil	Rationale/Comment
Supervision—inadequate	CI	AARC, 1991[1]	Org	
Training—prolonged periods	P	Kisner and Colby, 1996[4]	PT	Avoid prolonged periods of resistive training for inspiratory muscles. The diaphragm cannot completely rest to recover from a session of resistance exercise. Accessory muscle use during inspiration (neck muscles) is a sign the diaphragm is beginning to fatigue.[4]

BREATHING EXERCISES

Procedural issues related to inspiration, expiration, and deep breathing during breathing exercises as noted below.

PROCEDURAL CONCERNS

Issue	LOC	Sources	Affil	Rationale/Comment
Deep breathing—practice sessions	Advice	Kisner and Colby, 1996[4]	PT	Practice deep breathing for only three to four inspirations and expirations at a time to avoid hyperventilation.
Expiration—forced: never allow	Advice			It increases turbulence in the airways, leading to bronchospasm and increased airway restriction.
Expiration—very prolonged: avoid	Advice			Do not allow patient to take a very prolonged expiration. It can lead to the patient gasping for the next inspiration. Breathing then becomes irregular and inefficient.
Inspiration with accessory muscles: avoid	Advice			Do not initiate inspiration with accessory muscles and the upper chest. Upper chest should be quiet during breathing.

Pursed-Lip Breathing

Pursed lip breathing is a method of controlling respiration by exhaling through pursed lips (e.g., the lips gathered into a wrinkle or pucker). The technique is thought to increase airway pressure and keep bronchioles open so that gas exchange and breathing improves.[5]

PROCEDURAL CONCERNS

Issue	LOC	Sources	Affil	Rationale/Comment
Expirations—forced	P	Kisner and Colby, 1996[4]	PT	Avoid forced expiration with pursed-lip breathing. It increases turbulence
	Advice	McConnell, 1999[5]	Nurs	in the airways and restricts the small bronchioles.
Expirations—without abdominals	Advice	McConnell, 1999[5]	Nurs	Do not exhale without contracting the abdominal muscles.

REFERENCES

1. AARC: Clinical practice guideline, incentive spirometry. Respir Care 36:1404-1405, 1991.
2. Peruzzi WT, Smith B: Bronchial hygiene therapy. Crit Care Clin 11(1):79-96, 1995.
3. Pullen RL Jr: Clinical do's and don'ts: Teaching bedside incentive spirometry. Nursing 33(8):24, 2003.
4. Kisner C, Colby LA: Therapeutic exercise: foundations and techniques, ed 3. Philadelphia: F.A. Davis; 1996.
5. McConnell EA: Teaching pursed-lip breathing. Nursing 29(9):18, 1999.

35.2 Coughing (Cough Therapy)

OVERVIEW. A cough (reflex) is the expulsion of air from the lungs, performed in a noisy, sudden manner.[1] The sequence involves a brief inspiration, glottis closure, an expiratory muscle contraction (i.e., abdominals), increased pressures within the thorax and abdomen, the opening of the epiglottis, and the expulsion of air and sometimes foreign matter and sputum. It is used to clear secretions from the main bronchi and trachea.[2]

SUMMARY: CONTRAINDICATIONS AND PRECAUTIONS. Five sources cited a total of 14 concerns for cough (therapy). Sources cited anywhere from one to seven concerns. The largest proportion of concerns were procedural (e.g., hand placements for assisted coughs) and circulatory. Many concerns related to the Valsalva maneuver that accompanies a cough, which can stress the vascular system (ICP, eye surgery, aneurysm) or musculoskeletal system (spinal instability, back pain). One source mentioned the concern for spreading airborne infection (i.e., TB). The most frequently cited concerns were coughing in persons with a history of aneurysm.

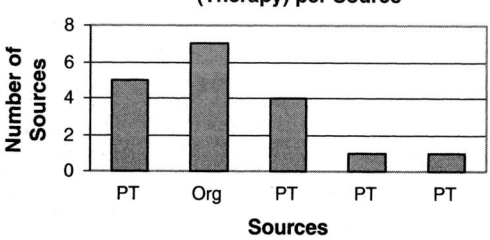

Number of Concerns for Cough (Therapy) per Source

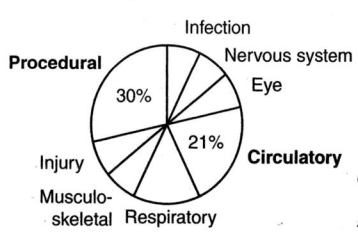

Proportion of Concerns for Cough (Therapy) Based on ICD

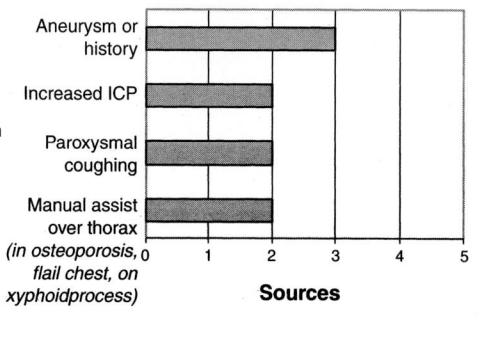

Top Concerns for Cough (therapy)

CONTRAINDICATIONS AND PRECAUTIONS

COUGHING

A00–B99 CERTAIN INFECTIONS AND PARASITIC DISEASES

Issue	LOC	Sources	Affil	Rationale/Comment
Infectious disease	CI	AARC, 1993[3]	Org	Inability to control possible transmission of infection by droplets (e.g., *M. tuberculosis*).

G00-G99 DISEASES OF THE NERVOUS SYSTEM

Issue	LOC	Sources	Affil	Rationale/Comment
Intracranial pressure—increased	RCI	AARC, 1993[3]	Org	
	CI	Pauls and Reed, 2004[4]	PT	

H00-H59 DISEASES OF THE EYE

Issue	LOC	Sources	Affil	Rationale/Comment
Eye surgery— recent	CI	Pauls and Reed, 2004[4]	PT	**In 2002, Obuchowska et al[5] described an 84-year-old female who developed a massive suprachoroidal hemorrhage when she had an unexpected Valsalva-induced cough during cataract surgery that resulted in sudden increased venous pressure and vessel wall rupture.**

I00-I99 DISEASES OF THE CIRCULATORY SYSTEM

Issue	LOC	Sources	Affil	Rationale/Comment
Aneurysm history and forceful coughing	CI	Pauls and Reed, 2004[4]	PT	Have these patients huff several times to clear the airways.
	RCI	AARC, 1993[3]	Org	
	P	Kisner and Colby, 1996[6]	PT	
Coronary artery perfusion—reduced	RCI	AARC, 1993[3]	Org	I.e., acute coronary infarction.
CVA history and forceful coughing	Avoid	Kisner and Colby, 1996[6]	PT	Have these patients huff several times to clear the airways.
	P			

J00-J99 DISEASES OF THE RESPIRATORY SYSTEM

Issue	LOC	Sources	Affil	Rationale/Comment
Pneumonectomy—recent	CI	Pauls and Reed, 2004[4]	PT	Note: No rationales provided.
Subcutaneous emphysema	CI			

M00-M99 DISEASES OF THE MUSCULOSKELETAL SYSTEM

Issue	LOC	Sources	Affil	Rationale/Comment
Cough in spinal disorders	Advice/red flag	Musnick and Hall, 2005[7]	MD	Coughing increases intra-abdominal and thoracic pain and may cause mechanical exacerbation of spinal pain condition. Consider having physician try to control the coughs.

Issue	LOC	Sources	Affil	Rationale/Comment
Unstable head/neck/spine injury—acute	RCI	AARC, 1993[3]	Org	

PROCEDURAL CONCERNS

Issue	LOC	Sources	Affil	Rationale/Comment
Paroxysmal coughing—uncontrolled	CI Avoid P	Pauls and Reed, 2004[4] Kisner and Colby, 1996[6]	PT PT PT	Avoid uncontrolled coughing spasms. Spasm of multiple coughs can lead to fatigue, bronchospasm, and airway closure.
Posture		Kisner and Colby, 1996[6]	PT	Patient should cough while in a somewhat erect posture.
Manual-assisted cough—pressure over the epigastric area	CI	AARC, 1993[3]	Org	**In the following:** • Abdominal aortic aneurysm • Abdominal pathology (acute) • Bleeding diathesis • Hiatal hernia • Pneumothorax—untreated • Pregnancy • Regurgitation/aspiration (increased potential) • Unconscious patients with unprotected airway

Continued

Issue	LOC	Sources	Affil	Rationale/Comment
Manual-assisted cough—with pressure over the thoracic cage	CI Avoid	AARC, 1993[3] Imle, 1987[8]	Org —	**In the following:** • Flail chest • Xyphoid process (direct pressure over) • Osteoporosis

Note: AARC uses the terminology "direct cough," which includes forced expiratory techniques (such as huff coughing) and manually assisted coughing.

REFERENCES

1. Dorland's illustrated medical dictionary, ed 24. Philadelphia: W.B. Saunders; 1965.

2. Thomson A, Skinner A, Piercy J: Tidy's physiotherapy, ed 12. Oxford: Butterworth-Heinemann; 1991.

3. AARC: Clinical practice guideline, direct cough. Respir Care 38:495-499, 1993.

4. Pauls JA, Reed KL: Quick reference to physical therapy, ed 2. Austin (TX): Pro-Ed; 2004.

5. Obuchowska, I, Mariak Z, Stankiewicz A: Massive suprachoroidal hemorrhage during cataract surgery: case report (in Polish—from abstract). Klin Oczna 104(5-6):406-410, 2002.

6. Kisner C, Colby LA: Therapeutic exercise: foundations and techniques, ed 3. Philadelphia: F.A. Davis; 1996.

7. Musnick D, Hall C: Red flags: potentially serious symptoms and signs in exercising patients. In: Hall CM, Brody LT, eds: Therapeutic exercise: moving toward function. Philadelphia: Lippincott Williams & Wilkins; 2005.

8. Imle, PC: Physical therapy and respiratory care for the patient with acute spinal cord injury. Phys Ther Health Care 1:45, 1987

36.1 Percussion and Vibration of the Chest

OVERVIEW. Percussion is a manual technique of administering rhythmic, alternating, cupped-hand movements over lung segments to dislodge and mobilize secretions that adhere to lung tissue. Vibration is a technique of administering small-amplitude rapid shaking over lung tissue to mobilize secretions.[1] In both techniques, forces are applied over the thorax.

SUMMARY: CONTRAINDICATIONS AND PRECAUTIONS. Seven sources cited a total of 46 concerns for percussion and vibration of the chest. Concerns ranged from 5 to 34 per source, with a physical therapist citing the largest number and another three physical therapy sources citing the fewest number. The largest proportion of concerns was related to diseases of the respiratory system (>25% of concerns). The most frequently cited concern was osteoporosis of the ribs and hemoptysis. The AARC listed two absolute contraindications: active hemorrhaging with hemodynamic instability and unstable spinal injury.

OTHER CONCERNS: INTRAVENTRICULAR HEMORRHAGES IN PREMATURE INFANTS. In a 1987 RCT, Raval et al[2] reported a higher incidence of IVH (grade 3 and 4) in preterm infants, less that 2000 g, with respiratory distress syndrome who received vibration, percussion, postural drainage, and suctioning than in controls who received only suctioning. In a 1998 case control design (chart review), Harding et al[3] noted that of 454 infants, 13 preterm babies who had received two to three times as many chest PT treatments in the second to fourth week of life as compared with controls had encephaloclastic porencephaly (a form of brain damage).

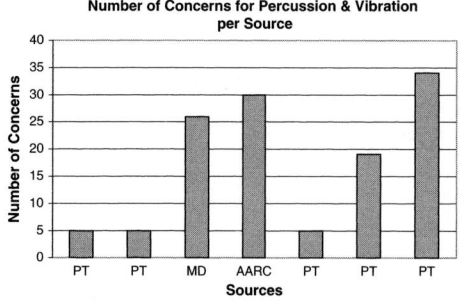

Number of Concerns for Percussion & Vibration per Source

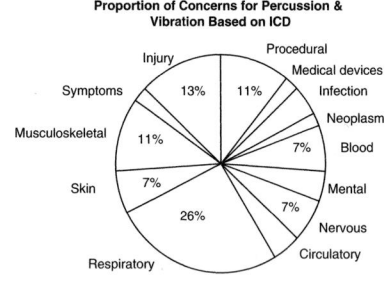

Proportion of Concerns for Percussion & Vibration Based on ICD

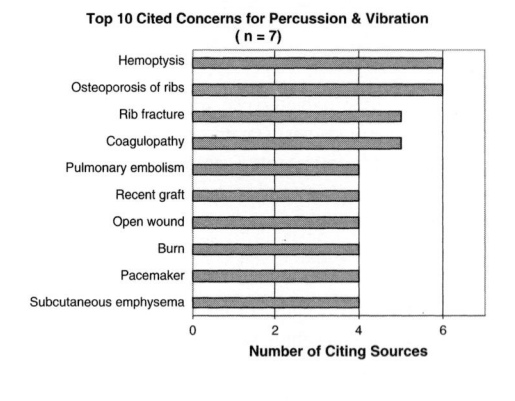

Top 10 Cited Concerns for Percussion & Vibration (n = 7)

CONTRAINDICATIONS AND PRECAUTIONS

A00-B99 CERTAIN INFECTIONS AND PARASITIC DISEASES

Issue	LOC	Sources	Affil	Rationale/Comment
Pulmonary tuberculosis—active	CI	Webber, 1988[4]	PT	
	Not use	Anderson and Innocenti, 1987[5]	PT	
Pulmonary tuberculosis—suspected	CI	Peruzzi and Smith, 1995[6]	MD	
	RCI	AARC, 1991[7]	Org	
	CI/P	Downs, 1996[8,a]	PT	

a, General note: Downs' recommendations[8] state that risks and benefits need to be weighed; guidelines pertain to thoracic external manipulation including percussion, shaking, and high-velocity chest compression, noting that vibration may be tolerated better; guidelines include their postural drainage CIs.

C00-C97 NEOPLASM

Issue	LOC	Sources	Affil	Rationale/Comment
Bone—metastases	P	Webber, 1988[4,a]	PT	The condition may lead to fragile ribs.[9]
	P	Sciaky et al, 2001[9,b]	PT	
	Careful	Anderson and Innocenti, 1987[5,b]	PT	
Tumor—obstructing airway	P	Sciaky et al, 2001[9]	PT	

a, If affecting ribs or vertebral column, treatment must be gentle; b, Over ribs.

D50-D89 DISEASES OF BLOOD AND BLOOD FORMING ORGANS AND CERTAIN DISORDERS

Issue	LOC	Sources	Affil	Rationale/Comment
Coagulopathies	CI	Peruzzi and Smith, 1995[6,a]	MD	
	P	AARC, 1991[7]	Org	
	CI/P	Sciaky et al, 2001[9]	PT	
	CI	Downs , 1996[8]	PT	
		Starr, 2001[10,b]	PT	

Continued

Issue	LOC	Sources	Affil	Rationale/Comment
Hemorrhage (active) with hemodynamic instability	P	Peruzzi and Smith, 1995[6]	MD	**See Hammon and Martin.[11]**
	ACI	AARC, 1991[7]	Org	
	CI/P	Downs, 1996[8]	PT	
Platelet count <200,000 per mm³	RCI	Sciaky et al, 2001[9]	PT	

a, If severe or uncontrolled; b, Increased partial thromboplastin time (PPT), increased prothrombin time (PT), platelet count <50,000. General note: Starr's guidelines are not meant to be inclusive and pertain to percussion and shaking; increased tolerance may be attainable in some situations through modification.

F00-F99 MENTAL AND BEHAVIORAL DISORDERS

Issue	LOC	Sources	Affil	Rationale/Comment
Anxiety—nervous	CI/P	Downs, 1996[8]	PT	Patients may not tolerate the procedure.
	RCI	AARC, 1991[7]	Org	
	P	Sciaky et al, 2001[9]	PT	
Confused—combative patients	CI	Peruzzi and Smith, 1995[6]	MD	
	RCI	AARC, 1991[7]	Org	
	CI/P	Downs, 1996[8,a]	PT	

a, Confused.

G00-G99 DISEASES OF THE NERVOUS SYSTEM

Issue	LOC	Sources	Affil	Rationale/Comment
Epidural spinal anesthesia or infusion—recent	RCI	AARC, 1991[7]	Org	
	CI/P	Downs, 1996[8]	PT	
Intracranial pressure—increased	CI	Peruzzi and Smith, 1995[6]	MD	Or other unstable intracranial pathology.
	RCI	AARC, 1991[7,a]	Org	
	CI/P	Downs, 1996[8,a]	PT	
Seizure disorder	P	Sciaky et al, 2001[9]	PT	

a, >20 mm.

I00-I99 DISEASES OF THE CIRCULATORY SYSTEM

Issue	LOC	Sources	Affil	Rationale/Comment
Hemodynamic status, unstable	CI	Sciaky et al, 2001[9]	PT	Note: Cardiac patients tend to tolerate treatment poorly. In CHF, do not position in Trendelenburg because of increased respiratory distress and cardiac dysrhythmia with the head down. Also, increased venous return to a failing heart can lead to increased pulmonary edema.[12] **Hammon et al[13] monitored 72 ICU patients during postural drainage with chest percussion and reported 18 patients developing major arrhythmias, 18 developing minor arrhythmias, and 46 none. Increased age and acute cardiac status were significantly associated with risk.**
Pulmonary embolism	CI	Peruzzi and Smith, 1995[6]	MD	Note: In this potentially fatal condition, blood supply to lung parenchyma is obstructed as a result of a blood clot lodged in the pulmonary artery.[14]
	CI/P	Downs, 1996[8]	PT	
	RCI	AARC, 1991[7]	Org	
	RCI	Sciaky et al, 2001[9]	PT	

Issue	LOC	Sources	Affil	Rationale/Comment
Bronchopleural fistula	CI	Peruzzi and Smith, 1995[6]	MD	A bronchopleural fistula may be a complication of lung surgery with a breakdown of the bronchial stump. There is a concern of "spill-over" of infected fluid into the remaining lung, so instruct patient to sit up or turn onto operated side.[5]
	RCI	AARC, 1991[7]	Org	
	CI/P	Downs, 1996[8]	PT	
Bronchospasms—uncontrolled	CI/P	Downs, 1996[8]	PT	
	P	Sciaky et al, 2001[9]	PT	
Empyema	RCI	AARC, 1991[7]	Org	Note: Empyema is a localized collection of pus in the pleural cavity.
	CI/P	Downs, 1996[8]	PT	
End-stage lung disease	Caution	Downs, 1996[8]	PT	Due to risk of hemoptysis.
Hemoptysis	CI/P	Downs, 1996[8,a]	PT	**In 1979, Hammon and Martin[11] reported a 51-year-old man with squamous cell carcinoma and possible pneumonia who received percussion with bronchial drainage and suffered a fatal, massive hemoptysis with exsanguination.**
	RCI	AARC, 1991[7,a]	Org	
	CI	Webber, 1988[4]	PT	
	RCI	Sciaky et al, 2001[9]	PT	
	Not use	Anderson and Innocenti, 1987[5,b]	PT	
	P	Starr, 2001[10]	PT	
Hypoxemia may develop	CI	Peruzzi and Smith, 1995[6]	MD	**Connors et al[15] found a significant decrease in PaO_2 following chest percussion in 10 acute nonsurgical pulmonary hospitalized patients who produced little or no mucoid sputum.**

Continued

Issue	LOC	Sources	Affil	Rationale/Comment
Pulmonary contusion	CI	Peruzzi and Smith, 1995[6]	MD	
	RCI	AARC, 1991[7]	Org	
	CI/P	Downs, 1996[8]	PT	
Pulmonary edema—associated with CHF	RCI	AARC, 1991[7]	Org	Note: Pulmonary edema is a potentially life-threatening excessive amount of fluid in the lung's air spaces and/or interstitial tissues that limits space available for gas exchange.[14]
	CI/P	Downs, 1996[8]	PT	
Pneumothorax, tension (untreated)	RCI	Sciaky et al, 2001[9]	PT	
Pleuritic pain (acute)	CI	Webber, 1988[4]	PT	
	Not use	Anderson and Innocenti, 1987[5]	PT	
Pleural effusions (large) or undrained empyema	CI	Peruzzi and Smith, 1995[6]	MD	Note: In pleural effusion, there is excess fluid in the pleural space.
	RCI	AARC, 1991[7]	Org	
	CI/P	Downs, 1996[8,c]	PT	
Subcutaneous emphysema	CI	Peruzzi and Smith, 1995[6]	MD	No rationale provided. Subcutaneous emphysema is a condition where air or other gas appears where it is not normally seen and may be due to infection (i.e., gangrene), weakness in structural organ continuity (e.g., pulmonary), or rupture of tissue (e.g., alveoli).[16] Large air leaks may suggest a disruption of the bronchus, and massive subcutaneous emphysema may suggest the drainage capacity of a chest tube is exceeded by the air loss from lung into the pleural cavity.[17]
	CI/P	Downs, 1996[8,c]	PT	
	RCI	AARC, 1991[7]	Org	
	RCI	Sciaky et al, 2001[9]	PT	

a, Active; b, Severe; c, Large.

L00-L99 DISEASES OF THE SKIN AND SUBCUTANEOUS TISSUE

Issue	LOC	Sources	Affil	Rationale/Comment
Myocutaneous flap procedure on thorax—recent	CI	Peruzzi and Smith, 1995[6]	MD	
	CI/P	Downs, 1996[8]	PT	
	RCI	Sciaky et al, 2001[9]	PT	
Skin graft—recent	CI	Peruzzi and Smith, 1995[6]	MD	
	CI/P	Downs, 1996[8,a]	PT	
	RCI	AARC, 1991[7]	Org	
	RCI	Sciaky et al, 2001[9]	PT	
Skin infection—on thorax	CI	Peruzzi and Smith, 1995[6]	MD	
	CI/P	Downs, 1996[8,a]	PT	
	RCI	AARC, 1991[7]	Org	

a, On thorax.

M00-M99 DISEASES OF THE MUSCULOSKELETAL SYSTEM AND CONNECTIVE TISSUE

Issue	LOC	Sources	Affil	Rationale/Comment
Degenerative bone disease	P	Starr, 2001[10]	PT	
Flail chest	CI	Peruzzi and Smith, 1995[6]	MD	Flail chest is characterized by a paradoxical mobility of the chest during respirations, attributed to multiple rib factures.
	P	Starr, 2001[10]	PT	

Continued

Issue	LOC	Sources	Affil	Rationale/Comment
Osteomyelitis	CI	Peruzzi and Smith, 1995[6]	MD	
	RCI	AARC, 1991[7,d]	Org	
	CI/P	Downs, 1996[8,e]	PT	
Osteoporosis—ribs	CI	Peruzzi and Smith, 1995[6]	MD	Webber notes that if osteoporosis affects the ribs or vertebral column, treatment must be gentle.[4] **In 1985, Koo et al**[18] **reported a very-low-birth-weight female infant with pulmonary atelectasis who received chest percussion (via rubber conductive face mask), chest vibration (battery operated), and passive exercise. She was later diagnosed with demineralized ribs, multiple scapula fractures, rickets, radius and left ulnar shaft fractures, osteopenia, and left hand and wrist fracture.** In a 2002 retrospective chart review, Chalumeau et al[19] noted five male infants with one to five rib fractures between the third and eighth ribs who had received daily chest PT about 1 month earlier.
	CI/P	Downs, 1996[8,a]	PT	
	RCI	AARC, 1991[7]	Org	
	P	Webber, 1988[4,d]	PT	
	P	Sciaky et al, 2001[9,a]	PT	
	Careful	Anderson and Innocenti, 1987[5,a,b]	PT	
Spinal surgery—recent	CI	Peruzzi and Smith, 1995[6]	MD	
	CI/P	Downs, 1996[8]	PT	
	RCI	AARC, 1991[7,c]	Org	

a, Body area not specified; b, Only for percussion; c, Or acute spinal injury, e.g., laminectomy; d, Rib or vertebra; e, Ribs.

R00-R99 SYMPTOMS AND SIGNS

Issue	LOC	Sources	Affil	Rationale/Comment
Pain—chest wall	CI	Peruzzi and Smith, 1995[6,a]	MD	
	RCI	AARC, 1991[7]	Org	
	CI/P	Downs, 1996[8]	PT	

S00-T98 INJURY, POISONING, AND CERTAIN OTHER CONSEQUENCES OF EXTERNAL CAUSES

Issue	LOC	Sources	Affil	Rationale/Comment
Burns	CI	Peruzzi and Smith, 1995[6]	MD	
	CI/P	Downs, 1996[8]	PT	
	RCI	AARC, 1991[7]	Org	
	RCI	Sciaky et al, 2001[9]	PT	
Rib fracture	CI	Peruzzi and Smith, 1995[6]	MD	
	CI/P	Downs, 1996[8,a]	PT	
	RCI	AARC, 1991[7,a]	Org	
	P	Starr, 2001[10]	PT	
	P	Sciaky et al, 2001[9]	PT	
Soft tissue injury—to thorax	CI	Peruzzi and Smith, 1995[6]	MD	

Continued

Issue	LOC	Sources	Affil	Rationale/Comment
Spinal injury—unstable	CI	Peruzzi and Smith, 1995[6]	MD	
	CI/P	Downs, 1996[8,c]	PT	
	ACI	AARC, 1991[7]	Org	
Surgical wound or healing	RCI	AARC, 1991[7]	Org	
	CI/P	Downs, 1996[8,b]	PT	
Wounds—open	CI	Peruzzi and Smith, 1995[6]	MD	
	CI/P	Downs, 1996[8]	PT	
	RCI	AARC, 1991[7]	Org	
	RCI	Sciaky et al, 2001[9]	PT	

a, With or without flail chest; b, Spinal; c, Head/neck, until spinal injury is stable.

Y70-Y82 MEDICAL DEVICES

Issue	LOC	Sources	Affil	Rationale/Comment
Pacemakers	CI	Peruzzi and Smith, 1995[6]	MD	Recent permanent pacemaker; temporary transvenous pacemaker.
	RCI	AARC, 1991[7]	Org	
	P	Sciaky et al, 2001[9]	PT	
	CI/P	Downs, 1996[8]	PT	

PROCEDURAL CONCERNS/MISCELLANEOUS CONCERNS

Issue	LOC	Sources	Affil	Rationale/Comment
Aged	CI/P	Downs, 1996[8]	PT	The elderly person may not tolerate chest PT. **See Hammon**
	RCI	AARC, 1991[7]	Org	**et al[13] above.**
	CI/P	Downs, 1996[8]	PT	
Anterior lobes in pediatrics	Caution	Downs, 1996[8]	PT	Due to risk of gastroesophageal reflux.
Positioning—reverse	RCI	AARC, 1991[7]	Org	
Positioning—Trendelenburg, if this	RCI	AARC, 1991[7]	Org	
posture is contraindicated	CI/P	Downs, 1996[8]	PT	
Unnecessary service	CI	Peruzzi and Smith, 1995[6]	MD	Provide service no longer than necessary (weigh risk/benefits). **See Connors et al[15] above.**

NEONATES: PERCUSSION CHEST PT BRONCHIAL DRAINAGE

Issue	LOC	Sources	Affil	Rationale/Comment
Apnea and bradycardia	P	Crane, 1981[20]	PT	
Arrhythmias—cardiac	P			
Chest tube	P			

Continued

Issue	LOC	Sources	Affil	Rationale/Comment
Fragile skin	P			
Hemoptysis	ACI			
Hyperactive airways	P			
Irritability—continuous (during procedure)	P			
Osteoporosis	P			
Persistent fetal circulation (pulmonary hypertension in a newborn—may not tolerate)	P			
Pneumothorax—untreated	ACI			
Rib fracture	ACI			
Rickets	P			
Subcutaneous emphysema	P			
Surgery—thoracic/abdominal (recent)	P			

NEONATES: VIBRATION CHEST PT BRONCHIAL DRAINAGE

Issue	LOC	Sources	Affil	Rationale/Comment
Apnea and bradycardia	P	Crane, 1981[20]	PT	
Hemoptysis	ACI			

Irritability—continuous during procedure	P
Fragile skin	P
Persistent fetal circulation	P
Pneumothorax—tension (untreated)	ACI

ADVERSE EVENTS

Source	Background	Therapy	Outcome	Follow-up/Interpretation
Chalumeau et al, 2002[19] **Chest PT and rib fractures in infants** Retrospective (chart review) Pediatr Radiol	All cases of rib fractures occurring after chest PT for bronchiolitis or pneumonia were identified over a 4-year period at three Parisian university hospitals.	Five male infants (median age 3 months) were identified between June 1996 and December 1999 with one to five rib fractures between the third and eighth ribs. Four were lateral and one posterior. All had received daily chest PT 1 month before rib fracture detected.	Prevalence after chest PT was estimated to be 1 in 1000 infants hospitalized with bronchiolitis or pneumonia.	The authors believe chest PT can be a rare but potential cause of rib fractures in infants, which should be distinguished from child abuse.

Continued

Source	Background	Therapy	Outcome	Follow-up/Interpretation
Dabezies and Warren, 1997[21] **Chest PT (risk factor), rickets, and fractures** Retrospective (chart review) Clinical Ortho and Related Research	In a chart review over a 42-month period between August 1989 and January 1993, 247 charts were reviewed with very-low-birth-weight cases.	Of 247 very-low-birth-weight cases identified, 26 (10.5%) infants had rickets (mean age 75 days) with fractures.	These 26 infants had 98 fractures (54 rib, 13 radial, 10 humeral, 8 ulnar, 4 metacarpal 3 clavicular, 5 femur, 1 fibular). With early recognition, treatment included metabolic therapy, splinting but not casting.	The authors advise very gentle passive range of motion and only doing postural drainage and vibration. Risk factors include physical therapy with passive motion, chest percussion therapy, hepatobiliary disease, total parenteral nutrition, diuretic therapy. Rib fractures were associated with vigorous chest physical therapy.
Hammon and Martin, 1979[11] **Chest PT and fatal pulmonary hemorrhage** Case report Phys Ther	A 51-year-old man with squamous cell carcinoma of right upper lobe mainstem bronchus and trachea was treated with a split course of radiation (4000 rads, 4 weeks)	Three weeks following therapy, the man was hospitalized for possible anaerobic pneumonia (sputum: dark red, many red and white blood cells with "mixed flora"). Treatment involved IV penicillin and bronchial drainage with percussion. On the first session (CPT), bright red blood expectorated.	Fatal pulmonary hemorrhage.	The exact cause of the fatal pulmonary hemorrhage was not determined. The authors (1) believe CPT appeared to have worsened bleeding via percussion, dislodging clots and allowing the free flow of blood; (2) indicated contraindication to percussion (bronchial drainage may also be CI) in patients with significant hemoptysis; and (3) believe the

On day 4, hemoglobin fell from 10.6 to 8.2 g/100 ml (given 2 units of packed cells).

On day 13, he spiked fever of 39 °C (102.2 °F) (started on clindamycin).

On day 15, hemoglobin was 9.1 g/100 ml) and clot factor was normal.

On day 16, during bronchial drainage, the patient suffered massive hemoptysis with exsanguination and died (autopsy refused).

Trendelenburg position may have helped to dislodge clots due to the increased blood and pressure to involved areas.

Harding et al, 1998[3]
Chest PT and encephaloclastic porencephaly
Case control design (chart review)
J Pediatr

Of 454 infants (<1500 g) between 1992 to 1994, 13 preterm baby cases were identified with encephaloclastic porencephaly (a form of brain damage) (24 to 27 weeks' gestation; birth weight 680 to 1090 g); they were matched with 26 controls for weight and gestation.

Chest PT was administered to cases by an experienced PT or a PT-trained neonatal nurse. Treatment involved positioning and percussion with a Laerdahl mask in two to three areas for 2 to 3 minutes, followed by lavage and suctioning. Babies were not placed in a head-down position. Frequency: every 2 to 8 hours.

Cases received two to three times as many chest PT treatments in the second to fourth week of life as compared to controls ($P < .001$).

No further cases noted once the practice of chest PT for very-low-birth-weight babies in the first month of life stopped.

The authors believe encephaloclastic porencephaly may be a complication of chest PT in extremely preterm infants.

Continued

Source	Background	Therapy	Outcome	Follow-up/Interpretation
Koo et al, 1985[18] **Percussion, osteopenia, and fractures** Case report Am J Dis Child	A female infant (680 g birth wt; 26 weeks' gestation) presented with a history of prolonged ventilatory support and pulmonary atelectasis.	She was administered chest percussion (via rubber conductive face mask), chest vibration (via battery operated vibrator) for pulmonary atelectasis, and passive exercise to minimize increased tone.	Chest x-rays revealed skeletal abnormalities at 15 weeks' postnatally with demineralized ribs, multiple scapula fractures, rickets, radius and left ulnar shaft fractures, osteopenia, and left hand and wrist fractures.	The authors believe fractures are likely due to the physical manipulation of demineralized bone. Infants with very low birth weight are at risk for osteopenia, with about 30% developing rickets. Avoid physiotherapy (overzealous passive exercise and chest percussion) until data on benefits are available.
Phillips and Lee, 1990[22] **IV catheter, prematurity, and fracture** Case Series BMJ	Girl (690 g, 25 weeks' gestation) presented with severe hyaline membrane disease (on prolonged ventilation), septicemia, patent ductus arteriosus, hydrocephalus with IVH, on parenteral and nasojejunal feeding.	At 10 weeks, an intravenous catheter was inserted into vein of left dorsal wrist. Soft tissue swelling was noted and x-rays showed distal metaphyses fractures of radius and ulna (with no loss of bone density or cortical thinning). (Serum phosphate was mildly elevated at 1.69 mmol/L.)	She was treated with immobilization and calcium, phosphate, and vitamin D supplements. Healing occurred (no duration noted).	Premature infants <28 weeks, even without definitive evidence of bone disease, are at risk of fractures. Handle premature infants with care during minimally invasive procedures (i.e., starting an intravenous infusion) to avoid trauma-related long bone fractures.

A boy (980 g; 29 weeks' gestation) presented with hyaline membrane disease, persistent ductus arteriosus, nasojejunal tube feedings. On day 5, he was given intravenous infusion at the left foot, which was stabilized.

Swelling of the left thigh occurred over the next 24 hours and x-rays showed distal metaphysis and midshaft left femur fractures (with normal cortical density). Serum alkaline phosphatase was elevated (975 IU/L at 3 wks) and serum phosphate was low (0.7 mmol/L).

Both fractures healed following immobilization.

Raval et al, 1987[2]
Chest PT and IVH
RCT
J Perinatol

20 preterm respiratory distress syndrome (RDS) infants less than 2000 g with endotracheal intubation were randomly assigned to group 1 ($n = 10$, receiving vibration, percussion, postural drainage and suctioning) or group 2 ($n = 10$, suctioning only).

Details: Group 1—in head-up position and head-down position—percussed 10 sec, vibrated 2 sec at anterior, lateral, posterior of right and left chest. Duration 2-3 minutes. Suctioning three times at 50-100 mm Hg negative pressure for 10-15 sec. All procedures repeated every 2-3 hours for first 24 hours of life.

Higher incidence of IVH (grade 3 and 4) in group 1 (5 vs 0) ($P < .05$). No significant difference in pH, Po_2/Fio_2 ratio and Pco_2 between groups; no differences in $TcPo_2$ or amount of secretions between groups.

Serial ultrasound recommended before and after CPT in larger population to better elucidate causal relationship between CPT and IVH. CPT in first 24 hours of life offered no benefit to premature RDS infants and may potentially cause severe IVH grades.

REFERENCES

1. Kisner C, Colby LA: Therapeutic exercise: foundations and techniques, ed 3. Philadelphia: F.A. Davis; 1996.
2. Raval D, Yeh TF, Mora A, et al: Chest physiotherapy in preterm infants with RDS in the first 24 hours of life. J Perinatol 7(4):301-304, 1987.
3. Harding JE, Miles FK, Becroft DM, et al: Chest physiotherapy may be associated with brain damage in extremely premature infants. J Pediatr 132(3 Pt 1):440-444, 1998.
4. Webber BA: The Brompton hospital guide to chest physiotherapy, ed 5. Oxford: Blackwell Scientific; 1988.
5. Anderson JM, Innocenti DM: Techniques used in chest physiotherapy. In: Downie PA, editor: Cash's textbook of chest, heart, and vascular disorders for physiotherapists, ed 4. Philadelphia: J.B. Lippincott; 1987.
6. Peruzzi WT, Smith B: Bronchial hygiene therapy. Crit Care Clin 11(1):79-96, 1995.
7. AARC: Clinical Practice Guidelines. Available at: http://www.rcjournal.com/online_resources/cpgs/cpg_index.asp. Accessed November 16, 2005.
8. Downs AM: Physiological bases for airway clearance techniques. In: Frownfelter D, Dean E, eds: Principle and practice of cardiopulmonary physical therapy, ed 2. St. Louis: Mosby; 1996.
9. Sciaky A, Stockford J, Nixon E: Treatment of acute cardiopulmonary conditions. In Hillegass EA, Sadowsky HS, eds: Essentials of cardiopulmonary physical therapy, ed 2. Philadelphia: W.B. Saunders; 2001.
10. Starr JA: Chronic pulmonary dysfunction. In O'Sullivan SB, Schmitz TJ, eds: Physical rehabilitation and treatment, ed 4. Philadelphia: F.A. Davis; 2001.
11. Hammon WE, Martin RJ: Fatal pulmonary hemorrhage associated with chest physical therapy. Phys Ther 59(10):1247-1248, 1979.
12. Irwin S, Tecklin JS: Cardiopulmonary physical therapy. St. Louis: Mosby; 1995.
13. Hammon WE, Connors AF Jr, McCaffee R: Cardiac arrhythmia during postural drainage and chest percussion of critically ill patients. Chest 102(6):1336-1341, 1992.
14. Goodman CC: The respiratory system. In: Goodman CC, Boissonnault WG, Fuller KS, eds: Pathology: implications for the physical therapist, ed 2. Philadelphia: Saunders; 2003.
15. Connors AF Jr, Hammon WE, et al: Chest physical therapy. The immediate effect on oxygenation in acutely ill patients. Chest 78(4):559-564, 1980.

16. Samlaska CP, Maggio KL: Subcutaneous emphysema. Adv Dermatol 11:117-151, 152, 1996.

17. Fishman AD, Elias JA, Fishman JA, et al: Fishman's manual of pulmonary diseases and disorders, ed 3. New York: McGraw-Hill; 2002.

18. Koo WW, Oestreich AE, Sherman R, et al: Radiological case of the month. Osteopenia, rickets, and fractures in preterm infants. Am J Dis Child 139(10):1045-1046, 1985.

19. Chalumeau M, Foix-L'Helias L, Scheinmann P, et al: Rib fractures after chest physiotherapy for bronchiolitis or pneumonia in infants. Pediatr Radiol 32 (9):644-647, 2002.

20. Crane L: Physical therapy for neonates with respiratory dysfunction. Phys Ther 61(12):1764-1773, 1981.

21. Dabezies EJ, Warren PD: Fractures in very low birth weight infants with rickets. Clin Orthop Rel Res 335:233-239, 1997.

22. Phillips RR, Lee SH: Fractures of long bones occurring in neonatal intensive therapy units. BMJ 301:225-226, 1990.

36.2 Suctioning

OVERVIEW. Airway suction is used to help remove bronchial secretions using a suction pump.[1] Concerns appear related to equipment used, how the technique is applied, and the medical status of the patients.

SUCTIONING: GUIDELINES

Issue	LOC	Sources	Affil	Rationale/Comment
Arrhythmias—hemodynamically significant	Advice	Peruzzi and Smith, 1995[2]	MD	
Force of catheters	P	Young, 1984[3]	PT	Never force catheters into airways with repeated jabbing movements. Lung perforation can occur if catheters are introduced too deeply.

Continued

Issue	LOC	Sources	Affil	Rationale/Comment
Frequent suctioning	P			Mucosal trauma from catheter contact has been noted even during one catheter insertion. Do not suction routinely but only as necessary.
Hyperinflation of lungs with 100% O_2	P			It can change blood acid-base levels and affect stability of severely ill patients. It may result in high positive intrathoracic pressures in neonates. Administer with care and by experienced staff.
Hypoxemia	Advice	Peruzzi and Smith, 1995[2]	MD	
Larger catheters	P	Young, 1984[3]	PT	Large-diameter catheters wedged into segmental bronchi of similar dimension can lead to airway collapse and atelectasis.
Laryngospasm or vocal cord injury—through vocal cords	Advice	Peruzzi and Smith, 1995[2]	MD	
Negative pressures—high	P	Young, 1984[3]	PT	Higher levels of vacuum pressure are more likely to cause tissue damage.
Positioning	P			Consider preparation and position of patient. There is less risk of vomit inhalation if nonintubated patients are positioned side-lying or with head turned to one side.
Prolonged suction	P			Prolonged suctioning induces hypoxia. Limit suctioning to 30 sec (15 sec in neonates). Hyperinflating lungs with O_2 or room air before or after suctioning reduces risk of hypoxia.
Sudden movements and resistance by patient—avoid	P			Sudden movements or resistance can increase risk of trauma.

SUCTION IN NEONATES

Issue	LOC	Sources	Affil	Rationale/Comment
Endotracheal suctioning—deep • Recent tracheoesophageal fistula repair	ACI	Crane, 1981[4]	PT	
Endotracheal suctioning—deep • Untreated pneumothorax	ACI			
Hyperactive gag	P			
Apnea	P			
Bradycardia	P			

REFERENCES

1. Doran BRH: Intensive Therapy—Apparatus. In Downie PA, editor: Cash's textbook of chest, heart, and vascular disorders for physiotherapists, ed 4. Philadelphia: J.B. Lippincott; 1987.
2. Peruzzi WT, Smith B: Bronchial hygiene therapy. Crit Care Clin 11(1):79-96, 1995.
3. Young CS: Recommended guide lines for suction. Physiotherapy 70(3):106-108, 1984.
4. Crane L: Physical therapy for neonates with respiratory dysfunction. Phys Ther 61(12):1764-1773, 1981.

37   POSTURAL DRAINAGE (BRONCHIAL DRAINAGE)

OVERVIEW. Postural drainage is the therapeutic use of positioning to drain the tracheobronchial tree so that secretions can then be eliminated either through coughing or suctioning.[1]

SUMMARY: CONTRAINDICATIONS AND PRECAUTIONS. Five sources cited a total of 35 concerns for postural drainage. Concerns ranged from 9 to 17 per source, with the American Association of Respiratory Care (AARC) citing the largest number. The largest proportion of concerns were related to circulatory, respiratory, and injury problems. The two most frequently cited concerns (four of five sources) were hemoptysis and pulmonary edema. The AARC cited three absolute contraindications: recent head injuries, neck injuries until stabilized, and hemorrhages with hemodynamic instability.

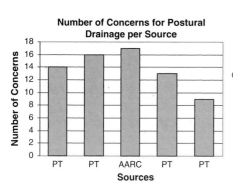

Number of Concerns for Postural Drainage per Source

Proportion of Concerns for Postural Drainage Based on ICD

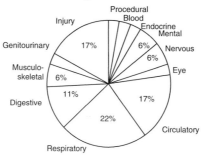

Top 8 Cited Concerns for Postural Drainage (n = 5)

POSTURAL DRAINAGE: GENERAL

D50-D89 DISEASES OF BLOOD AND BLOOD-FORMING ORGANS AND CERTAIN DISORDERS

Issue	LOC	Sources	Affil	Rationale/Comment
Hemorrhage (severe hemoptysis)—copious	CI	Webber, 1988[2,a]	PT	This is not the same as lightly blood-streaked sputum.
	ACI	AARC, 1991[3,b]	Org	
	CI/P	Downs, 1996[4,b]	PT	

a, Recent; b, With hemodynamic instability. General note: In Downs' guidelines, clinicians must weigh risks and benefits of postural drainage.[4]

E00-E90 ENDOCRINE, NUTRITIONAL, AND METABOLIC DISEASES

Issue	LOC	Sources	Affil	Rationale/Comment
Obesity, massive	P	Sciaky et al, 2001[5]	PT	

F00-F99 MENTAL AND BEHAVIORAL DISORDERS

Issue	LOC	Sources	Affil	Rationale/Comment
Confused patient	RCI	AARC, 1991[3]	Org	Position changes may not be tolerated.
	CI/P	Downs, 1996[4]	PT	
Nervous patient	CI/P	Downs, 1996[4,a]	PT	If agitated or upset from therapy.
	RCI	AARC, 1991[3]	Org	

a, Anxious.

G00-G99 DISEASES OF THE NERVOUS SYSTEM

Issue	LOC	Sources	Affil	Rationale/Comment
Cerebral edema	CI	Webber, 1988[3]	PT	
Intracranial pressure—increased	RCI	AARC, 1991[3,a]	Org	
	CI/P	Downs, 1996[4,a]	PT	
	RCI	Sciaky et al, 2001[5]	PT	

a, >20 mm Hg.

H00-H59 DISEASES OF THE EYE

Issue	LOC	Sources	Affil	Rationale/Comment
Eye surgery—post	RCI	Sciaky et al, 2001[5]	PT	Some associated edema may occur with tipping.[6] Danger of fluid
	CI	Anderson and Innocenti, 1987[6]	PT	accumulation behind the eye.[7]

100-199 DISEASES OF THE CIRCULATORY SYSTEM

Issue	LOC	Sources	Affil	Rationale/Comment
Aneurysm	CI	Webber, 1988[2,a]	PT	An aortic aneurysm's arterial wall is placed under tension when in a tipped position.[7]
	CI	Anderson and Innocenti, 1987[6,b]	PT	
Arrhythmia—cardiac	CI	Anderson and Innocenti, 1987[6]	PT	Some positions would increase myocardial oxygen demands, leading to an increase sensitivity to abnormal rhythms.[6]
Cardiovascular instability	CI	Webber, 1988[2,c]	PT	**Hammon et al[8] monitored 72 ICU patients during postural drainage with chest percussion and reported 8 patients developing major arrhythmias, 18 developing minor arrhythmias, and 46 none. Increased age and acute cardiac status were significantly associated with risk.**
	RCI	Sciaky et al, 2001[5,d]	PT	
Cerebral vascular accidents	CI	Anderson and Innocenti, 1987[6]	PT	ICP would increase.
Hypertension—severe	CI	Webber, 1988[2]	PT	Tipping would increase venous return and could overload the heart.[6]
	CI	Anderson and Innocenti, 1987[6]	PT	
Pulmonary embolism	CI/P	Downs, 1996[4]	PT	In this potentially fatal condition, blood supply to lung parenchyma is obstructed as a result of a blood clot lodged in the pulmonary artery.[9]
	RCI	AARC, 1991[3]	Org	

a, Cerebral and aortic aneurysms; b, Aortic; c, With arrhythmias or pulmonary edema; d, Hemodynamic instability.

Issue	LOC	Sources	Affil	Rationale/Comment
Asthma—acute	P	Webber, 1988[2]	PT	Dyspnea may increase and position may need to be modified.
Bronchopleural fistula	RCI	AARC, 1991[3]	Org	Bronchopleural fistula may be a complication of lung surgery
	CI/P	Downs, 1996[4]	PT	with a breakdown of the bronchial stump. There is a concern of "spill-over" of infected fluid into the remaining lung, so instruct to sit up or turn onto operated side.[6]
Emphysema—severe	P	Webber, 1988[2]	PT	Dyspnea may increase.[7] Positions may need to be modified.
	CI	Anderson and Innocenti, 1987[6,a]	PT	
Empyema	RCI	AARC, 1991[3]	Org	Empyema is a localized collection of pus in the pleural
	CI/P	Downs, 1996[4]	PT	cavity.[6]
Hemoptysis	RCI	AARC, 1991[3]	Org	If patient coughs up blood, treatment should be
	P	Sciaky et al, 2001[5]	PT	immediately stopped.[7] **In 1979, Hammon and**
	CI	Anderson and Innocenti, 1987[6,b]	PT	**Martin[10] reported a 51-year-old man with**
	CI/P	Downs, 1996[4]	PT	**squamous cell carcinoma and possible pneumonia, who received percussion with bronchial drainage and suffered a fatal, massive hemoptysis with exsanguination.**

Continued

Issue	LOC	Sources	Affil	Rationale/Comment
Pleural effusion—large	CI/P	Downs, 1996[4]	PT	Effusion may spread throughout pleura with positioning.
	RCI	AARC, 1991[3]	Org	
	P	Sciaky et al, 2001[5]	PT	
Pneumothorax	CI	Anderson and Innocenti, 1987[6,c]	PT	This is an acute emergency and postural drainage is not indicated.[6] Without an intercostal drain, the condition may lead to cardiac embarrassment and arrest if tipped. Treatment can begin once tube is inserted and patient is stable.
Pulmonary edema	RCI	AARC, 1991[3,d]	Org	Edema collects in the dependent area and can lead to extreme dyspnea and a worsening of the condition.[6]
	CI	Anderson and Innocenti, 1987[6]	PT	
	CI/P	Downs, 1996[4,d]	PT	
	P	Sciaky et al, 2001[5]	PT	

a, Surgical; b, Severe; c, Tension; d, With associated CHF.

K00-K93 DISEASES OF THE DIGESTIVE SYSTEM

Issue	LOC	Sources	Affil	Rationale/Comment
Ascites—massive	P	Sciaky et al, 2001[5]	PT	

Esophageal anastomosis—postoperative	RCI	Sciaky et al, 2001[5,a]	PT	In esophagectomy, drainage positions can strain the anastomosis.[7] Gastric juices may affect the suture line.[6] For postesophagectomy, with undue stress on the anastomosis, tipping may cause regurgitation.[6]
	CI	Anderson and Innocenti, 1987[6]	PT	
Hernia—diaphragmatic	RCI	Sciaky et al, 2001[5]	PT	Tipping may lead to regurgitated gastric juices.[6,7]
	CI	Anderson and Innocenti, 1987[6]	PT	
	CI	Webber, 1988[2,b]	PT	
Gastric reflux—esophageal-related	CI	Webber, 1988[2]	PT	

a, Recent; b, Diaphragm-related gastric reflux.

M00-M99 DISEASES OF THE MUSCULOSKELETAL SYSTEM AND CONNECTIVE TISSUE

Issue	LOC	Sources	Affil	Rationale/Comment
Laminectomy—recent	CI/P	Downs, 1996[4,a]	PT	Take care to properly roll (log roll) and correctly align.
	RCI	AARC, 1991[3]	Org	
Spinal fusion—recent	RCI	Sciaky et al, 2001[5]	PT	

a, Recent spinal surgery.

N00-N99 DISEASES OF THE GENITOURINARY SYSTEM

Issue	LOC	Sources	Affil	Rationale/Comment
Peritoneal dialysis—during the filling cycle	CI	Anderson and Innocenti, 1987[6]	PT	Tipping may cause respiratory distress because the diaphragm's descent is impeded during the filling phase of dialysis.

S00-T98 INJURY, POISONING, AND CERTAIN OTHER CONSEQUENCES OF EXTERNAL CAUSES

Issue	LOC	Sources	Affil	Rationale/Comment
Burns—facial	CI	Anderson and Innocenti, 1987[6]	PT	Facial edema may increase during tipping.
Head trauma—recent	RCI	Sciaky et al, 2001[5]	PT	ICP would increase.[6]
	CI	Anderson and Innocenti, 1987[6]	PT	
	ACI	AARC, 1991[3]	Org	
Neck injury—until stabilized	ACI	AARC, 1991[4]	Org	
	CI/P	Downs, 1996[4,a]	PT	
Rib fracture—with or without flair chest	RCI	AARC, 1991[3]	Org	
	CI/P	Downs, 1996[4]	PT	
Spinal injury—recent	RCI	Sciaky et al, 2001[5]	PT	
	RCI	AARC, 1991[3]	Org	
	CI/P	Downs, 1996[4]	PT	
Surgical wound/healing tissue	RCI	AARC, 1991[3]	Org	
	CI/P	Downs, 1996[4]	PT	

a, Head and neck injuries until stabilized.

Issue	LOC	Sources	Affil	Rationale/Comment
Aged	CI/P	Downs, 1996[4]	PT	If agitated or upset from therapy. **See Hammon and Martin[10] (above).**
	RCI	AARC, 1991[3]	Org	

SPECIFIC POSITIONAL CONCERNS DURING POSTURAL DRAINAGE

Trendelenburg Position Postural Drainage

E00-E90 ENDOCRINE, NUTRITIONAL, AND METABOLIC DISEASES

Issue	LOC	Sources	Affil	Rationale/Comment
Obesity	RP	Starr, 2001[11,a]	PT	

a, General note: Starr's list is not meant to be inclusive; RP = relative precaution.

G00-G99 DISEASES OF THE NERVOUS SYSTEM

Issue	LOC	Sources	Affil	Rationale/Comment
Epidural narcotic anesthetic—ongoing infusion	CI	Peruzzi and Smith, 1995[12]	MD	
Intracranial pressure—increased	CI	Peruzzi and Smith, 1995[12]	MD	
	RCI	AARC, 1991[3,a]	Org	
	CI/P	Downs, 1996[4]	PT	
Neurosurgical procedure—recent	CI	Peruzzi and Smith, 1995[12]	MD	
	ACI	Crane, 1981[13]	PT	
	RCI	AARC, 1991[3]	Org	

a, >20 mm Hg.

H00-H59 DISEASES OF THE EYE

Issue	LOC	Sources	Affil	Rationale/Comment
Eye surgery—recent	CI	Peruzzi and Smith, 1995[12]	MD	ICP increases and may affect site.
	ACI	Crane, 1981[13,a]	PT	
	RCI	AARC, 1991[3]	Org	

a, Neonates.

Issue	LOC	Sources	Affil	Rationale/Comment
Aneurysm—cerebral artery (unclipped)	CI	Peruzzi and Smith, 1995[12]	MD	
	RCI	AARC, 1991[3]	Org	
Cardiovascular instability	ACI	Crane, 1981[13,a,b]	PT	
CHF	P	Crane, 1981[13,c]	PT	In cardiac insufficiency, the heart would have to work harder against
	RP	Starr, 2001[11]	PT	gravity to pump blood to the legs when in a tipped position.[7]
Hemorrhage—intracranial	ACI	Crane, 1981[12,a]	PT	
Hypertension—uncontrolled	CI	Peruzzi and Smith, 1995[12]	MD	
	RCI	AARC, 1991[3]	Org	
	CI/P	Downs, 1996[4]	PT	
	RP	Starr, 2001[11,d]	PT	
Persistent fetal circulation	P	Crane, 1981[13,a]	PT	

a, Neonates; b, Acute CHF; c, Treated; d, Control not specified.

Issue	LOC	Sources	Affil	Rationale/Comment
Aspiration risk	CI	Peruzzi and Smith, 1995[12]	MD	I.e., tube feeding; after recent meal, esophageal surgery; altered airway
	RCI	AARC, 1991[3]	Org	protective reflexes; decreased mental status.
	CI/P	Downs, 1996[4,d]	PT	

Continued

Issue	LOC	Sources	Affil	Rationale/Comment
Hemoptysis—recent	ACI	Crane, 1981[13,a]	PT	
	RCI	AARC, 1991[3,b]	Org	
	CI/P	Downs, 1996[4,b]	PT	
Pneumothorax	ACI	Crane, 1981[13,a,c]	PT	
Pulmonary edema	CI	Peruzzi and Smith, 1995[12]	MD	
	RP	Starr, 2001[11]	PT	
Respiratory failure—severe	P	Crane, 1981[13,a]	PT	

a, Neonates; b, Gross and related to lung CA with radiation or surgery; c, Untreated; d, Unprotected airway.

K00-K93 DISEASES OF THE DIGESTIVE SYSTEM

Issue	LOC	Sources	Affil	Rationale/Comment
Abdominal distension	CI	Peruzzi and Smith, 1995[12]	MD	
	RCI	AARC, 1991[3]	Org	
	CI/P	Downs, 1996[4]	PT	
	RP	Starr, 2001[11]	PT	
Esophageal surgery	RCI	AARC, 1991[3]	Org	
Recent esophageal anastomosis	CI/P	Downs, 1996[4]	PT	
Gastroesophageal reflux risk	CI	Peruzzi and Smith, 1995[12]	MD	
Hernia, hiatal	RP	Starr, 2001[11]	PT	

R00-R99 SYMPTOMS, SIGNS, AND ABNORMAL CLINICAL AND LABORATORY FINDINGS (NOT ELSEWHERE CLASSIFIED)

Issue	LOC	Sources	Affil	Rationale/Comment
Apnea	P	Crane, 1981[13,a]	PT	
Bradycardia	P	Crane, 1981[13,a]	PT	
Nausea	RP	Starr, 2001[11]	PT	
Shortness of breath, worse in Trendelenburg	RP	Starr, 2001[11]	PT	

a, Neonate.

PROCEDURAL CONCERNS

Issue	LOC	Sources	Affil	Rationale/Comment
Food consumption, recent	RP	Starr, 2001[11]	PT	

Reverse Trendelenburg Position for Postural Drainage

I00-I99 DISEASES OF THE CIRCULATORY SYSTEM

Issue	LOC	Sources	Affil	Rationale/Comment
Hemodynamic instability—other	CI	Peruzzi and Smith, 1995[12]	MD	

Continued

Issue	LOC	Sources	Affil	Rationale/Comment
Hypotension	CI	Peruzzi and Smith, 1995[12]	MD	
	RCI	AARC, 1991[3]	Org	
Medication—vasoactive	RCI	AARC, 1991[3]	Org	

Prone Positioning for Bronchial Drainage

Issue	LOC	Sources	Affil	Rationale/Comment
Chest tube	P	Crane, 1981[13,a]	PT	
Nasal CDAP—continuous distending airway pressure	ACI	Crane, 1981[13,a]	PT	
Pneumothorax—untreated	ACI			

a, Neonates.

REFERENCES

1. Eisenberg MG: Dictionary of rehabilitation. New York: Springer; 1995.
2. Webber BA: The Brompton hospital guide to chest physiotherapy, ed 5. Oxford: Blackwell Scientific; 1988.
3. AARC: Clinical practice guidelines. Available at: http://www.aarc.org. Accessed November 16, 2005.
4. Downs AM: Physiological bases for airway clearance techniques. In: Frownfelter D, Dean E, eds: Principle and practice of cardiopulmonary physical therapy, ed 2. St. Louis: Mosby; 1996.

5. Sciaky A, Stockford J, Nixon E: Treatment of acute cardiopulmonary conditions. In Hillegass EA, Sadowsky HS, eds: Essentials of cardiopulmonary physical therapy, ed 2. Philadelphia: W.B. Saunders; 2001.

6. Anderson JM, Innocenti DM: Techniques used in chest physiotherapy. In Downie PA, editor: Cash's textbook of chest, heart, and vascular disorders for physiotherapists, ed 4. Philadelphia: J.B. Lippincott; 1987.

7. Thomson A, Skinner A, Piercy J: Tidy's physiotherapy, ed 12. Oxford: Butterworth-Heinemann; 1991.

8. Hammon WE, Connors AF Jr, McCaffee R: Cardiac arrhythmia during postural drainage and chest percussion of critically ill patients. Chest 102(6):1336-1341, 1992.

9. Goodman CC: The respiratory system. In: Goodman CC, Boissonnault WG, Fuller KS, eds: Pathology: implications for the physical therapist, ed 2. Philadelphia: Saunders; 2003.

10. Hammon WE, Martin RJ: Fatal pulmonary hemorrhage associated with chest physical therapy. Phys Ther 59(10):1247-1248, 1979.

11. Starr JA: Chronic pulmonary dysfunction. In: O'Sullivan SB, Schmitz TJ, eds: Physical rehabilitation and treatment, ed 4. Philadelphia: F.A. Davis; 2001.

12. Peruzzi WT, Smith B: Bronchial hygiene therapy. Crit Care Clin 11(1):79-96, 1995.

13. Crane L: Physical therapy for neonates with respiratory dysfunction. Phys Ther 61(12):1764-1773, 1981.

Section G   INTEGUMENT REPAIR AND PROTECTION TECHNIQUES

38   WOUND CARE

OVERVIEW. Wound care may incorporate debridement techniques. Debridement is the procedure of removing devitalized tissue (and foreign matter) from a wound. Moist devitalized tissue supports the growth of pathological organisms, initiates an inflammatory response, and retards wound healing. The removal of devitalized tissue is considered necessary for wounds to heal.[1]

In this section, debridement concerns for autolytic, enzymatic, mechanical (wet-to-dry gauze dressings, wound irrigation, whirlpool, dextromoners), and sharp techniques are reviewed. The sources included one governmental/agency, three physical therapy, and one nursing. Wound cleaning solvents and dressing issues are also briefly addressed.

CONTRAINDICATIONS AND PRECAUTIONS

DEBRIDEMENT

Autolytic Debridement (AD)

Autolytic debridement uses moisture-retentive synthetic dressing, permitting devitalized tissue to self-digest from enzymes normally in the wound. AD is indicated when the patient may not tolerate other forms of debridement and would not become infected if the wound was not debrided using faster methods. AD takes longer than other methods.[1]

General note: Stable heel ulcers. The AHCPR1 panel's opinion is that stable heel ulcers with a dry eschar do not need to be debrided if they do not have drainage, fluctuance, erythema, or edema because they provide a natural protective cover. These stable heel ulcers with dry eschar should be monitored daily and must be debrided if signs of pressure ulcer complications appear.

Issue	LOC	Sources	Affil	Rationale/Comment
Dressing, hydrocolloid or hydrogel wafer • Wound infection (documented) • Wound—dry gangrene (documented) • Wound—dry ischemic (documented) • Cellulitis	CI	Bates-Jensen, 1998[2]	PT	Do not use hydrocolloid or hydrogel wafer dressings on cellulitis, documented wound infection, dry gangrene, or dry ischemic wounds unless vascular consult is obtained and circulatory status is determined.
Dressing, transparent film • Wounds—dry gangrene • Wound—dry ischemic	CI			Do not use transparent film dressings on dry gangrene or dry ischemic wounds unless vascular consult and circulatory status is determined.
Maceration—periwound	P	Ramundo and Wells, 2000[3]	Nurs	Periwound maceration may occur because of wound exudate contact with intact skin. Consider barriers (film, skin) to surround skin. Change dressing at appropriate intervals.
Ulcers—infected	CI	AHCPR, 1994[1]	Agency	AD is contraindicated if ulcer is infected.

PROCEDURAL CONCERN

Issue	LOC	Sources	Affil	Rationale/Comment
Dressing—appropriate	P	Ramundo and Wells, 2000[3]	Nurs	Dressing—must choose most appropriate dressing based on wound and patient's status.

Enzymatic Debridement

Topical debriding enzymatic agents are applied to the wound surface of devitalized tissue and are considered if ulcer is not infected, individuals are in LTC facilities or at home or if surgery cannot be tolerated.[1]

S00-T98 INJURY, POISONING, AND CERTAIN OTHER CONSEQUENCES OF EXTERNAL CAUSES

Issue	LOC	Sources	Affil	Rationale/Comment
Wound—clean **Wound—dry gangrene** **Wound—dry ischemic**	CI	Bates-Jensen, 1998[2]	PT	Do not use on clean wounds, dry gangrene, or dry ischemic wounds unless vascular consultation or an ankle-brachial index is obtained and circulatory status is determined.

PROCEDURAL CONCERNS

Issue	LOC	Sources	Affil	Rationale/Comment
Agents—containing petrolatum	Advice	Loehne, 2002[4]	PT	Petrolatum may retard wound healing because viable cells are not bathed in oil base mediums. Discontinue agents containing petrolatum after wound has no more necrotic tissue.

Mechanical Debridement

Mechanical debridement uses some outside force to remove dead tissue such as (1) wet-to-dry dressings, (2) hydrotherapy, (3) wound irrigation, and (4) dextranomers.

Wet-to-Dry Gauze Dressings

Wet-to-dry gauze dressings removes necrotic tissue nonselectively that has dried and adhered to gauze.[4]

D50-D89 DISEASES OF BLOOD AND BLOOD-FORMING ORGANS AND CERTAIN DISORDERS

Issue	LOC	Sources	Affil	Rationale/Comment
Anticoagulant therapy	Do not use	Loehne, 2002[4]	PT	

S00-T98 INJURY, POISONING, AND CERTAIN OTHER CONSEQUENCES OF EXTERNAL CAUSES

Issue	LOC	Sources	Affil	Rationale/Comment
Wounds—clean	CI	Bates-Jensen, 1998[2]	PT	Do not use wet-to-dry gauze dressings on a clean wound because healthy tissue will be debrided.[2] Patients may need to be premedicated for pain before debridement.

PROCEDURAL CONCERNS

Issue	LOC	Sources	Affil	Rationale/Comment
Analgesia—adequate	Recommended	AHCPR, 1994[1]	Agency	Adequate analgesia is needed for this procedure.
Gauze dressings	CI	Ramundo and Wells, 2000[3]	Nurs	This is a controversial debridement method.[3] Some experts believe gauze dressings to be contraindicated. Limit their use to heavily necrotic wounds and stop when viable tissue is present.
Nonselective method	Disadvantage	AHCPR, 1994[1]	Agency	This method could potentially traumatically remove viable granulation tissue and new epithelial tissue.
Saline on gauze—excessive	P	Ramundo and Wells, 2000[3]	Nurs	Avoid excessive saline on gauze because it can lead to maceration of periwound tissue and prevent drying out of the dressing.[3]

Wound Irrigation

Wound irrigation is used to soften eschar and debride wounds.[1]

D50-D89 DISEASES OF BLOOD AND BLOOD-FORMING ORGANS AND CERTAIN DISORDERS

Issue	LOC	Sources	Affil	Rationale/Comment
Anticoagulants—pulsatile high-pressure lavage	P	Ramundo and Wells, 2000[3]	Nurs	

Vulnerable Biological Tissue

Issue	LOC	Sources	Affil	Rationale/Comment
Bone—pulsatile high-pressure lavage	P	Ramundo and Wells, 2000[3]	Nurs	Monitor for bleeding and avoid structures noted under issue column; **see**
Blood vessels	P			**Adverse Event section.**
Exposed muscle	P			
Exposed tendons	P			
Graft sites	P			

PROCEDURAL CONCERNS

Issue	LOC	Sources	Affil	Rationale/Comment
Enclosed area—pulsatile high-pressure lavage	P	Ramundo and Wells, 2000[3]	Nurs	Treat in an enclosed area, separate from other patients (to avoid contamination with mist).[3]
Irrigation pressures, excessive	Information CI	AHCPR, 1994[1] Sussman, 1998[5]	Agency PT	Some devices produce too much pressure and can damage healthy tissue. Safe and effective pressures range from 4 to 15 psi; pressures >15 psi may "cause trauma and drive bacteria into the tissue." Use gentle irrigation on clean wounds and vigorous irrigation on necrotic wounds. Mechanical wound irrigation is applied during dressing changes to all wounds.[5]
Protective equipment	P	Ramundo and Wells, 2000[3]	Nurs	Use protective equipment. Bacteria may disseminate over a wide area under the fluid pressure (high pressure irrigation; 8 to 12 psi), exposing provider and patient to contaminates.[3]

Whirlpool

Clean pressure ulcers with whirlpool when there is exudate, slough, or necrotic tissue. Discontinue whirlpool when the ulcer is clean.[1]

E00-E90 ENDOCRINE, NUTRITIONAL, AND METABOLIC DISEASES

Issue	LOC	Sources	Affil	Rationale/Comment
Diabetes	P	Ramundo and Wells, 2000[3]	Nurs	These patients may have an inability to detect changes in temperature due to autonomic and sensory neuropathies.
Diabetic, callus formation on plantar surface of feet	CI CI	Sussman, 1998[5] Loehne, 2002[4]	PT PT	Callus will soften and subsequent pressure during standing will lead to skin breakdown and a portal for infection (i.e., non-necrotic neuropathic foot ulcers).[4]
Diabetic ulcers—non-necrotic	P	Sussman, 1998[5]	PT	Callus often surrounds the ulcer and will soften and macerate. This tissue will not tolerate pressure, the wound will enlarge, and moisture retention under the callus may be source of infection.

F00-F99 MENTAL AND BEHAVIORAL DISORDERS

Issue	LOC	Sources	Affil	Rationale/Comment
Lethargy	CI	Sussman, 1998[5]	PT	
	CI	Loehne, 2002[4]	PT	
Unresponsiveness	CI	Sussman, 1998[5]	PT	
	CI	Loehne, 2002[4]	PT	

I00-I99 DISEASES OF THE CIRCULATORY SYSTEM

Issue	LOC	Sources	Affil	Rationale/Comment
Cardiovascular or pulmonary function—compromise	CI	Sussman, 1998[5]	PT	Water temperatures should not exceed 38° C due to added load to heart (dilating vessels, increased return to heart, and increased cardiac output).[5]
	CI	Loehne, 2002[4]	PT	
Phlebitis—acute	CI	Sussman, 1998[5]	PT	
	CI	Loehne, 2002[4]	PT	
Venous insufficiency leg ulcers with edema	P	Loehne, 2002[4]	PT	Water temperatures should not exceed local skin temperatures (34° C for patients with PVD).[5]
	P	Ramundo and Wells, 2000[3]	Nurs	Avoid dependent LE positioning in warm water because of increased venous hypertension and increased swelling.[1]
				Vasodilation, congestion, and edema may occur with venous ulcers because of dependency of leg and whirlpool.

K00-K93 DISEASES OF THE DIGESTIVE SYSTEM

Issue	LOC	Sources	Affil	Rationale/Comment
Incontinence of feces—if whirlpool is contaminated	CI	Sussman, 1998[5]	PT	
		Loehne, 2002[4,a]	PT	

a, Full-body whirlpool.

L00-L99 DISEASES OF THE SKIN AND SUBCUTANEOUS TISSUE

Issue	LOC	Sources	Affil	Rationale/Comment
Skin grafts—new	P	Sussman, 1998[5]	PT	New skin grafts will not tolerate high shear forces and turbulence.
	P	Loehne, 2002[4]	PT	
Tissue flaps—new	P	Sussman, 1998[5]	PT	New tissue flaps are sensitive to shear forces. Vasoconstriction may occur if temperatures result in chilling.
	P	Loehne, 2002[4]	PT	

M00-M99 DISEASES OF THE MUSCULOSKELETAL SYSTEM AND CONNECTIVE TISSUE

Issue	LOC	Sources	Affil	Rationale/Comment
Contractures—fetal posture	P	Sussman, 1998[5]	PT	The patient may not be able to be safely positioned in a whirlpool.

N00-N99 DISEASES OF THE GENITOURINARY SYSTEM

Issue	LOC	Sources	Affil	Rationale/Comment
Incontinence of urine—if whirlpool is contaminated	CI	Sussman, 1998[5]	PT	
		Loehne, 2002[4,a]	PT	
Renal failure	CI	Loehne, 2002[4]	PT	

a, Full-body whirlpool.

R00-R99 SYMPTOMS, SIGNS

Issue	LOC	Sources	Affil	Rationale/Comment
Dry gangrene	CI	Sussman, 1998[5]	PT	Don't soften. It serves to wall off tissue, and softening will decrease the barrier and allow infection/
	CI	Loehne, 2002[4]	PT	organisms to enter body.
Edema—moderate to severe	CI	Sussman, 1998[5]	PT	
	CI	Loehne, 2002[4,a]	PT	
Febrile conditions	CI	Sussman, 1998[5]	PT	$>101.9°$ F[4]
	CI	Loehne, 2002[4]	PT	

a, Extremity.

S00-T98 INJURY, POISONING, AND CERTAIN OTHER CONSEQUENCES OF EXTERNAL CAUSES

Issue	LOC	Sources	Affil	Rationale/Comment
Burns	Advice	Helm, 1982[6]	MD	There is the potential for hypotension, electrolyte imbalance, and wound contamination from bowel flora. Many burn centers use nonimmersion techniques.
				During the convalescent phase of burn care, as wounds close and grafts stabilize, whirlpool is avoided due to drying or injuring effect of fragile newly healed skin.
Maceration	CI	Sussman, 1998[5]	PT	Maceration is damage to new epithelium from either wound exudate leakage or the use of a product that moistens the skin.[7]
	CI	Loehne, 2002[4]	PT	
Wounds—clean, granulated	P	Sussman, 1998[5]	PT	Clean granulated wounds can easily be traumatized by force of mild agitation.
	P	Loehne, 2002[4]	PT	
Wounds—epithelializing	P	Sussman, 1998[5]	PT	Epithelialization starts immediately following trauma in an effort to close the wound. This tissue can be traumatized by mild whirlpool agitation; reduce aeration.[7]
	P	Loehne, 2002[4]	PT	

Issue	LOC	Sources	Affil	Rationale/Comment
Premedication	P	Loehne, 2002[4]	PT	Some patients may require premedication.
Temperatures—extreme, avoid if sensory loss	P	Sussman, 1998[5]	PT	Avoid extreme temperatures if the patient has sensory loss (i.e., alcoholic or diabetic-related neuropathy). Also see Hydrotherapy.
Temperature—optimal is 37° C	Advice	Sussman, 1998[5]	PT	A temperature of 37° C is optimal for epithelial cell migration, mitotic cell division, and leukocytic activity.
Whirlpool—discontinuing	Recommendation/guideline	AHCPR, 1997[1]	Agency	Discontinue when wound is clean, because the risk of trauma to regenerating tissue from high-pressure water jets (positioned too closely to the wound) in the whirlpool outweighs the wound cleaning benefits.

Dextranomers

Dextranomers are beads that absorb exudate, bacteria, and other debris when poured into the wound bed.[1]

Issue	LOC	Sources	Affil	Rationale/Comment
Slick (slippery) floor surface	Information	AHCPR, 1994[1]	Agency	If beads spill onto the floor, they can create a safety hazard because they produce a slick floor surface.

Sharp Debridement

Sharp debridement is used when there is an urgent need for debridement, such as when there is advancing cellulitis or sepsis. The technique is used to convert necrotic wound to a clean wound quickly and involves the use of scalpel, scissors, or other sharp instrument to remove devitalized tissue.[1]

S00-T98 INJURY, POISONING, AND CERTAIN OTHER CONSEQUENCES OF EXTERNAL CAUSES

Issue	LOC	Sources	Affil	Rationale/Comment
Dry gangrene	CI	Bates-Jensen, 1998[2]	PT	Do not use on dry gangrene. Must be kept dry as they may autoamputate (i.e., digits) before a more proximal surgical amputation.
	CI	Loehne, 2002[4]	PT	Do not use unless vascular consultation or ankle-brachial index obtained and circulatory status determined.[2]
Wound—clean	CI	Bates-Jensen, 1998[2]	PT	Do not use on clean wounds. A noninfected heel ulcer covered with dry eschar offers natural wound protection.[4]
	CI	Loehne, 2002[4]	PT	Do not use unless vascular consultation or ankle-brachial index obtained and circulatory status determined.[2]
Wound—dry ischemic	CI	Bates-Jensen, 1998[2]	PT	Do not use on dry ischemic wounds unless vascular consultation or ankle-brachial index obtained and circulatory status determined.[2]
Wound—nondraining wounds with severely limited perfusion	Do not debride	Loehne, 2002[4]	PT	They will develop necrosis.
Wounds—tunneling or undermining	CI			The wound (base) cannot be visualized.

D50-D89 DISEASES OF BLOOD AND BLOOD-FORMING ORGANS, AND CERTAIN DISORDERS

Issue	LOC	Sources	Affil	Rationale/Comment
Anticoagulant therapy	P	Loehne, 2002[4]	PT	
Clotting mechanism—impaired	Avoid	Loehne, 2002[4]	PT	Assess medications (heparin, warfarin, NSAIDs, antibiotics), thrombocytopenia,
	P	Ramundo and Wells, 2000[3]	Nurs	liver function, vitamin K deficiency, malnutrition.
Low platelet count	P	Loehne, 2002[4]	PT	

Vulnerable Biological Tissue

Issue	LOC	Sources	Affil	Rationale/Comment
Bone/tendon exposure—impending	CI	Bates-Jensen, 1998[2]	PT	
Fascial plane—close to	CI			

PROCEDURAL CONCERNS

Issue	LOC	Sources	Affil	Rationale/Comment
Clinical skills, decreased	Guideline	AHCPR, 1994[1]	Agency	One must have the necessary skill or knowledge of what is being cut.
	CI	Bates-Jensen, 1998[2]	PT	
Fatigue of practitioner or patient	P	Loehne, 2002[4]	PT	
Licensing requirements—satisfied	Guideline	AHCPR, 1994[1]	Agency	Extensive wounds are typically débrided in the operating room. Smaller wounds may be done at bedside.

WOUND CLEANING SOLUTIONS

Wounds heal better (optimized) and have lower potential for infection when all wastes, exudate, and necrotic tissue are removed from the wound.

PROCEDURAL CONCERNS

Issue	LOC	Sources	Affil	Rationale/Comment
Normal saline to clean ulcers	Recommendation	AHCPR, 1994[1]	Agency	For most pressure ulcers, use normal saline to clean a wound because it is physiologic (will not harm tissue).
Risk benefits	Recommendation			Need to weigh benefits of a clean wound with the risk of potential trauma to the wound bed as a result of cleaning.

| Skin cleaners or antiseptic agents | Do not use | | | Skin cleaners or antiseptic agents contain chemicals that are cytotoxic to normal tissue or human fibroblasts and should be avoided (e.g., do not use iodine, iodophor, sodium hypochlorite solution, hydrogen peroxide, acetic acid, Betadine, Hibiclens, pHisoHex, benzalkonium chloride, Granulex). |

DRESSINGS

Dressings are used to maintain the physiologic integrity of the ulcer so that it protects the wound and provides ideal hydration. They should be biocompatible. Wound cavities are loosely filled with dressing material to prevent the development of abscesses (from walled-off areas).

PROCEDURAL CONCERNS

Issue	LOC	Sources	Affil	Rationale/Comment
Cardinal rule: "Keep ulcer tissue moist and surrounding intact skin dry"	Recommendation	AHCPR, 2004[1]	Agency	The reason is that intact skin is more susceptible to injury with moisture. The drainage from the wound and the treatment solutions may damage unprotected intact skin. Choose an appropriate dressing that will keep ulcer tissue moist and surrounding intact skin dry.
Overpacking a wound	Do not			Overpacking a wound may cause additional trauma by increasing pressure on the tissue.

ADVERSE EVENTS

LITIGATION

Year, State	History	Location	Device	Complication	Comments/Award
1997, Florida[8] **Debridement and osteomyelitis**	Plaintiff was s/p comminuted fracture distal left tibia due to fall from roof (1993) s/p grafting and metallic plate and screw fixation.	3 months later, PT. 15 minutes of whirlpool therapy and wound débridement.	Four days after treatment, fever; diagnosed wound infection—possible osteomyelitis; hospitalized 1 month for IV antibiotics and skin graft for open wound.	Claimed PT unauthorized and negligent wound débridement exposed hardware and led to osteomyelitis; defendant claimed preexisting infection and unhealed wound, negligent surgeon care, and patient failed to stop smoking.	$646,000 gross verdict; plaintiff 20% at fault.

Note: Awards and settlements do not necessarily prove a cause-effect relationship between equipment or therapy and injury.

REFERENCES

1. AHCPR: Treatment of pressure ulcers, clinical guideline No 15 (AHCPR Publication No. 95-0652), December 1994.
2. Bates-Jensen BM: Management of necrotic tissue. In: Sussman C, Bates-Jensen BM, eds: Wound care: A collaborative practice manual for physical therapists and nurses. Gaithersburg (MD): Aspen; 1998.

3. Ramundo J, Wells J: Wound debridement. In Bryant RA: Acute and chronic wounds: nursing management, ed 2. St Louis: Mosby; 2000.

4. Loehne HB: Wound debridement and irrigation. In: Kloth LC, McCulloch JM, eds: Wound healing alternatives in management, ed 3. Philadelphia: FA Davis; 2002.

5. Sussman C. Whirlpool. In: Sussman C, Bates-Jensen BM, eds: Wound care: A collaborative practice manual for physical therapists and nurses. Gaithersburg (MD): Aspen; 1998. pp 621-642.

6. Helm PA, Kevorkian CG, Lushbaugh M, et al: Burn injury: rehabilitation management in 1982. Arch Phys Med Rehabil 63:6-16, 1982.

7. Sussman C, Bates-Jensen BM: Wound healing physiology and chronic wound healing. In: Sussman C, Bates-Jensen BM, eds: Wound care: A collaborative practice manual for physical therapists and nurses. Gaithersburg (MD): Aspen; 1998.

8. Medical malpractice, verdicts, settlements, and experts, October 1997, p 40, loc 2.

SECTION H   ELECTROTHERAPEUTIC MODALITIES

39   BIOFEEDBACK

OVERVIEW. Biofeedback is a treatment that uses a device that provides visual and auditory representations of physiologic events that are not normally perceived by the individual. With training, biofeedback permits the individual to voluntarily control responses. An example is the use of EMG signals to help patients initiate or control motor activity (e.g., activate muscle contraction or reduce muscle tension).[1]

SUMMARY: CONTRAINDICATIONS AND PRECAUTIONS. Seven sources cited a total of nine concerns for biofeedback. Concerns ranged from one to two per source. Sources' clinical backgrounds varied (therapists, physicians, psychology, and athletic training). The largest proportion of concerns was related to instrumentation safety. The most frequently cited concern (two sources) was potential tissue injury from excessive motion or tension during a training session (i.e., exceeding the limits of the musculoskeletal system). Other concerns include skin irritation from electrode gel, and prescribing the intervention to inappropriate patients (i.e., patients with receptive aphasia).

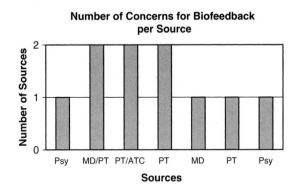

Number of Concerns for Biofeedback per Source

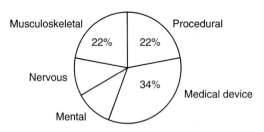

Proportion of Concerns for Biofeedback Based on ICD

CONTRAINDICATIONS AND PRECAUTIONS

F00-F99 MENTAL AND BEHAVIORAL DISORDERS

Issue	LOC	Sources	Affil	Rationale/Comment
Psychiatric disorders (some)	Caution	Green and Shellenberger, 1999[2]	Psy	No explanation or data.

G00-G99 DISEASES OF THE NERVOUS SYSTEM

Issue	LOC	Sources	Affil	Rationale/Comment
Aphasia—receptive	CI	Tan, 1998[3]	MD/PT	Patients need to follow directions.

M00-M99 DISEASES OF THE MUSCULOSKELETAL SYSTEM AND CONNECTIVE TISSUE

Issue	LOC	Sources	Affil	Rationale/Comment
Muscle contraction—when it would damage tissue	CI CI	Starkey, 1999[4] Prentice, 2002[5]	ATC PT/ATC	Avoid undue muscle tension that may affect graft or other tissue restriction.
Range of motion—exceeded	P	Starkey, 1999[4]	ATC	When prescribed range of motion is exceeded.

MEDICAL DEVICES

Issue	LOC	Sources	Affil	Rationale/Comment
Electrical connections—faulty, makeshift	Caution	Basmajian, 2005[6]	MD	Faulty connections between recording and computer devices using a 110V or 220V power source may expose patient and clinician to risk. Use a qualified technician to configure electrical systems.
Gels—adhesive or coupling	Advice	Prentice, 2002[5]	PT/ATC	Adhesive may irritate skin.
Limb load monitor—limitations	Advice	Fagerson and Krebs, 2001[7]	PT	Torsional and shear forces are not typically monitored in these devices.

PROCEDURAL CONCERNS

Issue	LOC	Sources	Affil	Rationale/Comment
Medication levels—adjust accordingly	Caution	Schwartz, 1995[8]	—	Monitor condition and adjust medication levels accordingly. Relaxation responses may induce homeostatic changes that require adjustments in the medication (i.e., insulin, hypertensive medications).
Patient selection—appropriate	Advice	Tan, 1998[3]	MD/PT	Selection criteria: • Potential for voluntary control • Well motivated • Cooperative • Follow directions

REFERENCES

1. Bottomley JM: Quick reference dictionary for physical therapy. Thorofare (NJ): Slack; 2000.
2. Green JA, Shellenberger R: Biofeedback therapy. In Jonas WB, Levin JE, eds: Essentials of complementary and alternative medicine. Philadelphia: Lippincott Williams & Wilkins; 1999.
3. Tan JC: Practical manual of physical medicine and rehabilitation: diagnostic, therapeutic, and basic problems. St. Louis: Mosby; 1998.
4. Starkey C: Therapeutic modalities. Philadelphia: FA Davis; 1999.
5. Prentice WE: Therapeutic modalities for physical therapists, ed 2. New York: McGraw-Hill; 2002.

6. Basmajian JV: Biofeedback in physical medicine and rehabilitation. In: Delisa JA, editor: Physical medicine and rehabilitation: principles and practices, ed 4, vol 1. Philadelphia: Lippincott Williams & Wilkins; 2005.
7. Fagerson TL, Krebs DE: Biofeedback. In: O'Sullivan SB, Schmitz TJ, eds: Physical rehabilitation: assessment and treatment, ed 4. Philadelphia: FA Davis; 2001.
8. Schwartz MS: Biofeedback: a practitioner's guide, ed 2. New York: Guilford; 1995.

40   IONTOPHORESIS

OVERVIEW. Iontophoresis is the use of electrical current to transcutaneously deliver ions into the body.[1] The issues below relate specifically to iontophoresis. Because iontophoresis uses electric currents, electrical stimulation concerns also apply[2,3] **(also see Electrical stimulation).**

SUMMARY: CONTRAINDICATIONS AND PRECAUTIONS. Six sources cited a total of 18 concerns for iontophoresis. Concerns ranged from one to eight per source with a physical therapist citing the largest number and a physical therapist/athletic trainer citing the fewest. The largest proportion of concerns was procedural (60%). The most frequently cited concern was substance-related allergies.

SUMMARY: ADVERSE EVENTS. Health devices[4] reports both burns and shocks occurring during iontophoresis treatment.

Number of Concerns for Iontophoresis per Source

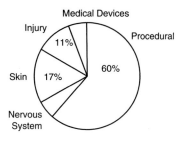

Proportion of Concerns for Iontophoresis Based on ICD

Top 5 Cited Concerns for Iontophoresis (n = 6)

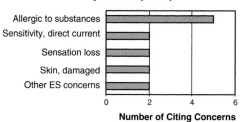

G00-G99 DISEASES OF THE NERVOUS SYSTEM

Issue	LOC	Sources	Affil	Rationale/Comment
Sensation absent	CI/caution	Ciccone, 1995[5]	PT	Monitor more frequently if sensation is not normal.[3]
	Safety rules	Cummings, 1991[3]	PT	

L00-L99 DISEASES OF THE SKIN AND SUBCUTANEOUS TISSUE

Issue	LOC	Sources	Affil	Rationale/Comment
Scars—recent	CI/never	Cummings, 1991[3]	PT	Scar tissue may not possess normal sensation.[3]
Sensitivity/allergies—to substance used	Investigate	Mehreteab and Holland, 2006[2]	PT	• Iodine (seafood sensitivity or reactive to intravenous pyelogram)[6]
	CI	Ciccone, 1995[5]	PT	• Hydrocortisone (if gastritis)[6] • Salicylates (if aspirin reactions)[6]
	Do not use	Kahn, 2000[6]	PT	• Metals (if sensitive to copper, zinc, magnesium)[6]
	CI (never use)/safety rules	Cummings, 1991[3]	PT	• Odor of mecholyl (if asthma)
	CI	Prentice, 2002[7]	PT/ATC	
Sensitivity—direct current	CI	Ciccone, 1995[5]	PT	Direct current can lead to excessive skin irritation.
	Investigate	Mehreteab and Holland, 2006[2]	PT	

S00-T98 INJURY, POISONING, AND CERTAIN OTHER CONSEQUENCES OF EXTERNAL CAUSES

Issue	LOC	Sources	Affil	Rationale/Comment
Injury (acute)/bleeding (in area of treatment)	CI	Mehreteab and Holland, 2006[2]	PT	
Skin—damaged	CI	Ciccone, 1995[5]	PT	Current concentrates in areas of least resistance such as cuts and bruises.[2] Electrochemical
	Avoid	Mehreteab and Holland, 2006[2]	PT	(not thermal) burns can result if the electrode is placed over a skin defect (i.e., shaved skin where resistance is lower).[5]

Y70-Y82 MEDICAL DEVICES

Issue	LOC	Sources	Affil	Rationale/Comment
Pacemaker	CI	Ciccone, 1995[5]	PT	Also other implanted electrical device.[3]

PROCEDURAL CONCERNS

Issue	LOC	Sources	Affil	Rationale/Comment
Administering two chemicals under same electrode	P/not advised	Kahn, 2000[6]	PT	The mutual repulsion of the chemicals may reduce penetration. (An exception is Iodex with methylsalicylate.)
Administering two ions with opposite polarity within same sessions	P/not advised			The second ion may reverse initial deposits; also a possible undesired synthesis of an antagonistic ion may occur. Consider alternative medication.
Administering iontophoresis after another physical agent	P	Cameron, 2003[1]	PT	The physical agent may alter skin permeability. Heat can also lead to increased vasodilation and accelerate the dispersal of the medication.

Continued

Issue	LOC	Sources	Affil	Rationale/Comment
Communication—burn discomfort	Safety rules			Patients must report burning or pain to therapist immediately.
Current—gradually change	Safety rules			Slowly increase and decrease current at beginning and end of session, respectively.
DC generator reliability	Safety rules			To enable current density calculations under each electrode.
Electrode contact	Safety rules			Electrodes must be in good contact and in constant pressure with skin.
Electrode soaking	Safety rules			Electrodes must be evenly and thoroughly soaked with water (tap), saline, or ion solution.
Electrodes (metal)—skin contact	CI/never			Shocks may occur if the leads are secured or removed from the patient while the unit is on. Never rearrange/remove electrodes without first switching off unit completely. **The journal *Health Devices* noted a hospital that reported two cases of skin reddening under the negative electrode during iontophoresis therapy and shocks. Shocks may have been caused by removing the electrode before the unit was turned off.**
Electrodes—removing/rearranging	Safety rules			
	Safety rules			
Other conditions where electrical stimulation is CI	CI	Mehreteab and Holland, 2006[2]	PT	
	CI/safety rules	Cummings, 1991[3,a]	PT	

a, Follow general rules.

ADVERSE EVENTS

Source	Background	Therapy	Outcome	Follow-up/Interpretation
Safety Report, 1997[4] **Skin redness and electric shock and Iontophoresis** Report, descriptive Health Dev	A hospital reported two cases of skin reddening under the negative electrode during iontophoresis therapy and shocks when the unit was turned off. The units were examined and working properly.	Reddening of skin is produced by increased blood flow due to the passage of electric current through the skin. Electrochemical (not thermal) burns can result if the pH increases or decreases beyond the range skin can tolerate, if current is too high or duration too long, or if electrode is placed over skin defect (i.e., shaved skin where resistance is lower). Shocks may occur if the leads are secured or removed from the patient while the unit is on, or if the unit is not first adjusted to zero output before turning it on or off, or if the device is defective. Still, minor shock can occur at the end of the procedure due to increased skin sensitivity from the electrolysis at the electrode.	Shocks in the two cases may have been caused by removing the electrode before the unit was turned off.	Read the manual. Do not place electrode over skin defects. Ensure good contact. Patient should report pain or burning sensation. Current should be minimal (e.g., zero) before unit is turned on or off. Attach electrodes and lead wires before turning on unit. Do not remove electrodes or lead wires until unit is turned off. Have unit inspected if problems occur.

REFERENCES

1. Cameron MH: Physical agents in rehabilitation: from research to practice. St. Louis: Saunders; 2003.
2. Mehreteab TA, Holland T: Iontophoresis. In: Hecox B, Mehreteab TA, Weisberg J, et al, eds: Integrating physical agents in rehabilitation. Upper Saddle River (NJ): Pearson Prentice Hall; 2006.
3. Cummings J: Iontophoresis. In Nelson RM, Currier DP, eds: Clinical electrotherapy, ed 2. Norwalk (CT): Appleton & Lange; 1991.
4. Anonymous: Lesions and shocks during iontophoresis. Health Dev 26(3):123-125, 1997.
5. Ciccone CD: Iontophoresis. In Robinson AJ, Snyder-Mackler L, eds: Clinical electrophysiology: electrotherapy and electrophysiologic testing, ed 2. Baltimore: Williams & Wilkins; 1995.
6. Kahn J: Principles and practice of electrotherapy, ed 4. New York: Churchill Livingstone; 2000.
7. Prentice WE: Therapeutic modalities for physical therapists, ed 2. New York: McGraw-Hill; 2002.

41   ELECTRICAL STIMULATION

41.1   Electrical Safety

OVERVIEW. McConnell[1] provides practical, nontechnical advice to clinicians to lessen the risk of electric shock with patients (**also see Hydrotherapy, Biofeedback).**

PROCEDURAL CONCERNS

Issue	LOC	Source	Affil	Rationale/Comment
Damaged electrical components	Advice	McConnell, 1996[1]	Nurs	**Do not use equipment with:** • Loose connections • Cracked, frayed, broken cords/cables • Broken knobs and switches • Damaged three-pronged plugs • Liquid/wet material on electrical equipment
Dropped equipment	Advice			Internal component may be damaged and pose a safety concern. Return any dropped equipment; add note and date of incident.
"Electrically sensitive patients"—identifying	Advice			Follow facilities policies for managing these patients. Examples: • Wet skin • Impaired skin integrity • Pacemakers
Expiration date of equipment—check	Advice			Check expiration date of safety equipment. Return outdated equipment.

Continued

Issue	LOC	Source	Affil	Rationale/Comment
Fluids that conduct electricity	Advice			Assess patient's environment for fluids that conduct electricity. Examples: • Urine • Blood • Water
High current equipment	Advice			In order to prevent circuit overload, plug devices that require high current (i.e., ventilator) into separate outlets.
Inappropriate electrical components	Advice			Examples: • Two-pronged plugs • Extension cords that bypass a ground wire
Removing plug from outlets	Advice			Grasp the plug, not the cord, when pulling (removing) a plug from an outlet. Otherwise, you may break the ground connection.
Smoking or sparks—equipment	Advice			If equipment smokes or sparks, turn off device immediately.
Tingling sensations reported—when equipment on	Advice			If patient feels a tingling sensation, turn off device immediately. Note: You do not want the patient to unintentionally become part of a circuit.
Turning off equipment before unplugging	Advice			Otherwise, resulting sparks can cause fires.

REFERENCES

1. McConnell EA: Clinical do's & don'ts: Ensuring electrical safety. Nursing 26(10):20, 1996.

41.2 Electrical Stimulation

(TRANSCUTANEOUS ELECTRICAL NERVE STIMULATION [TENS]; NEUROMUSCULAR ELECTRICAL STIMULATION)

OVERVIEW. Electrical stimulation (ES) uses alternating or direct current to accomplish various therapeutic aims including (1) to increase strength and endurance of innervated muscle (NMES), (2) to modulate pain (TENS), (3) to reduce edema (HVPC) and enhance healing, and (4) to stimulate denervated muscle (DC). It is also used (5) to deliver transdermal drugs using direct current (see Iontophoresis) and (6) to activate muscles during functional activities (see Functional electrical stimulation).[1]

The literature tends to treat electrical stimulation either in general terms, or alternatively, addresses motor (NEMS, or powered muscle stimulator) and pain modulation (TENS) modality concerns separately (as the FDA does).[2,3] In this text, I differentiate among NMES, ES, and TENS concerns.

SUMMARY: CONTRAINDICATIONS AND PRECAUTIONS. Thirteen sources together identify a total of 71 concerns for electrical stimulation (TENS, ES, and NMES). These concerns are listed under 16 categories. The largest number of concerns is noted as follows: For NMES, the FDA identifies 26 concerns. For TENS, the FDA and a PT both identify 14 concerns. And for ES, a PT identifies 14 concerns. The top three concerns, with all sources combined ($N = 13$), are pacemaker devices (92%), pregnancy (92%), and carotid sinus stimulation (85%).

GUIDELINE SIMILARITIES AND DIFFERENCES. NEMS, ES, and TENS shared some concerns: *demand pacemakers, pregnancy,* and treatments over the *carotid sinus.* On the other hand, modality-specific concerns were also apparent in this sample. For example, TENS had distinct concerns for undiagnosed pain, suppression of protective sensory mechanisms, and narcotic/drug use. This would make sense because TENS is used primarily for pain control. Also noteworthy, procedural concerns appear more common during TENS use (17 procedural concerns) than for NEMS (6 procedural concerns). In contrast, NEMS guidelines contain more motion-related concerns such as thrombophlebitis, fractures, hemorrhaging, the operation of machinery (e.g., driving), and conditions where movement is contraindicated. Again, this seems logical, in that NEMS affects muscle contraction.

OTHER ISSUES. (1) **Cross-infection:** In a 2000 laboratory-based study, Lambert et al[4] sampled microorganisms on suction cups and sponges used during interferential therapy and demonstrated the possibility of cross infection in a healthy volunteer. (2) **Partially denervated muscle and direct current:** In a 1979 *Nature* publication, Brown and Holland[5] reported that direct current interfered with sprouting in partially denervated muscle. In a critique, one source[1] argued that the parameters used in Brown and Holland's study were unlike those used in patients treated with denervated muscle. (3) **Brachial plexus injury:** In 1986, Mubarak and Wyatt[6] reported a 13-year-old white girl with idiopathic scoliosis who received electrical stimulation to the trunk for scoliosis and subsequently experienced upper/middle brachial plexus injury possibly from stimulus-related shoulder girdle hyperextension near the thoracic outlet. (4) **RA:** In 1981, Griffin and McClure[7] reported a 43-year-old female with RA who experienced a possible circulatory-related exacerbation of her symptoms following TENS use.

Notes: A few sources make recommendations for more than one modality. For NMES: only two sources apply, FDA used the term "powered muscle stimulator." Abbreviations in table: T = transcutaneous neuromuscular stimulation (TENS); M = neuromuscular electrical stimulation (NMES); E = electrical stimulation (general, not specified).

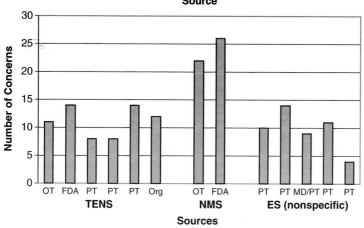

Number of Concerns for Electrotherapy per Source

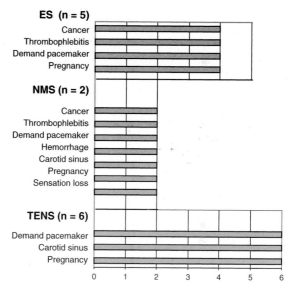

Top Concerns for ES, NMS, and TENS

CONTRAINDICATIONS AND PRECAUTIONS

A00-B99 CERTAIN INFECTIONS AND PARASITIC DISEASES

Issue	LOC	Sources	Affil	Rationale/Comment
Infections—active; TB	CI (M)	Bracciano, 2000[8]	OT	

C00-C97 NEOPLASMS

Issue	LOC	Sources	Affil	Rationale/Comment
Tumors—malignant	Warning (M)	FDA, 1999[2]	Gov	ES can increase local blood flow, enhancing tissue growth and metastasis. The FDA[2]
	P (E)	Shapiro, 2003[1]	PT	concern is the use of powered muscle stimulators over or proximal to cancerous
	CI (E)	Tan, 1998[9]	MD/PT	lesions (do not use).
	CI (M)	Bracciano, 2000[8]	OT	For cancer patients, informed consent is needed.[8]
	CI/P (E)	Mehreteab and Holland, 2005[10]	PT	
	Inappropriate (E)	Packman-Braun, 1992[11]	PT	

D50-D89 DISEASES OF BLOOD AND BLOOD-FORMING ORGANS AND CERTAIN DISORDERS

Issue	LOC	Sources	Affil	Rationale/Comment
Hemorrhage—active	CI (E)	Kahn, 2000[12]	PT	
	CI (E)	Tan, 1998[9]	MD/PT	
	CI (M)	Bracciano, 2000[8]	OT	
Hemorrhage tendency	Caution (M)	FDA, 1999[2]	Gov	Stimulation at the motor level can lead to bleeding if tissue is vulnerable.[10]
	CI/P (E)	Mehreteab and Holland, 2005[10]	PT	

E00-E90 ENDOCRINE, NUTRITIONAL, AND METABOLIC DISEASES

Issue	LOC	Sources	Affil	Rationale/Comment
Obese patients	CI (M)	Bracciano, 2000[8]	OT	It may be difficult to reach target tissue with intensity levels the patient could tolerate if excessive
	Inappropriate (E)	Packman-Braun, 1992[11]	PT	adipose tissue is present.

F00-F99 MENTAL AND BEHAVIORAL DISORDERS

Issue	LOC	Sources	Affil	Rationale/Comment
Incompetent; mentation impaired	P (T)	Mannheimer and Lampe, 1984[13]	PT	An incompetent patient may be unable to manage TENS. Also, reliable feedback on stimulation level of ES may be a problem for incompetent or young people.[8] Prevent output parameters from being adjusted by taping the dial settings in place.[13] With regard to the issue of impaired mentation, patients must be able to communicate discomfort to ensure that maximal ES currents are not exceeded. Use lowest effective currents.[1]
	P (T)	Gersh, 1992[14]	PT	
	CI (T,M)	Bracciano, 2000[8]	OT	
	P (E)	Shapiro, 2003[1]	PT	
	CI/P (E)	Mehreteab and Holland, 2005[10]	PT	
Psychological states	P (T)	AAMI, 1986[15]	Org	TENS outcome can be influenced by psyche.
Reliability—patient and/or attendant	Consider (E)	Packman-Braun, 1992[11]	PT	Reliable cooperation is important if the unit will be used at home.

G00-G99 DISEASES OF THE NERVOUS SYSTEM

Issue	LOC	Sources	Affil	Rationale/Comment
CNS disorders	CI (T)	Bracciano, 2000[8]	OT	
Cell body pathologies	CI (M)	Bracciano, 2000[8]	OT	I.e., polio.

Epilepsy/seizure disorder	Caution (M)	FDA, 1999[2]	Gov	FDA cautions use of muscle stimulator if epilepsy is suspect or diagnosed. Avoid TENS stimulation to head and neck areas.[8,10]
	CI (E)	Tan, 1998[9]	MD/PT	
	CI (T)	Bracciano, 2000[8]	OT	
	Inappropriate (E)	Packman-Braun, 1992[11]	PT	
Muscle-nerve junctions	CI (M)	Bracciano, 2000[8]	OT	I.e., myasthenia gravis.
Myelin sheath pathologies	CI (M)	Bracciano, 2000[8]	OT	I.e., multiple sclerosis.
Neuropathy—peripheral	CI (M)	Bracciano, 2000[8]	OT	I.e., diabetic neuropathy.[8]
	Inappropriate (E)	Packman-Braun, 1992[11,a]	PT	
Sensation impaired—area	Caution (M)	FDA, 1999[2]	Gov	Patients must be capable of feeling pain so that maximal ES currents are not exceeded.[1] Tan[9] states this is particularly important when using direct current because electrochemical burns can result. **In a 1999 survey, Partridge and Kitchen[16] reported 87 local adverse effects to interferential therapy including burns and rashes, suggesting that caution should be used in using these devices in neurologic patients.**
	P (E)	Shapiro, 2003[1]	PT	
	P/Extreme caution (T)	Kahn, 2000[12]	PT	
	CI (E)	Tan, 1998[9]	MD/PT	
	Caution (M)	Bracciano, 2000[8]	OT	
	CI/P (E)	Mehreteab and Holland, 2005[10]	PT	

a, PNS not intact; unless utilizing direct current.

100-199 DISEASES OF THE CIRCULATORY SYSTEM

Issue	LOC	Sources	Affil	Rationale/Comment
Arrhythmias	CI (E)	Shapiro, 2003[1]	PT	Stimulation may compromise cardiac function. Consult with physician.
Cardiac disease/history	Caution (M)	FDA, 1999[2]	Gov	The issue is to minimize the risk of current conducting to the vagus nerve and
	P (E)	Shapiro, 2003[1]	PT	thoracic organs. The FDA[2] cautions if disease is suspected.
Hypertension	CI (M)	Bracciano, 2000[8]	OT	
Hypotension	CI (M)	Bracciano, 2000[8]	OT	
Thrombophlebitis/thrombosis	Warning (M)	FDA, 1999[2]	Gov	ES may increase the risk of embolism.
	CI (E)	Shapiro, 2003[1]	PT	
	CI (E)	Kahn, 2000[12,a]	PT	
	CI (E)	Tan, 1998[9]	MD/PT	
	CI (M)	Bracciano, 2000[8,b]	OT	
	CI/P (E)	Mehreteab and Holland, 2005[10]	PT	
Varicose veins	Warning (M)	FDA, 1999[2]	Gov	

a, Phlebitis; b, PVD concern.

L00-L99 DISEASES OF THE SKIN AND SUBCUTANEOUS TISSUE

Issue	LOC	Sources	Affil	Rationale/Comment
Allergic skin reactions • To gel, electrode, or tape	P (M) P (T) Inappropriate (E)	FDA 1999[2] Gersh, 1992[14] Packman-Braun, 1992[11]	Gov PT PT	Skin irritation, ulceration, or hypersensitivity may occur from stimulation, gel, or tape.[2,11] Try alternative medium such as non–propylene glycol gels or conductive polymer electrodes. Try other electrode placements. Try other electrodes such as karaya or conductive polymer electrodes. **In a 1991 case report, Marren et al[17] reported a 35-year-old man who used TENS 16 hours/day for 18 months for low back pain relief and developed a florid eczema beneath the electrode pads at 9 months due to a methacrylate allergy. In a 1994 case report, Dwyer et al[18] reported on a 45-year-old man who used TENS for 8 months and exhibited eczematous patches from the propylene glycol gel used under the electrodes.**
Skin conditions	CI (M)	Bracciano, 2000[8]	OT	E.g., eczema, psoriasis, acne, dermatitis.
Skin, fragile	Inappropriate (E)	Packman-Braun, 1992[11]	PT	Skin may become irritated or ulcerated from gels or tape.

N00-N99 DISEASES OF THE GENITOURINARY SYSTEM

Issue	LOC	Sources	Affil	Rationale/Comment
Menstruating uterus	Caution (M)	FDA, 1999[2]	Gov	Note: Obviously not a disease.

O00-O99 PREGNANCY, CHILDBIRTH, AND PUERPERIUM

Issue	LOC	Sources	Affil	Rationale/Comment
Birth, during (TENS)	Warning (T)	FDA, 1998[3]	Gov	Safety of TENS during birth has not been established.
	Warning (T)	AAMI, 1986[15]	Org	
Over abdomen or lumbar area in pregnancy	P (T)	Gersh, 1992[14]	PT	The effects of ES on fetal development are not known. Also, the effects of TENS is not known.[13] Motor stimulation may induce uterine contractions.
	CI (E)	Shapiro, 2003[1,c]	PT	
	CI (E)	Tan, 1998[9]	MD/PT	
	P (T)	Mannheimer and Lampe, 1984[13]	PT	
	CI/P (E)	Mehreteab and Holland, 2005[10,d]	PT	
Pregnancy	Warning (T)	FDA, 1998[3]	Gov	The safety of TENS during pregnancy has not been established. Also see FDA and AAMI warnings under During birth.
	P (M)	FDA, 1999[2]		
	Warning (T)	AAMI, 1986[15]	Org	
	P/Caution (T)	Kahn, 2000[12,b]	PT	
	CI (T, M)	Bracciano, 2000[8,a]	OT	
	Inappropriate (E)	Packman-Braun, 1992[11]	PT	

a, CI in the first trimester; b, Except for TENS use in pregnancy: during labor and delivery for labor pain or meralgia paresthetica; c, Pelvic area concern; ES is used for pain control during uncomplicated labor and delivery; d, In first trimester directly over pregnant uterus.

Q00-Q99 CONGENITAL MALFORMATIONS, DEFORMITIES, AND CHROMOSOMAL ABNORMALITIES

Issue	LOC	Sources	Affil	Rationale/Comment
Muscular dystrophy	CI (M)	Bracciano, 2000[8]	OT	Muscle pathology.

R00-R99 SIGNS AND SYMPTOMS

Issue	LOC	Sources	Affil	Rationale/Comment
Infection	Warning (M)	FDA, 1999[2]	Gov	
Inflammation, areas	Warning (M)	FDA, 1999[2]	Gov	
Swollen—over	Warning (M)	FDA, 1999[2]	Gov	

S00-T98 INJURY, POISONING, AND CERTAIN OTHER CONSEQUENCES OF EXTERNAL CAUSES

Issue	LOC	Sources	Affil	Rationale/Comment
Fracture—fresh	CI (E)	Kahn, 2000[12]	PT	Important to avoid unwanted motion.
	CI (E)	Tan, 1998[9]	MD/PT	
Skin damage, lesions, or irritation, open wounds	P T, Warning (M)	FDA, 1998, 1999[2,3]	Gov	Motor stimulation can interfere with healing of tissue. Skin damage has lower tissue impedance, resulting in increased current delivery and pain. (ES is used over open wounds for healing with appropriate parameters.) Persistent use of TENS over irritated skin can lead to injury from long-term application at site of electrode.[15]
	Warning (T)	AAMI, 1986[15]	Org	
	P (E)	Shapiro, 2003[1]	PT	
	CI (T)	Gersh, 1992[14,a]	PT	
	Inappropriate (E)	Packman-Braun, 1992[11]	PT	
	CI/P (E)	Mehreteab and Holland, 2005[10]	PT	

a, Open wounds.

MEDICAL DEVICES

Issue	LOC	Sources	Affil	Rationale/Comment
Bladder stimulators—near	CI (M)	Bracciano, 2000[8]	OT	
Demand-type cardiac pacemakers	CI (T)	FDA, 1998[3]	Gov	TENS applications at the thorax or lumbosacral region can affect demand pacemakers. **Eriksson et al,[19] in a 1978 study of eight patients with pacemakers, reported that TENS units interfered with synchronous cardiac pacemakers (i.e., those that are ventricular inhibited,**
	CI (M)	FDA, 1999[2]	Gov	
	CI (E)	Shapiro, 2003[1]	PT	
	P/not use (T, E)	Kahn, 2000[12]	PT	

	CI (T)	Mannheimer and Lampe, 1984[13]	Org	
	CI (T)	AAMI, 1986[15]	Org	
	CI (T)	Gersh, 1992[14]	PT	
	CI (T,M)	Bracciano, 2000[8]	OT	
	Inappropriate (E)	Packman-Braun, 1992[11]	PT	
	CI/P (E)	Mehreteab and Holland, 2005[10]	PT	
Diathermy device—near	CI (M)	Bracciano, 2000[8]	OT	
Implantable cardioverter defibrillators (ICDs) with TENS users	RCI (T)	Philbin et al, 1998[22]	MD	
Metal—superficial, pins, plates, or hardware	CI (M)	Bracciano, 2000[8]	OT	

ventricular triggered, or atrial synchronous). On the other hand, Shade,[20] in a 1985 case report, described one 74-year-old man with a temporary pacemaker who was monitored closely using TENS for 1 hour continuously. Electrodes were kept about 4 inches away from the cardiac area and no interference with the demand pacemaker or with the patient's cardiac rhythm was noted. In 1996, Sliwa and Marinko[21] reported an ECG artifact from TENS applied at the thoracic and lumbar region, which was interpreted as a cardiac pacemaker malfunction.

Far-field potentials from TENS units can lead to "oversensing" and shocks (i.e., inappropriately administered therapy) by ICDs. **In 1998, Philbin et al[22] reported an 80-year-old woman with ventricular tachycardia who was fitted with an ICD. Her subsequent use of TENS created a signal that the ICD interpreted as VF, the criteria for shock therapy. Philbin et al[22] suggest reprogramming the sensitivity of the ICDs or altering the vector of TENS delivery to possibly ameliorate the problem.**

VULNERABLE BIOLOGICAL TISSUES

Issue	LOC	Sources	Affil	Rationale/Comment
Carotid sinus—over Any electrode placed with current to carotid sinus (anterior neck region)	CI (T)	FDA, 1998[3]	Gov	Stimulation of the vasovagal reflex can lead to a hypotensive response, arrhythmia,[8] or cardiac arrest.[13]
	Warning (M)	FDA, 1999[2]		
	CI (T)	Gersh, 1992[14]	PT	
	CI (E)	Shapiro, 2000[1]	PT	
	P/ Not use (T)	Kahn, 2000[12]	PT	
	CI (E)	Tan, 1998[9]	MD/PT	
	CI (T)	Mannheimer and Lampe, 1984[13]	PT	
	Warning (T)	AAMI, 1986[15]	Org	
	CI (T,M)	Bracciano, 2000[8]	OT	
	CI/P (E)	Mehreteab and Holland, 2005[10]	PT	
Eye—over (electrodes over the eyes)	P (T)	Gersh, 1992[14]	PT	Reasons include the concern that ES can injure eye structures, or that the effects of TENS over the eye are unknown.[10]
	P (T)	Mannheimer and Lampe, 1984[13]	PT	
	CI (T)	Bracciano, 2000[8]	OT	
	CI/P (E)	Mehreteab and Holland, 2005[10]	PT	
Heart (over/near) <u>in cardiac patient</u> (also across chest area)	P (T)	Gersh, 1992[14]	PT	Generally not recommended, but possibly use on an individual case basis if vigilant continuous cardiac monitoring employed and emergency assistance is available.
	CI (E)	Tan, 1998[9]	MD/PT	
	P (T)	Mannheimer and Lampe, 1984[13]	PT	
	CI (T)	Bracciano, 2000[8]	OT	
	CI/P (E)	Mehreteab and Holland, 2005[10,b]	PT	

Mouth—over	Warning (M)	FDA, 1999[2]	Gov	Breathing difficulties with powered muscle stimulators.
Mucosal lining—internal use	P (T)	Mannheimer and Lampe, 1984[13]	PT	The concern is possible damage or poor tolerance of the mucosal lining from
	CI (T)	Bracciano, 2000[8]	OT	stimulation.
	P (T)	Gersh, 1992[14]	PT	
	CI/P (E)	Mehreteab and Holland, 2005[10]	PT	
Neck—anterior	CI (T)	Bracciano, 2000[8]	OT	Powered muscle stimulators may cause severe spasms of the larynx and
	CI (T)	FDA, 1998[3]	Gov	pharynx, resulting in a closed airway or breathing difficulty. Furthermore,
	Warning (M)	FDA, 1999[2]	Gov	TENS in the vicinity of the carotid sinus (neck area) can lead to a hypotensive response.
Phrenic nerve—near	CI (M)	Bracciano, 2000[8]	OT	**In 1996, Mann[23] reported a 70-year-old UK man presenting with severe unstable angina who experienced respiratory compromise following TENS use over the chest area to control angina.** Note: Electrodes were placed over the chest; it is not known if the phrenic nerve was implicated.
Thoracic region—over	CI (M)	Bracciano, 2000[8]	OT	Same.
Transcerebral current flow—	CI (T)	FDA, 1998[3]	Gov	
through the head	Warning (M)	FDA, 1999[2]		
Transcranial or upper cervical	P (T)	Gersh, 1992[14]	PT	In epilepsy, electrical stimulation can potentially induce seizures.[10]
application in people with	P (T)	Mannheimer and Lampe, 1984[13]	PT	
CVA, TIA, or seizures	CI/P (E)	Mehreteab and Holland, 2005[10,a]	PT	
Transthoracically	Warning (M)	FDA, 1999[2]	Gov	Current traveling to heart may cause cardiac arrhythmias.

a, In epilepsy; b, Across chest.

PROCEDURAL CONCERNS

Issue	LOC	Sources	Affil	Rationale/Comment
Children	Warning (T)	FDA, 1998[3]	Gov	Keep out of children's reach.
	P (M)	FDA, 1999[2]	Gov	
	P (T)	AAMI, 1986[15]	Org	
	CI (T)	Bracciano, 2000[8]	OT	
Drug use	P (T)	AAMI, 1986[14]	Org	TENS outcomes can be influenced by drug use.
Electrical components: secure lead wires, electrodes, and potentiometers • In disoriented, cognitively impaired, and young children	P (T)	Gersh, 1992[14]	PT	
Electrode contact area—small	P (T)	Gersh, 1992[14]	PT	Burns can occur because current density is too high between or under electrodes. For TENS, contact size should be at lease 4 cm^2 and at a distance of at least the electrode's diameter.
Electrode contact—uneven • Due to uneven gelling or uneven body contour	P (T)	Gersh, 1992[14]	PT	Micropunctate electrothermal burns may occur if current is unevenly distributed under electrodes due to poor contact. Conform electrode to body surface and evenly apply gel to electrode.
Electrode—metal directly on skin or not fully "inserted"	P (T)	AAMI, 1986[15]	Org	Contact with the metal can lead to burns (TENS).
Electrocution	Warning (T)	FDA, 1998[3]	Gov	A TENS unit capable of delivering a charge per pulse of 25 microcoulombs or more is sufficient to cause electrocution. Cardiac arrhythmias can be caused by current of this magnitude flowing through the thorax. (You must not allow current flow through the thorax.)

Interelectrode distance—short	P (T)	Gersh, 1992[14]	PT	See comments above regarding burns.
Long-term use and skin irritation at site of TENS	P (T)	FDA, 1998[3]	Gov	**See Allergic skin reactions.**
Long-term effects of chronic ES unknown	Warning (M)	FDA, 1999[2]	Gov	
Machinery operations during muscle stimulation	P (M)	FDA, 1999[2]	Gov	Do not stimulate muscle while driving, operating machinery, or involved in tasks where involuntary movement would place patient at risk.
Malfunctions—other electronic monitoring equipment	Warning (T)	FDA, 1998[3]	Gov	ECG and other electronic monitoring equipment including alarms may not operate correctly during TENS application.
Medical condition that contraindicates muscle	Inappropriate (E)	Packman-Braun, 1992[11]	PT	An example is motor stimulation following recent surgery where contraction would interfere with healing.[2]
contraction or movement	Caution (M)	FDA, 1999[2]	Gov	
(i.e., phlebitis; PROM precautions following joint surgery)	CI/P (E)	Mehreteab and Holland, 2005[10]	PT	
Narcotic medications use	P/Extreme caution (T)	Kahn, 2000[12]	PT	

Continued

Issue	LOC	Sources	Affil	Rationale/Comment
Other warnings and TENS • Physician supervision • TENS has no curative value • Not effective for central pain	Warning (T) P (T)	FDA, 1998[3] AAMI, 1986[15]	Gov Org	The AAMI distinguishes between TENS effects on peripheral pain compared to central pain (for which it is not effective).
Shearing forces between skin and tape	P (T)	Gersh, 1992[14]	PT	Shearing leads to skin irritation. Try other tapes (e.g., use straps or self-adhering electrodes). Take care when placing and removing tape from skin.
Sports with TENS	P (T)	Kahn, 2000[12]	PT	Athletes are not permitted to play under the influence of TENS. Also relevant to animal competition.
Suppression of protective mechanisms with TENS	Warning (T) P (T) Warning (T)	FDA, 1998[3] Kahn, 2000[12] AAMI, 1986[15]	Gov PT Org	TENS may suppress sensation of pain that serves a protective function.[15]
Qualified pain management person	P (T,M)	FDA, 1998, 1999[2,3]	Gov	For TENS, effectiveness is dependent on patient selection by a qualified pain management person. For muscle stimulation, electroplacement and parameters should be determined by the prescribing practitioner.[2]
Undiagnosed pain syndromes and TENS	CI (T) P (T) P/not use (T)	FDA, 1998[3] AAMI, 1986[15] Kahn, 2000[12]	Gov Org PT	Pain provides important information when formulating a diagnosis. Masking pain may interfere with diagnostics.
Use recommended leads and electrodes	P (M)	FDA, 1999[2]	Gov	Use equipment recommended by the manufacturer.

ADVERSE EVENTS

Source	Background	Therapy	Outcome	Follow-up/Interpretation
Dwyer et al, 1994[18] **Propylene glycol TENS gel and hypersensitivity** Case report Contact Derm	A 45-year-old man presented with posttraumatic pain in his left shoulder.	He used TENS for 8 months for pain relief and had a 3-month history of skin reaction to TENS.	Positive eczematous patches were noted at the site of electrode application. Patch tests revealed hypersensitivity to gel containing propylene glycol.	The patient changed the gel type without further complication.
Eriksson et al, 1978[19] **Pacemakers and TENS interference** Descriptive Lancet	Eight patients (no details) with pacemakers were evaluated for interference from a TENS unit. Pacemaker types: 6 synchronous pacemakers 4 ventricular-inhibited 1 ventricular-triggered 1 atrial synchronous 2 fixed-rate pacemakers	TENS interference was evaluated under four conditions (with surface electrodes of TENS units placed): (1) thoracic, (2) paravertebral lumbar, (3) lumbar-sciatic, and (4) distal lower limb. The TENS unit (model not indicated) was administered with a constant current at 0.2 ms^2 pulses, 10-100 Hz, and with short trains of pulses (between 1 and 10 Hz) with current up to 40 mA (2500 ohm external load).	TENS totally blocked ventricular-inhibited pacemakers in all four patients (TENS at 1-3 Hz with current intensities about 20-40 mA). TENS triggered the ventricular pacemaker at frequencies >2 Hz and led to heart rates up to 130 bpm. TENS triggered the atrial synchronous pacemaker up to 150 bpm.	The authors considered TENS contraindicated in patients with synchronous cardiac pacemakers (those that are ventricular inhibited, ventricular triggered, or atrial synchronous). Mechanism: Synchronous pacemaker cannot "separate" electrical signals (which are externally applied) from spontaneous heart activity. Notes: TENS units were from 1970s; small descriptive study.

Continued

Source	Background	Therapy	Outcome	Follow-up/Interpretation
Glotzer et al, 1998[24] **ICD malfunction and EMS** Case series Pacing and clinical electrophysiology (PACE)	A 55-year-old man with idiopathic dilated cardiomyopathy and a history of cardiac arrest presented with an ICD (Guardian #4204; Telectronics Pacing Systems) and an epicardial rate sensing lead (#033-572) to detect and treat ventricular rates > 182 beats/min for 8 of 10 beats.	Three years later, he received EMS (Rich-Mar VI) for low back pain with electrodes placed on either side of his spine on his low back. (Specs: frequencies 1-60 pps; biphasic wave with intensity from 0 to 25 V. Settings were maximal voltage tolerated with frequency set at 60 pps.)	The ICD sensed the EMI from the EMS and delivered a 20-J shock.	The authors state that EMI with ICDs may not be universal during EMS therapy. They speculate that EMI may be related to older ICD sensing leads that were of the epicardial type. Based on available data, the authors suggest that prior to EMS therapy, ICD should be inactivated.
	A 70-year-old man presented with nonischemic cardiomyopathy and a nonsustained polymorphic ventricular tachycardia correlated with presyncope symptoms.	Following consent, this patient was stimulated with EMS (highest tolerated intensity, 50 Hz; intensity range 0-100 mA; asymmetric biphasic or symmetrical biphasic waveforms) with electrodes near the heart (left shoulder, upper back, and abdomen) as well as the low back. He was scheduled for EMS.	During EMS, the ICD sensed normally, but the therapy function of electric shock was disabled.	EMS did not interfere with ICD functioning in one patient.

	An ICD (Medtronic Jewl #7219C) was implanted in his left pectoral region and connected to an endocardial lead.	Note: He had been receiving Empi FOCUS (neuromuscular stimulator therapy) to the forearm.		
Griffin and McClure, 1981[7] **RA, exacerbation and TENS** Case report Phys Ther	A 43-year-old female with RA had a 2-year history of joint pain and swelling.	She was treated in a Hubbard tank followed by 2 days of TENS (electrodes on dorsal and ventral proximal to wrists with duration 0 on dial, frequency at "3" on dial (10-25 pulses/sec).	TENS was applied for 10 minutes on the first day followed by 3 hours of relief and then 30 minutes of numbness in the right wrist and distally. The next day, her pain returned with a "slightly funny feeling" in hands. The following day, TENS was applied for 15 to 20 minutes with electrodes on acupuncture sites [Li4, Sj5, Si4 (Right) and Li4, Sj5 (Left)]. After 1 hour, she experienced sharp pains in her hands and fingers lasting 5 minutes. That evening, she noted pain in her right hand spreading to her right shoulder, described as "deep, like in the bone," which	The authors suggested an association between these events and TENS use, cited literature of increased blood flow with electrical stimulation, and postulated that stimulus parameters (duration; frequency) interacted with patient's condition. The author cautions use of TENS in patients with involvement of the sensory and peripheral vascular system. RA patients should be informed about possible side effects. Responses should be monitored for 24 hours.

Continued

Source	Background	Therapy	Outcome	Follow-up/Interpretation
Lambert, 2000[4] **Contaminated sponges and cups used in ES** Laboratory and pretest-posttest, one subject J Hosp Infect	Study of microorganism growth and cross-contamination from interferential therapy equipment.	Suction cups and sponges and the water reservoir from an interferential therapy machine (no model details) were sampled for microorganisms 20 times before and after clinical use. To assess cross-infection potential, one healthy volunteer was exposed to a culture of *S. epidermidis* on the forearm, had two sterile suction cups and sponges secured directly over the site for 5 minutes, and then secured one of the cup and sponges to his opposite forearm.	lasted the night. The next morning she had swollen, painful fingers and wrist and distended superficial veins in her hands and forearms that lasted 2 days. Microorganisms were isolated from suction cups and sponges before clinical use: >500 colony-forming units (cfu) organisms (coagulase negative staphylococci; *Pseudomonas* spp, *Acinetobacter* spp, *Pasteurella* spp, *Rhodoterula* spp). Contamination significantly increased following clinical use. *Pseudomonas aeruginosa* was found in the water reservoir. For the cross-infection experiment, suction cups and sponges were contaminated with *S. epidermidis* from the first forearm and showed	The author found that disinfection of sponges and suction cups with 70% isopropyl alcohol after patient treatments can decrease transmission of microorganisms. Alternatively, disposable electrodes could be used.

			a significant number of these microorganisms transferred (mean 120 cfu/sample) to the opposite forearm site when the suction cup location was switched.	
Mann, 1996[23] **Respiratory compromise and TENS** Case report J Accident Emerg Med	A 70-year-old UK man presented with a history of ischemic heart disease and severe unstable angina that was refractory to pharmacological therapy.	He used TENS for 1 year with electrodes secured anterioposteriorly across his chest wall to control angina. Upon ambulance transportation to a medical appointment, his chest pain became severe and TENS current was increased to 50 mA (maximal setting).	At the ER, the patient was unable to speak, respiration rate was 25 per minute, and breathing was shallow with minimal air entry. ECG was not possible due to TENS interference. His chest wall movement virtually ceased with tetanic paralysis (uncoordinated sustained muscular contraction).	Upon removal of the TENS electrodes, the patient immediately exhaled, and within a few minutes, a normal respiratory pattern returned. His diagnosis was respiratory compromise.
Marren et al, 1991[17] **Methacrylate allergy and TENS gel** Case report Contact Derm	A 35-year-old man had a history of chronic LBP and two unsuccessful laminectomies.	He used TENS 16 hours/day for 18 months for pain relief. At 9 months, he developed dermatitis beneath the electrode pads.	He was diagnosed with florid eczema due to a methacrylate allergy. The patient was not sensitive to the gel, nickel, rubber, or adhesive tape.	He was successfully treated with Granuflex hydrocolloid dressings.

Continued

Source	Background	Therapy	Outcome	Follow-up/Interpretation
Mubarak and Wyatt, 1986[6] **Brachial plexus injury and ES** Case report Spine	A 13-year-old white girl with idiopathic scoliosis (right thoracic 28 degrees, left lumbar 35 degrees; hypokyphosis 20 degrees), Risser sign of 2, 1 year postmenarche; no back pain or neurologic involvement.	She was treated with dual channel Scolitron electrical stimulator; electrode placements: (thoracic) medial to left scapula, lateral to the inferior angle of the left scapula, and (lumbar) below the right scapula. It was used throughout the night at 70 mA. At 3 weeks, she noted tingling and numbness of her right hand and discomfort in her limb. Over the next 3 weeks, she noted progressive weakness of her right shoulder/elbow (i.e., lifting objects). After continuing 6 weeks with ES, she experienced right shoulder pain and sought help.	She was diagnosed with an upper and middle trunk brachial plexus injury. Proximal UE strength 2/5 to 4/5, EMG decreased AP. Scolitron was discontinued and strength returned 1 month later. Scolitron was reintroduced but resulted in immediate paresthesia and pain again. Changing the thoracic electrode placement to a more lateral scapular position presented no problems.	The authors caution of the potential serious complications of neurostimulators. The authors believe medial electrode placement in a thin, hypermobile, hypokyphotic patient led to excessive hyperextension of the right shoulder girdle, injuring the plexus at the thoracic outlet (similar to the Adson maneuver of extending the shoulder, which can stress the plexus when testing for thoracic outlet syndrome).
Partridge and Kitchen, 1999[16] **Neurologic risk with ES** Descriptive (survey) Physiotherapy	Questionnaires were sent to 200 physiotherapists at NHS hospitals in England and Wales over an 18-month period.	148 of 200 questionnaires returned with 36.5% adverse reports related to interferential therapy. (SWD, pulsed EM, US, UVL, laser.)	87 local adverse effects included: burns, blisters, rashes, bruising, swelling, and increased pain. 98 general adverse effects included general malaise, nausea, vomiting, faintness, and migraine headaches.	General consensus to use most electrotherapy with extreme caution if preexisting neurologic damage (i.e., decreased skin sensitivity or cognition).

Philbin et al, 1998[22] **Pacemakers and TENS interference** Case report Pacing Clin Electrophysiol	An 80-year-old woman with a history of CAD, bypass grafting, chronic AF, mitral regurgitation, and profound presyncope with VT was fitted with an ICD (CPT generator model 1762; Cardiac Pacemaker Inc, St Paul, MN).	Two weeks after implantation, the ICD administered four discrete shocks to the patient. No cardiac or physical changes were found, but the patient did report using a TENS unit for severe arthritic pain (prescribed by her primary care physician).	Inspection of intracardiac electrograms revealed that the ICD sensed tachycardia when the true heart rate was 50 beat/min. TENS was creating signals that the ICD sensed as ventricular depolarization, and interpreted as VF (the criteria for shock therapy).	The authors regard TENS as an RCI in patients with ICDs.
Rasmussen et al, 1988[25] **No interference of pacemaker and ES** Within subject Mayo Clin Proc	51 patients, ages 33 to 96 (32 men; 19 women), who used one of five types of permanent cardiac pacemakers (20 different models) were randomly selected from an outpatient clinic or hospital (patients were all non–pacemaker dependent with an escape rhythm > 30 beats/min).	TENS (Dynex II) was administered for 2 minutes at four sites (lumbar, cervical, left leg, lower ipsilateral arm) in each patient. Dosage: pulse width of 40, rate of 110, comfortable intensity, stimulation range 2 to 60 Hz.	The authors believe TENS can be safely used with most patients using permanent cardiac pacemakers. For patients using dependent pacemaker, monitor with a short interrupted period during the first application. The authors suggest not placing TENS electrodes parallel to pacemaker electrode vector (i.e., over right ventricle and pulse generator) because this placement was not tested and safety has not been verified.	

Continued

Source	Background	Therapy	Outcome	Follow-up/Interpretation
Shade, 1985[20] **No pacemaker malfunction and TENS** Case report Phys Ther	A 74-year-old man (200 lb) presented with metastatic CA, right traumatic AKA 1971, chronic heart failure, bronchitis, asthma, questionable MI in 1971, and a temporary pacemaker. Pain locations included left lateral chest, anterior nipple, and posterior to spine. The patient requested TENS for pain relief.	He was evaluated for TENS using ECG in an intensive care unit. TENS (rate, width, amplitude was set at 5) frequency was set at 35 pulse/sec, two electrodes placed parallel to the spinal cord 2 inches laterally at the 5th and 19th thoracic levels. Two electrodes were placed near the midaxillary line at the 5th and 10th intercostal areas (electrodes kept about 4 inches away from cardiac area).	No interference of the demand pacemaker or of the patient's cardiac rhythm was noted while wearing TENS for 1 hour continuously.	The author states that the patient used TENS with a temporary cardiac pacemaker successfully with ECG interference indicating that with close monitoring, some patients with cardiac pacemakers may be able to use TENS. Note: This is a case report. Note: Demand pacemakers are sensitive to external interference in the 50- to 60-Hz frequency range. The frequency range of TENS is 12 to 100 Hz.
Zugerman, 1982[26] **Contact dermatitis and TENS gel** Case report J Am Acad Dermatol	A 33-year-old white woman presented with a history of chronic, intractable lumbar pain due to a minor MVA. She was not responsive to analgesics or antiinflammatory agents and tried TENS in Feb 1981.	She immediately noted a rash under the electrodes on her back. After a month, she switched from the conductive gel to a nonconductive sterile surgical lubricant (Surgilube) but continued to present with a rash as well as eroded papules.	Her diagnosis was allergic contact dermatitis with small papular lesions suggesting micropunctate burns. Patch tests were positive for propylene gel. Treatment involved topical corticosteroids, skin hygiene, and electrode replacement, changes in	Alternatives for allergic patients include interface pads (karaya gum or synthetic gum with sodium chloride added), polysulfonic acid adhesive backing, and a stainless steel foil electrode with foam insulation (Medtronic Inc).

TENS (Neuromod # 7728 Comfort Burst dual-channel stimulator; Medtronic Inc), black rubber electrodes, and conductive jelly (Neuromod TENS gel containing 17% propylene gel).

electrode placement, and changes in the type of conductive jelly.
Note: The low conductive properties of Surgilube led to erratic electrical conduction and micropunctate skin burns.
Propylene gel is a common ingredient in conductive gels (of the 1980s) causing contact dermatitis.

Mercaptobenzothiazole, nickel, and adhesive tape are less common causes for allergic reactions with TENS use.

REFERENCES

1. Shapiro S: Electrical currents. In: Cameron MH: Physical agents in rehabilitation: from research to practice. St. Louis: Saunders; 2003. pp 216-259.
2. U.S. Food and Drug Administration: Guidance document for powered muscle stimulator 510 (k) s. Center for Device and Radiological Health, http://www.fda.gov/cdrh/mdr/. Accessed November 7, 2005.
3. U.S. Department of Health: FDA Guidance for TENS 510(K) Content UD, Department of Health draft August 1994, reformatted October,29, 1998.
4. Lambert I, Tebbs SE, Hill D, et al: Interferential therapy machines as possible vehicles for cross-infection. J Hosp Infect 44:59-64, 2000.
5. Brown MC, Holland RL: A central role for denervated tissues in causing nerve sprouting. Nature 282:724-726, 1979.
6. Mubarak SJ, Wyatt MP: Brachial plexus palsy resulting from the use of surface electrical stimulation in the treatment of idiopathic scoliosis. Spine 11(10):1053-1055, 1986.

7. Griffin JW, McClure M: Adverse responses to transcutaneous electrical nerve stimulation in a patient with rheumatoid arthritis. Phys Ther 61(3):354-355, 1981.

8. Bracciano AG: Physical agent modalities: theory and application for the occupational therapist. Thorofare (NJ): Slack; 2000.

9. Tan JC: Practical manual of physical medicine and rehabilitation: diagnostics, therapeutics, and basic problems. St. Louis: Mosby; 1998.

10. Mehreteab TA, Holland T: Clinical application of electrical stimulation. In: Hecox B, Mehreteab TA, Weisberg J, eds: Integrating physical agents in rehabilitation. Upper Saddle River (NJ): Pearson Prentice Hall; 2006.

11. Packman-Braun R: Electrotherapeutic application for the neurologically impaired patient. In Gersh MR, editor: Electrotherapy in rehabilitation. Philadelphia: FA Davis; 1992.

12. Kahn J: Principles and practice of electrotherapy, ed 4. New York: Churchill Livingstone; 2000.

13. Mannheimer JS, Lampe GN: Clinical transcutaneous electrical nerve stimulation. Philadelphia: FA Davis; 1984.

14. Gersh MR: Transcutaneous electrical nerve stimulation (TENS) for management of pain and sensory pathology. In: Gersh MR, editor: Electrotherapy in rehabilitation. Philadelphia: FA Davis; 1992.

15. Association for the Advancement of Medical Instrumentation: American national standards for transcutaneous electrical nerve stimulators, Biomed WL 26A849ac. 1986 Arlington, VA, 1986, Association for the Advancement of Medical Instrumentation.

16. Partridge CJ, Kitchen SS: Adverse effects of electrotherapy used by physiotherapists. Physiotherapy 85:298-303, 1999.

17. Marren P, DeBerker D, Powell S: Methacrylate sensitivity and transcutaneous electrical nerve stimulation (TENS). Contact Dermatitis 25:190-191, 1991.

18. Dwyer CM, Chapman RS, Forsyth A: Allergic contact dermatitis from TENS gel. Contact Dermatitis 30:305, 1994.

19. Eriksson MA, Schuller J, Sjolund BH: Letter: Hazard from transcutaneous nerve stimulation in patients with pacemakers. Lancet 1:1319, 1978.

20. Shade SK: Use of transcutaneous electrical nerve stimulation for a patient with a cardiac pacemaker: a case report. Phys Ther 65(2):206-208, 1985.

21. Sliwa JA, Marinko MS: Transcutaneous electrical nerve stimulator-induced electrocardiogram artifact: a brief report. Am J Phys Med Rehabil 75(4):307-309, 1996.

22. Philbin DM, Marieb MA, Aithal KH, et al: Inappropriate shocks delivered by an ICD as a result of sensed potentials from a transcutaneous electronic nerve stimulation unit. Pacing Clin Electrophysiol 21:2010-2011, 1998.

23. Mann CJ: Respiratory compromise: a rare complication for transcutaneous electrical nerve stimulation for angina pectoris. J Accident Emerg Med 13:68-69, 1996.

24. Glotzer TV, Gordon M, Sparta M, et al: Electromagnetic interference from a muscle stimulation device causing discharge of an implantable cardioverter defibrillator: epicardial bipolar and endocardial bipolar sensing circuits are compared. PACE 21:1996-1998, 1998.

25. Rasmussen MJ, Haves DL, Vlietstra RE, et al: Can TENS be safely used in patients with permanent cardiac pacemakers? Mayo Clin Proc 63:443, 1988.

26. Zugerman C: Dermatitis from transcutaneous electric nerve stimulation. J Am Acad Dermatol 6(5):936-939, 1982.

41.3 Functional Electrical Stimulation

OVERVIEW. Functional electrical stimulation (FES) is the use of electrical stimulation to activate several muscles in a coordinated sequence for the purpose of achieving a functional goal such as walking or grasping.[1] Its concerns in assisting individuals with spinal cord injuries (i.e., paraplegia) to ambulate will be discussed below. Note: In addition to electro-stimulation contraindications, specific FES concerns relate to the physiological and physical demands placed on some body systems (e.g., cardiac system, musculoskeletal system) during the act of walking.

SUMMARY: CONTRAINDICATIONS AND PRECAUTIONS. Five sources cited a total of 31 concerns for FES. Concerns ranged from 5 to 14 per source with an engineer citing the largest number. The largest proportion of concerns generally related to musculoskeletal problems (e.g., contractures, osteoporosis). The most frequently cited concerns were the presence of flaccid paralysis or severe spasticity. Uncontrolled hypertension was cited as an absolute CI.

OTHER ISSUES. Autonomic dysreflexia has been reported during FES in persons with spinal cord injuries.[2]

E00-E90 ENDOCRINE, NUTRITIONAL, AND METABOLIC DISEASES

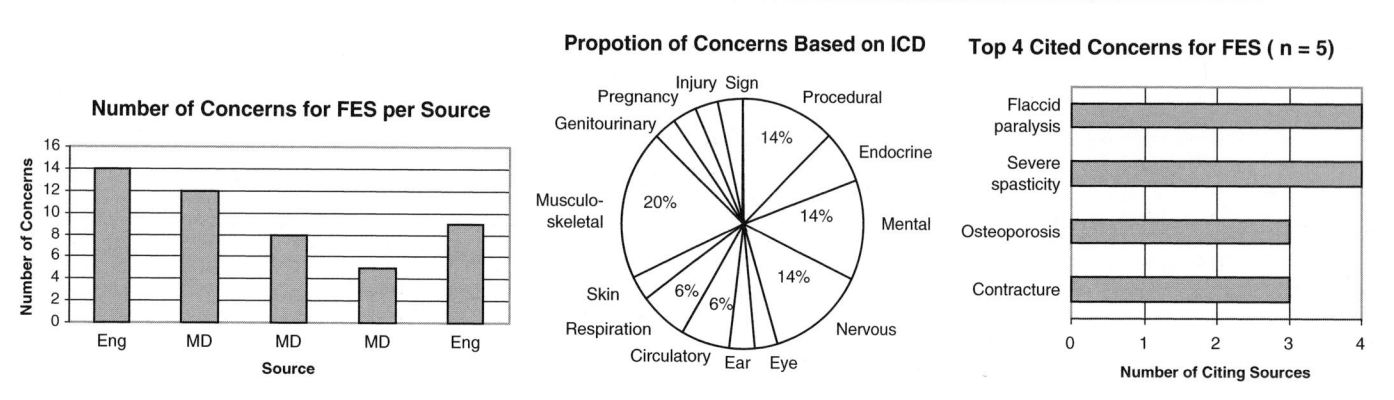

Number of Concerns for FES per Source

Propotion of Concerns Based on ICD

Top 4 Cited Concerns for FES (n = 5)

Issue	LOC	Sources	Affil	Rationale/Comment
Metabolic disturbances	CI	Kralj and Bajd, 1989[3]	Engineer	Also other involvement from damage to an autonomous system. No rationale provided.
Obesity	CI	Kralj and Bajd, 1989[3]	Engineer	Note: No rationale provided.
	CI	Graupe and Kohn, 1997[4,a,b,c]	Engineer	

a, For functional neuromuscular stimulation of unbraced, short distance ambulation in traumatic paraplegia; b, Morbid obesity; c, Rationale for CI is need for good cardiovascular status because the effort (O_2 testing) to stand and ambulate during FNS is 6 times normal.

F00-F99 MENTAL AND BEHAVIORAL DISORDERS

Issue	LOC	Sources	Affil	Rationale/Comment
Educational/mental level inadequate	CI	Kralj and Bajd, 1989[3]	Engineer	Note: No rationale provided.
Drug/alcohol abuse	RCI	Philip, 1987[5,a]	MD	Patient may be unreliable or manipulative in program.
Motivation level	Candidate selection	Chae, 2005[6]	MD	The candidate must desire an increased level of independence.
MMPI high score	RCI	Philip, 1987[5]	MD	The MMPI is an antisocial-sociopathic index.

a, Functional electrical stimulation as active physical therapy. He uses medical criteria (MC) to minimize risk during FES.

G00–G99 DISEASES OF THE NERVOUS SYSTEM

Issue	LOC	Sources	Affil	Rationale/Comment
Flaccid paraplegia	Candidate selection	Chae, 2005[6,a]	MD	A prerequisite for stimulation is an upper motor neuron lesion. Persons with flaccid paralysis (i.e., cauda equina lesions; alpha motor neuron lesions) are not suitable (not successful) for FES. Peripheral denervation requires higher FES intensities and longer stimulation durations. The lowest level of injury for FES should be T11/12.[3]
	CI	Turk and Obreza, 1985[7]	MD	
	MC	Philip, 1987[5]	MD	
	CI	Kralj and Bajd, 1989[3]	Engineer	
Spasticity—severe	CI	Turk and Obreza, 1985[7]	MD	Spastic activity may oppose prescribed computer-generated pattern and shut down during the FES.
	MC	Philip, 1987[5]	MD	
	CI	Kralj and Bajd, 1989[3]	Engineer	Muscles spasms need to be infrequent or controlled.[5]
	Candidate selection	Chae, 2005[6,b]	MD	
High lesions	CI	Turk and Obreza, 1985[7]	MD	C4/5 is the upper limit needed to allow diaphragmatic drive (C3-4-5) for aerobic activities.
	MC	Philip, 1987[5]	MD	
Sitting balance— inadequate	CI	Kralj and Bajd, 1989[3]	Engineer	

a, Intact lower motor neuron; b, Spasticity needs to be controlled.

H00-H59 DISEASES OF THE EYE

Issue	LOC	Sources	Affil	Rationale/Comment
Vision—poor/impaired	CI	Kralj and Bajd, 1989[3]	Engineer	Independence may be limited.[4]
	CI	Graupe and Kohn, 1997[4,a]	Engineer	

a, May be CI.

H60-H95 DISEASES OF THE EAR AND MASTOID PROCESS

Issue	LOC	Sources	Affil	Rationale/Comment
Hearing—poor	CI	Kralj and Bajd, 1989[3]	Engineer	Note: No rationale provided.

I00-I99 DISEASES OF THE CIRCULATORY SYSTEM

Issue	LOC	Sources	Affil	Rationale/Comment
Cardiac pathology	CI	Kralj and Bajd, 1989[3]	Engineer	Need for good cardiovascular status due to the high physical demands of ambulation.[4]
	CI	Graupe and Kohn, 1997[4]	Engineer	
Hypertension—uncontrolled	ACI	Philip, 1987[4]	MD	Also, consult with a cardiologist if CAD or angina.

J00-J99 DISEASES OF THE RESPIRATORY SYSTEM

Issue	LOC	Sources	Affil	Rationale/Comment
Respiratory infection—intercurrent	CI	Philip, 1987[5]	MD	Also, consult with pulmonary physician if COPD.
Respiratory pathology	CI	Kralj and Bajd, 1989[3]	Engineer	Physical demands of ambulation are high.[4]
	CI	Graupe, 1997[4]	Engineer	

L00-L99 DISEASES OF THE SKIN AND SUBCUTANEOUS TISSUE

Issue	LOC	Sources	Affil	Rationale/Comment
Skin disorder under area of electrodes	CI	Philip, 1987[5]	MD	Also, consult dermatology if chronic skin diseases.
	CI	Graupe and Kohn, 1997[4]	Engineer	

M00-M99 DISEASES OF THE MUSCULOSKELETAL SYSTEM AND CONNECTIVE TISSUE

Issue	LOC	Sources	Affil	Rationale/Comment
Contractures	CI	Turk and Obreza, 1985[7]	MD	Tightness will limit standing and walking. The contractures need to be corrected.[6]
	Candidate selection	Chae, 2005[6]	MD	
	CI	Graupe and Kohn, 1997[4,c]	Engineer	
Degenerative joint disease— moderate to severe	CI	Philip, 1987[5]	MD	Unclear if FES programs may lead to a Charcot joint.

Heterotopic ossification	CI	Turk and Obreza, 1985[7]	MD	Joint ossification.
	CI	Kralj and Bajd, 1989[3]	Engineer	
Osteoporosis	MC	Philip, 1987[5,a]	MD	SCI patients with severe osteoporosis (due to disuse) are
	CI	Kralj and Bajd, 1989[3]	Engineer	predisposed to fractures.[5]
	CI	Graupe and Kohn, 1997[4]	Engineer	
Spinal deformity	CI	Graupe and Kohn, 1997[4,b]	Engineer	Spinal deformity compromises standing ability and may require too much effort from the UEs for stability.
Spinal mobility—poor; shortened extremities	CI	Turk and Obreza, 1985[7]	MD	

a, Severe; b, Severe scoliosis; c, Irreversible contracture.

N00-N99 DISEASES OF THE GENITOURINARY SYSTEM

Issue	LOC	Sources	Affil	Rationale/Comment
Urinary tract infections—intercurrent	CI	Philip, 1987[5]	MD	Also, consult with urologist if chronic renal disease.

O00-O99 PREGNANCY, CHILDBIRTH, AND PUERPERIUM

Issue	LOC	Sources	Affil	Rationale/Comment
Pregnancy	CI	Graupe and Kohn, 1997[4]	Engineer	Note: Possibly related to high physical demands (oxygen) for ambulating.

S00-T98 INJURY, POISONING, AND CERTAIN OTHER CONSEQUENCES OF EXTERNAL CAUSES

Issue	LOC	Sources	Affil	Rationale/Comment
Pressure ulcers	CI	Kralj and Bajd, 1989[3]	Engineer	High-grade sores require surgery first.

SIGNS AND SYMPTOMS

Issue	LOC	Sources	Affil	Rationale/Comment
General state—poor	CI	Turk and Obreza, 1985[7]	MD	

PROCEDURAL CONCERNS/MISCELLANEOUS CONCERNS

Issue	LOC	Sources	Affil	Rationale/Comment
Age	CI	Turk and Obreza, 1985[7]	MD	
Hypersensitivity to electrical current	CI	Kralj and Bajd, 1989[3]	Engineer	
Support, attendant	Candidate selection	Chae, 2005[6]	MD	Support is needed because individuals generally require assistance to don the devices.
Vitals signs—monitor	MC/general rule	Philip, 1987[5]	MD	Monitor cardiac and vitals signs during FES program.

Terminate exercise beyond these levels:

Systolic BP not >180 mm Hg and not <80 mm Hg

Diastolic BP not >120 mm Hg and not <50 mm Hg

HR not >160 bpm and not <50 bpm

Also, monitor level of consciousness (i.e., visual acuity), fatigue, diaphoresis, grip. Inquire "How do you feel?" **Ashley[2] reported autonomic dysreflexic blood pressure responses in 10 individuals with high SCI during 30-minute FES-assisted leg extension exercises used to improve cardiovascular fitness. Upon stimulation, systolic BP immediately increased. In two persons, SBP >200 mm Hg. The authors caution SCI above T6 during FES exercise. In a proposed mechanism, ES is perceived as noxious below the level of the lesion, causing massive sympathetic response, vasoconstriction, and hypertension.**

REFERENCES

1. Tan JC: Practical manual of physical medicine and rehabilitation: diagnostics, therapeutics, and basic problems. St. Louis: Mosby; 1998.
2. Ashley EA, Laskin JJ, Olenik LM, et al: Evidence of autonomic dysreflexia during functional electrical stimulation in individuals with spinal cord injuries. Paraplegia 31(9):593-605, 1993.
3. Kralj A, Bajd T: Functional electrical stimulation: standing and walking after spinal cord injury. Boca Raton (FL): CRC; 1989.
4. Graupe D, Kohn KH: Transcutaneous functional neuromuscular stimulation of certain traumatic complete thoracic paraplegics for independent short-distance ambulation. Neurol Res 19(3):323-333, 1997.
5. Phillips CA: Medical criteria for active physical therapy: Physician guidelines for patient participation in a program of functional electrical rehabilitation. Am J Phys Med 66(5):269-286, 1987.
6. Chae J, Triolo RS, Kilgore K, et al: Functional neuromuscular stimulation. In: Delisa JA, editor: Physical medicine and rehabilitation: principles and practices, ed 4, vol 1. Philadelphia: Lippincott Williams & Wilkins; 2005.
7. Turk R, Obreza P: Functional electrical stimulation as an orthotic means for the rehabilitation of paraplegia. Paraplegia 23(6): 344-348, 1985.

42   CRYOTHERAPY (COLD THERAPY)

OVERVIEW. Cryotherapy involves the application of cold substances for the purposes of reducing blood flow and tissue metabolism and increase pain thresholds. Agents include cold packs, ice massage, and vapo-coolant spray.[1]

SUMMARY: CONTRAINDICATIONS AND PRECAUTIONS. Nine sources cited a total of 30 concerns for cryotherapy. Concerns ranged from 4 to 13 per source, with a physical therapist citing the greatest number. The largest proportion of concerns is contained within skin or circulatory categories (each 17% of concerns). The most frequently cited concerns were Raynaud's phenomenon and circulatory impairment. It is noteworthy that only 55% of sources cited impaired sensation as a concern.

Notes: (1) Although not routinely listed under contraindication guidelines, protocols for cryotherapy generally limit its use to short durations (i.e., 15 to 20 minutes). Proulx[2] describes a 79-year-old man who self-administered ice packs unremittingly for 3 days to his toe and subsequently sustained frostbite.

(2) Sources used a variety of terms to describe cold sensitivity: urticaria, sensitivity to cold, cold intolerance, cold hemoglobinuria, and cryoglobulins. In 1962, Shelley and Caro[3] classified three main types of cold sensitivity: (1) Cold urticaria from cold-induced histamine release, (2) cold hemoglobinuria with the presence of cold agglutinins and hemolysis, and (3) presence of cryoglobulins that precipitate when blood is chilled.

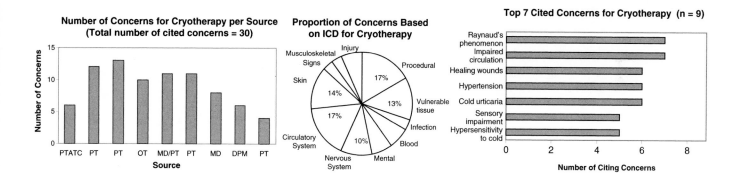

Number of Concerns for Cryotherapy per Source (Total number of cited concerns = 30)

Proportion of Concerns Based on ICD for Cryotherapy

Top 7 Cited Concerns for Cryotherapy (n = 9)

CONTRAINDICATIONS AND PRECAUTIONS FOR CRYOTHERAPY

A00-B99 CERTAIN INFECTIONS AND PARASITIC DISEASES

Issue	LOC	Source	Affil	Rationale/Comment
Infection	CI	Bell and Prentice, 2002[4]	PT/ATC	Note: Reason for rationale or type of infection not specified.

D50-D89 DISEASES OF BLOOD AND BLOOD-FORMING ORGANS AND CERTAIN DISORDERS

Issue	LOC	Source	Affil	Rationale/Comment
Cryoglobulinemia	CI	von Nieda and Michlovitz, 1996[5]	PT	In cryoglobulinemia, an abnormal blood protein gels at low temperatures, leading to ischemia or gangrene. This condition may be associated with rheumatic disease, systemic lupus erythematosus, chronic liver disease, some viral bacterial infections.[1]
	CI	Cameron, 2003[1]	PT	
	P/Avoid	Bracciano, 2000[6]	OT	
	CI/P	Tan, 1998[7]	MD/PT	
Paroxysmal cold hemoglobinuria	CI	von Nieda and Michlovitz, 1996[5]	PT	Blood is noted in urine following cold exposure. Hemoglobin is released from lysed red blood cells.[1] Cold autoantibodies called Donath-Landsteiner antibodies attach to cells at low temperatures (4° C) and undergo hemolysis when cells are then placed at 37° C for 1 hour.[8]
	CI/P	Tan, 1998[7]	MD/PT	
	CI	Cameron, 2003[1]	PT	

F00-F99 MENTAL AND BEHAVIORAL DISORDERS

Issue	LOC	Source	Affil	Rationale/Comment
Aversion to cold	CI	von Nieda and Michlovitz, 1996[5]	PT	Consider the patient's psychological responses to cold because it may work against goals of reducing pain or increasing relaxation.
Mentation impaired	P	Cameron, 2003[1]	PT	The patient may not be capable of responding (and communicating)
	CI/P	Tan, 1998[7]	MD/PT	discomfort.[1] Note: Sleeping states can affect responsiveness: **In 1996,**
	CI	Hecox and Sanko, 2006[10]	PT	**Gamble and Bonnecarre describe a 37-year-old black man who**
	CI/P	Basford, 2005[11,a]	MD	**sustained a third-degree burn (frostbite) while sleeping for**
				3 hours with an application of dry ice to his back.[9]

a, If unable to communicate or respond to pain. If unresponsive, do not treat.

G00-G99 DISEASES OF THE NERVOUS SYSTEM

Issue	LOC	Source	Affil	Rationale/Comment
Regenerating peripheral nerve—over	CI	Cameron, 2003[1]	PT	Cold application may delay nerve regeneration (local vasoconstriction; altered nerve conduction with reduced temperature).
	CI	Hecox and Sanko, 2006[10]	PT	Inquire about nerve damage or symptoms (numbness, tingling sensations).[1] New neural tissue has reduced tensile strength.[10]

Continued

Issue	LOC	Source	Affil	Rationale/Comment
Sensation impaired	P	Cameron, 2003[1]	PT	Insensate skin must be closely monitored because of the burn risk.
	CI	Bell and Prentice, 2002[4]	PT/ATC	Assess pain and temperature sensation and monitor physical signs
	CI/P	Tan, 1998[7]	MD/PT	(color, wheals).
	CI	Hecox and Sanko, 2006[10,a]	PT	
	CI/P	Basford, 2005[11,b]	MD	
Thermoregulatory	P	von Nieda and Michlovitz, 1996[5]	PT	The very old and young individual may have impaired and immature
disorders	P	Cameron, 2003[1]	PT	thermoregulation capabilities, respectively. Monitor intensity and
• In very old and young	CI/P	Basford, 2005[11]	MD	duration of therapy closely. **In a 1977 longitudinal study of 47 elderly people, Collins et al[12] found a smaller body core shell temperature gradient during controlled, environmental temperature changes, when compared to young controls, over a 5-year period. This physiological response indicated progressive thermoregulatory impairment possibly due to an autonomic nerve function defect.**

a, Over anesthetic skin; b, Cutaneous insensitivity—do not treat.

I00-I99 DISEASES OF THE CIRCULATORY SYSTEM

Issue	LOC	Source	Affil	Rationale/Comment
Cardiac patients	P	Umphred, 1990[13,e]	PT	Cold stimulus may cause reflexive constriction of coronary arteries. Avoid
	CI	Hecox and Sanko, 2006[10,f]	PT	application of cold to the left shoulder of cardiac patients.[13]

Circulation impaired—also peripheral vascular disease	P	von Nieda and Michlovitz, 1996[5]	PT	As stated above, cold may increase vasoconstriction, may increase blood viscosity, and may aggravate already compromised circulation (e.g., peripheral vascular disease). Frostbite may occur as a result of an abnormal vascular response.[10] Monitor and adjust treatment parameters (intensity, duration).
	CI	Cameron, 2003[1]	PT	
	CI	Hecox and Sanko, 2006[10,g]	PT	
	P/Avoid	Bracciano, 2000[6]	OT	
	CI	Bell and Prentice, 2002[4,a]	PT/ATC	
	CI/P	Tan, 1998[7]	MD/PT	
	CI/P	Basford, 2005[11,h]	MD	
Hypertensive patients	P	von Nieda and Michlovitz, 1996[5]	PT	Systolic and diastolic pressure increase transiently with cold application. **Wolf and Hardy,[15] in a series of human studies, described a close correspondence of increased blood pressure with pain intensity experienced and degree of water temperature when subjects had their hand dipped in cold water (no higher than 18 °C) during repeated experiments.**
	P	Cameron, 2003[1]	PT	
	CI/P	Helfand, 1994[14]	DPM	
	Never	Bracciano, 2000[6]	OT	
	CI/P	Tan, 1998[7,b]	MD/PT	
	CI	Hecox and Sanko, 2006[10,b]	PT	
Peripheral vascular disease affecting <u>arterial circulation</u>	CI	von Nieda and Michlovitz,1996[5]	PT	Cold may worsen the circulation by increasing vasoconstriction and blood viscosity.
	CI/P	Helfand, 1994[14]	DPM	
	CI	Cameron, 2003[1]	PT	
	CI/P	Tan, 1998[7]	MD/PT	
Raynaud's phenomenon	CI	von Nieda and Michlovitz, 1996[5]	PT	Raynaud's phenomenon is a vasospastic disorder (chronic vasospasms) that is precipitated by cold or emotional stress. Cold agents only worsen vasoconstriction and can lead to ischemia and necrosis. **In a 1990 case report, Olive[16] described a 42-year-old woman with idiopathic**
	CI/P	Helfand, 1994[14]	DPM	
	CI	Cameron, 2003[1,c]	PT	
	CI	Hecox and Sanko, 2006[10]	PT	

Continued

Issue	LOC	Source	Affil	Rationale/Comment
	P/Avoid	Bracciano, 2000[6]	OT	**Raynaud's phenomenon who sustained fingertip necrosis after**
	CI/P	Tan[7]	MD/PT	**depressing and becoming exposed to cold temperatures from**
	CI/P	Basford, 2005[11,c]	MD	**the contents of an aerosol spray can.** The reaction can be associated
				with thoracic outlet syndrome, carpal tunnel syndrome, or trauma.[1]

a, Peripheral vascular disease; b, Severe HTN, monitored BP closely; c, Disease or phenomenon; d, Disease; e, Over left shoulder; f, Unstable cardiac conditions; g, Poor peripheral circulation; h, Ischemia.

L00-L99 DISEASES OF THE SKIN AND SUBCUTANEOUS TISSUE

Issue	LOC	Source	Affil	Rationale/Comment
Cold intolerance	CI	Cameron, 2003[1]	PT	Cold intolerance is characterized by severe pain, numbness, or color changes in
	CI/P	Tan, 1998[7]	MD/PT	response to cold that can occur in patients with rheumatic disease or after
	CI/P	Basford, 2005[11]	MD	accidents or surgical trauma to digits.[1]
Cold urticaria—cold	CI	von Nieda and Michlovitz, 1996[5]	PT	Cold hypersensitivity may present locally or systemically. (1) *Local responses*
hypersensitivity	CI	Cameron, 2003[1]	PT	include wheals (red raised centers with blanched centers on skin) due to
	CI	Hecox and Sanko, 2006[10,b]	PT	histamine release and generalized swelling of mucous membrane and viscera
	P/Avoid	Bracciano, 2000[6]	OT	in severe cases. (2) *Systematic responses* include flushed face, blood pressure
	CI/P	Tan, 1998[7]	MD/PT	drop, heart rate increase, and syncope.
	CI/P	Basford, 2005[11,b]	MD	Inquire if a rash and itching follow exposure to cold. Cameron suggests performing
				an ice-cube test on the patient to assess cold sensitivity (i.e., determining if

Hypersensitivity to cold	P	von Nieda and Michlovitz, 1996[5]	PT
	CI/P	Helfand, 1994[14]	DPM
	CI	Bracciano, 2000[6]	OT
	CI/P	Bell and Prentice, 2002[4]	PT/ATC
		Tan, 1998[7,a]	MD/PT
Skin conditions	CI	Bell and Prentice, 2002[4]	PT/ATC

a, Group of cold sensitivity conditions; b, Allergy or cold allergy.

ice massage for 3 minutes results in a wheal over the tested skin area).[1] If the patient is allergic or extra sensitive to cold, then it will be poorly tolerated.[10] **In a 1936 case series, Horton et al[17] described reactions of 22 patients with abnormal local and latent systemic responses to cold such as urticaria by immersing hands in cold water (8° C) for 6 minutes.**

Escher and Tucker[18] describe a healthy 25-year-old man who experienced severe urticarial lesions over his torso after running in 3° C weather and 25 mph winds with his top removed.

Assess sensitivity to cold by testing a small patient area first and note the response.[10] Note: An operational definition of "hypersensitivity to cold" to distinguish it from urticaria and cold intolerance (above) would be useful.

M00-M99 DISEASES OF THE MUSCULOSKELETAL SYSTEM AND CONNECTIVE TISSUE

Issue	LOC	Source	Affil	Rationale/Comment
Rheumatoid arthritis	CI/P	Helfand, 1994[14]	DPM	Patients with RA may have an associated concern of Raynaud's phenomenon, cryoglobulinemia, or cold intolerance.
				Schmidt et al,[19] citing experimental animal models of inflammation, stressed undesirable local cold responses in rheumatic disease, including increased synovial fluid viscosity (in certain cases), enhanced inflammation (prostaglandin mediated inflammations can be aggravated by cold), reduced circulation, and prolonged muscle cooling.

S00-T98 INJURY, POISONING, AND CERTAIN OTHER CONSEQUENCES OF EXTERNAL CAUSES

Issue	LOC	Source	Affil	Rationale/Comment
Healing wounds	P	von Nieda and Michlovitz, 1996[5]	PT	Cryotherapy can delay wound healing and reduce wound tensile strength as a result of a decreased blood supply. **In a 1959 animal study, Lundgred et al[20] demonstrated how the tensile strength of a rabbit's wound decreased 20% with exposure to lower temperatures for 5 days.**
	CI	Cameron, 2003[1,b]	PT	
	P/Avoid	Bracciano, 2000[6]	OT	
	CI	Bell and Prentice, 2002[4]	PT/ATC	
	CI/P	Tan, 1998[7,a]	MD/PT	Both metabolic activity and circulation are reduced. In addition, cutaneous thermal receptors may be damaged at the wound site and less protection of skin due to reduced insulation could result in excessive cooling.[1]
	CI	Hecox and Sanko, 2006[10,c]	PT	
				Avoid direct cold application over wound for initial 2- to 3-week healing period.[7]
Frostbite history	CI/P	Helfand, 1994[14]	DPM	Note: No rationale provided.

a, First 2-3 weeks of healing; b, Deep open wound; suggests using less intense cooling; c, Open wounds.

SIGNS AND SYMPTOMS

Issue	LOC	Source	Affil	Rationale/Comment
Cold pressor responses, severe	CI/P	Basford, 2005[11]	MD	A concern if it aggravates cardiovascular disease.

VULNERABLE BIOLOGICAL TISSUE

Issue	LOC	Source	Affil	Rationale/Comment
Ear (behind)—with repetitive icing	P	Umphred, 1990[13]	PT	It may lower blood pressure suddenly.
Facial area above the lips—over; i.e., forehead	P			Avoid icing the facial area above the lips (i.e., forehead) because it may lead to an unwanted ANS response.
Midline trunk—over	P			The midline trunk contains a high concentration of C fibers. Application may produce vasoconstriction and increased blood pressure. Avoid midline trunk.
Superficial peripheral nerve	P	von Nieda and Michlovitz, 1996[5]	PT	Cold may lead to nerve conduction blocks (including neuropraxia or axonotmesis) when applied over superficial nerves. **In a 1989 case report, Green et al[21]**
	P/Avoid	Bracciano, 2000[6]	OT	**described an 18-year-old college football player who sustained a peroneal nerve palsy following cryotherapy with compression (bandage). Also see Moeller et al[22] and Bassett et al[23] under Procedures.**

PROCEDURAL CONCERNS

Issue	LOC	Source	Affil	Rationale/Comment
Age—very young or elderly	CI/P/Monitor	Tan, 1998[7]	MD/PT	Cold can lead to skin burns.
Blood pressure—monitor	P	Bracciano, 2000[6]	OT	Monitor blood pressure because systolic and diastolic pressures may temporarily increase. **See Wolf and Hardy[15] above.**
Directly over skin—cold application	P	Bracciano, 2000[6]	OT	Never place a cold gel pack directly on skin because the interface may result in subfreezing temperatures, leading to frostbite. **Moeller et al,[22] in a case report, described a football player who sustained a common peroneal nerve injury proximal to the fibular head after he received an ice pack directly over bare skin without any subcutaneous fat protection. Bassett et al,[23] in a case series, reported six young male athletes who sustained a nerve palsy following crushed or cubed ice applied directly to the skin. O'Toole and Rayatt[24] described a 59-year-old woman who sustained a superficial partial-thickness burn after resting her calf skin directly over an ice pack for 20 minutes.** Monitor skin. Note: Although most authors don't include this issue in their formal list of precautions, it is generally mentioned under their procedure sections.
Quick movement following cold application	Counterproductive Caution	Hecox and Sanko, 2006[10] Bracciano, 2000[6,a]	PT OT	Controversial.[10] Cold slows nerve conduction and increases connective tissue viscosity. Protective mechanisms (sensation) may be reduced.[6] **In a 1997 quasi-experiment, Kauranen and Vanharanta[25]**

				found that 20 healthy female subjects performed significantly slower in movement speed ($P < .05$), tapping speed ($P < .001$), and delayed simple reaction times ($P < .05$) following 15-minute cold pack to the right hand.
Stretching following cold application	Great Care	Hecox and Sanko, 2006[10]	PT	Collagen's ability to elongate is reduced following cold applications. This event along with concomitant anesthesia may lead to tears in connective tissue with subsequent stretching.

a, Overuse.

MODALITY-SPECIFIC COLD CONCERNS

Vapocoolant Spray

Issue	LOC	Sources	Affil	Rationale/Comment
Avoid spraying eyes[a,b]	Advice	Hecox and Sanko, 2006[10]	PT	Drape face when treating neck area.
Avoid frosting skin[a,b]	Advice			Can lead to ulcerations. Avoid spraying more than 6 seconds. Massage area lightly if frosting occurs.[10]
Do not drop[a]	Advice			Explosive; also explosive when heated.
Highly flammable[a]	Advice			If heated.
Minimize inhalation of vapors[a,c]	P	Bell and Prentice, 2002[4,b]	PT/ATC	Especially when working at head and neck areas.[4]
	Advice	Hecox and Sanko, 2006[10]	PT	Inhalation of large amounts of ethyl chloride can lead to general anesthesia.[10]

a, Ethyl chloride; b, Spray and Stretch; c, Fluorimethane spray.

ADVERSE EVENTS

Source	Background	Therapy	Outcome	Follow-up/Interpretation
Bassett et al, 1992[23] **Ice on skin and nerve palsy** Case series Notes: Never apply ice directly to skin (except for ice massage). In persons with little subcutaneous fat, restrict use of ice to 20 minutes, use an insulator, and avoid compression when applying ice.	A 22-year-old male college football player sprained his right fibular collateral ligament during practice.	A bag of ice was applied directly to his lateral right knee for 30 to 45 minutes.	He later noted weakness and numbness. He was diagnosed with right peroneal nerve palsy. At 4 weeks, an EMG revealed axonotmesis.	He recovered after 6 months.
	A 21-year-old male college football player injured his left lateral leg during a game.	A bag of crushed ice was applied directly onto his leg using an elastic bandage.	The athlete noted numbness in the dorsal foot area and tested 4/5 muscle grade for extensor hallucis longus and peroneal muscles. He was diagnosed with a left peroneal nerve injury.	Sensation and motor power returned after 1 hour.
	A 24-year-old male professional basketball player complained of an aching left hip and knee after 40 minutes of play.	The following day, a crushed bag of ice was applied directly to the hip and knee for about 1 hour.	Upon removal, left anterior lateral thigh and dorsal foot numbness and complete foot drop were noted. He had a positive Tinel's sign over his left peroneal nerve at the fibular head area and over his lateral cutaneous femoral nerve. He was diagnosed with a left peroneal and lateral cutaneous femoral nerve injury	He missed the rest of the NBA season and recovered after 6 months.

A 21-year-old male college sprinter complained of slight pain at the left anterior superior iliac spine following a meet.	The following week, a bag of crushed ice was applied directly to the area for 20 minutes.	He noted numbness over the left lateral thigh, decreased sensation over the left lateral cutaneous femoral nerve, and a positive Tinel's sign. He was diagnosed with a left lateral cutaneous femoral nerve injury.	He recovered in 4 days.
A 20-year-old male college defensive tackle complained of nonspecific shoulder pain following a practice.	A bag of crushed ice was applied directly to the supraclavicular area (duration not reported).	He noted decreased sensation to pinprick (from left clavicle to anterior deltoid) and paresthesia over his left shoulder. He was diagnosed with a supraclavicular nerve injury.	Sensation returned after 3 weeks.
A 17-year-old male high school soccer player sustained a traction injury to his left anterior superior iliac spine with discomfort for 1 month.	A bag of ice cubes was applied directly to the area for 30 minutes.	He later noted numbness over the anteriolateral thigh and was diagnosed with an anterior cutaneous femoral nerve injury.	He recovered after 2 weeks.

Continued

Source	Background	Therapy	Outcome	Follow-up/Interpretation
Escher and Tucker, 1992[18] **Cold exposure and urticaria** Case report Phys Sports Med	A 25-year-old healthy man with exercise-induced asthma ran in 3° C (38° F) weather with 25 mph winds for 35 minutes. He removed his top for 5 minutes to cool down.	Within 2-3 minutes, he noted generalized pruritus and then severe urticarial lesions over his torso. He was also light-headed and anxious. Ten minutes after a warm shower, the pruritus and lesions resolved.	Treatment involved avoidance of cold exposure. If not possible, use prophylactic antihistamines. Testing: place an ice cube (0 to 4° C) on the skin for several seconds to 10 minutes and observe for urticarial wheals.	Urticarial lesions occurred in skin areas cooled by wind while running in cold weather.
Gamble and Bonnecarre, 1996[9] **Dry ice, prolonged contact, and frostbite** Case report Aviation Space Environ Med	A 37-year-old black man strained his back (left lumbar area) while lifting. While on a commercial airline, an attendant provided a cold pack (not telling the man that it was dry ice [frozen carbon dioxide] in a towel).	The man applied the dry ice and slept for 3 hours.	When he awoke, the site was darkened, numb, and blistered. He was diagnosed with a third-degree (full-thickness) frostbite burn (over 1.5% of his total body surface area).	He required two skin grafts.
Green et al, 1989[21] **Ice, body type and nerve palsy** Case report Phys Sports Med	An 18-year-old college wide receiver (football) who was 194 cm tall and weighed 80.5 kg twisted his right leg, straining the biceps femoris tendon and spraining the lateral collateral ligament.	The trainer gave the athlete an ice bag, over a towel, to the right knee for 20 minutes, which was held in place with an elastic bandage (for compression).	The athlete noted heaviness in the lower leg less than 20 minutes later. The ice bag was immediately removed. Drop foot was noted within 1 hour and loss of sensation was noted at the web space (between digits 1 and 2). DTRs were normal.	The authors believe ice with compression of the nerve by a bandage in an ectomorphic body type may have contributed to the palsy.

Horton et al, 1936[17]
Hypersensitivity and cold exposure
Case report
JAMA

22 patients, ages 15 to 59 years, with an abnormal reaction to cold exposure were followed at the Mayo Clinic over a 10-year period (11 males; 11 females). All were in good general health except one person with hyperthyroidism and another with osteitis deformans.

All patients demonstrated an abnormal reaction to cold. 14 had systematic reactions, 11 of whom developed syncope (2 patients were unconscious for >2 hours; 4 had to be rescued while swimming).
Symptoms included urticaria wheals primarily on the face, neck, and hands. One patient had dysphagia after drinking cold water/ice cream.

The athlete was diagnosed with peroneal nerve palsy. Six months later, atrophy of the right extensor digitorum brevis occurred; other muscles were slightly weak and sensation improved. At 7 months, he started (noncontact) football practices.
Symptoms were reproduced by immersing hands in water at 8° C for 6 minutes: Local responses included pallor, redness, and swelling. Latent, systemic response, after 3-6 minutes, included a flushed face, a sharp fall in BP, a rise in pulse rate, and a tendency toward syncope. Transitory recovery occurred after 10 to 15 minutes.

Authors caution against cryotherapy with compression, and to check patient every 5 to 10 minutes for distal signs of paresthesia or numbness.

The authors recommended desensitization as a treatment for hypersensitivity to cold.

Continued

Source	Background	Therapy	Outcome	Follow-up/Interpretation
Lundgred et al, 1959[20] **Cold and wound healing** Animal study Act Chirurg Scand	The wound tensile strength of albino rabbits was evaluated under lower environmental temperatures.	The environmental temperature was lowered from 20° C to 12° C.	Tensile strength of wounds decreased 20% after 5 days of temperature reduction.	The authors believe reflex vasoconstriction of skin was a primary factor in the impaired healing.
Moeller et al, 1997[22] **Ice, direct contact, and nerve palsy** Case report Clin J Sports Med	A 22-year-old football player presented with soreness of the left ankle (tender anterior talofibular ligament) and left distal hamstring.	The athlete self-administered, with the athletic trainer's recommendation, an ice pack over bare skin on the left ankle and rested for 20 minutes. The posterior distal left thigh rested over the ice pack.	Upon removal of the ice, the individual was unable to move the left foot (no sensory warning). Shortly afterward, minimal movement was possible. The following week, the foot moved against gravity and numbness was noted over the anterior lateral leg region. A 2/5 grade of dorsiflexion, eversion, great toe extension were noted. The athlete was diagnosed with a common peroneal nerve injury proximal to fibular head with axonotmesis due to cryotherapy.	Motor and sensory impairment were recovered 12 months following injury. The author cautions against cryotherapy treatments in patients with low body fat or in nerve areas not protected by subcutaneous tissue.
Olive, 1990[16] **Raynaud's, cold, and necrosis** Case report J Rheumatol	A 42-year-old woman with idiopathic Raynaud's phenomenon.	She was applying hair spray color to her child's costume, using the right index finger to depress the spray button.	A 0.5-cm, yellow indurated, depressed, macule developed. She was diagnosed with a localized necrosis of her fingertip. Laboratory measures indicated the product could get cold enough to cause vasospasms.	She healed without scarring within 2 weeks. The author suggests caution about cold injuries with some aerosol products in these patients.

O'Toole and Rayatt, 1999[24] **Ice, direct contact, and burn** Case report Br J Sports Med	A 59-year-old woman strained her calf muscle at gym while running. Staff provided an ice pack and instructed the client to apply it.	The woman applied the ice pack directly to the site without intervening material for 20 minutes while resting the calf over the pack.	A large blistered area formed over a 24-hour period. She was diagnosed with a superficial partial-thickness burn requiring treatment of the blister and dressing.	The burn healed in 10 days.
Parker et al, 1983[26] **Ice, prolonged contact, and palsy** Case Report Athl Train	A 15-year-old high school football player sustained a nonspecified injury that resulted in joint effusion.	The athlete was instructed to keep the ice pack on for the duration of the practice session (2 hours).	Upon removal of the ice, anesthesia was noted over the anterior lateral tibial muscles and left dorsal foot area. There was weakness in dorsiflexion, and an inability to extend the great toe. The athlete was diagnosed with superficial and deep peroneal nerve palsy.	He was treated with a foot drop brace and 10 days of electrical stimulation to the anterior lateral tibial musculature. After about 30 days, complete recovery of function and sensation occurred. The trainer subsequently modified the ice protocol by placing an iced elastic bandage between the ice and athlete's skin.
Proulx, 1976[2] **Ice, prolonged contact, and frostbite** Case report J Am Coll Emerg Physician	A 79-year-old man dropped a suitcase on his left great toe.	He self-administered ice packs unremittingly for 3 days. His toes were blistered, discolored, warm, "weeping," and had delayed refilling times.	The patient was diagnosed with frostbite and a fracture of his distal phalanx. His toenail fell off 2 days later. He recovered following débridement, elevation, non–weight-bearing,	Ice packs should be used episodically, not continually.

Source	Background	Therapy	Outcome	Follow-up/Interpretation
Stevens and D'Angelo, 1978[27] **Gel pack, direct contact, and frostbite** Case report N Engl J Med	A 35-year-old man with right epididymitis was told to apply ice as part of treatment.	He self-administered synthetic frozen gel pack to the area.	tetanus toxoid/immune globulin, and antibiotics. 10 days later, redness and erosion over the scrotum was noted. Prolonged direct contact of the cold pack with skin (improper) led to a diagnosis of superficial frostbite.	Warm soaks and topical steroid cream led to healing. The authors caution to wrap ice packs in towels; do not apply directly to the skin.

FOOD AND DRUG ADMINISTRATION REPORTS[28]: REFRIGERANT, TOPICAL (VAPOCOOLANT)

Date	Device	Event	Outcome
10/21/97	Ethyl chloride	A mother dropped a bottle of ethyl chloride. The neck of the bottle broke off; the contents escaped and hit the woman in the face and one eye.	She claimed the eye became red and blistered. She was diagnosed as having a chemical burn.

Note: FDA reports do not necessarily establish cause-effect relationships between equipment and injury. Incidences may be due to equipment or user error. Also, some reports are alleged by attorneys.

REFERENCES

1. Cameron MH: Physical agents in rehabilitation: from research to practice, ed 2. St. Louis: W.B. Saunders; 2003.
2. Proulx RP: Southern California frostbite. J Am Coll Emerg Phys 5(8):618, 1976.

3. Shelley WB, Caro WA: Cold erythema. JAMA 180:639-642, 1962.

4. Bell GW, Prentice WE: Infrared modalities. In Prentice WE, editor: Therapeutic modalities for physical therapists. New York: McGraw-Hill; 2002.

5. von Nieda K, Michlovitz SL: Cryotherapy. In: Michlovitz SL, editor: Thermal agents in rehabilitation, ed 3. Philadelphia: F.A. Davis; 1996.

6. Bracciano AG: Physical agent modalities: theory and application for the occupational therapist. Thorofare (NJ): Slack; 2000.

7. Tan JC: Practical manual of physical medicine and rehabilitation: diagnostics, therapeutics, and basic problems. St. Louis: Mosby; 1998.

8. Horwitz CA: Autoimmune hemolytic anemia. 3. Cold antibody type. Postgrad Med 66(4):189-193, 196-198, 200, 1979.

9. Gamble WB, Bonnecarre ER: Coffee, tea, or frostbite? A case report of inflight freezing hazard from dry ice. Aviat Space Environ Med 67(9):880-881, 1996.

10. Hecox B, Sanko JP: Cryotherapy. In: Hecox B, Mehreteab TA, Weisberg J, eds: Integrating physical agents in rehabilitation. Upper Saddle River (NJ): Pearson Prentice Hall; 2006.

11. Basford JR: Therapeutic physical agents. In: Delisa JA, editor: Physical medicine and rehabilitation: principles and practices, ed 4, vol 1. Philadelphia: Lippincott Williams & Wilkins; 2005.

12. Collins KJ, Dore C, Exton-Smith AN, et al: Accidental hypothermia and impaired temperature homeostasis in the elderly. BMJ 1(6057): 353-356, 1977.

13. Umphred DA, McCormack GL: Classification of common facilitatory and inhibitory treatment techniques. In: Umphred DA, editor: Neurological rehabilitation. St. Louis: Mosby; 1990.

14. Helfand AE: Physical modalities in the management of mild to moderate foot pain. Clin Podiatr Med Surg 11(1):107-123, 1994.

15. Wolf S, Hardy JD: Studies on pain. Observations on pain due to local cooling and on factors involved in the "cold pressor" effect. J Clin Invest 20:521-533, 1941.

16. Olive KE: Aerosol spray can induced cold injury in a patient with Raynaud's phenomenon. J Rheumatol 17(4):556-557, 1990.

17. Horton BT, Brown GE, Roth GM: Hypersensitiveness to cold with local and systemic manifestation of a histamine-like character: its amenability to treatment. JAMA 107:1263, 1936.

18. Escher S, Tucker A: Preventing, diagnosing, and treating cold urticaria. Phys Sport Med 20(12):73-84, 1992.

19. Schmidt KL, Ott VR, Rocher G, et al: Heat, cold and inflammation. Z Rheumatol 38:391-404, 1979.

20. Lundgred C, Murren A, Zederfeldt B: Effects of cold vasoconstriction on wound healing in the rabbit. Acta Chirurg Scand 118:1, 1959.

21. Green GA, Zachazewski JE, Jordan SE: Peroneal nerve palsy induced by cryotherapy. Phys Sport Med 17 (9):63-70, 1989.

22. Moeller JL, Monroe J, McKeag DB: Cryotherapy induced common peroneal nerve palsy. Clin J Sports Med 7(3):212-216, 1997.

23. Bassett FH, Kirkpatrick JS, Engelhardt DL, et al: Cryotherapy induced nerve injury. Am J Sports Med 22:516-528, 1992.

24. O'Toole G, Rayatt S: Frostbite at the gym: a case report of an ice pack burn. Br J Sports Med 33(4):278-279, 1999.

25. Kauranen K, Vanharanta H: Effects of hot and cold packs on motor performance of normal hands. Physiotherapy 83(7):340-344, 1997.

26. Parker JT, Small NC, Davis DG: Cold induced nerve palsy. Athl Train 18:76-77, 1983.

27. Steven DM, D'Angelo JA: Frostbite due to improper use of frozen gel pack. N Engl J Med 299(25):1415, 1978.

28. U.S. Food and Drug Administration: Center for Device and Radiological Health. Available at: http://www.fda.gov/cdrh/mdr/. Accessed November 7, 2005.

43 DIATHERMY

OVERVIEW. Diathermy (or "through heating") employs physical agents that convert high-frequency electric current or electromagnetic waves to deep heat to promote healing.[1-3] Heat is generated in tissue by its resistance to the passage of the high-frequency EM energy.[4] Shortwave diathermy converts non-ionizing radiation (radio waves) between 10 and 100 MHz, with a commonly used frequency at 2712 MHz, to deep-heat tissue. Microwave diathermy uses non-ionizing electromagnetic radiation between 300 and 300,000 MHz with a commonly used frequency of 2450 MHz.[1-3] Note: Sound waves may also be considered a form of diathermy but are discussed elsewhere (**see Therapeutic ultrasound**).

SUMMARY: CONTRAINDICATIONS AND PRECAUTIONS. Six sources cited a total of 47 concerns for diathermy. Concerns ranged from 12 to 26 per source with a physician citing the greatest number. The largest proportion of concerns is contained under medical devices (e.g., metal, contact lenses, leads), procedural, and vulnerable tissue categories. The most frequently cited concerns were malignancy, impaired circulation or sensation, implanted metal, cardiac pacemakers, and hemorrhaging. The FDA warns about the presence of implanted leads (from stimulators) because of lead-related fatalities reported with diathermy use.

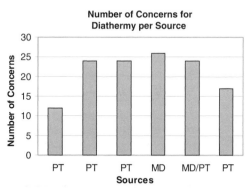

Number of Concerns for Diathermy per Source

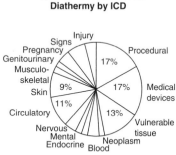

Proportion of Concerns for Diathermy by ICD

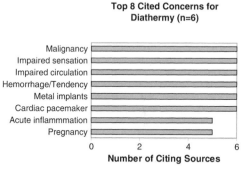

Top 8 Cited Concerns for Diathermy (n=6)

CONTRAINDICATIONS AND PRECAUTIONS

C00-C97 NEOPLASMS

Issue	LOC	Sources	Affil	Rationale/Comment
Malignancy area	CI /P	Docker et al, 1992[5,a]	PT	Cancer cells can proliferate at 40 to 41°C, which are the temperatures
	CI	Cameron et al, 2003[3,c]	PT	used in rehabilitation.
	CI/P/Avoid	Kloth and Ziskin, 1996[6,b]	PT	
	CI/P	Tan, 1998[2]	MD/PT	
	CI	Day and Katz, 2006[7]	PT	
	CI/P	Basford, 2005[8]	MD	

a, Continuous SWT 27.12 MHz; Precaution noted as "special precaution"; CI unless part of cancer treatment; b, CSWD; c, contraindications for thermotherapy also apply to diathermy in this chapter.

D50-D89 DISEASES OF BLOOD AND BLOOD-FORMING ORGANS, AND CERTAIN DISORDERS

Issue	LOC	Sources	Affil	Rationale/Comment
Hemorrhage	CI/P	Docker et al, 1992[5]	PT	Temperature elevation will lead to arteriole dilation, increased blood flow,
	CI	Cameron et al, 2003[3]	PT	and a tendency to bleed in patients with bleeding disorders.
	CI/P	Tan, 1998[2]	MD/PT	
	CI	Day and Katz, 2006[7]	PT	
	CI/P	Basford, 2005[8,a]	MD	

Hemophilia, bleeding tendencies	CI/P/Avoid	Kloth and Ziskin, 1996[6]	PT	
	CI/P	Tan, 1998[2]	MD/PT	
	CI	Cameron et al, 2003[3]	PT	
	CI	Day and Katz, 2006[7]	PT	

a, Acute.

E00-E90 ENDOCRINE, NUTRITIONAL, AND METABOLIC DISEASES

Issue	LOC	Sources	Affil	Rationale/Comment
Obesity	CI/P	Docker et al, 1992[5]	PT	Fat is poorly vascularized and can lead to burns. Diathermy using capacitive plate applicators may heat excess fat.[3]
	P	Cameron et al, 2003[3]	PT	For obese patients, consider magnetic field over capacitor applicator where subcutaneous fat heats more easily than muscle tissue.

F00-F99 MENTAL AND BEHAVIORAL DISORDERS

Issue	LOC	Sources	Affil	Rationale/Comment
Mentation impaired	CI	Cameron et al, 2003[3]	PT	There may be an inability to communicate or respond to pain (i.e., dementia, coma).[2]
	CI/P	Tan, 1998[2]	MD/PT	
	CI	Day and Katz, 2006[7]	PT	
	CI/P	Basford, 2005[8]	MD	

G00-99 DISEASES OF THE NERVOUS SYSTEM

Issue	LOC	Sources	Affil	Rationale/Comment
Sensation area impaired	CI /P	Docker et al, 1992[5]	PT	An example is a person with a spinal cord injury. Exposure levels
	CI/P/Avoid	Kloth and Ziskin, 1996[6]	PT	depend on patient's ability to communicate a comfortable level
	CI	Cameron et al, 2003[3]	PT	of warmth. Apply only mild to moderate doses and check patient
	CI/P	Tan, 1998[2]	MD/PT	and equipment frequently if pain and temperature sense are
	CI	Day and Katz, 2006[7]	PT	diminished.[6]
	CI/P	Basford, 2005[8]	MD	
Thermal regulation impaired	P	Cameron et al, 2003[3]	PT	
	CI/P	Tan, 1998[2]	MD/PT	
	CI/P	Basford, 2005[8]	MD	

I00-I99 DISEASES OF THE CIRCULATORY SYSTEM

Issue	LOC	Sources	Affil	Rationale/Comment
Angina, unstable	CI/P	Basford, 2005[8]	MD	
Blood pressure, unstable	CI/P			
Cardiac insufficiency	P	Cameron et al, 2003[3]	PT	
	CI/P	Basford, 2005[8,b]	MD	

Circulation impaired	P	Cameron et al, 2003[3]	PT	Compromised circulation may not meet increased metabolic
	CI/P	Tan, 1998[2]	MD/PT	demands on tissue that is heated.
	CI	Day and Katz, 2006[7]	PT	
	CI/P	Docker et al, 1992[5,a]	PT	
	CI/P/Avoid	Kloth and Ziskin, 1996[6,a]	PT	
	CI/P	Basford, 2005[8,a]	MD	
Thrombophlebitis	CI	Cameron et al, 2003[3]	PT	

a, Ischemia concerns; b, Heart failure (decompensated) within 6-8 weeks of a myocardial infarct.

L00-L99 DISEASES OF THE SKIN AND SUBCUTANEOUS TISSUE

Issue	LOC	Sources	Affil	Rationale/Comment
Atrophic skin	CI/P	Tan, 1998[2]	MD/PT	Prolonged steroids may cause atrophic skin.
	CI/P	Basford, 2005[8]	MD	
Blisters	CI/P	Basford, 2005[8]	MD	Microwaves selectively heat water.
Scar tissue	CI/P	Tan, 1998[2,a]	MD/PT	
	CI/P	Basford, 2005[8]	MD	
Infected skin	CI/P	Tan, 1998[2,a]	MD/PT	

a, Immature scar.

M00-M99 DISEASES OF THE MUSCULOSKELETAL SYSTEM AND CONNECTIVE TISSUE

Issue	LOC	Sources	Affil	Rationale/Comment
Infection, joint	CI/P	Basford, 2005[8]	MD	Microwaves selectively heat water.

N00-N99 DISEASES OF THE GENITOURINARY SYSTEM

Issue	LOC	Sources	Affil	Rationale/Comment
Menstruating	CI	Tan, 1998[2]	MD/PT	Note: Obviously not a "disease." Menstruating females should be warned that menstrual
	P	Day and Katz, 2006[7]	PT	flow may temporarily increase following treatment to the low back.[6]
	CI/P	Kloth and Ziskin, 1996[6]	PT	

O00-O99 PREGNANCY, CHILDBIRTH, AND PUERPERIUM

Issue	LOC	Sources	Affil	Rationale/Comment
Pregnancy	CI /P	Docker et al, 1992[5]	PT	Maternal hyperthermia may lead to abnormal fetal development. Anomalies have been
	CI/P/Avoid	Kloth and Ziskin, 1996[6]	PT	noted in rat fetuses exposed to frequency of 27.12 MHz due to hyperthermia. The
	CI	Cameron et al, 2003[3]	PT	diathermy field cannot be constrained to a body region. Inquire if patient is pregnant
	CI	Tan, 1998[2]	MD/PT	or trying to get pregnant. Also note, pregnant clinicians may be at risk. **From a case**
	CI	Day and Katz, 2006[7]	PT	**series, Rubin[9] reported a 21-year-old woman with chronic pelvic inflammatory**

				disease who received eight microwave exposures during the first 59 days of pregnancy and aborted on the 67th day. She later received treatments during the first half of her menstrual cycle, conceived, and delivered a normal infant at term. Nonthermal pulsed shortwave diathermy to pregnant patients is also a concern because the effects of EM energy on fetal development are not known.[1]
Vaginal electrodes to women who are pregnant	CI/P/Avoid	Kloth and Ziskin, 1996[6]	PT	It is not known if amniotic fluid is selectively heated with these electrodes. Temperatures of 39.8° C or more can damage a human fetus.

R00-R99 SYMPTOMS, SIGNS

Issue	LOC	Sources	Affil	Rationale/Comment
Acutely inflamed tissue	CI/P/Avoid	Kloth and Ziskin, 1996[6]	PT	Superimposing an inflammatory process (heat) on an existing inflammatory process may lead to tissue necrosis.
	CI	Cameron et al, 2003[3]	PT	
	CI/P	Tan, 2003[2]	MD/PT	
	CI	Day and Katz, 2006[7]	PT	
	CI/P	Basford, 2005[8]	MD	

Continued

Issue	LOC	Sources	Affil	Rationale/Comment
Edema	P	Cameron et al, 2003[3]	PT	Microwaves selectively heat water.[8]
	CI/P	Tan, 1998[2]	MD/PT	
	CI/P	Basford, 2005[8]	MD	
Fever	CI	Day and Katz, 2006[7]	PT	
	CI	Kloth and Ziskin, 1996[6]	PT	

S00-T98 INJURY

Issue	LOC	Sources	Affil	Rationale/Comment
Acute injury	CI	Cameron et al, 2003[3]	PT	
	CI/P	Tan, 1998[2]	MD/PT	
	CI/P	Basford, 2005[8]	MD	
Wounds—open	CI /P	Docker et al, 1992[5]	PT	Use extreme caution.
	P	Cameron et al, 2003[3]	PT	
	CI/P	Tan, 1998[2]	MD/PT	

Issue	LOC	Sources	Affil	Rationale/Comment
Contact lenses	CI/P/Avoid	Kloth and Ziskin, 1996[6]	PT	Energy fields concentrate and may potentially lead to excessive heating of ciliary
	CI	Tan, 1998[2]	MD/PT	bodies. Remove contact lenses. **In an in vitro study, Scott[10] showed that shortwave fields emitted in the anterior posterior plane heated up a perforation on a Perspex contact lens.**
Electromagnetic medical devices in the vicinity—other	CI/P/Avoid	Kloth and Ziskin, 1996[6]	PT	Electromagnetic interference (EMI) from diathermy may cause other electromedical
	P	Cameron et al, 2003[3]	PT	devices to malfunction. Examples include EEGs, EKG, EMG instruments; unshielded
	CI/P	Docker et al, 1992[5]	PT	cardiac pacemakers, TENS, muscle stimulators, electrophrenic pacers, cerebellar and
	CI	Day and Katz, 2006[7,d]	PT	urinary bladder stimulators, watches,[6] computers, and computer-controlled devices.[1] Consider using other equipment at least 3 m and preferably 5 m from diathermy.[5]
Implanted leads—or systems containing leads Cardiac pacemakers Defibrillators Cochlear implants Bone growth stimulators Deep brain stimulators Spinal cord stimulators Other nerve stimulators	Safety notice	FDA, 2002[11]	Gov	Do not use shortwave or microwave diathermy on patients with any implanted metallic lead or system that contains a lead (i.e., cardiac pacemakers, defibrillators, cochlear implants, bone growth stimulators, deep brain stimulators, spinal cord stimulators, other nerve stimulators).[11] **Nutt et al[12] reported a case of a 70-year-old man with Parkinson's disease who had undergone DBS (with leads in place) and sustained lesions to the pons, midbrain, cerebral peduncles and internal capsule following exposure to diathermy administered by an oral surgeon.** Leads are often left after implants are removed. Do not apply diathermy unless absolutely sure implants and all leads are entirely removed.

Continued

Issue	LOC	Sources	Affil	Rationale/Comment
Intrauterine contraceptive devices *with copper* (metal)	P	Cameron et al, 2003[3,a]	PT	These devices contain metal and slightly heat up.
	CI	Tan, 1998[2]	MD/PT	Inquire if patient is wearing a copper-bearing contraceptive device.[3]
	CI/P	Kloth and Ziskin, 1996[6]	PT	
	CI/P	Basford, 2005[8,g]	MD	
Metal—metal implants; external metal	CI /P	Docker et al, 1992[5]	PT	Avoid metal. Diathermy heats metal, which then can cause burns because of
	CI/P/Avoid	Kloth and Ziskin, 1996[6]	PT	subsequent transfer of heat to adjacent tissue. Remove jewelry from area.
	CI	Cameron et al, 2003[3]	PT	Very small fillings in the head are not significant. Nonthermal pulsed shortwave
	CI	Tan, 1998[2,b]	MD/PT	diathermy may also be a problem for metal or metal implants that form a
	CI	Day and Katz, 2006[7]	PT	closed loop (e.g., metal used to repair some fractures) because current can flow
	CI/P	Basford, 2005[8,e]	MD	through the loop and develop heat.[3] For continuous SWD, remove and place any
				metallic objects outside the EM field (internal, external, surgically implanted
				devices; metal includes jewelry, zippers, metal in treatment table and chairs,
				intrauterine devices with metal).[6] **The journal *Health Devices*[13] published**
				a report of a mattress (containing metal) that began to smoke and
				burn while a patient received diathermy.
Neural stimulators	CI	Tan, 1998[2]	MD/PT	EMI can cause malfunctions in neural stimulators. Burning sensation can occur
Transcutaneous, cutaneous stimulator	CI	Cameron et al, 2003[3,c]	PT	under the electrodes whether or not the stimulator device is turned on.
	CI/P	Kloth and Ziskin, 1996[6]	PT	
Muscle stimulator	CI/P	Basford, 2005[8,f]	MD	
Electrophrenic stimulator				
Cerebral stimulator				
Urinary bladder stimulator				

Pacemakers—cardiac	CI /P	Docker et al, 1992[5]	PT	A strong electromagnetic field can affect the performance of pacemakers. In addition, metal pacemaker components can heat up, with the risk greatest when the thorax is treated. Nonthermal pulsed shortwave diathermy is also a CI around cardiac pacemakers because it emits EMI that can interfere with the functioning of the pacemaker.[1] Kloth and Ziskin suggest choosing a nonelectromagnetic thermal agent.[6] **In a 1965 animal report, Lichter and Borrie[14] described how a sheep's pacemaker went into a high-frequency response with the heart subsequently fibrillating following exposure to shortwave diathermy. In a review, Jones[15] found 49 cases of ventricular fibrillation and 391 cases of other physiologic dysfunctions occurring in patients with cardiac pacemakers due to EMI. One noted source of interference was shortwave diathermy.**
	CI	Cameron et al, 2003[3]	PT	
	CI	Tan, 1998[2]	MD/PT	
	CI	Day and Katz, 2006[7,d]	PT	
	CI	Kloth and Ziskin, 1996[6]	PT	
	CI/P	Basford, 2005[8,d]	MD	
Pumps, implanted	CI/P	Basford, 2005[8]	MD	

a, Thermal and nonthermal diathermy; b, Surgical implants (metal not specified), SWD and MWD share same CIs; c, Thermal and nonthermal pulsed shortwave diathermy; d, Any pacing device, also concern for others in vicinity with pacemakers; e, Jewelry or metal implants; f, Stimulators; g, IUDs, small clips. Note: The FDA's safety notice is included because of the specific and grave issue surrounding leads, but because it is used once, it is not included as a source in my descriptive statistics.

VULNERABLE BIOLOGICAL TISSUE

Issue	LOC	Sources	Affil	Rationale/Comment
Epiphyses—growing	CI/P/Avoid	Kloth and Ziskin, 1996[6]	PT	Significant temperature increases at the epiphyses, at intensities that cause pain, can
	CI	Cameron et al, 2003[3]	PT	disturb bone growth in children. Because the effect of nonthermal pulsed shortwave
	CI	Day and Katz, 2006[7]	PT	diathermy on skeletally immature patients is not known, use with these device
	CI/P	Basford, 2005[8]	MD	parameters is also precautionary.[3] **Doyle and Smart,[16] in an animal experiment**
				of 20 rats, 21 to 70 days old and similar controls exposed to shortwave
				diathermy (27.12 MHz) to knee epiphyses, showed significant (average
				1.4 mm) growth in all treated limbs. The increased blood flow, creating
				hyperemia, may have stimulated growing epiphyses.
Eyes	CI/P/Avoid	Kloth and Ziskin, 1996[6]	PT	Tissues with high fluid volume have a higher dielectric constant and conductivity,
	CI	Cameron et al, 2003[3]	PT	resulting in selective absorption of energy, overheating of fluids, and burning of
	CI	Day and Katz, 2006[7]	PT	adjacent tissues. Space-occupying lesions (i.e., protruded nucleus pulposus) may
	CI/P	Basford, 2005[8]	MD	result in swelling and congestion around lesions. Testes are more susceptible
Fluid-filled joints	CI/P/Avoid	Kloth and Ziskin, 1996[6]	PT	because of their superficial locations/vulnerability to stray radiation. **Daily**
	CI/P	Basford, 2005[8]	MD	**et al[17] reported that 7 of 17 albino rabbits and 3 of 17 pigmented**
Gonads—testes or	CI/P/Avoid	Kloth and Ziskin, 1996[6]	PT	**rabbits developed cataracts following microwave 2- to 5-inch exposure**
ovaries	CI	Cameron et al, 2003[3,a]	PT	**distances to eye tissue at 75% output (94 watts) for 10 to 30 minutes.**
	CI	Day and Katz, 2006[7,a]	PT	
	CI/P	Basford, 2005[8]	MD	
Moist skin	CI/P	Basford, 2005[8]	MD	
Space-occupying lesions	CI/P/Avoid	Kloth and Ziskin, 1996[6]	PT	

a, Testes.

PROCEDURAL CONCERNS

Issue	LOC	Sources	Affil	Rationale/Comment
Hazards to pregnant therapists	CI	Day and Katz, 2006[7a]	PT	Avoid operating the unit if pregnant. The source cites a study where MWD operation by pregnant PTs was associated with an increased miscarriage risk.
Hazards to therapist	Advice	Kloth and Ziskin, 1996[6]	PT	Day and Katz[7] noted the literature on the occupational hazards of stray radiation to be equivocal, but cite recommendations by others such as to remain with 1 m of the unit for short periods only (ordinary prudent practice); to remain at least 1 m from continuous SWD and 0.5 m from MWD or pulsed SWD; to remain at least 1 m from continuous SWD, 0.5-0.8 m from pulsed condenser field SWD, and 0.2 m from pulsed inductive field SWD.[7] Kloth and Ziskin[6] note that overexposure of therapist from CSWD is not possible if distance between therapist and applicator is 20 cm or more. Some stray radiation concerns include an association between heart disease and male PTs using SWD, a reduced number of rats (radio frequency radiation exposed) that became pregnant, and a link between brain cancer development and portable cellular phone use (no proven definitive relationship).[7]
Moist dressings or clothing	CI/P/Avoid Concern	Kloth and Ziskin, 1996[6] Tan, 1998[2]	PT MD/PT	Surface moisture can focus heat, leading to overheating. To reduce the risk of excessive heating of surface moisture, use toweling (terrycloth) that absorbs surface perspiration or wide spacing between the diathermy applicator and the skin.[6]

Continued

Issue	LOC	Sources	Affil	Rationale/Comment
Perspiration	CI/P	Docker et al, 1992[5]	PT	Water is preferentially heated with diathermy. Keep skin dry to minimize heating of perspiration.
	Concern	Tan, 1998[2]	MD/PT	
	CI/P/Avoid	Kloth and Ziskin, 1996[6]	PT	
Position of limb: dependent with edema	CI/P	Tan, 1998[2]	MD/PT	
Synthetic material—over (nylon, foam rubber, plastics)	CI/P/Avoid	Kloth and Ziskin, 1996[6]	PT	Synthetic materials near unshielded cables may be a fire hazard. Examples include some pillows, pillowcases, clothing, coverings, and foam rubber. Keep unshielded cables and wires away from synthetics.
Topical counterirritant applied—over	P	Cameron et al, 2003[3]	PT	Same concern as for superficial heat. Vascular system is already dilated from ointment.
Training of personnel	CI/P	Docker et al, 1992[5]	PT	

a, The source[3] makes some mention of risks and precautions for pregnant therapists, p 397.

NONTHERMAL PULSED SHORTWAVE DIATHERMY

Issue	LOC	Sources	Affil	Rationale/Comment
Internal organ—diseased (over)	CI	Cameron et al, 2003[3]	PT	
Pacemakers, electronic devices, metal implants	Warning (avoid)			EM radiation can interfere with pacemaker function. The EM field can also interfere with other medical internal or external equipment on the area. Furthermore, metal can become hot if it forms a closed loop.

Pregnancy	P			The effects of electromagnetic energy from nonthermal diathermy on the fetus or skeletally immature persons are not known.
Skeletally immature patients	P			
Substitute for conventional therapy for treating edema and pain	CI			For use as an adjunct to other therapies.

PULSED RADIO FREQUENCY RADIATION (PRFR): NONTHERMAL EFFECTS

Issue	LOC	Source	Affil	Rationale/Comment
Cancerous tissue; pregnant uterus	CI/P/Avoid	Kloth and Ziskin, 1996[6]	PT	"Prudent to avoid..."
Electromedical/electronic devices	CI/P/Avoid			As noted above.

OTHER NOTES: DIATHERMY

Issue	LOC	Source	Affil	Rationale/Comment
Calibrate		Docker et al, 1992[5]	PT	(Continuous SWT 27.12 MHz)
Maintenance service regularly, i.e., every 6 months				

Continued

Issue	LOC	Source	Affil	Rationale/Comment
Minimize exposure—operator should				Exposure to EM fields in the radiofrequency range of 10–400 MHz should not exceed 1 mW/cm. Stay at least 1 meter from applicator and lead during operation. Extra caution for pregnant operators.
Shock hazards		Arledge, 1978[18]	PT	Check for cracks or faulty wiring insulation between drum plates of drum-type applicators because contact with exposed wiring can result in a shock and burn. Never assume hospital maintenance will be conducted or is conducted for all hazardous areas.
Terminate treatment if signs of distress		Docker et al, 1992[5]	PT	(Continuous SWT 27.12 MHz)
Treatment area—keep dry at all times				
Use minimal dosage required to achieve desired benefit				
Visually inspect for damage: applicators, leads, electrodes routinely				

ADVERSE EVENTS

Source	Background	Therapy	Outcome	Follow-up/Interpretation
Jones, 1976[15] **Electromagnetic interference, diathermy, and cardiac pacemaker malfunction** Review Phys Ther	A review was conducted from 1949 to 1973 of EMI in patients with cardiac pacemakers because some frequencies from the electromagnetic spectrum can disrupt and interfere with cardiac pacemaker function and induce fibrillations.	49 cases of ventricular fibrillation occurred in patients due to EMI. The most common sources were autotransformers, faulty pacemakers, competitive rhythms, ECG, and current leakage. 391 cases of other physiologic dysfunctions (i.e., erratic pacing, inhibition, marked interference, cessation of pacemaker activity) were due to EMI. Interference was most commonly attributed to shortwave diathermy (85), electric razors (83), food mixers (59), hairdryers (54), and vacuum cleaners (41).	The distance of electromedical equipment when interference occurred ranged from contact to 458 cm (highest incidence was from contact to 31 cm).	Demand and atrial synchronous pacemakers are least resistant to EMI. Recommendations: • Shortwave diathermy, microwave diathermy, and electrical stimulators interfered with pacemaker function and should not be used with patients using cardiac pacemakers. • Caution using other electromedical apparatus in patients with cardiac pacemakers. Test equipment for leakage. All equipment should be grounded. • PTs should recognize signs and symptoms of cardiac pacemaker failure, remove electromedical equipment from area, and administer lifesaving measures.

Continued

Source	Background	Therapy	Outcome	Follow-up/Interpretation
Lichter and Borrie, 1965[14] **Shortwave diathermy and pacemaker malfunction** Animal study (case report) BMJ	Experiment 7, Sept 14, 1964 A sheep had a bipolar catheter electrode inserted into its right ventricle (through the right external jugular vein).	The sheep's heart was controlled by an IME pacemaker at 140 beats per minute with a 4-volt pulse. A shortwave diathermy machine used in physiotherapy (Liebel Flarsheim Co) had its condenser applicator placed across the sheep's right hind thigh with the output capacity increasing to 300 Watts at 27.12 Mc/sec.	The pacemaker immediately went into a high-frequency response, and the heart subsequently fibrillated.	
Nutt et al, 2001[12] **Diathermy, deep brain stimulator, and brain damage** Case report Neurology	A 70-year-old man with Parkinson's disease for 18 years underwent DBS for moderate improvement of PD and to reduce the need for dopaminergic medications. The DBS was equipped with bilateral quadripolar electrodes (Medtronics) and ITREL # 7424 implanted pulse generators (IPGs).	19 months following surgery, he underwent extraction of all maxillary teeth and returned to the oral surgeon the following day for diathermy in order to hasten recovery. Diathermy was administered with an induction coil applied on one cheek at 95 µs pulses, 4000 Hz, and a power setting of 10 (Magnatherm International Medical Electronics Ltd; model 1000; 27.120 MHz frequency range).	The patient was hospitalized with decerebrate posturing, bilateral Babinski signs, and an unremarkable CT scan. Upon transfer to another hospital, MRI (3 days after diathermy) revealed bilateral, symmetrical T2 lesion in the tegmentum of the pons and midbrain, cerebral peduncles, and posterior limbs of the internal capsule. At the 6th day of hospitalization he was	The authors state: The diagnosis was attributed to tissue damage around the electrodes induced by diathermy. The RF (diathermy) current may have heated the edema near the electrode. The most likely path was conduction through the bony structures of the skull base (maxillary application).

30 minutes later (the patient was now drowsy), the other cheek was heated. After another 30 minutes, the patient was unarousable, unresponsive to pain, and presented with small pupils.

anarthric, withdrew from pain, had roving eye movements, and occasionally opened his eyes.
On day 18, he was discharged to a long-term skilled nursing facility, and on day 32 after diathermy, MRI revealed a T2 signal in the immediate vicinity of the electrodes.

Health Devices, 1988[13]
Metal mattress, diathermy, and smoke
Report/descriptive
Health Dev

A hospital reported that a mattress, upon which a patient was receiving diathermy, began to smoke and burn.

The mattress was conductive (type used in surgery) and absorbed radiofrequency energy, leading to a dangerous temperature rise and diminished energy delivery to the patient. In this case, the unit's cables rested on the mattress, resulting in overheating.

All metal should be removed from treatment area during diathermy. Replace conductive mattresses with nonconductive ones on treatment tables.

FOOD AND DRUG ADMINISTRATION REPORT[11]

Date	Device	Event	Outcome
FDA, 2002[11] Patient Safety News **DBS, diathermy, and death** Online	Diathermy treatment can lead to heating at the interface between the body and the neurostimulator electrode of a neurostimulator and cause tissue damage, permanent damage, and even death.	In 2001, two patients with implanted deep brain stimulators received diathermy treatment and subsequently died as a result of severe brain damage from energy when the lead electrodes were implanted in the brain. (One patient was treated with diathermy after oral surgery [reported in this book—note no mention of patient death], whereas the other patient was treated for diathermy for chronic scoliosis.)	Medtronic issued an alert and other manufacturers, Cyberonics and Advanced Neuromodulation Systems, have also issued warnings. The FDA warns that patients with these devices should not be treated with diathermy, even if the implanted device is turned off or is implanted but no longer in use. Any implant is of concern including those used for brain, spinal cord, peripheral nerves, or sacral nerves.

Note: FDA reports do not necessarily establish cause-effect relationships between equipment and injury. Incidences may be due to equipment or user error. Also, some reports are alleged by attorneys.

REFERENCES

1. Eisenberg MG: Dictionary of rehabilitation. New York: Springer; 1995.

2. Tan JC: Practical manual of physical medicine and rehabilitation: diagnostics, therapeutics, and basic problems. St. Louis: Mosby; 1998.

3. Cameron MH, Perez D, Otáno-Lata S: Electromagnetic radiation. In: Cameron MH: Physical agents in rehabilitation: from research to practice. St. Louis: Saunders; 2003. pp 369-413.

4. Prentice WE, Draper DO: Shortwave and microwave diathermy. In: Prentice WE, editor: Therapeutic modalities for physical therapists, ed 2. New York: McGraw-Hill; 2002.

5. Docker M, Bazin S, Dyson M, et al: Guidelines for the safe use of continuous shortwave therapy equipment. Physiotherapy 78:755-757, 1992.

6. Kloth LC, Ziskin MC: Diathermy and pulsed radio frequency radiation. In: Michlovitz SL, editor: Thermal agents in rehabilitation, ed 3. Philadelphia: F.A. Davis; 1996.

7. Day MJ, Katz JS: Diathermy. In: Hecox B, Mehreteab TA, Weisberg J, eds: Integrating physical agents in rehabilitation. Upper Saddle River (NJ): Pearson Prentice Hall; 2006.

8. Basford JR: Therapeutic physical agents. In: Delisa JA, editor: Physical medicine and rehabilitation: principles and practices, ed 4, vol 1. Philadelphia: Lippincott Williams & Wilkins; 2005.

9. Rubin A, Erdman WJ: Microwave exposure of the human female pelvis during early pregnancy and prior to conception. Am J Phys Med 38:219-220, 1959.

10. Scott BO: Effects of contact lenses on shortwave field distribution. Br J Ophthalmol 40:696-697, 1956.

11. U.S. Food and Drug Administration: FDA Public Health Notification: Diathermy Interactions with Implanted Leads and Implanted Systems with Leads: Available at: http://www.fda.gov/cdrh/psn/show4.html. Accessed November 14, 2005.

12. Nutt JG, Anderson VC, Peacock JH, et al: DBs and diathermy interaction induces severe CNS damage. Neurology 56:1384-1386, 2001.

13. Shortwave diathermy units. Health Dev 17(8):247, 1988.

14. Lichter I, Borrie J: Radio-frequency hazards with cardiac pacemakers. BMJ 5449(1):1513-1518, 1965.

15. Jones SL: Electromagnetic field interference and cardiac pacemakers. Phys Ther 56(9):1013-1018, 1976.

16. Doyle JR, Smart BW: Stimulation of bone growth by shortwave diathermy. J Bone Joint Surg 45A:15-24, 1963.

17. Daily L Jr, Wakim KG, Herrick JF, et al: The effect of microwave diathermy on the eye: an experimental study. Am J Ophthalmol 35:1001-1017, 1952.

18. Arledge RL: Prevention of electric shock hazards in physical therapy. Phys Ther 58(10):1215-1217, 1978.

44   HYDROTHERAPY

INCLUDES FULL BODY IMMERSION; WHIRLPOOL EXCLUDES DEBRIDEMENT/WOUND CARE (SEE DEBRIDEMENT)
EXCLUDES AQUATIC THERAPY (SEE AQUATIC THERAPY)

OVERVIEW. Hydrotherapy is water treatment used for exercises, pain management, and wound care[1] and includes whirlpool, pool therapy, and contrast baths. Hydrotherapy benefits are derived from its cleansing action, buoyancy properties (reduced weight bearing), hydrostatic pressure effects (improved venous return), and psychological effects.

Sources generally recommend monitoring patient vital signs (because of patients' inability to lose heat while in water if fully immersed), check temperature levels, clean tanks, and caution to never leave patient unattended during or after hydrotherapy.[2,3] Note: (1) Because of the potential for cross-contamination, aspiration, drowning, cardiovascular stress, and burns (in heated water), patient screening is required. (2) If hydrotherapy is used in conjunction with hot or cold water, then superficial heat and cryotherapy concerns also apply, respectively.[3-5]

SUMMARY: CONTRAINDICATIONS AND PRECAUTIONS. Five sources cited a total of 48 concerns for hydrotherapy. Several of these concerns were temperature related. Concerns ranged from 19 to 28 per source, with physical therapists citing the greatest number. The largest proportion of concerns fell within the ICD categories of circulatory, skin, mental/behavioral, or nervous system. The most frequently cited concerns in this sample were malignancy and sensory impairments. In addition, 10 other frequently cited concerns included bowel incontinence, urinary incontinence, pulmonary disease, cardiac insufficiency, impaired circulation, skin infection, mental impairment, epilepsy, and fever (mentioned by 80% of sources). The concerns below include both full body and local immersion (for local concerns, also see Debridement section in Wound Care).

OTHER ISSUES: ELECTROLYTE IMBALANCES IN BURNS, SLIPS, AND FALLS, AND HAIR ENTANGLEMENT. (1) Said and Hussein,[6] in a 1987 case series, reported on two brothers who sustained partial-thickness burns and subsequently developed hyponatremia while immersed in a whirlpool filled with tap water. (2) In a 1994 Missouri lawsuit,[7] a man with arthritis was awarded $47,773.90 after he slipped and fractured his patella while being assisted out of a whirlpool bath. (3) The CPSC[8] reported 43 incidences of hair getting sucked into suction fittings of spas, whirlpools, or hot tubs, including 12 deaths (the head of victim was trapped underwater).

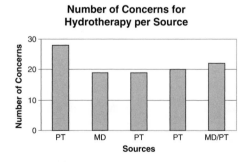

Number of Concerns for Hydrotherapy per Source

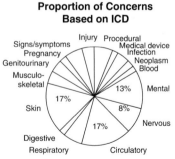

Proportion of Concerns Based on ICD

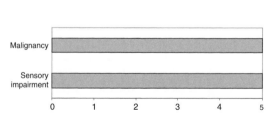

Top 2 Concerns for Hydrotherapy (N = 5)

CONTRAINDICATIONS AND PRECAUTIONS FOR HYDROTHERAPY

A00-B99 CERTAIN INFECTIONS AND PARASITIC DISEASES

Issue	LOC	Source	Affil	Rationale/Comment
Infectious conditions spread by pool water	CI Concern	Cameron, 2003[4,a,b] Basford, 2005[9,c]	PT MD	Infectious conditions that may spread by water. Consider using a Hubbard tank, where water is changed between patients, instead of the pool.[4] **In 1981, McGuckin et al[10] reported an outbreak of *Pseudomonas aeruginosa* in 10 postsurgical patients who had received hydrotherapy in a hospital during a time when disinfection procedures were not in place. Also see Schlech et al[11] below.**
Tuberculosis	CI CI/P	Walsh, 1996[3] Tan, 1998[5]	PT MD/PT	

a, Also precaution for local immersion of an infected area; b, General thermotherapy concerns are included in this hydrotherapy section; c, Disease transmission concern.

C00-C97 NEOPLASMS

Issue	LOC	Source	Affil	Rationale/Comment
Malignancy[a]	CI CI/P CI CI CI/P	Cameron, 2003[4,a] Tan, 1998[5] Walsh, 1996[3] Hecox and Leinanger, 2006[2,b] Basford, 2005[9]	PT MD/PT PT PT MD	Heat may enhance activity and movement of malignant cells.

a, Thermotherapy; b, Skin and lymphatic cancer—safety not yet determined.

D50-D89 DISEASES OF BLOOD AND BLOOD-FORMING ORGANS AND CERTAIN DISORDERS

Issue	LOC	Source	Affil	Rationale/Comment
Danger of hemorrhaging	RCI	Hecox and Leinanger, 2006[2,a]	PT	Heat can increase bleeding.
	CI	Walsh, 1996[3]	PT	
	CI/P	Basford, 2005[9,b]	MD	

a, Relative to heat intensity and immersion degree; b, Hemorrhage or bleeding disorder.

F00-F99 MENTAL AND BEHAVIORAL DISORDERS

Issue	LOC	Source	Affil	Rationale/Comment
Alcohol ingestion	P	Cameron, 2003[4]	PT	Alcohol reduces judgment and enhances a hypotensive response, both of which pose safety concerns. Inquire if the patient has ingested alcohol in the past several hours.
Confusion or disorientation	P			Disoriented patients may be unsafe in water. Determine if the patient is alert and oriented to time, person, and place. Also, for local application, burns can occur if patient's communications about discomfort are not reliable. Use water at body temperature and monitor closely.

Continued

Issue	LOC	Source	Affil	Rationale/Comment
Fear of water	P	Cameron, 2003[4]	PT	Fearful patients will probably refuse full immersion. Consider local
	CI	Hecox and Leinanger, 2006[2]	PT	immersion (extremity tank), nonimmersion technique, or land exercises.[4]
Mental disorder—severe	CI/P	Tan, 1998[5]	MD/PT	Do not use Hubbard tank.
Mentation impaired	P	Cameron, 2003[4]	PT	If hot water used and the patient cannot communicate discomforts.
	CI/P	Tan, 1998[5]	MD/PT	
	CI	Hecox and Leinanger, 2006[2]	PT	
	CI/P	Basford, 2005[9,a]	MD	
Suicidal patients	CI	Cameron, 2003[4]	PT	Check chart because there is an increased risk of drowning.

a, Inability to communicate or respond to pain.

G00-G99 DISEASES OF THE NERVOUS SYSTEM

Issue	LOC	Expert	Affil	Rationale/Comment
Epilepsy	CI	Cameron, 2003[4,f]	PT	There is a greater risk of drowning during an attack. Do not use a
	CI/P	Tan, 1998[5,f,g]	MD/PT	Hubbard tank for patients with uncontrolled epilepsy.[5]
	Concern	Basford, 2005[9,e]	MD	
	CI	Walsh, 1996[3,g]	PT	

Multiple sclerosis—in *warm or hot water*	P Advice	Cameron, 2003[4] Tan, 1998[5]	PT MD/PT	Temperatures above 31° C (88° F) may lead to increased fatigue and weakness in persons with MS. For pool therapy, temperatures of 84° F or less are recommended for persons with MS.[5] **In a 1937 descriptive study of 21 patients with multiple sclerosis, Simons[12] reported that 62% became weaker, 24% were unchanged, and 14% improved with heat. Berger and Sheremata[13] in 1983 reported four patients with MS who presented with new, prolonged neurological signs following tests in a hot bath.**
Sensation impaired[a]	P CI/P CI CI CI/P	Cameron, 2003[4,b] Tan, 1998[5] Walsh, 1996[3] Hecox and Leinanger, 2006[2,b] Basford, 2005[9,c]	PT MD/PT PT PT MD	Burns occur if water is too hot in insensate patients. Monitor water temperature.[4] **In a 1995 case report, Hwang et al[14] describe a 39-year-old person with paraplegia who was insensate below the T12 level and sustained bilateral fourth-degree burns to the distal third of the legs and feet and subsequent bilateral BKAs following débridement in scalding hydrotherapy water. Check water temperature with hand.**
Thermal regulation impairment—*in very warm or hot water*	P CI/P CI/P	Cameron, 2003[4] Tan, 1998[5,d] Basford, 2005[9,d]	PT MD/PT MD	These individuals can experience thermal shock if fully immersed in warm or hot water because convection and sweating may be impaired. Very young and elderly may have associated thermoregulation problems. Cameron suggests limiting warm water application to small body areas.[4]

a, Hot water; b, Thermal sensation decreased; c, Cutaneous insensitivity; d, From neuroleptics; e, Hot water–related seizures; f, Severe epilepsy; g, Uncontrolled epilepsy.

100-199 DISEASES OF THE CIRCULATORY SYSTEM

Issue	LOC	Source	Affil	Rationale/Comment
Blood pressure, unstable	CI	Walsh, 1996[3]	PT	Do not place patient in a Hubbard tank.[5]
	CI/P	Tan, 1998[5]	MD/PT	
	CI/P	Basford, 2005[9]	MD	
Cardiac instability	CI	Cameron, 2003[4]	PT	Full immersion in water may overload heart. This concern is specific to Hubbard and Pool.[4]
	CI/P	Basford, 2005[9,f]	MD	
Cardiac insufficiency/dysfunction	CI	Hecox and Leinanger, 2006[2,c]	PT	Cardiac patients may have difficulty adapting to changes for thermal homeostasis as heat dissipation requirements are increased. Consider limiting the maximum immersion time to 10 minutes initially.[3]
	P	Walsh, 1996[3]	PT	
	P	Cameron, 2003[4,a]	PT	
	CI/P/Concern	Basford, 2005[9,e]	MD	
Cardiac medication—cardiac, antihypertensives	P	Cameron, 2003[4]	PT	Some medications can affect a patient's response to exercise.
Circulation impaired—peripheral vascular disease	CI	Hecox and Leinanger, 2006[2,b]	PT	For hot water applications, there is a risk of burns if the patient's circulation cannot adequately dissipate heat from the heated tissue. Examples include persons with diabetes or arteriosclerosis. Avoid temperatures >95° F.[2]
	P	Cameron, 2003[4]	PT	
	CI/P	Tan, 1998[5]	MD/PT	
	CI/P	Basford, 2005[9,d]	MD	
Hypotensive patients	CI	Hecox and Leinanger, 2006[2,b]	PT	Blood pressure problems may be exacerbated by full immersion in cold or hot water.
Hypertensive patients	P	Walsh, 1996[3]	PT	As stated above for cardiac patients, there is an increased demand on cardiovascular (and pulmonary) systems and increased heat dissipation requirements. Limit maximum immersion time to 10 minutes initially.
	CI	Hecox and Leinanger, 2006[2,b]	PT	

Thrombophlebitic area	CI	Cameron, 2003[4]	PT	If hot water is used, thermotherapy concerns apply because of the increased risk of dislodging the clot with enhanced circulation.[4] Also, mechanical stimuli may cause dislodgment.[2]
	CI	Hecox and Leinanger, 2006[2,a]	PT	
				Imai et al,[15] in a 1998 case report, describe a 37-year-old hypertensive man who, after alternating between a hot sauna and cold water bathing for 2 hours, had an MI, possibly (speculated) due to plaque rupture/thrombosis from a coronary artery spasm.

a, Hot water; b, Severe impairment, e.g., arterial sclerosis, diabetes; c, Significant; d, Ischemia; e, Heart failure (decompensated) within 6-8 weeks of a myocardial infarction. Note: Cardiac disease may not be an absolute contraindication; f, Unstable angina.

J00-J99 DISEASES OF THE RESPIRATORY SYSTEM

Issue	LOC	Source	Affil	Rationale/Comment
Pulmonary disease	P	Walsh, 1996[3,a]	PT	Full immersion increases the work of breathing because of a poor ability to resist hydrostatic pressures while immersed.[5] Monitor for respiratory distress.
	P	Cameron, 2003[4]	PT	
	Caution	Tan, 1998[5]	MD/PT	
	CI	Hecox and Leinanger, 2006[2,b]	PT	
Upper respiratory infection	CI/P	Tan, 1998[5]	MD/PT	Do not use a Hubbard tank if patient has an upper respiratory infection.[5]
Vital capacity <1000 mL	Caution	Walsh, 1996[3]	PT	See above.
	P	Cameron, 2003[4]	PT	
	Caution	Tan, 1998[5]	MD/PT	

a, Cardiopulmonary patients; b, Significant respiratory dysfunction.

K00-K93 DISEASES OF THE DIGESTIVE SYSTEM

Issue	LOC	Source	Affil	Rationale/Comment
Bowel incontinence	CI	Cameron, 2003[4]	PT	The concern centers around wound contamination because wounds can be infected from patient's feces. Use of a Hubbard tank for patients with incontinence is not recommended.[5] Consider using a nonimmersion technique if patient is bowel incontinent and has wounds.[4]
	CI	Hecox and Leinanger, 2006[2]	PT	
	CI	Walsh, 1996[3]	PT	
	CI/P	Tan, 1998[5]	MD/PT	

L00-L99 DISEASES OF THE SKIN AND SUBCUTANEOUS TISSUE

Issue	LOC	Source	Affil	Rationale/Comment
Hypersensitivity, thermal	CI	Hecox and Leinanger, 2006[2]	PT	E.g., cold urticaria (if neutral water is not used).
Maceration around wound	CI	Cameron, 2003[4]	PT	Immersion can increase maceration and enlarging the size of a wound. Consider a nonimmersion technique.
Skin, atrophic	CI/P	Tan, 1998[5]	MD/PT	For hot water.[5]
	CI/P	Basford, 2005[9]	MD	
Skin conditions, some	CI	Hecox and Leinanger, 2006[2]	PT	Hydration may exacerbate some conditions and remove the skin's natural moisture. Conditions include atopic eczema, ichthyosis, and senile or winter pruritus. Note: Ichthyosis is hypertrophy of the "horny" skin layer with characteristic scaliness, dryness, and roughness.[16]

Skin graft, near—recent[b]	Advice	Walsh, 1996[3]	PT	Agitators should be minimal or turned off. Skin grafts are delicate 3 to 5 days
	P	Cameron, 2003[4]	PT	following grafting and possess inadequate capillary infiltration to offer nutritional support to the graft.[3] Also, grafts may not have sufficient vascularization to tolerate extreme water temperatures. Consider directing agitators away from the graft and using neutral or mild water temperatures.[4]
Skin infection	CI	Walsh, 1996[3]	PT	The concern is cross contamination via the medium of water.
	CI	Hecox and Leinanger, 2006[2,a]	PT	A Hubbard tank is not recommended.[5]
	CI/P	Tan, 1998[5]	MD/PT	
Scar, immature	CI/P	Tan, 1998[5]	MD/PT	For hot water.[5]
	CI/P	Basford, 2005[9,c]	MD	
Tissue flaps	Advice	Walsh, 1996[3,b]	PT	If water is too cold or patient has chills, vasoconstriction may occur with ischemia, leading to a loss of the tissue flap. Too much agitation (agitator) can also affect the site.

a, Surface infections (includes fungal); b, Local concern; c, Scar tissue.

M00-M99 DISEASES OF THE MUSCULOSKELETAL SYSTEM AND CONNECTIVE TISSUE

Issue	LOC	Source	Affil	Rationale/Comment
Musculoskeletal impairments	P	Cameron, 2003[4]	PT	Marked impairments (strength, balance, endurance, range of motion) can be unsafe (i.e., drowning). Cameron[4] suggests providing 1:1 supervision or secure patient with equipment so the head remains above water.
RA—acute	CI	Hecox and Leinanger, 2006[2]	PT	Heat is CI in the acute stage.

N00-N99 DISEASES OF THE GENITOURINARY SYSTEM

Issue	LOC	Source	Affil	Rationale/Comment
Incontinence, urinary	P	Cameron, 2003[4]	PT	Urinary tract infections can occur in catheterized patients who are fully immersed.[4] Also, there can be contamination of the water.[2]
	CI	Walsh, 1996[3]	PT	
	CI/P	Tan, 1998[5]	MD/PT	
	CI	Hecox and Leinanger, 2006[2]	PT	
Sperm count, reduced	Safety concern	Basford, 2005[9]	MD	Source notes reduced sperm counts after repeated or isolated sauna exposures.

O00-O99 PREGNANCY, CHILDBIRTH, AND PUERPERIUM

Issue	LOC	Source	Affil	Rationale/Comment
Pregnancy—in *very warm or hot water*	P/Avoid	Cameron, 2003[4]	PT	Full heat immersion with heating can lead to maternal hyperthermia and harm to the fetus. Inquire if patient is pregnant or is trying to become pregnant.[4] The heat in the water that is sufficient to raise a patient's core temperature to more than 102° F (38.9° C) for 20 minutes may harm a fetus.[2] A concern is Hubbard tank use during the first trimester.[2] Consider using only normal water temperatures in this population.[4] **Mulunsky et al,[17] in a 1992 prospective study of 23,491 women, reported that exposure to hot tub,**
	Special consideration	Hecox and Leinanger, 2006[2]	PT	
	Safety concern	Basford, 2005[9,a]	MD	

sauna, and fever in the first trimester of pregnancy were associated with increase risk of neural tube defects in the fetus. Edwards,[18] in a 1967 animal experiment, reported that 33% of impregnated guinea pigs exposed to 111-113° F temperatures, 1 hour/day for 8 days, had offspring with fetal malformations.

In 1993, Mottola et al[19] reported an animal experiment in which pregnant rats that swam and exercised in 37.6° C water 1 hour/day, 5×/week, had the greatest number of abnormal fetuses and the greatest number of abnormalities when compared with three rat control groups.

a, Early pregnancy.

R00-R99 SYMPTOMS, SIGNS, AND ABNORMAL CLINICAL AND LABORATORY FINDINGS (NOT ELSEWHERE CLASSIFIED)

Issue	LOC	Source	Affil	Rationale/Comment
Edema	CI/P	Tan, 1998[5]	MD/PT	If hot water is used, the heat can increase edema in a dependent
	P	Cameron, 2003[4]	PT	limb. **In a 1970 quasi-experiment, Magness et al[20] found**
	CI/P	Basford, 2005[9]	MD	**that patients (mostly orthopedic) who received whirlpool in 100 to 104° F temperatures, with their limbs dangling, developed edema in that limb.**

Continued

Issue	LOC	Source	Affil	Rationale/Comment
Febrile episode—acute	CI/P	Tan, 1998[5]	MD/PT	
	CI	Walsh, 1996[3]	PT	
	CI	Hecox and Leinanger, 2006[2]	PT	
	Concern	Basford, 2005[9,b]	MD	
Inflammation—acute	CI/P	Tan, 1998[5]	MD/PT	For hot water. Heat would aggravate the inflammatory process.
	CI	Cameron, 2003[4]	PT	
	CI	Walsh, 1996[3,a]	PT	
	CI/P	Basford, 2005[9]	MD	

a, See thermotherapy precautions; b, Systematic hyperthermia.

S00-T98 INJURY, POISONING, AND CERTAIN OTHER CONSEQUENCES OF EXTERNAL CAUSES

Issue	LOC	Source	Affil	Rationale/Comment
Injury—acute	CI/P	Tan, 1998[5]	MD/PT	For hot water.
	CI	Cameron, 2003[4]	PT	
	CI/P	Basford, 2005[9]	MD	
Wounds—open or discharging	CI/not	Tan, 1998[5]	MD/PT	For pool therapy, there should be no open or discharging wounds.

Y70-Y82 MEDICAL DEVICES

Issue	LOC	Source	Affil	Rationale/Comment
Metal in area	P	Cameron, 2003[4]	PT	For hot water.

PROCEDURAL CONCERNS/MISCELLANEOUS

Issue	LOC	Source	Affil	Rationale/Comment
Counterirritant, topical/liniment/ heat rub applied over area	P CI	Cameron, 2003[4] Walsh, 1996[3]	PT	If hot water is used, burns can result if a heat ointment is also applied. Vessels are already vasodilated from the ointment.
Elderly	P	Walsh, 1996[3]	PT	Increased demands are placed on the elderly patient's cardiovascular and pulmonary systems and heat dissipation requirements. Limit maximum immersion time to 10 minutes initially.[3]
Position of upper limb, dependent	P	Walsh, 1996[3]	PT	**See Magness et al.[20]** Edema can form in the dependent hand when heated water is used. Avoid a dependent position of hand; perform active ROM if possible; pad tank edge to avoid constricting lymphatic and vascular circulation.

Note: Also see summary for precautions such as monitoring vitals, monitoring water temperatures, and never leaving a patient alone.

For Contrast Bath

Issue	LOC	Source	Affil	Rationale/Comment
Cardiovascular problems	CI	Hecox and Leinanger, 2006[2]	PT	
Hemorrhage, tendency	CI			
Hypersensitivity, temperature	CI			
Peripheral vascular disease	CI	Walsh, 1996[3,a]	PT	
	CI	Hecox and Leinanger, 2006[2,b]	PT	
Pregnancy	CI	Hecox and Leinanger, 2006[2]	PT	
Sensation loss	CI			
Small vessel disease	CI	Walsh, 1996[3]	PT	Examples include diabetes, arteriosclerotic endarteritis, and Buerger's disease.
	CI	Tan, 1998[5]	MD/PT	Other cold and heat concerns also apply with this modality.[5]

Note: Hecox and Leinanger indicated that both heat and cold contraindications apply to contrast baths.
a, For water temperatures higher than 40° C; b, E.g., arterial sclerosis.

Nonimmersion Hydrotherapy Techniques

Issue	LOC	Source	Affil	Rationale/Comment
Maceration	P	Cameron, 2003[4]	PT	Avoid maceration by wetting intact skin (around wound).
Nonimmersion	Disadvantages			Nonimmersion fails to address buoyancy, hydrostatic, or temperature (superficial heating) benefits that are found in immersion hydrotherapy.

Whirlpool Tank

Issue	LOC	Source	Affil	Rationale/Comment
Adequate grounding of all exposed metal surfaces	Shock hazards P	Arledge, 1978[21] Walsh, 1996[3]	PT PT	Electrical shorts will result in electrical current flowing through the plumbing to the earth ground. Otherwise, both patient and staff can be shocked. Never assume hospital maintenance is being conducted for all hazardous areas.
Allergies to cleaning solution	Care	Hecox and Leinanger, 2006[2]	PT	Check if patient is allergic to any solutions or additives.
Clean whirlpool tank and turbines after each use	P	Walsh, 1996[3]	PT	Scrubbing alone will not eradicate contaminants on edges, drains, overflow pipes, thermometers, and agitators (these are areas frequently contaminated).

Agitators

Issue	LOC	Source	Affil	Rationale/Comment
Adequate electrical installation	P	Hecox and Leinanger, 2006[2]	PT	Hospital-grade plugs; fail-safe hospital-grade receptacles; ground fault interrupters (GFI) on new equipment.
Agitator must be secured OUTSIDE the tank	P			Electrocution may result if agitator (live motor) falls into tank.
Do not clog/plug opening	P			Appendages or bandages may plug agitator opening.
Electrical wiring must be insulated	P			To avoid shock.
Monitor for current leaks at least every 6 months	P			
Person inside tank must never turn on or off agitator switch	P	Hecox and Leinanger, 2006[2]	PT	If ground is inadequate, shock or electrocution is possible. Cover switches with plastic or rubber.
	Advice	Arledge, 1978[21]	PT	

ADVERSE EVENTS

Source	Background	Therapy	Outcome	Follow-up/Interpretation
Edwards, 1967[18] **Pregnancy, heat, and fetal abnormalities** Animal experiment (randomized) Arch Pathol	90 impregnated guinea pigs were randomly allocated into treatment or control groups (subjects were matched for weight)	The experimental group was placed in an egg incubator 1 hour daily for 8 consecutive days at temperatures ranging from 111 to 113 °F. Rectal temperatures increased to 110 °F on average. Of heated females, 16% died; 17% aborted.	Abnormalities were noted in 58 of the 173 newborns from the experimental (heated females) group and 1 of 31 from the control females. Fetal malformations included microcephaly, abdominal wall defects, amyoplasia, talipes conditions (hind limb joints fixed in flexion or extension), cataracts, lateral forefoot digit hypoplasia (small), dental defects (failure of incisors to erupt).	Defects were noted more in the brain and musculoskeletal systems. The tissue was more susceptible to small brain size when heated in early gestation.
Imai et al, 1998[15] **Cardiac, heat, and cold** Case report Cardiology	A 37-year-old Japanese man (172 cm height; 60 kg weight) smoked 1½ packs of cigarettes per day for 20 years. He was not hypertensive.	In an effort to lose weight, the man alternated between a hot sauna and cold water bathing repeatedly for 2 hours.	He felt chest pain for 2 hours and discomfort for the entire night. Two days later, tests indicated elevated serum cardiac enzymes and changes on EKG. He was diagnosed with an acute MI. On day 11, cardiac catheterization revealed mild stenosis in the infarct-related artery, suggesting plaque in the proximal portion of the left anterior descending artery.	The authors underscore the danger of rapid cooling after sauna bathing in patients with coronary risk factors. They postulated that the MI was attributed to plaque rupture/thrombosis as a result of a coronary artery spasm (induced by alpha-adrenergic receptors during alternating heating and cooling).

Magness et al, 1970[20] **Edema, heat, and limb dependency** Quasi-experiment: Nonequivalent pretest, posttest Arch Phys Med Rehab	Normal arms (22 male, 23 female) and 20 patient arms were immersed for 30 minutes. Patient characteristics: 7 UE fracture; 5 RA reconstruction; 2 RA, 2 shoulder-hand; 1 obstructive lymphedema; 1 epicondylitis; 1 laceration.	Arms were immersed in very warm to hot water for 30 minutes and allowed to passively dangle while an agitator was on. Water temperatures: Normal arms (92 to 112° F) Patient arms (100 to 104° F)	Normal arm edema significantly increased after whirlpool ($P < .001$) in normal arms (regression slope was 5.34 mL/°F). Patient arm volume increases were greater than the normal ($P < .01$ with statistical correction).	Avoid hot whirlpool temperatures if edema formation prevention is an important goal. If heat is needed, elevate limb, and encourage active motion with a different heat modality (e.g., hot pack). Note: Controls were not patients.
McGuckin et al, 1981[10] **Spread of infection and hydrotherapy** Epidemiological investigation Arch Phys Med Rehab	A hospital gynecological oncology unit reported increased postoperative cases with new wound infections.	Eleven cases were identified within a 2-week period with positive cultures of *Pseudomonas aeruginosa* (this organism proliferates in warm, moist environments outside a host). Of the 11 cases, 10 had received hydrotherapy, which represented 55% (10 of 18) of those who received hydrotherapy over the 2-week period.	The investigation revealed that the hospital ran out of sodium hypochlorite during this time period and it was therefore not used during the hydrotherapy disinfection procedures.	No additional cases reported when use of sodium hypochlorite resumed in subsequent weeks.

Continued

Source	Background	Therapy	Outcome	Follow-up/Interpretation
Said and Hussein, 1987[6] **Hyponatremia, burns, and whirlpool** Case series Burns	A 20-year-old male Saudi patient presented with 55-60% partial-thickness burns at the head, neck, anterior chest wall, arms, and legs as a result of a house fire. An 18-year-old male (brother of the above case) presented with 35% partial-thickness burns.	During hospitalization, he received daily hydrotherapy for 1 hour in a 1200-L whirlpool tank using tap water. On day 11, drowsiness, anorexia, nausea, confusion, poor skin turgor, and dehydration were noted. Serum sodium and potassium levels were 113 mmol/L and 6-8 mmol/L, respectively. Hyponatremia was noted on day 13 of hospitalization with serum sodium 120 mmol/L. He then received a 1-hour whirlpool treatment. Following treatment, sodium levels dropped further, to 113 mmol/L.	The patient was treated with IV 5% NaCl for 6 hours and maintained on a 9% saline infusion. The whirlpool contained no (0 mmol/L) sodium. When 124 mmol/L sodium was added to whirlpool water, serum sodium and potassium was generally maintained. He was treated with 5% NaCl for 6 hours to partially correct hyponatremia. When 120 mmol/L of sodium was added to whirlpool, serum sodium was maintained in this patient.	In burn patients, hyponatremia occurs from submersion in tap water baths. The burned skin acts as a dialyzing membrane. Once sodium is added to the water, the movement of sodium across the burned skin stopped. The authors recommend adding sodium chloride to whirlpool water to address this potentially lethal problem.
Schlech et al, 1986[11] **Pool infections** Epidemiology Can Med Assoc J	Epidemiological report of an infection in a physical therapy department affecting therapists, inpatients, and outpatients.	A rash (e.g., tender erythematous papules over abdomen and trunk in index case) was noted in 5 of 11 physiotherapists (45%) using a newly constructed (6-month-old) outpatient pool	*Pseudomonas folliculitis* was the cause. Risk factors for the infection were not identified using this case-control design, but physiotherapists did frequent the pool more often than the patients.	Note on pool history: Automatic chlorination broke; instead, chlorination was performed manually and haphazardly twice a day on average.

Mottola et al, 1993[19]
Pregnancy, warm water exercise, and fetal deformity
Animal experiment
Int J Sports Med

Pregnant rats (about 36 days old; Sprague-Dawley type) with prior training (6 weeks), were randomly assigned to four groups: (during days 1-18 of gestation)
1. Cool water (34.6° C): exercise 1 hour daily for 5×/ week
2. Warm water (37.6° C): exercise 1 hour daily for 5×/week
3. Warm controls: only immersed to the neck level 1 hour daily for 5×/week
4. Cool controls who received no swimming or immersion

in their department. Of 17 who did not use the pool, none developed the rash ($P < .005$). The infection was also noted in 6 of 29 outpatients, 4 of 12 inpatients, and 1 of 4 surgical wounds.

Maternal body temperature of the warm water swim group elevated 2.3° C (within the teratogenic range) ($P < .01$) compared to controls.

No further cases were reported following hyperchlorination (residual-free chlorine concentration 3 to 4 ppm) and repairs (structural) to the pool.

Of 90 fetuses analyzed, 24 were abnormal.
The warm water swim group had the greatest number of abnormal fetuses (14 of 24) (other groups had 4 or fewer) and the greatest number of abnormalities (20 of 31) (other groups had 4 or fewer).
Abnormalities included 9 with microencephaly, 3 with narrow cerebral hemispheres, 2 with enlarged ventricles of the brain, 2 with enlarged right cerebral hemisphere, 2 with small/irregular heart shape, 1 with microphthalmia, and 1 with large head.

An improperly installed filtering system was not operating properly. Organic debris was found in the pool and accumulated around peeling sealant.

The authors suggest that swimming (immersion plus exercise) in warm water should be avoided during gestation due to potential teratogenic effects.

U.S. CONSUMER PRODUCT SAFETY COMMISSION[8]

Event	Background	Recommendations
Body part entrapment	Since 1990, 74 incidences (with 2 disembowelments and 13 deaths) occurred whereby the body was entrapped by strong drain suction in pools, wading pools, spas, and hot tubs.	CPSC standards require down-shaped drain outlets and 2 outlets of each pump to reduce suction power if one drain becomes blocked. Warn of drain covers in spas, hot tubs, and whirlpools resulting in hair entanglement and body part entrapment.
Child drownings	CPSC reports move than 800 deaths in spas and hot tubs since 1990 (a fifth were in children under age 5)	There is a need for locked safety covers or constant adult supervision.
Hair entanglement	There have been 43 incidences with 12 deaths. Children play "hold your breath the longest." Hair gets sucked into suction fittings in the spa, hot tub, or whirlpool resulting in the head being held under water.	This occurs when hair became entangled in drain covers. Get drain covers that meet CPSC standards. Warn of drain covers in spas, hot tubs, and whirlpools resulting in hair entanglement and body part entrapment.
Hot tub temperatures	CPSC reports several cases of extremely hot water (about 110° F) that led to drowsiness and unconsciousness and then drowning. High temperatures can also raise body temperature and lead to heat stroke and death.	Spa water temperatures should never exceed 104° F. Pregnant women and young children should consult with their physicians.

Year and State	History	Location	Device	Complication	Award and Comments
1994 Missouri[7] **Fall in hydrotherapy** Dec 1994, p 45, loc 4	A man with lower extremity arthritis slipped while being assisted out of a whirlpool bath by staff.	Outpatient physical therapy.	He sustained a patella fracture.	The plaintiff required surgery and eventually removal of the patella.	A jury found against the defendant (medical center). Award: $47,773.90

REFERENCES

1. Eisenberg MG: Dictionary of rehabilitation. New York: Springer; 1995.
2. Hecox B, Leinanger PM: Hydrotherapy. In: Hecox B, Mehreteab TA, Weisberg J, eds: Integrating physical agents in rehabilitation. Upper Saddle River (NJ): Pearson Prentice Hall; 2006.
3. Walsh MT: Hydrotherapy: the use of water as a therapeutic agent. In: Michlovitz SL, editor: Thermal agents in rehabilitation, ed 3. Philadelphia: F.A. Davis; 1996.
4. Cameron MH: Physical agents in rehabilitation: from research to practice. St. Louis: Saunders; 2003.
5. Tan JC: Practical manual of physical medicine and rehabilitation: diagnostics, therapeutics, and basic problems. St. Louis: Mosby; 1998.
6. Said RA, Hussein MM: Severe hyponatraemia in burn patients secondary to hydrotherapy. Burns 13(4):327-329, 1987.
7. Medical malpractice verdicts, settlements and experts, Dec 1994, p 45 loc 4.
8. Consumer Product Safety Commission: Spas, hot tubs, and whirlpools. Available at: http://www.cpsc.gov/cpscpub/pubs/5112.pdf. Accessed November 26, 2005.

9. Basford JR: Therapeutic physical agents. In: Delisa JA, editor: Physical medicine and rehabilitation: principles and practices, ed 4, vol 1. Philadelphia: Lippincott Williams & Wilkins; 2005.

10. McGuckin MB, Thorpe RJ, Abrutyn E: Hydrotherapy: An outbreak of *Pseudomonas aeruginosa* wound infections related to Hubbard tack treatments. Arch Phys Med Rehab 62:283-285, 1981.

11. Schlech III, Simonsen N, Sumarah R, et al: Nosocomial outbreak of *Pseudomonas aeruginosa* folliculitis associated with a physiotherapy pool. Can Med Assoc J 134:909-913, 1986.

12. Simons DJ: A note on the effect of heat and of cold upon certain symptoms of multiple sclerosis. Bull Neurol Inst N Y 6:385-386, 1937.

13. Berger JR, Sheremata WA: Persistent neurological deficit precipitated by hot bath test in multiple sclerosis. JAMA 249(13):1751-1753, 1983.

14. Hwang JCF, Himel HN, Edlich RF: Bilateral amputation following hydrotherapy tank burns in a paraplegic patient. Burns 21(1):70-71, 1995.

15. Imai Y, Nobuoka S, Sagashima J, et al: Acute myocardial infarction induced by alternating exposure to heat in a sauna and rapid cooling in cold water. Cardiology 90(4):299-301, 1998.

16. Dorland's illustrated medical dictionary, ed 24. Philadelphia: Saunders; 1965.

17. Milunsky A, Ulcickas M, Rothman KJ, et al: Maternal heat exposure and neural tube defects. JAMA 268(7):882-885, 1992.

18. Edwards MJ: Congenital defects in Guinea pigs following induced hyperthermia during gestation. Arch Pathol 84:42-48, 1967.

19. Mottola MF, Fitzgerald HM, Wilson NC, et al: Effect of water temperature on exercise-induced maternal hyperthermia on fetal development in rats. Int J Sports Med 14(5), 248-251, 1993.

20. Magness JL, Garrett TR, Erickson DJ: Swelling of the upper extremity during whirlpool baths. Arch Phys Med Rehab 51(5):297-299, 1970.

21. Arledge RL: Prevention of electric shock hazards in physical therapy. Phys Ther 58(10):1215-1217, 1978.

45 | LIGHT AGENTS

45.1 Cold LASER

OVERVIEW. LASER stands for light amplification by stimulated emission of radiation. Cold (low power) lasers use less than 60 mW of power and produce little or no thermal response. The He-Ne cold laser has generated interest in physical therapy because of its purported wound healing and analgesic effects (when used over acupuncture or trigger points).[1-5] Users must obtain an investigational device exemption from the FDA for this class III medical device. In 2002, the FDA approved its use for carpal tunnel syndrome.[5,6]

SUMMARY: CONTRAINDICATIONS AND PRECAUTIONS. Six sources cited a total of 23 concerns for cold laser. Concerns ranged from 3 to 13 per source, with a physical therapist citing the largest number. The largest proportion of concerns were listed under skin, vulnerable tissue, or procedural categories. Many concerns are inadequately explained for cold laser; perhaps the basis for some concerns is a lack of information on its effects on tissue.[3] The most frequently cited concern was irradiating the eyes (a concern well supported by evidence), use during pregnancy, and application near cancerous lesions.

Number of Concerns for Cold Laser per Source (n = 6)

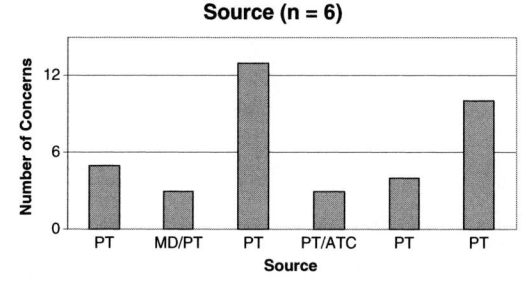

Proportion of Concerns Based on ICD for Cold Laser

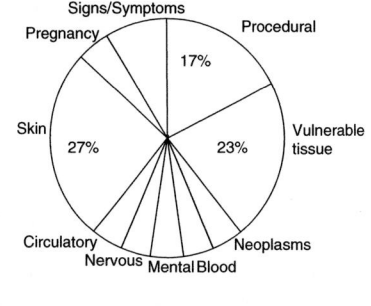

Top 3 Concerns for Cold Laser (n = 6)

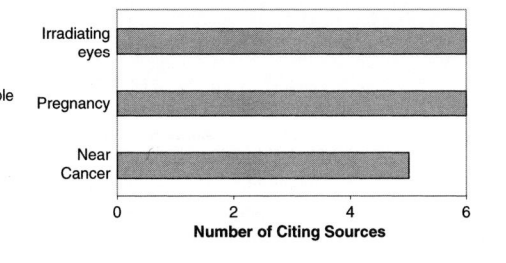

CONTRAINDICATIONS AND PRECAUTIONS

C00-C97 NEOPLASMS

Issue	LOC	Source	Affil	Rationale/Comment
Cancerous lesions—near	CI	Snyder-Mackler and Collender, 1996[1]	PT	Cold laser may increase tissue metabolism[5] and enhance and spread cancer.
	CI	Tan, 1998[2]	MD/PT	
	P	Cameron et al, 2003[3]	PT	
	CI	Saliba and Foreman-Saliba, 2002[4]	PT/ATC	
	CI	Weisberg and Adams, 2006[5]	PT	

D50-D89 DISEASES OF BLOOD AND BLOOD-FORMING ORGANS

Issue	LOC	Source	Affil	Rationale/Comment
Hemorrhagic region—over	CI	Cameron et al, 2003[3]	PT	Cold laser may cause vasodilation and bleeding in hemorrhagic areas.[3,5] **In a case**
	CI	Weisberg and Adams, 2006[5,a]	PT	**series, Gabel[7] reports on bruising in two female athletes following laser and exercise, suggesting that treatment may have led to increased tissue permeability.**

a, Active or suspected bleeding.

F00-F99 MENTAL AND BEHAVIORAL DISORDERS

Issue	LOC	Source	Affil	Rationale/Comment
Confused patients	P	Cameron et al, 2003[3]	PT	Confused patients may not be able to report discomfort.

G00-G99 DISEASES OF THE NERVOUS SYSTEM

Issue	LOC	Source	Affil	Rationale/Comment
Sensation impaired	P	Cameron et al, 2003[3]	PT	Patients with diminished sensation may be unable to report discomfort. **Bliddal et al[8] and Waylonis et al[9] each reported patients who communicated sensory complaints during laser treatments.**

I00-I99 DISEASES OF THE CIRCULATORY SYSTEM

Issue	LOC	Source	Affil	Rationale/Comment
In cardiac patients, over heart, vagus nerve, sympathetic regions	P	Cameron et al, 2003[3]	PT	Neurogenic responses (altered conduction) may stress a diseased heart.

L00-L99 DISEASES OF THE SKIN AND SUBCUTANEOUS TISSUE

Issue	LOC	Source	Affil	Rationale/Comment
Dry skin, extra—over	P	Kahn, 2000[10]	PT	
Eschar, thick—over	P			
Infected skin—over	P	Cameron et al, 2003[3]	PT	Cold laser may increase circulation to area.
Photosensitive skin—over	CI	Kahn, 2000[10]	PT	
Photosensitized from medication	CI			
Scar tissue—over considerable	P			

O00-O99 PREGNANCY, CHILDBIRTH, AND PUERPERIUM

Issue	LOC	Source	Affil	Rationale/Comment
Pregnant woman	CI	Snyder-Mackler and Collender, 1996[1]	PT	The effects of cold laser during pregnancy are not known.[10]
	CI	Tan 1998[2,a]	MD/PT	The endocrine system may be stimulated (effects also unknown).[5]
	P	Cameron et al, 2003[3]	PT	
	CI	Kahn, 2000[10]	PT	
	CI	Saliba and Foreman-Saliba, 2002[4,a]	PT/ATC	
	CI	Weisberg and Adams, 2006[5]	PT	

a, Concerns during first trimester.

R00-R99 SYMPTOMS, SIGNS, AND ABNORMAL CLINICAL AND LABORATORY FINDINGS (NOT ELSEWHERE CLASSIFIED)

Issue	LOC	Source	Affil	Rationale/Comment
Fever	P	Cameron et al, 2003[3]	PT	Fear of worsening condition.
Infection—active	P	Kahn, 2000[10]	PT	

VULNERABLE BIOLOGICAL TISSUE

Issue	LOC	Source	Affil	Rationale/Comment
Cornea/eye—directly into	CI	Snyder-Mackler and Collender, 1996[1]	PT	Never direct laser into the eye or along the axis of the beam
	CI	Tan, 1998[2]	MD/PT	because retinal lesions and burns can occur. There is also
	CI	Cameron et al, 2003[3]	PT	potential for damage to the cornea.[5]
	CI	Kahn, 2000[10]	PT	Safety glasses are recommended to avoid exposure from reflection.[4]
	CI	Saliba and Foreman-Saliba, 2002[4]	PT/ATC	Patients and clinicians should opaque wear goggles (specific for
	CI	Weisberg and Adams, 2006[5]	PT	wavelength). **In an animal study, Ham et al[11] reported irreversible retinal burn damage in the monkey at about 7 mW after direct eye exposure to He-Ne laser**.
Endocrine glands—directly over	CI	Cameron et al, 2003[3]	PT	The concern is the possibility of cellular effects that the laser may have on endocrine function.
Epiphyseal areas in growing children—over	P			
Fontanels of children, unclosed—over	CI	Snyder-Mackler and Collender, 1996[1]	PT	
Testicular region—over	P	Cameron et al, 2003[3]	PT	The effect of cold laser application over the testes is not known.

a, Gonads.

PROCEDURAL CONCERNS

Issue	LOC	Source	Affil	Rationale/Comment
Age—extreme	P	Kahn, 2000[10]	PT	
Medicated—heavily	P			
Radiotherapy—within past 4-6 months	CI	Cameron et al, 2003[3]	PT	Radiated tissue may be more vulnerable to cancer and burns.
Syncope following treatment lasting >5 minutes	CI	Saliba and Foreman-Saliba, 2002[4]	PT/ATC	If syncope lasts more than 5 minutes after application, do not give further treatments.

ADVERSE EVENTS

Source	Background	Therapy	Outcome	Follow-up/Interpretation
Bliddal et al, 1987[8] **Laser, RA, and burning sensations** RCT (Double blind) Scand J Rheumatol	18 patients with RA (11 class II, 7 class III; ages 41-79) were recruited from an outpatient clinic. Duration of illness ranged from 1 to 21 years.	Patients were randomly assigned to either a laser or placebo group; treated left and right second MCP joint (index) for 5 minutes with slow semicircular back-and-forth movements on joint line 3 alternate days/ week for 3 weeks followed by 4 weeks of observation (area 0.5 cm^2; 6 J/cm^2)	Adverse effect: Three patients complained of burning sensation from laser treatment group at the joint line.	Burning stopped within a few hours. (Two of these patients showed improved joint ability scores, and the other patient showed reduced pain.)

Continued

Source	Background	Therapy	Outcome	Follow-up/Interpretation
		(laser type: C biotronic laser; continuous He-Ne laser; 633 nm, 10 mW) with pen applicator.		
Ham et al, 1970[11] **Lasers and retinal burns** Animal study (pretest-posttest) Arch Ophthalmol	The eyes of 25 rhesus monkeys were exposed to He-Ne radiation (632.8 nm). Equipment: CW laser (Spectra-physics #125). Max output 80 mW; beam diameter about 2 mm at 2 sigma points and divergence of 0.7 milliradian; exposure times ranged from 15 msec to 1000 msec.	The fundus of eyes (rhesus monkeys) were photographed prior to and after exposure (16 exposures). The beam of light was directed into 25 eyes. The image size was 298 μ and exposure time ranged from 125 msec to 3 sec.	He-Ne burn thresholds on the retina of mammalian eyes were noted by 24 hours via fundus photography (in 6 of 16 exposures) or by opthalmoscopic exam.	"The data indicate that for worst case accidental exposure to He-Ne lasers (whole beam entering eye and focused on minimal spot size) the threshold power for irreversible burn damage in the monkey is about 7 mW at the cornea." "Until more reliable data are forthcoming, the He-Ne total power entering the human eye should be limited to 1 mW or less."
Gabel, 1995[7] **Laser and bruising with exercise** Case series Aust J Physiother	Two female long-distance runners and Scottish country dancers (no demographics) presented with soleous (lateral mid-belly) subacute strains toward the end of their training session. There was pain on	Both patients were treated with low-level laser therapy (904-nm gallium arsenide laser; LTU Mark 1) 4 days after injury. Parameters: 1 mW average power, 1 W peak power, 6-mm-diameter probe, 2.44 J cm^{-2} energy density, for 11.5 min. Seven to 8 spots (1 cm apart) received 0.03 to 0.15 J.	Follow-up revealed bruising at the sites of laser spot application that was more defined at the sites receiving higher laser dosages. (Bruising occurred the morning following treatment.) Less discomfort was noted during the training.	The author believed the laser increased permeability of soft tissue structures, and the subsequent exercise moved a possible intramuscular hematoma to a more superficial location where it became visible.

walking and running (greater at toe off).

Both patients also performed calf stretches and resumed training within 4 hours of treatment.

Over the next week, two to three additional laser treatments were administered with no further side effects noted.

Alternative mechanisms for the bruising include (1) weakening connective tissue by the laser, (2) increasing the local pain threshold, allowing exercise beyond the typical point of pain, or (3) pressure from examiner palpation or the laser probe during application.

Note: One patient in the placebo group, who received NO laser, complained of a dramatic increase in symptoms by the eighth session and dropped out of the study.

Waylonis et al, 1988[9]
Laser side effects and fibromyalgia (fibrositis; myofascial pain syndrome)
Experiment: crossover, double blind
Arch Phys Med Rehab

A total of 62 patients with fibromyalgia were randomly assigned to one of four groups. There were 6 males and 56 females.

Groups were given two sessions of five treatments of laser, placebo, or crossed over with both, with session separated by 6 weeks. There was a 120-day long-term follow-up period. Pain was measured with a McGill Pain Questionnaire.

Laser (Dynatronic 1120) was applied to 12 acupuncture points for 15-second durations at the hand (Ho ku), cervical, dorsal, and shoulder area.

Seven patients dropped out of the study.

Aside from the main findings of no significant difference for this population using acupuncture points with laser, a few side effects are reported below.

In the placebo group: Two patients complained of increased pain.

In the laser group: Two patients complained of numbness and tingling and another patient had a temporary skin rash.

REFERENCES

1. Snyder-Mackler L, Collender SL: Therapeutic uses of light in rehabilitation. In: Michlovitz SL, editor: Thermal agents in rehabilitation, ed 3. Philadelphia: F.A. Davis; 1996.

2. Tan JC: Practical manual of physical medicine and rehabilitation: diagnostics, therapeutics, and basic problems. St. Louis: Mosby; 1998.

3. Cameron MH, Perez D, Otaño-Lata S: Electromagnetic radiation. In: Cameron MH: Physical agents in rehabilitation: from research to practice. St. Louis: Saunders; 2003.

4. Saliba E, Foreman-Saliba S: Low-power lasers. In: Prentice WE, editor: Therapeutic modalities for physical therapists, ed 2. New York: McGraw-Hill; 2002.

5. Weisberg J, Adams D: Low-level laser therapy. In: Hecox B, Mehreteab TA, Weisberg J, eds: Integrating physical agents in rehabilitation. Upper Saddle River (NJ): Pearson Prentice Hall; 2006.

6. Basford JR: Therapeutic physical agents. In: Delisa JA, editor: Physical medicine and rehabilitation: principles and practices, ed 4, vol 1. Philadelphia: Lippincott Williams & Wilkins; 2005.

7. Gabel P: Does laser enhance bruising in acute sporting injuries? Aust J Physiother 41:273-275, 1995.

8. Bliddal H, Hellesen C, Ditleven P, et al.: Soft-laser therapy of rheumatoid arthritis. Scand J Rheumatol 16:225-228, 1987.

9. Waylonis GW, Wilke S, O'Toole D, et al.: Chronic myofascial pain management by low-output helium-neon laser therapy. Arch Phys Med Rehab 69(12):1017-1020, 1988.

10. Kahn J: Principles and practice of electrotherapy, ed 4. New York: Churchill Livingstone; 2000.

11. Ham WT Jr, Geeraets WJ, Mueller HA, et al.: Retinal burn thresholds for the helium-neon laser in the rhesus monkey. Arch Ophthalmol 84(6):797-809, 1970.

45.2 Ultraviolet (UV) Therapy

OVERVIEW. Ultraviolet therapy uses electromagnetic radiation beyond the violet end, acting to facilitate steroid metabolism, enhance vasomotor responses, and elicit bacteriocidal and antirachitic ("against rickets") effects.[1] Clinically, it is used to treat psoriasis (for nonacute stages by promoting exfoliation), acne vulgaris (by promoting exfoliation), uremic pruritus (by reducing skin itchiness in chronic renal failure), jaundice (by eliminating bilirubin in newborns), and wounds (by killing bacteria, boasting immune response and circulation).[2]

SUMMARY: CONTRAINDICATIONS AND PRECAUTIONS. Five sources cited 38 concerns for ultraviolet therapy. Concerns ranged from 13 to 25 per source, with a physical therapist citing the largest number. Most concerns fell under the ICD skin category. The most frequently cited concerns were the use of UV therapy on individuals with lupus erythematosus, pulmonary tuberculosis, or renal insufficiency. Other commonly cited concerns were eczema, acute psoriasis, hepatic insufficiency, photosensitive medications, hyperthyroidism, and diabetes. Conditions were often listed as concerns because of known photosensitivity, or poor tolerance of UV therapy. Sources generally noted the need for eye protection during UV therapy.

OTHER ISSUES: UV AND INFANTS. In 1992, Siegfried et al[3] reported a case series of two premature infants who received phototherapy (UVA) for neonatal jaundice and sustained phototherapy-induced erythema, one with second-degree burns after exposure to UVA without protective Plexiglas shields (see Thermotherapy for details).

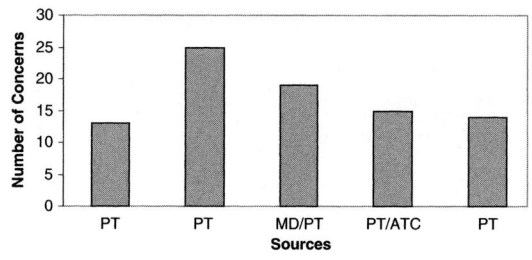

Number of Concerns per Source for Ultraviolet Therapy

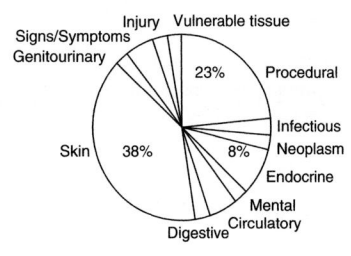

Proportion of Concerns for Ultraviolet Therapy Based on ICD

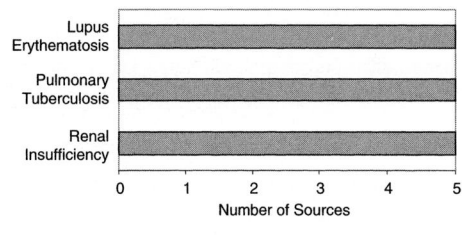

Top 3 Concerns for Ultraviolet Therapy (n = 5)

CONTRAINDICATIONS AND PRECAUTIONS

A00-B99 CERTAIN INFECTIONS AND PARASITIC DISEASES

Issue	LOC	Sources	Affil	Rationale/Comment
Pulmonary tuberculosis	P	Snyder-Mackler and Collender, 1996[4]	PT	Concern for exacerbating the infection.[2]
	CI	Cameron et al, 2003[5]	PT	
	Caution	Tan, 1998[6,a]	MD/PT	
	CI	Davis, 2002[7]	PT/ATC	
	CI/P	Weisberg and Balogun, 2006[2,b]	PT	

a, Active progressive TB; b, Active.

C00-C97 NEOPLASMS

Issue	LOC	Sources	Affil	Rationale/Comment
Cancer	P	Weisberg and Balogun, 2006[2]	PT	UV may lead to anemia.

E00-E90 ENDOCRINE, NUTRITIONAL, AND METABOLIC DISEASES

Issue	LOC	Sources	Affil	Rationale/Comment
Diabetes	P	Snyder-Mackler and Collender, 1996[4]	PT	Individuals with diabetes may not tolerate UV.
	Caution	Tan, 1998[6,a]	MD/PT	UV may cause itching due to interactions with insulin.[2]
	CI	Davis, 2002[7]	PT/ATC	
	CI/P	Weisberg and Balogun, 2006[2,b]	PT	
Hyperthyroidism	P	Snyder-Mackler and Collender, 1996[4]	PT	Hyperthyroidism (also thyrotoxicosis) is a condition with
	Caution	Tan, 1998[6]	MD/PT	excessive thyroid hormone secretion that elevates
	CI	Davis, 2002[7]	PT/ATC	metabolism in most systems, resulting in heat intolerance
	P	Weisberg and Balogun, 2006[2]	PT	and sensitivity to light.[8] UV may cause itching due to interactions with thyroid medications.[2]
Porphyria	CI	Tan, 1998[6]	MD/PT	Porphyria is a disturbance of porphyrin metabolism, often
	CI	Davis, 2002[7]	PT/ATC	with cutaneous manifestations. The variegata and
	CI	Weisberg and Balogun, 2006[2]	PT	erythropoietica forms present with photosensitivity.[9]

a, CI in severe diabetes; b, Acute.

F00-F99 MENTAL AND BEHAVIORAL DISORDERS

Issue	LOC	Sources	Affil	Rationale/Comment
Alcoholism	P	Weisberg and Balogun, 2006[2]	PT	Photochemical hypersensitivity.

I00-I99 DISEASES OF THE CIRCULATORY SYSTEM

Issue	LOC	Sources	Affil	Rationale/Comment
Arteriosclerosis—	Caution	Tan, 1998[6]	MD/PT	
advanced	CI	Davis, 2002[7]	PT/ATC	
Cardiac disease	CI	Cameron et al, 2003[5]	PT	Persons with cardiac disease may become worse with UV exposure.[5] Tolerance
	CI/P	Weisberg and Balogun, 2006[2,a]	PT	may be less.[2]

a, CI if severe.

K00-K93 DISEASES OF THE DIGESTIVE SYSTEM

Issue	LOC	Sources	Affil	Rationale/Comment
Hepatic insufficiencies	P	Snyder-Mackler and Collender, 1996[4]	PT	The condition of a person with liver disease may worsen with UV.[5]
	CI	Cameron et al, 2003[5,a]	PT	
	Caution	Tan, 1998[6,b]	MD/PT	
	CI	Davis, 2002[7]	PT/ATC	

a, Liver disease; b, Acute liver failure.

L00-L99 DISEASES OF THE SKIN AND SUBCUTANEOUS TISSUE

Issue	LOC	Sources	Affil	Rationale/Comment
Dermatitis—acute	P	Snyder-Mackler and Collender, 1996[4,a]	PT	
	CI	Weisberg and Balogun, 2006[2,c]	PT	
Dermatitis—generalized	CI	Davis, 2002[7]	PT/ATC	
	Caution	Tan, 1998[6]	MD/PT	
Eczema	P	Weisberg and Balogun, 2006[2,a]	PT	Eczema may be exacerbated. Note: Three sources specify acute.
	CI	Tan, 1998[6]	PT	
	P	Snyder-Mackler and Collender, 1996[4,a]	PT	
	CI	Davis, 2002[7,a]	PT/ATC	
Herpes simplex	P	Weisberg and Balogun, 2006[2]	PT	Herpes simplex may be exacerbated with UV.[2]
	CI	Tan, 1998[6]	MD/PT	
	CI	Davis, 2002[7]	PT/ATC	
Lupus erythematosus	CI/P	Weisberg and Balogun, 2006[2,b]	PT	UV may exacerbate lupus erythematosus.[2,5] Of SLE patients,
	CI	Tan, 1998[6]	MD/PT	45%[10] are photosensitive. **James et al[10] reported a**
	CI	Cameron et al, 2003[5]	PT	**39-year-old female with systemic lupus erythematosus**
	P	Snyder-Mackler and Collender, 1996[4]	PT	**and end-stage renal failure with hyperparathyroidism**
	CI	Davis, 2002[7]	PT/ATC	**who developed calciphylaxis (potentially life-threatening painful ischemic skin necrosis) following UV therapy for the treatment of pruritus.**

Continued

Issue	LOC	Sources	Affil	Rationale/Comment
Pellagra	CI	Tan, 1998[6]	MD/PT	Pellagra or vitamin B_3 deficiency (i.e., niacin) presents with
	CI	Davis, 2002[7]	PT/ATC	dermatitis, diarrhea, and dementia. Photosensitive eruptions
	CI	Weisberg and Balogun, 2006[2]	PT	and erythema over sun-exposed areas lead to hyperpigmentation, desquamation, and crusting.[11]
Photosensitivity	P	Cameron et al, 2003[5]	PT	Individuals with these characteristics (red hair, fair skin and hair)
	CI	Weisberg and Balogun, 2006[2]	PT	may have an exaggerated response to UV. (Modify: lower dose.)
Premature aging	P	Snyder-Mackler and Collender, 1996[3]	PT	
Psoriasis—acute	P	Weisberg and Balogun, 2006[2]	PT	Acute psoriasis may be exacerbated with UV.[2]
	CI	Tan, 1998[6]	MD/PT	
	P	Snyder-Mackler and Collender, 1996[4]	PT	
	CI	Davis, 2002[7]	PT/ATC	
Sarcoidosis	CI	Tan, 1998[6]	MD/PT	Sarcoidosis is a chronic progressive systemic granulomatous
	CI	Davis, 2002[7]	PT/ATC	reticulitis with hard tubercles affecting almost any tissue. In
	CI	Weisberg and Balogun, 2006[2]	PT	the skin, it presents as skin plaque and cancer.[11]
Scars	Caution	Tan, 1998[6]	MD/PT	Note: Scars may be insensate.
Skin—atrophic	Caution			
Skin cancer	P	Snyder-Mackler and Collender, 1996[4]	PT	UV irradiation causes DNA damage. With chronic exposure,
	CI	Cameron et al, 2003[5]	PT	photocarcinogenesis leads to skin cancers.[12] **In a review, patients with psoriasis who took oral methoxsalen and PUV A developed nonmelanoma skin cancer 5 to 10 years after first treatment.**[13]

Skin cancer, history	P	Weisberg and Balogun, 2006[2]	PT	May be more sensitive to UV. If treating, lower overall dosage.
Xeroderma pigmentosum	CI	Tan, 1998[6]	MD/PT	Xeroderma pigmentosum (xerotic = pigmented dark skin) is a
	CI	Davis, 2002[7]	PT/ATC	rare and fatal autosomal recessive condition characterized
	CI	Weisberg and Balogun, 2006[2]	PT	by photosensitivity and early onset of all major forms of skin
				cancer. Easily sunburned with mild sun exposure.[11]
				In a review of 830 published cases, Kraemer et al[14] reported 158 patients (19%) had abnormal reactions to sunlight and 378 (45%) had some form of malignant skin neoplasm.

a, Acute; b, CI for discoid lupus, P for systematic; c, Acute skin pathologies.

N00-N99 DISEASES OF THE GENITOURINARY SYSTEM

Issue	LOC	Sources	Affil	Rationale/Comment
Renal insufficiencies	P	Snyder-Mackler and Collender, 1996[4]	PT	Individuals with renal insufficiencies may not tolerate UV.
	CI	Cameron et al, 2003[5]	PT	
	Caution	Tan, 1998[6]	MD/PT	
	CI	Davis, 2002[7]	PT/ATC	
	P	Weisberg and Balogun, 2006[2]	PT	

R00-R99 SYMPTOMS, SIGNS

Issue	LOC	Sources	Affil	Rationale/Comment
Fair complexion	Caution	Tan, 1998[6]	MD/PT	Individuals with red or blond hair have exaggerated response to UV. If treatment
	P	Weisberg and Balogun, 2006[2]	PT	is necessary, use lower MED and treatment exposures on these individuals.[2]
Fever	CI	Cameron et al, 2003[5]	PT	The condition may worsen following UV exposure[5] and may elevate core
	CI	Weisberg and Balogun, 2006[2]	PT	temperature.[2]

S00-T98 INJURY, POISONING, AND CERTAIN OTHER CONSEQUENCES OF EXTERNAL CAUSES

Issue	LOC	Sources	Affil	Rationale/Comment
Burns/redness	P	Snyder-Mackler and Collender, 1996[4]	PT	

Vulnerable Biological Tissues

Issue	LOC	Sources	Affil	Rationale/Comment
Eyes	CI	Cameron et al, 2003[5]	PT	UV radiation can damage the cornea, eyelids, and lens (patient and clinician wear UV-opaque goggles throughout treatment) (also see procedural concerns). Based on epidemiological studies, cortical and posterior subcapsular type cataracts are associated with dose-related UVB exposure to the eyes.[15] **Hightower, in an animal study, demonstrated cataracts in cultured rabbit lenses exposed to low irradiation levels (1-2 mW/cm^2) within the 295-340 nm spectral range.[16]**

PROCEDURAL CONCERNS

Issue	LOC	Sources	Affil	Rationale/Comment
Age, infants or elderly	P	Weisberg and Balogun, 2006[2,a]	PT	Patient may have low tolerance.[2]
Chemotherapy, receiving	P			Patient may have low tolerance.[2]
Foods, ingestion	P			Ingestion of strawberries, eggs, or shellfish prior to treatment can lead to increased sensitivity to UV.
Photosensitive or interacting medications	P	Snyder-Mackler and Collender, 1996[4]	PT	The interaction of UV and photosensitive medication such as antibiotics and diuretics can cause general dermatitis and
	P	Cameron et al, 2003[5]	PT	itching, increase sensitivity to UV, and increase the risk of
	Caution	Tan, 1998[6]	MD/PT	burns. If the patient is taking photosensitive medications,
	P	Weisberg and Balogun, 2006[2,a]	PT	remeasure minimal erythemal dose (MED). Inquire if patients is taking sulfonamide, tetracycline, quinolone (antibiotics), gold-based medications (for RA), amiodarone hydrochloride, quinidines (for arrhythmias), phenothiazines (for anxiety), or psoralens (for psoriasis).[4] Also caution with use of cosmetics[6] **(also see footnote for some additional medications[2]).**
Protective (polarized) goggles	P	Snyder-Mackler and Collender, 1996[4]	PT	Patient and therapist must wear protective (polarized/UV
	Caution	Tan, 1998[6]	MD/PT	goggles) or cotton pledgets at all times.[6]
	Advice	Cameron et al, 2003[5]	PT	

Continued

Issue	LOC	Sources	Affil	Rationale/Comment
Recent x-rays to an area	P	Cameron et al, 2003[5]	PT	These irradiated areas may be more vulnerable to cancer development.[5] Also, there is cellular breakdown and inflammation in the epidermis similar to a first-degree burn. Avoid heat modalities.[17]
Repeated UV radiation when effects of previous dose still apparent	P			To minimize risk of burns, determine if the effects of a previous UV dose are still visible.
Superficial heat administered prior to UV	P	Weisberg and Balogun, 2006[2]	PT	
Shock hazards	Shock hazard	Arledge, 1978[18]	PT	Never assume hospital maintenance will be conducted or is conducted for all hazardous areas. On older ultraviolet lamps, a metal tape retrieving system may jam or break. If forced into the lamp and the tape touches the electrical wiring, a lethal shock can occur.

a, UV may heighten the medication effects of the following: sulfonamides, sulfonylurea, griseofulvin, tetracycline, quinine, endocrines, gold, other heavy metals, diuretics, insulin, phenothiazines, psoralens, tar. UV can cause blotching with birth control pill use.

REFERENCES

1. Bottomley JM: Quick reference dictionary for physical therapy. Thorofare (NJ): Slack; 2000.
2. Weisberg J, Balogun JA Ultraviolet radiation. In: Hecox B, Mehreteab TA, Weisberg J, eds: Integrating physical agents in rehabilitation. Upper Saddle River (NJ): Pearson Prentice Hall; 2006.

3. Siegfried EC, Stone MS, Madison KC: Ultraviolet light burn: a cutaneous complication of visible light phototherapy of neonatal jaundice. Pediatr Dermatol 9:278-282, 1992.

4. Snyder-Mackler L, Collender SL: Therapeutic uses of light in rehabilitation. In: Michlovitz SL, editor: Thermal agents in rehabilitation, ed 3. Philadelphia: F.A. Davis; 1996.

5. Cameron MH, Perez D, Otaño-Lata S: Electromagnetic radiation. In: Cameron MH, editor: Physical agents in rehabilitation: from research to practice. St. Louis: Saunders; 2003.

6. Tan JC: Practical manual of physical medicine and rehabilitation: diagnostics, therapeutics, and basic problems. St. Louis: Mosby; 1998.

7. Davis JM: Ultraviolet therapy. In: Prentice WE, editor: Therapeutic modalities for physical therapists, ed 2. New York: McGraw-Hill; 2002.

8. Goodman CC, Snyder TEK: The endocrine and metabolic systems. In: Goodman CC, Boissonnault WG, Fuller KS, eds: Pathology: implications for the physical therapist, ed 2. Philadelphia: Saunders; 2003.

9. Dorland's illustrated medical dictionary, ed 24. Philadelphia: Saunders; 1965.

10. James LR, Lajoie G, Prajapati D, et al: Calciphylaxis precipitated by ultraviolet light in a patient with end-stage renal disease secondary to systemic lupus erythematosus. Am J Kidney Dis 34(5):932-936, 1999.

11. Bolognia JC, Jarizzo JL, Rapini RP: Dermatology. Edinburgh, Scotland: Mosby; 2003.

12. Matsumura Y, Ananthaswamy HN: Toxic effects of ultraviolet radiation on the skin. Toxicol Appl Pharmacol 195(3):298-308, 2004.

13. Burns F: Cancer risk associated with therapeutic irradiation of skin. Arch Dermatol 125:979-981, 1989.

14. Kraemer KH, Lee MM, Scotto J: Xeroderma pigmentosum: Cutaneous, ocular, and neurologic abnormalities in 830 published cases. Arch Dermatol 123:241-250, 1987.

15. Taylor HR: The biological effects of ultraviolet-B on the eye. Photochem Photobiol 50(4):489-492, 1989.

16. Hightower K, McCready J: Physiological effects of UVB irradiation on cultured rabbit lens. Invest Ophthalmol Vis Sci 33(5):1783-1787, 1992.

17. Goodman CC, Snyder TEK: Problems affecting multiple systems. In: Goodman CC, Boissonnault WG, Fuller KS, eds: Pathology: implications for the physical therapist, ed 2. Philadelphia: Saunders; 2003.

18. Arledge RL: Prevention of electric shock hazards in physical therapy. Phys Ther 58(10):1215-1217, 1978.

46   SOUND AGENTS

46.1 Therapeutic Ultrasound

OVERVIEW. Therapeutic ultrasound is a physical agent that emits high frequency oscillations or sound waves (0.7 to 3.3 MHz frequency range) that penetrates tissue and produces deep heat. The clinical aim is to promote healing by softening scar tissue, increasing cell metabolism, and promoting nutrition. The agent has both a thermal and mechanical effect.[1] Because therapeutic ultrasound produces heat, tissues need to be capable of dissipating heat via adequate blood circulation.

SUMMARY: CONTRAINDICATIONS AND PRECAUTIONS. Eight sources cited a total of 37 concerns for therapeutic US. Concerns ranged from 7 to 23 per source with a physician citing the largest number and an OT citing the fewest number. The greatest percentage of concerns related to vulnerable tissue (e.g., over reproductive tissue, eyes, heart, or neural tissue). The most frequently cited concerns were neoplasm, pregnancy, and over the eye (cited by all 8 sources).

While not formally listed under contraindications, sources generally recommended the procedure of moving the sound head (i.e., avoid stationary transducers) to avoid increasing the risk of hot spots, unstable cavitation, blood cell stasis, or blood vessel damage to the endothelial cells. Pain from a stationary technique may suggest periosteal heating. In an in vivo 1974 study, Dyson[2] describes blood cell stasis (temporary blood flow arrest) and endothelial damage (permanent) in the blood vessels of a chick embryo treated with US using a stationary technique (minimum intensity <0.5 W/cm²; 3 MHz).[2]

OTHER ISSUES. In a case series, Gnatz[3] reported transient radicular symptoms in 36-year-old and 37-year-old females with lumbar disc herniations a few minutes following US treatment to lumbar paraspinals at 1.5-1.75 W/cm². The incidences were postulated to be due to heat-induced edema accumulation within a confined space.

Note: Several sources incorporates general thermotherapy concerns into their US guidelines.

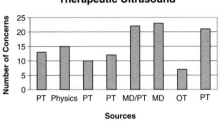

Number of Concerns per Source for Therapeutic Ultrasound

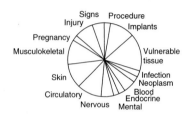

Proportion of Concerns for Therapeutic US Based on ICD

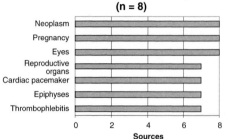

Top 7 Cited Concerns for Therapeutic US (n = 8)

A00-B99 CERTAIN INFECTIONS AND PARASITIC DISEASES

Issue	LOC	Source	Affil	Rationale/Comment
Infections/ Infectious conditions	CI	Oakley, 1978[4]	PT	Ultrasound may stimulate cell division. Also, US may spread infection.[6]
	CI	ter Haar et al, 1987[5]	Physics	
	CI	Sweitzer, 2006[6]	PT	
	CI/P	Basford, 2005[7]	MD	

C00-C97 NEOPLASMS

Issue	LOC	Source	Affil	Rationale/Comment
Tumor	CI	McDiarmid et al, 1996[8,a]	PT	US may increase growth rate and size of tumors. Furthermore, vibration may stimulate
	CI	ter Haar et al, 1987[5,b]	Physics	tissue to grow and encourage metastasis.[10] Increased cellular detachment and possible
	CI	Oakley, 1978[4]	PT	metastasis have been shown in in-vitro studies, and increased tumor growth has
	CI	Cameron, 2003[1,a]	PT	been noted in an in vivo study. **In a randomized animal experiment ($N = 76$),**
	CI	Tan, 1998[9,a]	MD/PT	**Sicard-Rosenbaum[11] found in an experimental group of mice injected with**
	CI/Avoid	Bracciano, 2000[10]	OT	**tumor cells and receiving 10 US treatments (continuous; 3 MHz, 1.0 W/cm^2),**
	CI	Sweitzer, 2006[6,b]	PT	**that subcutaneous murine tumors increased in both size (394 mm^3) and**
	CI/P	Basford, 2005[7]	MD	**weight (426 g).**

a, Malignant tissue; b, Malignant and benign.

D50-D89 DISEASES OF BLOOD AND BLOOD-FORMING ORGANS, AND CERTAIN DISORDERS

Issue	LOC	Source	Affil	Rationale/ Comment
Hemorrhage	CI/P	Tan, 1998[9]	MD/PT	
	CI/P	Basford, 2005[7,a]	MD	
Bleeding disorder—	CI/P	Tan, 1998[9]	MD/PT	US can increase capillary permeability and blood flow and promote bleeding.
tendency to bleed	CI	Sweitzer, 2006[6]	PT	
	CI/P	Basford, 2005[7]	MD	

a, Acute.

E00-E90 ENDOCRINE, NUTRITIONAL, AND METABOLIC DISEASES

Issue	LOC	Source	Affil	Rationale/Comment
Diabetes	CI	ter Haar et al, 1987[5]	Physics	The tissue may not be able to adequately dissipate heat in persons with diabetes.
	CI	Oakley, 1978[4]	PT	Also, there is a slight reduction in blood sugar during insonation. If treating, give low intensity and short dosage and encourage rest after treatment.

F00-F99 MENTAL AND BEHAVIORAL DISORDERS

Issue	LOC	Source	Affil	Rationale/Comment
Communicate—	CI/P	Tan, 1998[9]	MD/PT	
inability	CI	Sweitzer, 2006[6]	PT	
	CI/P	Basford, 2005[7]	MD	

G00-G99 DISEASES OF THE NERVOUS SYSTEM

Issue	LOC	Source	Affil	Rationale/Comment
Pain/temperature	P	McDiarmid et al, 1996[8]	PT	Patient may not be able to inform the clinician when intensity is excessive
sensation impaired	CI	ter Haar et al, 1987[5,a]	Physics	(too hot) if sensation is impaired.
	CI/P	Tan, 1998[9]	MD/PT	

Continued

Issue	LOC	Source	Affil	Rationale/Comment
	CI	Sweitzer, 2004[6,b]	PT	
	CI/P	Basford, 2005[7]	MD	
Thermal regulation impaired	CI/P	Tan, 1998[9]	MD/PT	
	CI/P	Basford, 2005[7]	MD	

a, Diminished pain appreciation; b, Anesthesia or dysthesia concerns.

I00-I99 DISEASES OF THE CIRCULATORY SYSTEM

Issue	LOC	Source	Affil	Rationale/Comment
Blood vessels in poor condition	CI	Oakley, 1978[4]	PT	Vibration can cause rupture of vessel walls. Thrombi may loosen and form emboli.
Cardiac disease	CI	Oakley, 1978[4]	PT	Stimulation of afferent nerves, particularly the vagus nerve, could cause a change in cardiac rate. Don't treat over cervical ganglia, stellate ganglion, the thorax region of the heart, or the vagus nerve because a coronary reflex might result. Keep intensity low and duration time short in other areas because the heart receives fibers from both sympathetic and parasympathetic portions of the autonomic nervous system.
	CI	Sweitzer, 2006[6]	PT	
	CI	ter Haar et al, 1987[5]	Physics	
	CI/P	Basford, 2005[7,a]	MD	
Circulation/ischemia, impaired	CI/P	Tan, 1998[9]	MD/PT	Heat may not be adequately dissipated in PVD.[6]
	CI	Sweitzer, 2006[6]	PT	
	P	McDiarmid et al, 1996[8]	PT	
	CI/P	Basford, 2005[7]	MD	

Thrombophlebitis—	CI	McDiarmid et al, 1996[8]	PT	US applications may increase the possibility of dislodging a thrombus.
over/near	CI	ter Haar et al, 1987[5]	Physics	Vibrations can cause partial disintegration of clot, travel to a vital organ,
	CI	Oakley, 1978[4]	PT	resulting in obstructions in the brain, heart, or lungs.
	CI	Cameron, 2003[1]	PT	
	CI	Tan, 1998[9]	MD/PT	
	Care	Bracciano, 2000[10]	OT	
	CI	Sweitzer, 2006[6]	PT	

a, From thermotherapy concerns: unstable angina, unstable blood pressure, or decompensated heart failure (within 6-8 weeks of a myocardial infarction). Note: These are thermotherapy concerns that are added to US guidelines as author indicated.

L00-L99 DISEASES OF THE SKIN AND SUBCUTANEOUS TISSUE

Issue	LOC	Source	Affil	Rationale/Comment
Infected skin lesion	CI/P	Tan, 1998[9]	MD/PT	
Scar—immature	CI/P	Tan, 1998[9]	MD/PT	Reduced sensation may lead to burns (see Thermotherapy).
	CI/P	Basford, 2005[7]	MD	
Skin, atrophic	CI/P	Basford, 2005[7]	MD	
Skin graft— superficial	CI/P	Tan, 1998[9]	MD/PT	

M00-M99 DISEASES OF THE MUSCULOSKELETAL SYSTEM AND CONNECTIVE TISSUE

Issue	LOC	Source	Affil	Rationale/Comment
Osteoporosis	P	Sweitzer, 2006[6]	PT	Further information is needed to rule out the effects of US on demineralized bone.
Primary repair of tendon or ligament	P	Sweitzer, 2006[6,a]	PT	Also, early stage, partial tendon ruptures.
Sepsis, bone—acute	CI	ter Haar et al, 1987[5]	Physics	The concern is the spread of infection because there is no superficial escape route
	CI	Oakley, 1978[4]	PT	for pus.
	CI	Tan, 1998[9]	MD/PT	
Sepsis, soft tissue—acute	CI	ter Haar et al, 1987[5]	Physics	

O00-O99 PREGNANCY, CHILDBIRTH, AND PUERPERIUM

Issue	LOC	Source	Affil	Rationale/Comment
Pregnant uterus—over	CI	McDiarmid et al, 1996[8]	PT	Maternal hyperthermia (US near fetus leading to temperature elevations) is associated
	CI	ter Haar et al, 1987[5]	Physics	with fetal abnormalities (low birth weight, reduced brain size, orthopedic
	CI	Oakley, 1978[4]	PT	deformities). Also, the area is a fluid-filled cavity, which is avoided during US
	CI	Cameron, 2003[1]	PT	applications. Inquire if patient is pregnant or attempting to become pregnant.
	CI	Tan, 1998[9]	MD/PT	Avoid abdomen, pelvis, or lumbar or sacral areas of pregnant patients. **In a case**
	CI	Bracciano, 2000[10]	OT	**report, McLeod and Fowlow[12] described a 28-year-old female with left**
	CI	Sweitzer, 2006[6,a]	PT	**psoas bursitis who received 18 treatments of US between the 6th and**
	CI/P	Basford, 2005[7,b]	MD	**29th days after conception. (She was unknowingly pregnant.) Her baby**
				exhibited multiple dysmorphic features; delayed gross, fine, and
				receptive/expressive language; and growth below the 5th percentile.

a, The guideline does not include diagnostic ultrasound as a CI; avoid pelvis, abdomen and LS areas; b, Gravid uterus.

Issue	LOC	Source	Affil	Rationale/Comment
Edema	CI/P	Tan, 1998[9]	MD/PT	Heating can increase edema formation.
	CI/P	Basford, 2005[7]	MD	
Fever	CI	Sweitzer, 2006[6]	PT	Avoid adding to the heat of a systemic temperature.
Inflammation, acute	P	Cameron, 2003[1]	PT	The thermal effects of US can increase bleeding and edema in acutely inflamed tissue.
	CI/P	Tan, 1998[8]	MD/PT	Inquire about any trauma over the past 2 to 3 days.
	CI	Sweitzer, 2006[6]	PT	
	CI/P	Basford, 2005[7,a]	MD	

a, Acutely inflamed joints because of concern that intraarticular temperature elevations will lead to increased enzyme activity.

S00-T98 INJURY, POISONING, AND CERTAIN OTHER CONSEQUENCES OF EXTERNAL CAUSES

Issue	LOC	Source	Affil	Rationale/Comment
Fractures—over	P	Cameron, 2003[1]	PT	*High-intensity* US causes pain and may impair fracture healing.[1]
	P	Sweitzer, 2006[6,a]	PT	Low-intensity US over fracture sites may actually shorten fracture healing time.[1] McDiarmid[8] believes there is no reason to avoid fracture areas unless sensation is impaired.
Trauma— acute	P	Cameron, 2003[1]	PT	See Acute inflammation, above.
	CI/P	Tan, 1998[9]	MD/PT	
	CI/P	Basford, 2005[7]	MD	

a, Unhealed sites.

VALUNERABLE BIOLOGICAL TISSUES

Issue	LOC	Source		Rationale/Comment
Cervical and stellate ganglia	CI	Tan, 1998[9]	MD/PT	
	CI/P	Basford, 2005[7,f]	MD	
CNS tissue—over	CI	Oakley, 1978[4,a]	PT	US may damage nerve tissue, especially in areas not covered by bone. Avoid US over fluid-filled cavity (head). Inquire if patient had a laminectomy. **Borrelli et al[13] reported spinal cord damage (mainly periphery and ventrally) associated with paralysis in neonatal mice exposed to 1 MHz of unfocused continuous US at 40 to 289 W/cm² intensities over the lumbar area.**
	CI	Cameron, 2003[1]	PT	
	CI	Tan, 1998[9]	MD/PT	
	CI	Sweitzer, 2006[6,b]	PT	
	CI	Basford, 2005[7,e]	MD	
Epiphyseal areas in children—over	P/Caution	McDiarmid et al, 1996[8]	PT	Controversial. The concern is particularly for treatments at high intensities. There is some evidence of damage to epiphyseal plates (growth areas), bone demineralization, and bone growth retardation at US intensities above 3.0 W/cm² for 3 minutes or more with a stationary transducer. Determine if plate has closed and avoid high dosage over these growing epiphyseal plates.[1]
	CI	ter Haar et al, 1987[5]	Physics	
	P	Cameron, 2003[1]	PT	
	CI	Tan, 1998[9]	MD/PT	
	Avoid if possible	Bracciano, 2000[10]	OT	
	CI	Sweitzer, 2006[6]	PT	
	CI/P	Basford, 2005[7]	MD	
Eyes—over	CI	McDiarmid et al, 1996[8]	PT	The lens has a poor blood supply, so heat dissipation may be inadequate, resulting in cataracts. Also, avoid US over fluid-filled cavities. US may cause cavitation of ocular fluid and damage the eye and the retina.[1,6]
	CI	ter Haar et al, 1987[5]	Physics	
	CI	Oakley, 1978[4]	PT	
	CI	Cameron, 2003[1]	PT	
	CI	Tan, 1998[9]	MD/PT	
	CI	Bracciano, 2000[10]	OT	
	CI	Sweitzer, 2006[6]	PT	
	CI/P	Basford, 2005[7,d]	MD	

Heart—over	CI	McDiarmid et al, 1996[8]	PT	Avoid US directly over this area. ECG changes in dogs occurred after direct US
	CI	Bracciano, 2000[10]	OT	exposure to their heart (1.5 W/cm^2).[7]
	CI/P	Basford, 2005[7]	MD	
Reproductive organs—over	CI	ter Haar et al, 1987[5]	Physics	US may affect gamete development in women and men. Avoid US over fluid-filled
	CI	Oakley, 1978[4]	PT	cavities (i.e., testes). Temperature elevation of the testes can result in temporary
	CI	Cameron, 2003[1]	PT	sterility.[7]
	CI	Tan, 1998 (testes)[9,c]	MD/PT	
	CI	McDiarmid et al, 1996[8,c]	PT	
	CI	Bracciano, 2000 (testes)[10,c]	OT	
	CI/P	Basford, 2005[7,d]	MD	

a, US over the brain/head, over spinal cord without protection; b, Over spinal cord without bone protection; c, Over the testes; d, Fluid-filled cavities, concern for cavitation and heat damage; e, Over brain, spine (not high-intensity exposure), laminectomy sites; f, Cervical ganglion.

Y70-Y82 MEDICAL DEVICES

Issue	LOC	Source	Affil	Rationale/Comment
Breast implants	P	Cameron, 2003[1]	PT	High-intensity US may cause implant ruptures. Inquire if patient has a breast implant and avoid high dosages of US in that area.
Cardiac pacemakers— over	CI	McDiarmid et al, 1996[8]	PT	Direct exposure may interfere with electrical circuitry and functioning of the pacemaker. Some authors are concerned about mechanical/thermal damage to unit.
	CI	ter Haar et al, 1987[5]	Physics	
	CI	Oakley, 1978[4]	PT	
	CI	Cameron, 2003[1]	PT	

Continued

Issue	LOC	Source	Affil	Rationale/Comment
	CI	Tan, 1998[9]	MD/PT	
	CI	Sweitzer, 2006[6,b]	PT	
	CI/P	Basford, 2005[7,c]	PT	
Cement and plastic	CI	Cameron, 2003[1]	PT	US rapidly heats both cement (methylmethacrylate) and plastic joint components and may
prosthetic	CI	Tan, 19989	MD/PT	possibly cause loosening due to unstable cavitation in cement. High-density plastics
components	P	Sweitzer, 2005[6,a]	PT	(found in joint replacements) have a high coefficient of absorption.
				Inquire if patient has a plastic joint prosthesis and if it is cemented.[1]
Metal implants—	Caution	Tan, 1998[9]	MD/PT	Controversial—US does not appear to concentrate heat (metal does not rapidly heat)[1,9]
screws, plates,	P	Sweitzer, 2006[6]	PT	or loosen hardware[1] in animal studies.[6]
uncemented	CI/caution	ter Haar et al, 1987[5]	Physics	
prostheses	CI/P	Basford, 2005[7,d]	MD	

a, Plastic; b, Distal body sites are not CI if the pacemaker is unaffected by the sound field; c, Pacemakers; d, Comment that many clinicians avoid area because of concern for increased tissue temperatures.

PROCEDURAL CONCERNS

Issue	LOC	Source	Affil	Rationale/Comment
After/during treatment	CI	ter Haar et al, 1987[5]	Physics	Low-intensity ultrasound and ionizing radiation may interact with and affect surface of
by deep x-ray, radium,	CI	Oakley, 1978[4]	PT	tumor cells (wait 6 months). This concern does not include exposure to routine x-ray.[6]
or radioactive	CI	Sweitzer, 2006[6]	PT	
isotopes				

ADVERSE EVENTS

Source	Background	Therapy	Outcome	Follow-up/Interpretation
McLeod and Fowlow, 1989[12] **Birth defect and ultrasound** Case report Am J Med Genet	A 28-year-old female with left psoas bursitis received 18 therapeutic ultrasound treatments (0.5 W/cm^2 pulsed for 5 minutes).	The patient was later diagnosed as being pregnant, placing the 18 treatments between the 6th and 29th day after conception. Both parents were in generally good health.	A female infant was born at 37 weeks' gestation, birth wt 2100 g, length 43.5 cm, head circumference 28.5 cm. At 5 and 13 months multiple dysmorphic features were noted: large ears, epicanthic folds, low nasal bridge, mild micrognathia, high palate arch, widely spaced chest nipples, sacrum deviated to left and sacral agenesis, mild ventricular enlargement, and clinodactyly. At 21 months, 8- to 12-month, 7-month, and 10- to 12-month delays in gross, fine, and receptive/expressive language, respectively, were noted. Her growth was ranked below the 5th percentile for height, weight, and head circumference.	The authors believe the timing of therapeutic US treatments during fetal development was consistent with microcephaly and sacral agenesis, but that any thermal-related effects were not likely derived from pulsed US. Although ultrasound dosage was low and pulsed, US calibration was not performed frequently. Authors suggested further studies of multiple (additive effect) of US dosage using an animal model.

REFERENCES

1. Cameron MH: Physical agents in rehabilitation: from research to practice. St. Louis: Saunders; 2003.
2. Dyson M, Pond JB, Woodward B, Broadbent J: The production of blood cell stasis and endothelial damage in the blood vessels of chick embryos treated with ultrasound in a stationary wave field. Ultrasound Med Biol 63:133-138, 1974.
3. Gnatz SM: Increased radicular pain due to therapeutic ultrasound applied to the back. Arch Phys Med Rehabil 70(6):493-494, 1989.
4. Oakley EM: Dangers and contraindications of therapeutic ultrasound. Physiotherapy 64:173-174, 1978.
5. ter Haar G, Dyson M, Oakley EM: The use of ultrasound by physiotherapists in Britain, 1985. Ultrasound Med Biol 13(10):659-663, 1987.
6. Sweitzer RW: Ultrasound. In: Hecox B, Mehreteab TA, Weisberg J, eds: Integrating physical agents in rehabilitation. Upper Saddle River (NJ): Pearson Prentice Hall; 2006.
7. Basford JR: Therapeutic physical agents. In: Delisa JA, editor: Physical medicine and rehabilitation: principles and practices, ed 4, vol 1. Philadelphia: Lippincott Williams & Wilkins; 2005.
8. McDiarmid T, Ziskin MC, Michlovitz SL: Therapeutic ultrasound. In: Michlovitz SL, editor: Thermal agents in rehabilitation, ed 3. Philadelphia: F.A. Davis; 1996.
9. Tan JC: Practical manual of physical medicine and rehabilitation: diagnostics, therapeutics, and basic problems. St. Louis: Mosby; 1998.
10. Bracciano AG: Physical agent modalities: theory and application for the occupational therapist. Thorofare (NJ): Slack; 2000.
11. Sicard-Rosenbaum L, Lord D, Danoff JV, et al: Effects of continuous therapeutic ultrasound on growth and metastasis of subcutaneous murine tumors. Phys Ther 75:3-11, 1995.
12. McLeod DR, Fowlow SB: Multiple malformations and exposure to therapeutic ultrasound during organogenesis. Am J Med Genet 34(3): 317-319, 1989.
13. Borrelli MJ Frizzell LA Dunn F: Ultrasonically induced morphological changes in the mammalian neonatal spinal cord. Ultrasound Med Biol 12:285-295, 1986.

46.2 Phonophoresis

Phonophoresis uses sound energy (i.e., ultrasound) to introduce molecules (not ions) into the body.[1] The overall concern is patient sensitivity to the substances (molecules) used during phonophoresis. Note: Other ultrasound concerns probably also apply for this therapy.

L00-L99 DISEASES OF THE SKIN AND SUBCUTANEOUS TISSUE

Issue	LOC	Sources	Affil	Rationale/Comment
Allergies and sensitivities to substances	CI	Kahn, 2000[1]	PT	Some individuals are sensitive or may have systematic skin reactions to the following: • Iodine • Metal • Mecholyl (vasodilator) • Hydrocortisone (may be the novocaine) • Salicylates

REFERENCE

1. Kahn J: Principles and practice of electrotherapy, ed 4, New York: Churchill Livingstone; 2000.

47 THERMOTHERAPY

(Includes Hot Packs, Paraffin Wax, Infrared Lamps)

OVERVIEW. Thermotherapy comprises a number of physical agents that use superficial heat to increase soft tissue extensibility, reduce pain, improve circulation, and accelerate healing. Thermal therapy is believed to accomplish these goals by increasing blood flow (vasodilation), reducing alpha motor neuron firing rate, increasing pain threshold (gating effect; reduced ischemia), and increasing metabolic activity (increasing the availability of oxygen to tissue).[1] Note: Because thermotherapy produces heat, the tissue needs to be capable to dissipating the heat via adequate blood circulation, and the patient must be capable of informing the clinician (or escaping) if the modality gets too hot.

SUMMARY: CONTRAINDICATIONS AND PRECAUTIONS. Six sources cited a total of 31 concerns for thermotherapy. Concerns ranged from 8 to 18 per source, with a physician citing the largest number. The largest proportion of concerns related to the skin, procedural, and circulatory issues. The most frequently cited concerns were malignancy, hemorrhaging, impaired mentation or sensation, and acute inflammation.

OTHER ISSUES: POSSIBLE PROCEDURAL IRREGULARITIES CONTRIBUTING TO COMPLICATIONS. (1) Monitoring insulation: In a 1996 California lawsuit,[2] a 13-year-old girl received a $175,000 arbitration award after she sustained a third-degree arm burn from a hot pack that was inadequately insulated and not periodically monitored. (2) Monitoring excessive treatment: Waldorf et al[3] reported on a 46-year-old woman who developed erythema ab igne (hyperpigmentation) from using an electric heating pad 12 hours a day for about 6 weeks. (3) Monitoring paraffin temperatures: The FDA[4] reports14 incidences of paraffin wax device problems from September 1992 to January 2003. Of these, 10 reports were of wax becoming too hot. Five cases led to hand burns.

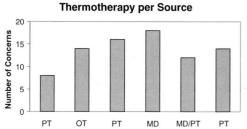

Number of Concerns for Thermotherapy per Source

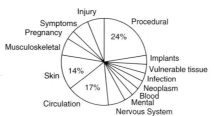

Proportion of Concerns Based on ICD

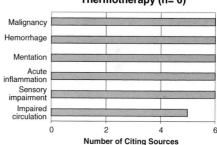

Top 6 Cited Concerns for Thermotherapy (n= 6)

CONTRAINDICATIONS AND PRECAUTIONS FOR SUPERFICIAL HEAT

A00-B99 CERTAIN INFECTIONS AND PARASITIC DISEASES

Issue	LOC	Source	Affil	Rationale/Comment
Infected areas—over	CI	Rennie and Michlovitz, 1996[5]	PT	Heat may help spread of infection. Cross-contamination can also occur (i.e., by exposing an open wound in a paraffin machine; by touching an open wound directly with a hot pack). Finally, some conditions (e.g., skin diseases) may be exacerbated with exposure to moist warm or hot heat.[7] **In a 2002 New York lawsuit,[8] a patient with a left knee replacement and an inflamed unclosed, oozing wound was awarded a $500,000 arbitration verdict after she received moist heat that led to a burn and a worsening of her inflammation.**
	CI	Bracciano, 2000[6]	OT	
	CI	Hecox and Sanko, 2006[7,a]	PT	

a, Local infection with hot pack.

C00-97 NEOPLASM

Issue	LOC	Source	Affil	Rationale/Comment
Malignancy	CI	Cameron, 2003[1]	PT	Increased circulation and metabolism generated from heat can increase the growth
	CI	Rennie and Michlovitz, 1996[5]	PT	rate or metastasis rate of cancer. In terminally ill cancer patients with informed
	CI/P	Tan, 1998[9]	MD/PT	consent, heat provides pain relief. The safety of heat with skin and lymphatic CA
	CI	Bracciano, 2000[6,a]	OT	has not been determined.
	CI	Hecox and Sanko, 2006[7,b]	PT	
	CI/P	Basford, 2005[10]	MD	

a, Tumors; b, Skin and lymphatic cancer; over malignancy for hot packs.

D50-89 DISEASES OF BLOOD AND BLOOD-FORMING ORGANS, AND CERTAIN DISORDERS

Issue	LOC	Source	Affil	Rationale/Comment
Hemorrhage—	CI	Cameron, 2003[1]	PT	Heat causes a vasodilatory response that can reopen a vascular lesion. Inquire about
recent or	CI	Rennie and Michlovitz, 1996[5]	PT	any bleeding disorders or bruising.
potential	CI/P	Tan, 1998[9]	MD/PT	
	CI	Bracciano, 2000[6]	OT	
	CI	Hecox and Sanko, 2006[7,a]	PT	
	CI/P	Basford, 2005[10,b]	MD	

a, Specified for hot pack; b, Or bleeding disorders.

F00-F99 MENTAL AND BEHAVIORAL DISORDERS

Issue	LOC	Source	Affil	Rationale/Comment
Mentation impaired	CI	Cameron, 2003[1,c]	PT	The patients must report if treatment is too hot to prevent burns and ensure
	CI/P	Tan, 1998[9]	MD/PT	a safe level heat level (e.g., in dementia, sensations may not be reported accurately).
	CI	Bracciano, 2000[6,a]	OT	
	CI	Hecox and Sanko, 2006[7]	PT	
	CI	Rennie and Michlovitz, 1996[5,b]	PT	
	CI/P	Basford, 2005[10]	MD	

a, Semicomatose; b, Unreliable situations such as language difficulties; c, Lack of ability to report heat sensation.

G00-99 DISEASES OF THE NERVOUS SYSTEM

Issue	LOC	Source	Affil	Rationale/Comment
Sensation impaired	CI	Cameron, 2003[1]	PT	The patients must perceive pain or heat threshold to prevent burns and ensure a safe
	CI/P	Tan, 1998[9]	MD/PT	heating level. Dysthesia can lead to burns.[7]
	CI	Rennie and Michlovitz, 1996[5]	PT	Consider testing temperature sensation using test tubes. With impaired areas, consider
	CI	Bracciano, 2000[6]	OT	applying heat proximally to insensate area. **Katcher and Shapiro,[11] in a 1987**
	CI	Hecox and Sanko, 2006[7,b]	PT	**retrospective chart review, found that of 37 patients with diabetes mellitus**
	CI/P	Basford, 2005[10,c]	MD	**who received burn therapy, 27% had LE burns related to sensory loss.**

Continued

Issue	LOC	Source	Affil	Rationale/Comment
				Bill et al[12] reported a case series involving a 32-year-old with L5-S1 spina bifida who required skin grafts due to burns on the feet caused by a heating pad. Also reported was a 39-year-old with insulin-dependent diabetes who sustained a full-thickness malleolus burn from a electric heating pad.
				Stevenson et al,[13] in a 1985 case series, reported on three women s/p breast reconstruction with flaps who sustained burns from placing a hot pack or pad over the area.
				Nahabedian and McGibbon[14] reported four additional cases with similar outcomes of treating reconstructed breast areas with a heat source, one of which was from sunbathing. (Also see Hwang under Hydrotherapy.)
Thermal regulation impaired	P CI/P CI/P	Cameron, 2003[1] Tan, 1998[9,a,d] Basford, 2005[10,d]	PT MD/PT MD	The patient with thermal regulation problems may not adequately vasodilate to keep an area from burning. The very young and old are particularly at risk.[1,7] Consider using lower heat, more insulation, and more frequent monitoring.[1]
				Simonsen et al,[15] in a 1995 case series, reported on second-degree burns sustained by two newborns treated with infrared heat lamps during resuscitation efforts.
				In a 1977 longitudinal study of 47 elderly people, Collins et al[16] found a smaller body core shell temperature gradient during controlled, environmental temperature changes when compared to young controls, over a 5-year period. This physiologic response indicated progressive thermoregulatory impairment possibly due to an autonomic nerve function defect.

a, Need to supervise children and elderly with heat because of this risk; b, Anesthesia or dysesthesia; c, Cutaneous insensitivity; d, Due to neuroleptics.

Issue	LOC	Source	Affil	Rationale/Comment
Angina, unstable	CI/P	Basford, 2005[10]	MD	
Blood pressure, unstable	CI/P			
Cardiac insufficiency	P	Cameron, 2003[1]	PT	Vasodilation, caused by heating, places greater demands on the heart (especially
	CI	Bracciano, 2000[6,a]	OT	if large body areas are heated). Monitor vital signs and discontinue treatment
	CI/P	Basford, 2005[10,d]	MD	if heart rate drops or fainting sensations occur.[1]
Circulation impaired	P	Cameron, 2003[1]	PT	This issue concerns heat dissipation ability. Circulation needs to be adequate in
	CI	Rennie and Michlovitz, 1996[5]	PT	order to dissipate heat generated from the heating source. Cold blood and
	CI/P	Tan, 1998[9]	MD/PT	sufficient oxygen may not be able to be shunted to heated area.[7] Inadequate
	CI	Hecox and Sanko, 2006[7]	PT	vasodilation and blood flow responses can lead to burns. In PVD, increasing
	CI/P	Basford, 2005[10,c]	MD	temperature and oxygen requirements may endanger exposed structures.[17]
				Balakrishnan et al,[18] in a case series, reported on a 20-year-old girl with spina bifida and a 62-year-old veteran with insulin-dependent diabetes, both of whom sustained burns in foot areas with impaired sensation and vasodilation ability during a bath.
				Also see Stevenson et al[13] and Nahabedian and McGibbon.[14]
Thrombophlebitic area	CI	Cameron, 2003[1]	PT	The concern centers around clots and what happens to them when exposed to
	CI	Bracciano, 2000[6,b]	OT	heat. Heating results in increased blood flow that can cause an existing blood clot
	CI	Hecox and Sanko, 2006[7,b]	PT	to dislodge and migrate proximally to a vital organ (resulting in illness or death).

a, People with advanced cardiac disease; b, Over area; c, Ischemia; d, Heart failure (decompensated) within 6-8 weeks of a myocardial infarction.

L00-99 DISEASES OF THE SKIN AND SUBCUTANEOUS TISSUE

Issue	LOC	Source	Affil	Rationale/Comment
Dermatological conditions—some	CI	Hecox and Sanko, 2006[7,a]	PT	Some skin conditions may respond poorly to moist heat.
Scar	CI/P	Tan, 1998[9,b]	MD/PT	Scars have reduced sensation.[7]
	CI/P	Basford, 2005[10]	MD	
Skin—atrophic	CI/P	Tan, 1998[9]	MD/PT	
	CI	Bracciano, 2000[6]	OT	
	CI/P	Basford, 2005[10]	MD	
Skin graft—superficial	CI	Bracciano, 2000[6]	OT	

a, Hot packs; b, Immature.

M00-99 DISEASES OF THE MUSCULOSKELETAL SYSTEM AND CONNECTIVE TISSUE

Issue	LOC	Source	Affil	Rationale/Comment
Repair of tendon or ligament—primary	CI	Bracciano, 2000[6]	OT	
Rheumatoid arthritis	CI			Vigorous heat may heighten enzyme activity and consequently increase joint inflammation.

O00-99 PREGNANCY, CHILDBIRTH, AND PUERPERIUM

Issue	LOC	Source	Affil	Rationale/Comment
Pregnancy	P	Cameron, 2003[1]	PT	Maternal hyperthermia can injure the fetus. Inquire if patient is pregnant or trying to become pregnant.[1] Avoid
	CI	Bracciano, 2000[6]	OT	full body immersion or heat directly to abdomen and low back/pelvis. Effects on fetus are not known.[6]
	CI	Hecox and Sanko, 2006[7,a]	PT	**In a retrospective study of eight maternal cases of *fever*-induced hyperthermia during early gestation from infections, similar clinical presentations were noted in infants: severe mental deficiency, seizure, hypotonia, impaired distal limb development, midface hypoplasia, microphthalmia.[19]**

a, Specified for hot packs over pelvis, low back, or abdominals in pregnancy.

R00-R99 SYMPTOMS, SIGNS

Issue	LOC	Source	Affil	Rationale/Comment
Edema	CI/P	Tan, 1998[9]	MD/PT	Heat may cause further edema to develop **(see Hydrotherapy).**
	P	Bracciano, 2000[6]	OT	
	CI/P	Basford, 2005[10]	MD	
Inflammation—acute	CI	Cameron, 2003[1]	PT	Heat enhances the inflammatory process by increasing blood flow,
	CI	Rennie and Michlovitz, 1996[5]	PT	increasing edema, and promoting bleeding, which can further delay
	CI/P	Tan, 1998[9]	MD/PT	healing.[1] Inquire if the patient injured the area over the past 2 to 3 days

Continued

Issue	LOC	Source	Affil	Rationale/Comment
	CI	Bracciano, 2000[6]	OT	and evaluate area for warmth, redness, and local swelling.[1,2] **See 2002**
	CI	Hecox and Sanko, 2006[7]	PT	**New York lawsuit.[8]**
	CI/P	Basford, 2005[10]	MD	

S00-98 INJURY, POISONING, AND CERTAIN OTHER CONSEQUENCES OF EXTERNAL CAUSES

Issue	LOC	Source	Affil	Rationale/Comment
Injury—acute	CI	Cameron, 2003[1]	PT	See Acute inflammation.
	CI/P	Tan, 1998[9]	MD/PT	
	CI	Bracciano, 2000[6]	OT	
	CI/P	Basford, 2005[10]	MD	
Wound—open (over)	P	Cameron, 2003[1]	PT	The issue concerns spreading infection via cross-contamination for some
(especially paraffin)	CI/P	Tan, 1998[9]	MD/PT	heat modalities (especially paraffin; pools). Also, open wounds have less
	CI	Hecox and Sanko, 2006[7,a]	PT	skin insulation and therefore are more susceptible to burns. In general, consider alternative heat modalities at lower heat intensities, with frequent patient monitoring, and with heat applications near but not directly over wound (also see Wound Care and Hydrotherapy for Water Treatment with Open Wounds). **See 2002 New York lawsuit.[8]**

a, CI for paraffin due to contamination of wound and tank; questionable for infrared due to drying out (moist environment better for wounds).

VULNERABLE BIOLOGICAL TISSUE

Issue	LOC	Source	Affil	Rationale/Comment
Eyes—for infrared therapy	CI	Cameron, 2003[1]	PT	Infrared irradiation causes optical damage (IR-opaque goggles should be worn by patient and therapist).

Y70-Y82 MEDICAL DEVICES

Issue	LOC	Source	Affil	Rationale/Comment
Metal in the area	P	Cameron, 2003[1]	PT	Metal gets very hot when heated because of its high thermal conductivity and specific heat and can therefore lead to burns. Inquire about any staples, bullet fragments, or jewelry that can place patient at risk. Consider lowering heat intensity, and monitoring frequently for burns.[1]

PROCEDURAL CONCERNS

Issue	LOC	Source	Affil	Rationale/Comment
Drain excess water	Advice	Basford, 2005[10]	MD	To reduce scalding from hot packs.
Falling asleep on top of a hot pack	Do not Advice	Hecox and Sanko, 2006[7] Basford, 2005[10,c]	PT MD	**Although outside thermotherapy's scope**, in a retrospective review of 80 fatal burns recorded at a California hospital over a 5-year period,

Continued

Issue	LOC	Source	Affil	Rationale/Comment
				Parks[20] described 26% with smoking-related burns, in which some occurred while sleeping. Also, in a 1996 California lawsuit,[21] a 56-year-old California woman contended she sustained second- and third-degree burns to her back when she lay on an uninsulated hot pack for 30 minutes.
Hot pack weight	CI/ Advice	Hecox and Sanko, 2006[7,b]	PT	If patient does not tolerate the weight of a hot pack on a body part, consider other
	Advice	Basford, 2005[10]	MD	thermotherapy options (e.g., infrared therapy).
Insulate pack—not wet	CI/P	Basford, 2005[10]	MD	To reduce risk of scalding from hot pack. Toweling should not be wet.
Position of limb: dependent limb with edema	P	Cameron, 2003[1]	PT	Heat increases edema in a dependent limb. Consider positioning (elevating) limb to counter edema tendency.[b] **See Hydrotherapy.**
Topical counterirritant	P	Cameron, 2003[1]	PT	Burns may occur if heat is applied to area already treated with a vasodilating ointment
recently applied over area— i.e., liniments/heat rubs	CI	Rennie and Michlovitz, 1996[5]	PT	because the vasculature may not be able to vasodilate further. Inquire if the patient uses a topical counterirritant ointment over the area such as menthol.[1]
Visual inspection of area	CI	Hecox and Sanko, 2006[7,a]	PT	If application blocks the visual inspection of an area.

a, For hot packs; b, CI if direct pressure of hot pack must be avoided; c, Hot packs should be on, not over, patients.

Paraffin Wax

Issue	LOC	Sources	Affil	Rationale/Comment
Blisters—extensive (in burns)	Delay	Helm et al, 1982[22]	MD	Paraffin may lead to further breakdown. Consider delaying treatment until skin becomes less fragile.
Contagious skin conditions, warts	P	Rennie and Michlovitz, 1996[5]	PT	Wax bath/tank could become contaminated. Cover area with a bandage or plastic film.

Fragile and trophic skin	CI	Head and Helm, 1977[23]	PT	
Infected skin lesions—over	CI	Rennie and Michlovitz, 1996[5.]	PT	Treatment may exacerbate the lesions.
Inflammation, acute—joint/tissue	Advice	Basford, 2005[10]	MD	Most clinicians will not prescribe. Increasing temperatures can increase intraarticular enzymatic activity.
Hypersensitive skin	CI	Head and Helm, 1977[23]	PT	Because temperature typically is 37-38° C.
Sensation reduced	CI			
Sustained stretching and paraffin—in burn contractures	P			Treatment may cause trauma and break down the immature scar.
Temperature—check	Advice	Basford, 2005[10]	MD	Check temperature prior to use to avoid burns. A solid film of wax around reservoir margins is a warning sign that temperature of the wax may be too high.
Wounds—open (over)	Do not use	Cameron, 2003[1]	PT	Wound and tank can become contaminated.[7] Also, risk of burning tissue.[1]
	CI	Rennie and Michlovitz, 1996[5]	PT	
	CI	Hecox and Sanko, 2006[7,a]	PT	

a, Also burn wounds.

ADVERSE EVENTS

Source	Background	Therapy	Outcome	Follow-up/Interpretation
Balakrishnan et al, 1995[18] **Burns and diabetes** Case series Burns	A 62-year-old veteran presented with insulin-dependent diabetes and a neuropathy (10 years) and reduced sensation. The ABI was 0.9.	The veteran used a foot bath for an infected callus.	The right foot was burned from the bath. Sensation was reduced over the burn site. Treatment involved excision and grafting.	Both cases involved neuropathies susceptible to burns. Impaired sensation and circulatory status increased the chance of ulceration.
	A 20-year-old woman with spina bifida presented with a pressure ulcer over her 5th metatarsal base due to a brace.	The ulcer was treated with foot baths and dressings. Foot discoloration occurred following the bath.	She was examined 5 days later. Dx: Deep burn to sole and partial burn to dorsum of the foot.	
Imai et al, 1998[24] **Alternating heat/cooling and heart attack** Case report Cardiology See Hydrotherapy for details	A 37-year-old Japanese man.	Alternated between hot sauna and cold water bathing repeatedly for 2 hours.	He felt chest pain and was diagnosed as having an MI.	The authors underscore danger of rapid cooling after sauna bathing in patients with coronary risk factors.
Katcher and Shapiro, 1987[11] **Burns and diabetes** Retrospective (chart review) J Fam Pract	A retrospective chart review was conducted on 37 patients with diabetes mellitus from four hospitals (1970-1985) who received burn therapy.	27% (10 of 37) had preventable LE burns related to sensory loss. Seven incidences involved the self-administered use of heat.	Five patients were burned by hot tap water during foot care. Two patients burned themselves with hot moist compresses/ heat pads.	The authors believe patients with diabetes need to be educated on burn risks.

			Three patients were burned while walking barefoot on hot sandy beaches or blacktop driveways.	
Mulunsky et al, 1992[25] **Neural tube fetal defects and hot tub** Prospective study (telephone interview) JAMA	23,491 women from the New England area with serum alpha-fetal protein screening or an amniocentesis took part in a prospective study.	The women were interviewed for environmental exposure to heat in their first trimester of pregnancy, and any relevant family, medical, genetic, diet, or medication history.	Exposure to hot tub, sauna, and fever in the first trimester of pregnancy was associated with increased risk of neural tube defects in fetus. (Multivariate adjusted RR were 2.8, 1.8, and 1.8, respectively.)	Hot tub had the strongest effect.
Nahabedian and McGibbon, 1998[14] **Burn, breast reconstruction, and heating pad** Case series Br Plast Surg	A 53-year-old female with a right modified radical mastectomy due to cancer underwent reconstruction 8 months later.	On night 6 postop, a heating pad was applied for discomfort.	The heat resulted in a full-thickness necrosis, requiring débridement and a split-thickness skin graft. She healed completely.	The authors argue that burns were a result of impaired thermoregulatory capacity of the transplanted tissue (vascular and neural components of skin so that flaps were not able to dissipate heat load).
	A 42-year-old with a right modified radical mastectomy due to cancer underwent flap reconstruction 1 year later.	The patient applied an electric heating pad to an indurated region (from fat necrosis).	The heat resulted in a partial-thickness burn over the midportion of her breast, which was confined to the flap area.	Factors include: Poor sensation Impaired vasodilation Inability to sweat

Continued

Source	Background	Therapy	Outcome	Follow-up/Interpretation
	A 37-year-old patient with radical mastectomy underwent a latissimus dorsi musculocutaneous flap.	Four years later, the patient received US treatment for a shoulder ailment and a heating pad over the previously reconstructed breast.	The heat resulted in a 5×2 cm partial-thickness burn over the flap area. She healed with wound care.	
	A 24-year-old patient with a left radical mastectomy due to cancer underwent flap reconstruction.	The patient was exposed to sunlight through a bathing suit.	The exposure resulted in a sunburn.	
Simonsen et al, 1995[15] **Infant burns and infrared heat** Case series Acta Paediatr	A 32-year-old Caucasian mother gave birth at term to an apparently dead male infant (2896 g). Apgar score 1 at 1 minute.	The infant was placed on resuscitation for 1 hour under a 250-W adjustable infrared heat lamp (to prevent hypothermia). Note: The restraint mechanism to prevent lamp from getting closer than 50-70 cm was missing.	The infant sustained second-degree burns and died, from unrelated causes, 3 hours after the cesarean section was performed.	The authors believe asphyxia and insufficient peripheral circulation (no pulse) combined with long heat exposure contributed to the burns.
	A 33-year-old Caucasian mother had a cesarean section 1 week post term. The infant was apparently dead at delivery with Apgar scores of 0 at 1 and 7 minutes.	Resuscitation was attempted for 100 minutes. Also, a 250-W adjustable infrared heat lamp was employed, not closer than 32 cm to the infant.	The infant sustained a second-degree burn and died 3 days later from unrelated causes.	The burns occurred when skin temperature was raised above the critical level of 44° C. The heat lamp may have been positioned too close to the infant in the first case.

Siegfried et al, 1992[26] **Burn, neonatal jaundice, and ultraviolet treatment** Case series Pediatr Dermatol	Two premature female infants: (1) 27 weeks, 930 g; (2) 30 weeks, 1615 g	Both received phototherapy for neonatal jaundice.	Both infants sustained phototherapy-induced erythema (one with second-degree burns) after exposure to UVA without protective Plexiglas shields.	Premature infants in the first 2 weeks of life are especially susceptible to UVA-induced erythema.
Stevenson et al, 1985[13] **Burn, insensate skin, and hot pack** Case series Ann Plast Surg	A 53-year-old female was s/p modified radical mastectomy due to carcinoma, 12 months of chemotherapy, and breast reconstruction using transverse rectus abdominis musculocutaneous flap with anesthetic skin.	Three weeks post reconstruction, the patient applied a hot pack over the graft for 40 minutes to reduce discomfort.	Blisters in the central portion of flap were noted the following day. Over the next 10 days, eschar formed and débridement was performed.	The authors report that flaps can have anesthetic areas and advise not to apply hot packs to insensate flaps. They suggest instead using water bottles filled with tap water.
	A 46-year-old female was s/p modified radical mastectomy due to breast cancer. She had reconstruction surgery 8 years later.	Seventeen days after surgery, she went to sleep on a heating pad.	On that morning, she noted a 2-cm red wound centrally located on the reconstruction site. Eschar formed by week 3 post burn, and the wound healed (reepithelialization) by week 4.	

Continued

Source	Background	Therapy	Outcome	Follow-up/Interpretation
	A 72-year-old female was s/p sternal staphylococcus infection following coronary artery bypass. At week 14, she received a left pectoralis major muscle flap over her sternum.	Four weeks after the flap transfer, the patient slept on a heating pad.	The following day, she noted a reddish area medial to her left nipple. The wound developed eschar and reepithelialized 14 days after the burn.	
Waldorf et al, 1971[3] **Erythema ab igne and electric heating pad** Case report JAMA	A 46-year-old woman sustained a thigh injury due to a fall (no fracture).	Local heating was advised. The patient applied an electric heating pad 12 hours a day and only removed the pad if heat became unbearable.	After 3 weeks, she noted retiform eruption sites on her body. She continued to apply heat for another 3 weeks. After discontinuation of heat, the eruptions slowly faded over a 6-month period, but a hyperpigmented atrophic lacework pattern at the site remained. Her diagnosis was erythema ab igne .	Erythema ab igne is a disorder of overexposure to heat that was common in 19th- and 20th-century Great Britain from exposure to heaters (central heating was not available). Once marks are noted, they are usually permanent. Histopathologically, they reveal thin epidermis, alterations in dermal elastic fibers, and flattening of rete ridges.

FDA[4] REPORTS FOR PARAFFIN BATH

14 Reports from 9/18/92 to 1/9/03

Date	Event
1/9/03	The bath overheated.
12/13/02	The drain heater coil overheated and the unit smoked.
4/18/02	The bath temperature was not regulated; a replacement thermostat corrected the problem.
4/3/02	Paraffin wax leaked onto the carpet.
1/13/98	The bath had a faulty thermostat; the wax reached a flash point and then caught fire. The incident was replicated by a biomedical department.
3/14/97	The bath provided insufficient heat.
4/02/02	The bath's temperature fluctuated from low to high.
2/28/01	The paraffin wax surface was too hot.
2/13/01	A wax burn was reported (minor hand burn).
2/6/01	A patient complained the wax was too hot and sustained a second-degree burn to the fingers. The device temperature read 155°. The PTA noticed that the machine switch had been switched to Start instead of Operate.
7/29/98	An individual sustained a second-degree burn on the left hand after using the device in hospital. The wound took 3 to 4 weeks to heal.
12/29/95	During therapy, a patient's right hand was dipped in paraffin and wrapped for 15 minutes. The next day, the patient returned with a dime-size blister that appeared to be a burn on the right finger.
2/15/95	The unit got too hot, and then not hot enough.
9/18/92	The temperature of the wax varied from one area of the unit to another.

Note: FDA reports do not necessarily establish cause-effect relationships between equipment and injury. Incidences may be due to equipment or user error. Also, some reports are alleged by attorneys.

LITIGATION

Year, State	Background	Treatment	Adverse Event	Verdict
1996 California[2] **Burn, inadequate insulation, and Hot pack**	A 13-year-old girl presented with a concussion and bruises due to a dune buggy accident.	Hot packs and TENS were administered to the neck and right arm by an employee of the physician (who had worked for 1 week). The hot pack with a cover was allegedly wrapped around patient's arm without additional insulation or toweling.	The patient and mother complained that the hot pack was too hot, but the patient was not checked until the pack was removed 15-20 minutes later. A white blister appeared on the arm and she was diagnosed with a third-degree burn with full-thickness skin loss that required a skin graft, revision, and steroid injections.	The patient's family contended the physician's employee was unlicensed, untrained, and unsupervised. $175,000 arbitration award.
1996 California[21] **Burn, inadequate insulation, and a hot pack**	A 56-year-old California woman contended she sustained 12- to 18-inch, second- and third-degree burns to her back.	She lay on a hot pack for 30 minutes without "wrapping" (insulation).	The plaintiff went to an emergency room 11 hours after the treatment and subsequently required plastic surgery.	A jury found for the defendant (physician), who claimed the burn was recent and self-administered at home.
2002 New York[8] **Inflamed, infected joint and hot pack**	A seamstress was s/p left knee replacement, débridement and knee manipulation (due to an oozing, unclosed	Physical therapy included moist heat applications. Oozing continued during rehabilitation.	Moist heat caused irritation and blisters and a second-degree burn. A *Staphylococcus aureus* infection in her knee joint required removal	The arbitrator found the patient had inflammation when the hot pack was applied, which resulted in a

wound and inability to bend her knee).

of the prosthetic meniscus and antibiotic therapy. The entire prosthesis became infected, was removed, and a second prosthesis was inserted. The infection continued and required removal of the second prosthesis, administration of antibiotics, and the insertion of a third prosthesis.

burn that exacerbated the inflammation. However, the infection after the second prosthesis insertion was due to a dog-related fall by the patient. $500,000 arbitration verdict.

Note: Awards and settlements do not necessarily prove a cause-effect relationship between equipment or therapy and injury.

REFERENCES

1. Cameron MH: Physical agents in rehabilitation: from research to practice. St Louis: Saunders; 2003.
2. Medical malpractice verdicts, settlements and experts, Feb 1996, p 27, loc 1.
3. Waldorf DS, Rast MF, Garofalo VJ: Heating-pad erythematous dermatitis "erythema ab igne," JAMA 218(11):1704, 1971.
4. U.S. Food and Drug Administration: Web page. Available at: http://www.FDA.gov.cdrh/mdr. Accessed: November 7, 2005.
5. Rennie GA, Michlovitz SL: Biophysical principles of heating and superficial heating agents. In: Michlovitz SL, editor: Thermal agents in rehabilitation, ed 3. Philadelphia: FA Davis; 1996.
6. Bracciano AG: Physical agent modalities: theory and application for the occupational therapist. Thorofare (NJ): Slack; 2000.
7. Hecox B, Sanko JP: Superficial thermotherapy. In: Hecox B, Mehreteab TA, Weisberg J, eds: Integrating physical agents in rehabilitation. Upper Saddle River (NJ): Pearson Prentice Hall; 2006.

8. Medical malpractice verdicts, settlements and experts, Feb 2002, p 51, loc 2.

9. Tan JC: Practical manual of physical medicine and rehabilitation: diagnostics, therapeutics, and basic problems. St Louis: Mosby; 1998.

10. Basford JR: Therapeutic physical agents. In: Delisa JA, editor: Physical medicine and rehabilitation: principles and practices, ed 4, vol 1. Philadelphia: Lippincott Williams & Wilkins; 2005.

11. Katcher ML, Shapiro MM: Lower extremity burns related to sensory loss in diabetes mellitus. J Fam Pract 24(2):149-151, 1987.

12. Bill TJ, Edich RF, Himel HN: Electric heating pad burns. J Emerg Med 12(6):819-824, 1994.

13. Stevenson TR, Hammond DC, Keip D, et al: Heating pad burns in anesthetic skin. Ann Plast Surg 15(1):73-75, 1985.

14. Nahabedian MY, McGibbon BM: Thermal injuries in autogenous tissue breast reconstruction. Br J Plast Surg 51(8):599-602, 1998.

15. Simonsen K, Graem N, Rothman LP, Degn H: Iatrogenic radiant heat burns in severely asphyxic newborns. Acta Paediatr 84(12):1438-1440, 1995.

16. Collins KJ, Dore C, Exton-Smith AN, et al.: Accidental hypothermia and impaired temperature homeostasis in the elderly. BMJ 1(6057):353-356, 1977.

17. Abramson DI: Physiologic basis for the use of physical agents in peripheral vascular disorders. Arch Phys Med Rehabil 46:216-244, 1965.

18. Balakrishnan C, Rak TP, Meininger MS: Burns of the neuropathic foot following use of therapeutic footbaths. Burns 21:622-623, 1995.

19. Smith DW, Clarren SK, Harvey MA: Hyperthermia as a possible teratogenic agent. J Pediatr 92(6):878-883, 1978.

20. Parks JG, Noguchi TT, Klatt EC. The epidemiology of fatal burn injuries. J Forens Sci 34(2):399-406, 1989.

21. Medical malpractice verdicts, settlements and experts, July 1996, p 47, loc 4.

22. Helm PA, Kevorkian CG, Lushbaugh M: Burn injury: rehabilitation management in 1982. Arch Phys Med Rehabil 63: 6-16, 1982.

23. Head MD, Helm PA: Paraffin and sustained stretching in the treatment of burn contractures. Burns 4:136-139, 1977.

24. Imai Y, Nobuoka S, Sagashima J, et al: Acute myocardial infarction induced by alternating exposure to heat in a sauna and rapid cooling in cold water. Cardiology 90(4):299-301, 1998.

25. Milunsky A, Ulcickas M, Rothman KJ, et al: Maternal heat exposure and neural tube defects. JAMA 268(7):882-885, 1992.

26. Siegfried EC, Stone MS, Madison KC: Ultraviolet light burn: a cutaneous complication of visible light phototherapy of neonatal jaundice. Pediatr Dermatol 9:278-282, 1992.

(Intermittent Compression Pumps)

OVERVIEW. Vasopneumatic compression devices (VCD) are a form of compression therapy that uses mechanical force from a pump to intermittently exerts external pressure on a body part (i.e., increasing hydrostatic pressure, milking effects on fluid). The device typically includes a chambered sleeve wrapped around the involved limb, a connecting elastic tube, and an electric pump.[1]

Vasopneumatic compression devices are used to treat lymphedema, reduce edema (due to venous insufficiency), help heal venous stasis ulcers (due to impaired circulation), prophylactically reduce the incidence of DVTs in postoperative patients, reshape residual limbs following amputation, and control hypertrophic scarring. Note: Because ICP can be applied at pressures that act as a tourniquet or induce fluid overload in some patients who have compromised cardiovascular systems, proper screening and monitoring are required.[2]

SUMMARY: CONTRAINDICATIONS AND PRECAUTIONS. Five sources cited a total of 16 concerns for vasopneumatic compression devices. Concerns ranged from 2 to 16 per source, with a physical therapist citing the largest number. Most concerns were circulatory (about 45%). The most frequently cited concerns were deep vein thromboses, congestive heart failure, and severe peripheral artery disease.

SUMMARY: ADVERSE EVENTS. Many of the reported compression device complications[3] (embolism-related deaths; palsies, pressure ulcers, compartment syndromes) stem from its use in DVT prophylaxis with surgical patients. In this protocol (compression lasts 12 seconds per minute, 40 mm Hg), calf compressions serve to reproduce leg contractions, promote venous return, and stimulate fibrinolysis for the prevention of thrombus formation.[2]

Number of Concerns for ICP per Source

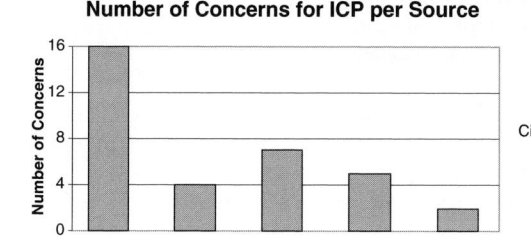

Proportion of Concerns Based on VCD

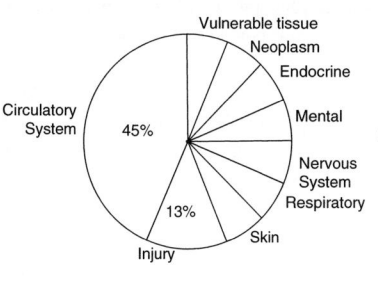

Top 6 Cited Concerns for VCD Therapy (n = 5)

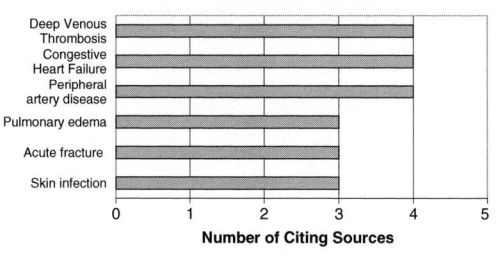

CONTRAINDICATIONS AND PRECAUTIONS

C00-C97 NEOPLASMS

Issue	LOC	Sources	Affil	Rationale/Comment
Cancer	P	Cameron, 2003[1]	PT	Controversial. There is a risk of increased metastases from compression and increased tumor growth from improved nutrition. If the patient is receiving chemotherapy, hormone therapy, or a biological response modifier for cancer, many feel ICP can be used. Some believe compression close to the cancer site should be avoided, and others think patients should be cancer-free for 5 years before providing compression (controversial).[1]

E00-E90 ENDOCRINE, NUTRITIONAL AND METABOLIC DISEASES

Issue	LOC	Sources	Affil	Rationale/Comment
Hypoproteinemia—significant	CI	Cameron, 2003[1]	PT	Inquire about serum protein levels, changes in diet, or weight loss. When serum protein is <2 g/dl, returning fluid to vessels during ICP can lead to cardiac and immunological dysfunction.

F00-F99 MENTAL AND BEHAVIORAL DISORDERS

Issue	LOC	Sources	Affil	Rationale/Comment
Mentation impaired	P	Cameron, 2003[1]	PT	The patient may not be able to communicate or recognize uncomfortable pressure levels. Consider using lower pressures and monitoring closely or, alternatively, using a compression garment.

G00-G99 DISEASES OF THE NERVOUS SYSTEM

Issue	LOC	Sources	Affil	Rationale/Comment
Sensation impaired	P	Cameron, 2003[1]	PT	The patient may not be able to recognize uncomfortable pressure levels. Consider using lower pressures and monitoring closely or, alternatively, using a compression garment.

I00-I99 DISEASES OF THE CIRCULATORY SYSTEM

Issue	LOC	Sources	Affil	Rationale/Comment
Congestive heart failure	CI	Lachmann et al, 1992[2]	MD	Increased venous return from ICP can overload an already compromised heart (that cannot
	CI	Cameron 2003[1]	PT	efficiently contract) and can increase pressure in lung capillaries in pulmonary edema
	CI	Hecox and Jacobs, 2006[4]	PT	where capillaries are already elevated. Inquire about lung or heart problems, or signs
	CI	Hooker, 2002[5]	PT/ATC	of bilateral LE swelling.
Deep vein thrombosis	CI	Lachmann et al, 1992[2,a]	MD	If a clot is already present, ICP can dislodge the clot, move it upstream, and impair
(acute/recent) or	CI	Cameron, 2003[1]	PT	circulation to vital organs (lung, heart, brain), causing morbidity (stroke) or death.[1,4]
thrombophlebitis	CI	Hecox and Jacobs, 2006[4]	PT	Inquire/evaluate for DVT and risk factors. **Over the past 10 years, the FDA[3] received**
	CI	Hooker, 2002[5]	PT/ATC	**seven reports of fatalities from pulmonary embolisms allegedly occurring**
				after DVT prophylactic use of pneumatic compression pumps.
Hypertension—	P	Cameron, 2003[1]	PT	ICP can contribute to already elevated blood pressure. Assess baseline blood pressure and
uncontrolled				monitor it during treatment. Discontinue ICP if blood pressure exceeds a limit set by physician.
Obstructed lymphatic or	CI	Cameron, 2003[1]	PT	If return is totally obstructed, the obstruction must be removed first (i.e., surgically) before
venous return	CI	Grieveson, 2003[6]	PT	ICP is administered. If partially obstructed, confirm (monitor) that ICP indeed reduces
	CI	Hecox and Jacobs, 2006[4,d]	PT	edema.[1]
Peripheral arterial disease	CI	Lachmann et al, 1992[2,b]	MD	An ankle-brachial pressure index <0.8 (low score) indicates obstruction to blood flow.
(severe)	CI	Cameron, 2003[1]	PT	ICP can further impair arterial circulation by closing down diseased vessels. Avoid
	CI	Grieveson, 2003[6]	PT	compression if ABI is <0.8 (i.e., systolic blood pressure at ankle is 80% < upper
	CI	Hecox and Jacobs, 2006[4]	PT	extremity). Inquire about peripheral artery disease, bypass surgeries, intermittent
				claudication, ulcers from artery disease, and the patient's ABI.

Pulmonary embolism	CI	Cameron 2003[1]	PT	
	CI	Hooker, 2002[5,c]	PT/ATC	
Stroke, TIAs, or other significant vascular insufficiencies	P	Cameron, 2003[1]	PT	ICP can alter brain circulation.

a, Suspected DVT; b, Leg ischemia due to PVD; c, Acute; d, Completely obstructed lymphatics or obstructed venous vessel.

J00-J99 DISEASES OF THE RESPIRATORY SYSTEM

Issue	LOC	Sources	Affil	Rationale/Comment
Pulmonary edema	CI	Lachmann et al, 1992[2]	MD	IPC moves fluid to an already overburdened area and can stress both the lungs and the heart.
	CI	Cameron, 2003[1]	PT	
	CI	Hecox and Jacobs, 2006[4]	PT	

L00-L99 DISEASES OF THE SKIN AND SUBCUTANEOUS TISSUE

Issue	LOC	Sources	Affil	Rationale/Comment
Skin infection— acute, local	CI	Cameron, 2003[1]	PT	The ICP's sleeve can promote moisture, increase temperatures, and promote microorganism growth.
	CI	Hecox and Jacobs, 2006[4]	PT	Consider using a single-use sleeve in persons with chronic infections to avoid cross-contamination
	CI	Hooker, 2002[5,a]	PT/ATC	or reinfection.[1]

a, Local superficial infection.

S00-T98 INJURY, POISONING, AND CERTAIN OTHER CONSEQUENCES OF EXTERNAL CAUSES

Issue	LOC	Sources	Affil	Rationale/Comment
Fracture—acute	CI	Cameron, 2003[1]	PT	ICP may displace the fracture,[5] aggravate the trauma site (increased bleeding
	CI	Hecox and Jacobs, 2006[4,a]	PT	and inflammation), and affect healing.[1]
	CI	Hooker, 2002[5]	PT/ATC	
Trauma—acute	CI	Cameron, 2003[1]	PT	IPC may further inflame the acute trauma site (see above).

a, Unstable and acute.

VULNERABLE BIOLOGICAL TISSUE

Issue	LOC	Sources	Affil	Rationale/Comment
Superficial peripheral nerves	P	Cameron, 2003[1]	PT	Superficial nerves are vulnerable to compressive injuries, particularly if the patient has lost weight. Monitor for sensation or motor loss if treating over a superficial nerve. **Lachmann et al[2] describes two men in their 60s who received IPC devices preoperatively for DVT prophylaxis and developed either peroneal neuropathies or compartmental syndrome with subsequent nerve palsy. In 2000, McGrory and Burke[7] reported a 79-year-old and a 63-year-old woman who both sustained peroneal nerve palsy following intermittent sequential pneumatic compression.**

Note: Lachmann et al's contraindications for IPC were written within the context of patients receiving the device at the calf during and after surgery as a DVT prophylaxis.

Source	Background	Therapy	Outcome	Follow-up/Interpretation
Lachmann et al, 1992[2] **Palsy, compartment syndrome, and IPC** Case series Arch Phys Med Rehabil	A 65-year-old man presented with atherosclerotic heart disease, hypertension, and diabetes. A CT scan revealed a mass at the head of his pancreas. A 62-year-old man with a diagnosis of recurrent transitional cell carcinoma of the bladder underwent radical cystectomy and ileal neobladder substitution (palliative).	He underwent a subtotal pancreatectomy secondary to adenocarcinoma. Preoperatively, he wore surgical stockings and IPCDs for DVT prophylaxis. The patient wore surgical stockings and underwent IPCD preoperatively (for DVT prophylaxis). He was also positioned in a lithotomy position during the 8-hour procedure.	Postoperatively, the man complained of sensation loss over the anterolateral legs and dorsal feet, and ambulated with a bilateral steppage gait. At 14 days postop, testing revealed bilateral peroneal neuropathies with denervation of the tibialis anterior, peroneus longus, and extensor halluis longus. Partial resolution of weakness was noted over the next 3 months, but he required a cane and AFOs for the remainder of his life. Postoperatively, he complained of LE pain, paresthesia, a swollen RLE, decreased sensation over the foot dorsum, and weakness of the ankle dorsiflexors and great toe. Compartmental pressures in lower leg ranged from 50 to 58 mmHg.	The envelope around the calf restricts the volume of the leg compartments, can increase intracompartmental pressures, and thus hasten compartment syndromes. Use IPCD with caution in surgical patients with cancer, peripheral neuropathy, weight loss, or if placed in a lithotomy position during the procedure. Suggested modifications to avoid complications include (1) leaving the fibular head area exposed during IPCD (so it is not compressed); (2) padding; (3) avoiding stretching foot abductors, adductors, hip adductors, hip hyperextension, and flexion >60 degrees while in lithotomy posture during surgery; and (4) avoiding leaning/resting objects on the patient's limb during surgery.

Continued

Source	Background	Therapy	Outcome	Follow-up/Interpretation
			He was diagnosed with acute compartmental syndrome, treated with a fasciotomy and shin grafts. After 2 weeks, he recovered motor power.	Consider alternative interventions including use of CPM, passive motion, electrical stimulation, and surgical stockings.

FOOD AND DRUG ADMINISTRATION REPORTS[3]

Fatalities: Pneumatic Compression Pump: Maude and MDR (JOW)

Note: the majority of these devices had been used during and after surgery to prevent the development of deep vein thrombosis.

Date	Device	Event	Outcome
4/29/04	Flowtron IPC	Three patients allegedly developed DVTs. One patient s/p gastric bypass surgery allegedly developed a pulmonary embolism.	Expired. No other information available.
12/18/00	Pulstar PAS II Pump antiembolism system	A patient s/p CVA connected the PAS tubing of a pneumatic compression device to a connector-compatible heparin-locked IV in the right ankle (a hypothesis), resulting in a massive air embolism.	Expired (misuse of device).
6/19/95	Plexipulse	A patient, s/p CVA, used a device to prevent a DVT and developed a pulmonary embolism.	Expired.
1/4/95	Flowtron DVT-AC500	A patient developed a pulmonary embolism 4 days following a surgery.	Expired.

2/4/94	Jobst Athromic Pump	A patient used a pump prophylactically during a surgery. Seven days after discharge, the patient may have developed a pulmonary embolism.	Expired.
8/11/93	Jobst System 7000 Pump	A patient with CHF was treated with a pump for pedal edema. He developed a DVT and a pulmonary embolism. The daughter alleges the device contributed to her father's death.	Expired. Note: Device labeling indicates CHF as a CI.
1/20/93	Jobst Athromic Pump	A 62-year-old male, s/p surgical correction of a bowel obstruction, was treated with antiembolism stockings and a pump to prevent DVTs. On day 7, he developed a pulmonary embolism.	Expired.
1991	Kendall SCD Sequential Compression Device	A 75-year-old female s/p surgery for a massive pelvic tumor had a septic episode. A pump was used bilaterally, and increased foot temperatures were noted after several days. Subsequently, she developed gas gangrene and underwent an AK amputation. Gangrene spread to the abdomen and she died 10 hours later.	Expired.

Note: FDA reports do not necessarily establish cause-effect relationships between equipment and injury. Incidences may be due to equipment or user error. Also, some reports are alleged by attorneys.

IPCD-Related Injuries

Date	Summary Outcomes
FDA, 11/12/97 to 6/29/04	During this 7-year period, the FDA has reported the following 24 nonlethal complications with IPCD: • 10 cases: skin ulcers, blisters, or redness • 5 cases: drop foot

Continued

Date	Summary Outcomes
	• 5 cases: pulmonary embolism (not deaths)
	• 1 case: stress fracture
	• 1 case: pedal edema due to incorrect application
	• 2 cases: unknown injury reported

Note: FDA reports do not necessarily establish cause-effect relationships between equipment and injury. Incidences may be due to equipment or user error. Also, some reports are alleged by attorneys.

REFERENCES

1. Cameron MH: Physical agents in rehabilitation: from research to practice. St. Louis: Saunders; 2003.
2. Lachmann EA, Rook JL, Tunkel R, et al: Complications associated with intermittent pneumatic compression. Arch Phys Med Rehabil 73(5):482-485, 1992.
3. U.S. Food and Drug Administration: Center for Device and Radiological Health [web page]. Available at: http://www.fda.gov/cdrh/mdr/. Accessed: November 7, 2005.
4. Hecox B, Jacobs LF: External compression. In: Hecox B, Mehreteab TA, Weisberg J, eds: Integrating physical agents in rehabilitation. Upper Saddle River (NJ): Pearson Prentice Hall; 2006.
5. Hooker DN: Intermittent compression devices. In: Prentice WE, editor: Therapeutic modalities for physical therapists, ed 2. New York: McGraw-Hill; 2002.
6. Grieveson S: Intermittent pneumatic compression pump settings for the optimum reduction of oedema. J Tissue Viability 13(3):98-110, 2003.
7. McGrory BJ, Burke DW: Peroneal nerve palsy following intermittent sequential pneumatic compression. Orthopaedics 23(10):1103-1105, 2000.

(Tilt Table, Prone Standers, Supine Standers, Stand-Up Wheelchairs)

OVERVIEW. Gravity-assisted compression devices (GACD) are devices that allow persons with disabilities to stand or achieve some level of assisted vertical orientation. The purposes include (1) accommodating their cardiovascular system to an upright posture following a period of bed rest (tilt tables), and (2) offering alternative positioning for children with disabilities (supine stander; prone stander), or providing standing support during vocational and avocational endeavors (stand-up type wheelchairs).[1,2] The device is typically comprised of a flat support surface, a foot support for weight bearing, straps and bolsters to secure and properly align the body, and either a manual or electric mechanism to raise and lower the individual to and from a vertical position.

SUMMARY: CONTRAINDICATIONS AND PRECAUTIONS. Published guidelines for GACDs are sparse. The two sources cited here express concern about standing an individual *too* upright in the device.[1,2] One source stressed the importance of monitoring vitals.[1] Warnings/cautions listed from a manufacturer's product guide[3,4] are also included below for a prone and supine stander.[3,4]

SUMMARY: ADVERSE EVENTS. The FDA[5] reported one death an five injuries between 1990 and 1998. Incidents often involved falls or trips while an individual was in the GACD.

Note: Perhaps (1) guidelines can emphasize supervision requirements while patients are on GACD (as reflected in product manuals); (2) weight-bearing precautions for persons with hip subluxations, hip dislocations, or severe osteoporosis are lacking and may be useful in future GAPD guidelines.

CONTRAINDICATIONS AND PRECAUTIONS

TILT TABLES

MEDICAL DEVICES

Issue	Level of Concern	Sources	Affil	Rationale/Comment
Chest strap	Caution	Pierson, 2002[1]	PT	Abdominal straps do not replace the use of a chest strap. Patients must have sufficient strength if chest strap is not used. Patients who lack sufficient trunk and hip extensor strength will fall forward.

PROCEDURAL CONCERNS

Issue	Level of Concern	Sources	Affil	Rationale/Comment
Full upright position— Avoid	Advice Avoid	Pierson, 2002[1] Minor and Minor, 1999[2]	PT PT	Avoid a fully upright position. At about 80 degrees of elevation, the patient may have a sensation of falling forward due to a shift in his or her center of gravity. Elevation to 70-80 degrees is sufficient.[1]
Tolerance—monitor • **Elevation intolerance** • **Postural hypotension** • **Autonomic hyperreflexia**	Caution	Pierson, 2002[1]	PT	Lower elevation if not tolerated. Signs of intolerance include loss of consciousness, tachycardia, drop in blood pressure (excessive), facial pallor, perspiration (excessive), nausea, dizziness, color/sensory changes in the LEs.
Vitals—monitor	Advice	Pierson, 2002[1]	PT	Monitor vital signs before and after each progression to a higher elevation.

Supine and Prone Standers: Sample User Manual Warnings/Concerns[3,4]

Issue	Level of Concern	Sources	Rationale/Comment
Product requires approval and guidance of qualified therapist or physician	Warning	Rifton Product Guide *E41 Large supine board or E59 Prone stander with tray*	
Supervision is required at all times	Warning		
Use of straps and supports requires supervision and cannot be used to replace a caregiver	Warning		Straps cannot replace a caregiver.
Use indoors only	Warning		
Armrests need to be securely tightened	Warning	Rifton Product Guide *E41 Large supine board*	The armrest has a "potential crush point."
Secure footrests	Warning		The footrest has a "potential crush point." Footrests should be adjusted in place before placing person in the device and before assuming a vertical position.
Secure telescoping legs	Warning	Rifton Product Guide *E41 Large supine board or E59 Prone stander with tray*	Use with telescoping legs in an extended position.
Secure headboard	Warning	Rifton Product Guide *Large supine board*	Headboard should be in place before patient assumes the horizontal position.
Stabilize supine unit during transfers	Caution	Rifton Product Guide *E41 Large supine board or E59 Prone stander with tray*	Transfers onto device—stabilize supine unit by locking all four caster weights to prevent rolling or unanticipated movements during the transfer.

Continued

Issue	Level of Concern	Sources	Rationale/Comment
Have two adults assist during transfers	Caution/ recommendation		For safety.
Keep all four casters locked at all times	Caution		Except when actually moving unit.
Maintenance	Recommended		Every month—check lubrication. Twice a year—lubricate casters. Periodically—inspect for missing parts, loose parts, breaks, and cracks.
Remove from service if condition makes operation unsafe	Recommended		
Surfaces not waterproof—do not use excessive water on wood	Recommended		
User modifications: If done, should be done by qualified, licensed professional who tests patient on equipment and certifies in writing that modifications are "safe and satisfactory"	Recommended ("urge")		Company cannot be responsible for user modifications.

I thank the Rifton Equipment Company for supplying me with their product guides for the E41 Large Supine Board and E59 50-inch Prone Stander with Tray.

ADVERSE EVENTS

FOOD AND DRUG ADMINISTRATION REPORTS[5]

Standing Frames

Date	Device	Event	Outcome
04/03/98	Rifton prone stander	A child was placed in the device. The child grabbed the Velcro restraint and pulled it open.	The child's head hit the concrete floor leading to vomiting and a laceration that required stitches. The head injury was not severe.
07/03/97	Midland standing frame	A 72 year-old woman who had been admitted for a left total hip prosthesis and experienced a subsequent CVA complication had sustained a toe injury following use of a standing frame.	Her right great toe was partially torn away. No details.
02/19/97	Chief SR stand recline power chair	The user was in a standing position when the chair tipped forward.	The user's knees were bruised. He was not wearing a seatbelt or chest harness, only a knee bolster.
3/09/91	Rifton E74 Small Freedom Stander	An angry child threw himself backward.	The device fell, and the child sustained a bump on the back of the head. Stable legs were added to the device later.
4/02/90	Rifton E74 Small Freedom Stander	A child was positioned in the device, leaned to hit a balloon, and tipped the device too far forward.	The child fell forward and hit mouth on floor.

Note: FDA reports do not necessarily establish cause-effect relationships between equipment and injury. Incidences may be due to equipment or user error. Also, some reports are alleged by attorneys.

Standing Frame Fatality

Date	Device	Event	Outcome
10/12/93	Rifton adjustable standing frame	A parent placed a 5-year-old with Rett syndrome in the device but did not secure the knee support and left the child unsupervised for an unknown period of time.	The child became entangled in the upper support strap and strangulated, resulting in death.

Note: FDA reports do not necessarily establish cause-effect relationships between equipment and injury. Incidences may be due to equipment or user error. Also, some reports are alleged by attorneys.

REFERENCES

1. Pierson FM, Fairchild SL: Principles and techniques of patient care, ed 3. Philadelphia: Saunders; 2002.
2. Minor MAD, Minor SD: Patient care skills, ed 4. Stamford (CT): Appleton & Lange; 1999.
3. Rifton E41 Large Supine Stander Board Product Guide, User Information HX 96 LCO 752 Revision AA, 1996.
4. Rifton E 59 50″ Prone Stander with Tray Product Guide, User Information VH97 LCO 752, 1998.
5. U.S. Food and Drug Administration: Center for Device and Radiological Health. Available at: http://www.fda.gov/cdrh/mdr/. Accessed: November 7, 2005.

50 CONTINUOUS PASSIVE MOTION

OVERVIEW. Continuous passive motion (CPM) devices provide uninterrupted, joint-passive range of motion over a controlled range and speed (slow) for up to 24 hours per day. The device is essentially a hinged, framelike machine with supports for the limb above and below the joint, a motor (A/C or battery), and controls for regulating the amount and speed of joint excursion. CPM was originally conceived to reduce the adverse effects of joint immobilization (i.e., adhesions, contracture formation, joint effusion, postoperative pain) by introducing *controlled* continuous passive motion *soon* after limb surgery. Concerns include the application of inappropriate forces that may either disrupt healing of tissue (skin, joint, bone, bleeding) or cause new injury (skin ulcers and nerve palsies).[1]

SUMMARY: CONTRAINDICATIONS AND PRECAUTIONS. Four sources cited a total of 12 concerns. Concerns ranged from one to four per source, with a physician and hand clinician citing the greatest number. Most concerns were musculoskeletal or skin related (abrasions). The most frequently cited concern was the presence of fractures. Other concerns cited by lone sources included the presence of joint infection, joint arthrosis, unstable joints, bleeding, and sensation loss.

OTHER ISSUES. The FDA[2] reports 25 CPM-related complications, some of which involve either a patient or a health professional getting an appendage (finger, foot, genitalia) caught in the moving parts of the CPM device.

Note: Entrapment issues, proper operation of units (watching out for erratic output), and adequate training (e.g., proper dosage and donning) could be highlighted in future published guidelines.

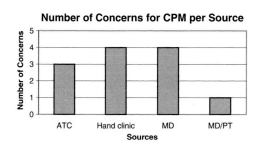

Number of Concerns for CPM per Source

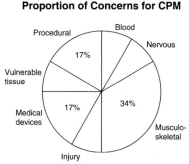

Proportion of Concerns for CPM

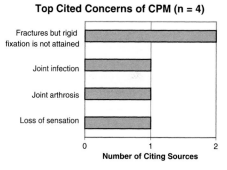

Top Cited Concerns of CPM (n = 4)

CONTRAINDICATIONS AND PRECAUTIONS

D50-D89 DISEASES OF BLOOD AND BLOOD-FORMING ORGANS AND CERTAIN DISORDERS

Issue	LOC	Sources	Affil	Rationale/Comment
Anticoagulation therapy	P	Starkey, 1999[3]	ATC	In 1985, Graham and Loomer[4] reported a 36-year-old woman who underwent ORIF for tibial plateau fractures, developed a deep vein thrombosis, was anticoagulated, and later developed an anterior compartment syndrome 24 hours after CPM was administered.

G00-G99 DISEASES OF THE NERVOUS SYSTEM

Issue	LOC	Sources	Affil	Rationale/Comment
Sensation loss	CI	Adam and Thompson, 1996[5]	Hand Clinic	A manufacturer's manual is cited.

M00-M99 DISEASES OF THE MUSCULOSKELETAL SYSTEM AND CONNECTIVE TISSUE

Issue	LOC	Sources	Affil	Rationale/Comment
Joint infection—active	CI	Adam and Thompson, 1996[5]	Hand Clinic	

Joint arthrosis—acute	CI			A manufacturer's manual is cited.
Joint—unstable/ insufficient soft tissue constraints (ligaments)	RCI	O'Driscoll and Giori, 2000[1]	MD	**In a 1994 Kansas lawsuit,[6] a 42-year-old patient with rheumatoid arthritis and s/p knee prosthesis was awarded $50,000 after CPM use led to a knee dislocation. The FDA[2] has also received three reports of dislocations in patients with hip or knee joint prostheses while using CPM.**
Translation of opposing bone—unwanted	CI	Starkey, 1999[3]	ATC	**See FDA report[2]; lawsuit[6]**

S00-T98 INJURIES

Issue	LOC	Sources	Affil	Rationale/Comment
Fracture—rigid fixation not attained	CI	Adam and Thompson, 1996[5]	MD	
	RCI	O'Driscoll and Giori, 2000[1]	MD	

Y70-Y82 MEDICAL DEVICES

Issue	LOC	Sources	Affil	Rationale/Comment
Restrictive (nonelastic) dressing on limb	P	O'Driscoll and Giori, 2000[1]	MD	Avoid circumferentially wrapped dressings on limbs during CPM. Abrasions can occur from the compressive and shear forces of restrictive nonelastic dressing against wounds. Consider elastic tub grip sleeve or fishnet that can freely move with the joint.

Continued

Issue	LOC	Sources	Affil	Rationale/Comment
Rubbing from straps and carriage	P	Starkey, 1999[3]	ATC	**In a 1998 Ohio lawsuit,[7] a 78-year-old male s/p knee replacement surgery received a $35,000 settlement after he sustained a heel ulcer while using CPM. The FDA also received two reports of abrasions caused by rubbing of the device on skin. Also see FDA reports.[2]**

VULNERABLE BIOLOGICAL TISSUE

Issue	LOC	Sources	Affil	Rationale/Comment
Nerves—peripheral (excessive pressure)	P	O'Driscoll and Giori, 2000[1]	MD	Patients may develop nerve compression palsies due to local pressure from a CPM device. The risk is increased if an anesthetic is used or if patient and staff fail to recognize pressure. Consider frequent adjustments in position and close monitoring. **The FDA received three reports of nerve palsy (peroneal) from pressure during CPM.**

PROCEDURAL CONCERNS

Issue	LOC	Sources	Affil	Rationale/Comment
Adjunct—use	Advice	Tan, 1998[8]	MD/PT	Only use CPM as an adjunct to an exercise program. It does not strengthen muscle.
Tension in the wound if swelling is already present	P	O'Driscoll and Giori, 2000[1]	MD	Do not use CPM through the joint's full range until swelling is reduced.

ADVERSE EVENTS

FOOD AND DRUG ADMINISTRATION REPORTS[2]

Powered Exerciser

Date	Device	Event	Outcome
2/12/01	Othologic CPM	A unit reportedly changed from 90 degrees abduction to 0 degrees. Patient underwent a second surgery that resulted in infection.	Infection
10/13/00	Optiflex CPM	Patient was s/p knee surgery and placed in the device while on morphine and asleep with a sheet covering the unit. Seven hours later, the right foot was found wedged under the carriage with a cut between the first and second toe that required 9 stitches. The staff could not visualize the patient and the patient could not respond to the pain.	Laceration
8/02/99	Legasus 10000X CPM	A patient got out of bed in the middle of the night and fell, tripped, or fainted onto a CPM left on the floor. The patient severed his ear and required surgery to reattach it.	Severed ear
4/09/99	8080 Hand and wrist CPM	A patient sustained a wrist fracture with the device under the supervision of a therapist. No details provided.	Wrist fracture
8/20/96	CPM (Smith and Nephew)	The CPM operated erratically and resulted in pain that required additional surgery.	Required surgery
6/14/96	Sutter Litelift	An attorney reports a 78-year-old woman with osteoporosis and s/p TKR surgery who on post-op day 3 was found to have dislocated her knee due to an anterior force acting on tibia.	Dislocated knee
7/21/95	Sutter Corp	Product liability—no information.	Not reported
2/03/95	Total CPM (Invacare)	The patient incorrectly set the CPM and overflexed the arm.	Ulna fracture
1/10/94	Stryker continuous passive motion leg exerciser	The skin at the base of an elderly patient's penis was caught in the hip hinge of the device resulting in a <2 cm abrasion.	Penile abrasion

Continued

Date	Device	Event	Outcome
9/17/93	Continuous passive motion (Smith and Nephew)	The CPM malfunctioned following R knee replacement surgery, resulting in a peroneal nerve injury.	Peroneal nerve injury
6/02/92	Stryker continuous passive motion	An 80-year-old woman's left foot became lodged between the leg carriage and base of the CPM device and sustained a chip fracture of the left metatarsal.	Metatarsal fracture
4/20/92	Smith and Nephew continuous passive motion	A man placed his finger in the gear of the CPM device (the shielded area was broken) and sustained a severe laceration of the right index finger.	Laceration
5/01/90	CPM 100 (Empi)	A patient sustained a hip dislocation. The details are in dispute, i.e., unit collapse versus jerky movements of the unit.	Hip dislocation
3/01/88	Richards Medical	The CPM device turned over on its side and dislocated the patient's hip.	Hip dislocation
4/16/86	Stryker Corp	A patient with knee surgery was using a CPM unit when an unknown individual allegedly turned the knee flexion control to a full 110 degrees, resulting in full knee flexion and a patella tendon rupture.	Patella tendon rupture
11/14/85	Sutter Biomechanical	A 19-year-old patient s/p surgery for a ruptured flexor tendon of the left hand used a CPM device attached to a wrist splint via a bracket. The device slipped off, stressed, and injured the surgical repair.	Re-injury of surgical repair
11/21/86	Richards Medical Patient guided knee exerciser	A 77-year-old female sustained a fractured femur with the exerciser.	Femoral fracture
6/25/86	Richards Medical Patient guided knee exerciser	An obese patient sustained a drop foot after the weight of his leg resulted in compression between the articulating frame and the leg near the peroneal nerve.	Nerve injury (peroneal)
5/07/86	Stryker Corp CPE	A nurse lifted a CPM unit by the frame instead of the handle. The frame separated from the nylon block and dropped on the nurse's foot resulting in a fracture.	Foot fracture
12/06/85	Richards Medical	Patient's leg became impinged on the moving parts of exerciser, resulting in bruises and cuts.	Leg laceration and bruise

6/11/85	Richards Medical	A patient with knee replacement surgery got his foot caught in the moving parts of the device's frame while sleeping.	Not reported
6/10/85	Richards Medical	A nurse placed her hand in the moving parts of a CPM unit while setting it up and sustained a laceration.	Hand laceration
4/15/85	Richards Medical	An obese patient s/p total knee replacement sustained an abrasion on the knee due to patient's knee rubbing on the hinge of exerciser. The physical therapist had changed setup procedures and had stopped using (wrapping) a towel as done previously.	Knee abrasion
4/09/85	Richards Medical	A patient with a total knee replacement was using unit for 4 hours. The hinge of the exerciser's articulating arm abraded the leg resulting in peroneal nerve damage and foot drop.	Peroneal nerve injury; abrasion
1/25/85	Richards Medical	A 92-year-old woman caught her contralateral leg in the moving frame, resulting in a fractured ankle that required surgery.	Ankle fracture

Note: FDA reports do not necessarily establish cause-effect relationships between equipment and injury. Incidences may be due to equipment or user error. Also, some reports are alleged by attorneys.

LITIGATION

Year, State	History	Location	Device	Complication	Comments/Award
1998, Ohio[7] **CPM and heel ulcer**	78-year-old man s/p knee replacement surgery	Doctors Hospital	Postop continuous passive motion machine	Heels were unprotected and ulcerated from rubbing on sheets while machine in use.	Claimed that nurse failed to pad heels to protect from injury Settlement $35,000

Continued

Year, State	History	Location	Device	Complication	Comments/Award
1994, Kansas[6] **CPM and knee dislocation**	42-year-old person with rheumatoid arthritis and femur fracture s/p knee prosthesis	Hospital and surgeon	Using CPM for 2½ hours	Knee dislocated and required replacement of knee prosthesis	Alleged that employees refused to turn off machine and machine was set incorrectly Net verdict $50,000 against hospital

Note: Awards and settlements do not necessarily prove a cause-effect relationship between equipment, therapy, and injury.

REFERENCES

1. O'Driscoll SW, Giori NJ: Continuous passive motion: theory and principles of clinical application. J Rehabil Res Dev 37(2):179-188, 2000.
2. U.S. Food and Drug Administration: Center for Device and Radiological Health. Available at: http://www.fda.gov/cdrh/mdr/. Accessed: November 7, 2005.
3. Starkey C: Therapeutic modalities for athletic trainers, ed 2. Philadelphia: FA Davis; 1999.
4. Graham B, Loomer RL: Anterior compartment syndrome in a patient with fracture of the tibial plateau treated by continuous passive motion and anticoagulants. Report of a case. Clin Orthop Rel Res 195:197-199, 1985.
5. Adam KM, Thompson ST: Continuous passive motion use in hand therapy. Hand Clin 12(1):109-127, 1996.
6. Medical malpractice verdicts, settlements, and experts, July 1994, p 43, loc 1.
7. Medical malpractice verdicts, settlements, and experts, February 1998, p 24, loc 2.
8. Tan JC: Practical manual of physical medicine and rehabilitation: diagnostics, therapeutics, and basic problems. St Louis: Mosby; 1998.

(Includes Mechanical and Inversion Traction)
(Excludes Manual Traction)

OVERVIEW. Traction is a modality that uses force to elongate soft tissue and separate bone surfaces at the joint. The aim is to address general joint hypomobility, reduce subacute inflammation, treat nerve root impingement, and treat disc herniations.

The proposed mechanisms for traction include (1) gating out pain transmissions, (2) interrupting the pain-spasm cycle, (3) reducing pressure on pain-sensitive structures (reducing the disc's bulge that compresses a nerve root), and (4) increasing the size of the foramen opening.[1]

Traction can be administered mechanically (using an electric motor), manually (using hands), and positionally. Mechanical traction devices typically include an electric motor, a cable, and a harness or device that is secured to the patient's body. Inversion traction is a special case of positional traction whereby individuals use their own body weight (often hanging upside-down from boots) to exert traction forces on the low back. This section will report on spinal traction applied mechanically or through inversion.[1]

SUMMARY: CONTRAINDICATIONS AND PRECAUTIONS. Ten sources cited a total of 51 concerns for spinal traction. Approximately 40 and 43 concerns are relevant to lumbar and cervical traction, respectively. Concerns ranged from 5 to 29 per source, with a physical therapist citing the greatest number. The largest proportion of concerns was musculoskeletal (24%). Whereas digestive (i.e., hernia, hemorrhoids, peptic ulcer) and respiratory concerns were particular to lumbar traction, TMJ, denture, and C1-C2 stability issues were particular to cervical traction. Overall, the most frequently cited concerns were malignancy, cardiovascular disease, and osteoporosis.

OTHER ISSUES.   The FDA[2] received nine reports of mechanical traction malfunctioning between February 1985 and July 2000 that allegedly have resulted in soft tissue injury, including increased symptoms, pain, and contusions. The devices exceeded the load setting, released cord tension unexpectedly, or fell from an unsecured position.

Notes: (1) Perhaps future published guidelines can emphasize periodic maintenance/calibration of mechanical traction units. (2) Technical note: some source variability may be attributed to regional traction concerns (i.e., cervical versus lumbar).

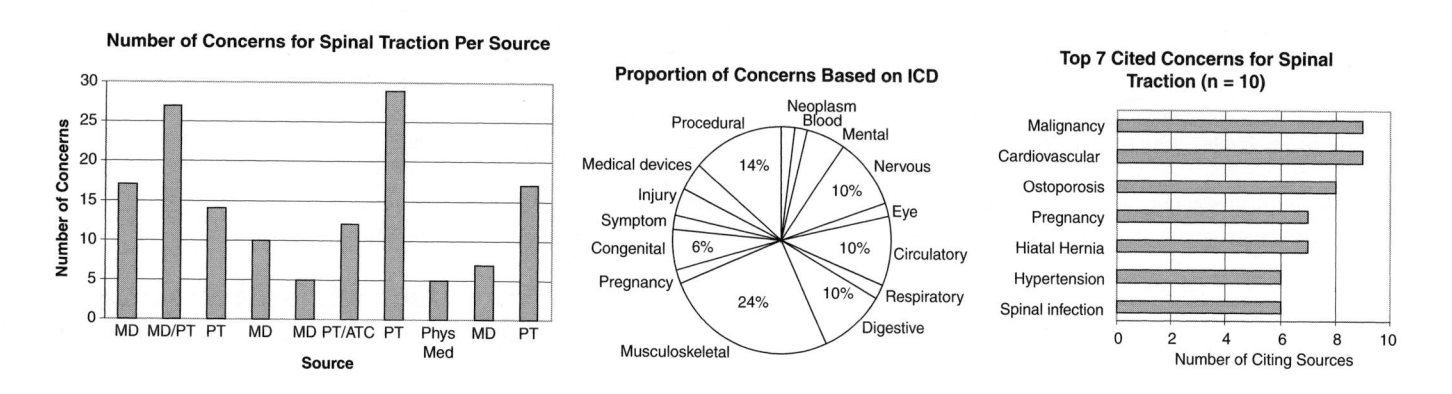

CONTRAINDICATIONS AND PRECAUTIONS FOR TRACTION

C00-C97 NEOPLASMS

Issue	LOC	Source	Affil	Rationale/Comment
Malignancy	CI	Judovich, 1952[3,a]	MD	Heavy traction can produce severe damage in presence of metastatic lesions.[3]
	CI	Hinterbuchner, 1985[4]	MD	**In a case report, LaBan and Meerschaert[10] describe a 77-year-old male**
	CI	Tan, 1998[5,e]	MD/PT	**with severe paravertebral, cervical, shoulder and anterior chest**
	CI	Geiringer and deLateur, 1990[6,a]	MD	**pain who became quadriparetic following intermittent overhead**
	CI	Pellechia, 1994[7,b]	PT	**cervical traction. A laminectomy revealed an extradural prostatic**
	CI	Hooker, 2002[8,c]	PT/ATC	**adenocarcinoma.** Judovick recommended roentgen studies of the cervical
	CI	Weisberg and Schmidt, 2006[9,c]	PT	spine, shoulder girdle, and chest on first visit and repeat x-rays if no improvement
	P	Cameron, 2003[1,c]	PT	because lesions may not be evident on initial x-rays (note 1952 publication).[3]
	CI	Yates, 1972[11,d]	MD	

a, Cervical traction; source may not have intended to provide a complete list of contraindications; b, Lumbar traction concern; c, Spinal tumors and cancers; d, Malignant deposits in vertebral disease; e, Lytic lesions.

D50-D89 DISEASES OF BLOOD AND BLOOD-FORMING ORGANS, AND CERTAIN DISORDERS

Issue	LOC	Source	Affil	Rationale/Comment
Bleeding disorders	CI	Tan, 1998[5]	MD/PT	**For inversion/gravity lumbar traction**

F00-F99 MENTAL AND BEHAVIORAL DISORDERS

Issue	LOC	Source	Affil	Rationale/Comment
Anxious patients	CI	Tan, 1998[5]	MD/PT	The patient may not be able to relax.
Claustrophobia	P	Cameron, 2003[1]	PT	Some patients may not tolerate the confined passive environment of mechanical traction. Consider positional or manual traction (less restrictive and no belts).[1]
Disorientation	P			Disoriented patients may move during treatment, get entangled in strapping, and alter traction forces. Consider manual traction.[1]

G00-G99 DISEASES OF THE NERVOUS SYSTEM

Issue	LOC	Source	Affil	Rationale/Comment
Cord compression	CI	Hinterbuchner, 1985[4]	MD	Never apply traction if signs of compression are noted. Typically, these cases require immobilization rather than mobilization.
	CI	Pellechia, 1994[7]	PT	Refer to neurology/neurosurgery. Cord compression may require surgical intervention.[4]
Resolution, complete—of severe pain with traction	P	Cameron, 2003[1]	PT	Complete resolution of pain during treatment may suggest that a nerve block occurred. Monitor neurologic signs (strength, sensation, deep tendon). If no neurologic changes occurred, consider lowering force and/or adjusting the direction of traction forces.[1] **In a 1962 case series, Eie[12] describes 12 patients with lumbar disc herniations who initially experienced symptomatic relief that was followed by neurologic deficits from nerve root compression following lumbar traction.**

Issue	LOC	Source	Affil	Rationale/Comment
				In Frazer's 1954 review,[13] he mentions six complications for traction in Europe, one of which involved leg paresis following the resolution of sciatica.
Root compression—4th sacral	CI	Tan, 1998[5,b]	MD/PT	For lumbar traction.[5,b] Paralysis of the bladder may result.
	CI	Hinterbuchner, 1985[4]	MD	
	CI	Yates, 1972[11,a]	MD	
Peripheralization of symptoms	CI	Cameron, 2003[1]	PT	Peripheralization suggests increased nerve compression (i.e., symptoms move from a central location to the peripherally, down the limb). If this occurs, either discontinue treatment or immediately modify treatment (lower the force, or adjust body position before reapplying traction) so that there is no longer peripheralization of symptoms.[1]
Spondylotic myelopathy	CI/P	Tan, 1998[5]	MD/PT	

a, For S3-4 root compression, if micturition is involved, immediate neurosurgical opinion is warranted; b, Lumbar traction concern for cauda equina compression.

H00-H59 DISEASES OF THE EYE

Issue	LOC	Source	Affil	Rationale/Comment
Glaucoma	CI	Tan, 1998[5]	MD/PT	For inversion/gravity lumbar traction. In a case report, Kobet[14] describes a 44-year-old highly myopic photographer with no past medical history of retinal disease who sustained a retinal tear from using an inversion device for 3 consecutive days for up to 5 minutes.

I00-I99 DISEASES OF THE CIRCULATORY SYSTEM

Issue	LOC	Source	Affil	Rationale/Comment
Aneurysm—aortic	CI	Hinterbuchner, 1985[4]	MD	**For lumbar traction.** An aneurysm is an abnormal dilation of a vessel with a diameter ≥50% of normal. The vessel is weak, results in a permanent sacklike structure and can rupture. (A thoracic aortic aneurysm can rupture under the force of elevated blood pressure.[15])
	CI	Tan, 1998[5]	MD/PT	
	CI	Yates, 1972[11]	MD	
	CI	Pellechia, 1994[7]	PT	
	CI	Weisberg and Schmidt, 2006[9,e]	PT	
Arteriosclerotic obstruction of carotid or vertebral arteries	CI	Tan, 1998[5]	MD/PT	**For cervical traction.** The concern is harness-related neck pressure and its impact on circulation in individuals with arteriosclerosis. Note: The common and internal carotid arteries, if stenosed, can lead to strokes and TIA affecting brain territories supplied by the middle and anterior arteries. One mechanism is embolization from atherosclerotic plaque. The vertebral-basilar circulation is also affected by atherosclerosis.[16]
	CI	Hinterbuchner, 1985[4]	MD	
	CI	Yates, 1972[11]		
Cardiovascular disease	CI	Hinterbuchner, 1985[4]	MD	Harness pressure is a concern in this population. For example, caution is advised because of the possibility of pelvic belt compression on the femoral artery in persons with cardiovascular disease during lumbar traction.[1] **In a 1954 review, Frazer[13] mentions six complications for traction in Europe, one of which involved a cardiovascular reaction in a patient with mitral disease.**
	CI	Tan, 1998[5]	MD/PT	
	CI	Geiringer and deLateur, 1990[6]	MD	
	CI	Pellechia, 1994[7]	PT	
	CI	Hooker, 2002[8,f]	PT/ATC	
	CI	Weisberg and Schmidt, 2006[9,d]	PT	
	P/Caution	Cameron, 2003[1,f]	PT	
	CI/Be careful	Frazer, 1954[13,a,h]	Phys Med	
	CI	Yates, 1972[11,i]	MD	

Hypertension	CI	Hinterbuchner, 1985[4]	MD	The side straps of a cervical halter may compress the jugular vein during cervical
	CI	Tan, 1998[5]	MD/PT	traction. Also, inversion traction can lead to an undesired increase in blood
	P	Judovich, 1952[3,b]	MD	pressure with body inversion in this population. **Vehr et al.[17] showed significant**
	CI	Cameron, 2003[1,c]	PT	**increases in systolic and diastolic blood pressures (average BP 146/97)**
	CI/Be careful	Frazer, 1954[13]	Phys Med[j]	**and no training effect in healthy male students who exercised using**
	CI	Pellechia, 1994[7,g]	PT	**inversion traction.**
				In a randomized experiment Haskvitz and Hanten[18] demonstrated
				significantly increased systolic and diastolic blood pressure in a group of
				young women without cardiovascular a history.
Vertebrobasilar arterial disease	CI	Geiringer and deLateur, 1990[6]	MD	**For cervical traction.** Neck pressure from a halter negatively affects
	CI	Tan, 1998[5]	MD/PT	circulation.[9] Note: The vertebral-basilar circulation, which supplies the cerebellum, medulla, and caudal pons, can be affected by atherosclerosis and embolic occlusion.[16]

Note: Classifying concerns under cardiovascular table is a challenge in that some sources note general vascular or cardiovascular concerns while others specify more local concerns involving the carotid or vertebral-basilar circulation.

a, Cardiac disturbance; b, Hypertension, strap concerns with cervical traction; c, Inversion traction in persons with uncontrolled hypertension; d, Peripheral vascular disease or uncontrolled cardiac disorder because of harness pressure concerns; e, Abdominal aneurysm; f, Vascular; g, Uncontrolled hypertension; h, Affiliation could not be determined from publication; i, Left ventricular heart failure; j, source read its published material about traction for backache at the Australian Association of Physical Medicine's annual meeting.

J00-J99 DISEASES OF THE RESPIRATORY SYSTEM

Issue	LOC	Source	Affil	Rationale/Comment
Lung disease— restrictive	CI	Tan, 1998[5,a]	MD/PT	Thoracic belts used in lumbar traction may constrict respiration. **Quain and Tecklin,[19] using a within-subjects design, demonstrated that mean respiration rate, vital capacity, and tidal volume can worsen in healthy volunteers who undergo lumbar traction in supine with a garment.**
	CI	Pellechia, 1994[7]	PT	
	CI	Hooker, 2002[8]	PT/ATC	
	CI	Weisberg and Schmidt, 2006[9,b]	PT	
	P/Caution	Cameron, 2003[1]	PT	

a, Other breathing disorders; b, Uncontrolled pulmonary disorders.

K00-K93 DISEASES OF THE DIGESTIVE SYSTEM

Issue	LOC	Source	Affil	Rationale/Comment
Hemorrhoids— gross	CI	Hinterbuchner, 1985[4]	MD	**For lumbar traction.** Note: Hemorrhoids are varicose veins in the perianal area that may be associated with any condition that increases intraabdominal pressure.[20] Harness pressure may increase abdominal pressure.
	CI	Pellechia, 1994[7]	PT	
	CI/Be careful	Frazer, 1954[13]	Phys Med	
Hernia—abdominal	CI	Pellechia, 1994[7]	PT	**For lumbar traction.**
Hernia—hiatus		Yates, 1972[11]	MD	**For lumbar traction.** Note: Hernias are acquired or congenital abnormal protrusion of an organ or tissue through a structure, leading to bulging, possible pain, and sometimes incarceration (irreducible) and strangulation. Intraabdominal pressure or activities involving the Valsalva maneuver can aggravate hernia conditions.[20]
	CI	Pellechia, 1994[7]	PT	
	CI	Hinterbuchner, 1985[4,a]	MD	

	CI	Tan, 1998[5,a]	MD/PT	Harness pressure increases abdominal pressure and may cause esophageal reflux in persons with hiatus hernia.[1]
	CI	Weisberg and Schmidt, 2006[9]	PT	
	P	Cameron, 2003[1]	PT	
	CI/Be careful	Frazer, 1954[13,b]	Phys Med	
Hernias—other	CI	Hinterbuchner, 1985[4]	MD	
	CI	Tan, 1998[5]	MD/PT	
Peptic ulcers— active	CI	Hinterbuchner, 1985[4]	MD	**For lumbar traction**
	Probable/CI	Frazer, 1954[13]	Phys Med	

Note: Digestive system concerns generally relate to lumbar traction use.
a, Also other hernias; b, Nonspecific.

M00-M99 DISEASES OF THE MUSCULOSKELETAL SYSTEM AND CONNECTIVE TISSUE

Issue	LOC	Source	Affil	Rationale/Comment
Dislocations—previous	CI	Cameron, 2003[1]	PT	Traction can further increase instability.
Displacement—annular fragment	P			Traction will not affect symptoms or alter the position of a loose fragment. An MRI or CT scan can reveal a detached annular fragment.
Hypermobility/instability—Joint	CI	Cameron, 2003[1]	PT	Traction can lead to further instability and aggravation in persons with
	CI	Hooker, 2002[8]	PT/ATC	hypermobility. Inquire about previous dislocations, C1-C2 instability,

Continued

Issue	LOC	Source	Affil	Rationale/Comment
	CI	Weisberg and Schmidt, 2006[9,g]	PT	RA, Down syndrome, Marfan's syndrome, pregnancy, lactation (high relaxin levels). Consider treating the hypomobile segment manually so as to localize the forces.[1] **(Also see Congenital diseases.)**
	CI	Tan, 1998[5]	MD/PT	
Infectious diseases of the spine	CI	Hinterbuchner, 1985[4]	MD	Muscle or ligament infections may result in structural weakness of the tissues.
	CI	Tan, 1998[5,a]	MD/PT	
	CI	Pellechia, 1994[7]	PT	
	CI	Weisberg and Schmidt, 2006[9]	PT	
	P	Cameron, 2003[1]	PT	
	CI	Hooker, 2002[8]	PT/ATC	
Inflammatory spondylitis	CI	Yates, 1972[11]	MD	For cervical traction including RA, psoriatic arthritis, ankylosing spondylitis. Atlantoaxial subluxation and pain are common complications.
Instability—ligamentous—cervical	CI	Tan, 1998[5]	MD/PT	**For cervical traction.**
Lumbago—acute (lumbar pain)	CI	Pellechia, 1994[7]	PT	**For lumbar traction.**
Osteoporosis	CI	Hinterbuchner, 1985[4]	MD	The concerns center around hazardous belt pressures.[1]
	CI	Yates, 1972[11,h]	MD	
	CI	Tan, 1998[5,c]	MD/PT	
	CI	Geiringer and deLateur, 1990[6,h,c]	MD	
	CI	Pellechia, 1994[7]	PT	
	CI	Hooker, 2002[8]	PT/ATC	
	CI	Weisberg and Schmidt, 2006[9,f]	PT	
	P	Cameron, 2003[1]	PT	

Protrusions—midline, of herniated disks	CI/great caution	Hinterbuchner, 1985[4]	MD	Applying traction to individuals with a midline disc protrusion can lead to cord damage.[4] Traction can increase symptoms when the nerve root compresses medially against the disk. MRI or CT scans can reveal protruding medial disks.
	P	Cameron, 2003[1]	PT	
	P	Judovich, 1952[3,d]	MD	
Rheumatoid arthritis	CI	Hinterbuchner, 1985[4]	MD	Concerns include instability, particularly at the C1-C2 joint.[1]
	CI	Pellechia, 1994[7]	PT	
	CI	Tan, 1998[5]	MD/PT	
	CI	Cameron, 2003[1]	PT	
	CI	Weisberg and Schmidt, 2006[9]	PT	
Structural diseases affecting the spine	P	Cameron, 2003[1]	PT	Diseased bone structures may not withstand traction forces.
	CI	Hooker, 2002[8,e]	PT/ATC	Inquire about possible bone/joint diseases such as cancer, infection, RA, osteoporosis, or the long-term use of steroids. Only treat/monitor with lower traction forces (i.e., manual traction).[1]
	CI	Yates, 1972[11,b]	MD	
Subluxation—Atlantoaxial with spinal cord compromise	CI	Tan, 1998[5]	MD/PT	
Temporomandibular joint problems	P	Cameron, 2003[1]	PT	**For cervical traction.** Halters that apply traction forces through the mandible can irritate current or preexisting TMJ problems. Inquire about TMJ problems. Consider an occipital halter that avoids compression through the mandible.[1] **In a 1997 Virginia lawsuit,[21] a woman with previous TMJ surgery was awarded a $600,000 verdict after receiving cervical traction with a chin strap that aggravated her preexisting TMJ problem.**
	CI	Weisberg and Schmidt, 2006[9]	PT	

a, Discitis and TB concerns; b, For lumbar traction, vertebral diseases such as Paget's disease, osteoporosis, osteomalacia, spondylitis, sepsis, or malignant deposits; c, Osteopenia; d, Cervical traction; e, Bone disease; f, Advanced spinal osteoporosis; g, Spinal hypermobility; h, Also menopausal and steroid osteoporosis for thoracic traction.

O00-O99 PREGNANCY, CHILDBIRTH, AND PUERPERIUM

Issue	LOC	Source	Affil	Rationale/Comment
Pregnancy	CI	Hinterbuchner, 1985[4]	MD	Relaxin levels during pregnancy or lactation are high and can lead to joint
	CI	Yates, 1972[11,a]	MD	hypermobility.[1] Also, harness pressures over the abdomen can be
	CI	Tan, 1998[5,a]	MD/PT	hazardous during pregnancy.[1,9]
	CI	Pellechia, 1994[7]	PT	
	CI	Hooker, 2003[8]	PT/ATC	
	CI	Weisberg and Schmidt, 2006[9]	PT	
	CI	Cameron, 2003[1]	PT	

a, Lumbar traction.

Q00-Q99 CONGENITAL

Issue	LOC	Expert	Affil	Rationale/Comment
Down syndrome	CI	Tan, 1998[5]	MD/PT	Concern for instability at the C1-C2 joint.[1]
	CI	Cameron, 2003[1]	PT	
Marfan's syndrome	CI	Cameron, 2003[1]	PT	Concern for instability at the C1-C2 joint.[1]
Spinal deformity—congenital	CI	Tan, 1998[5]	MD/PT	

R00-R99 SYMPTOMS, SIGNS, AND ABNORMAL CLINICAL AND LABORATORY FINDINGS (NOT ELSEWHERE CLASSIFIED)

Issue	LOC	Source	Affil	Rationale/Comment
Inflammation—acute	CI	Cameron, 2003[1]	PT	Treatment may further stress inflamed areas.[9] (Also see Injury, acute.)
	C	Tan, 1998[5]	MD/PT	
	P	Judovich, 1952[3]	MD	
	CI	Hooker, 2002[8]	PT/ATC	
	CI	Weisberg and Schmidt, 2006[9]	PT	

S00-T98 INJURY, POISONING, AND CERTAIN OTHER CONSEQUENCES OF EXTERNAL CAUSES

Issue	LOC	Source	Affil	Rationale/Comment
Fracture	CI	Hooker, 2002[8]	PT/ATC	
	CI	Cameron, 2003[1]	PT	
Injury—acute	CI	Cameron, 2003[1]	PT	Traction can stress and aggravate acutely inflamed tissue and/or will be
	CI	Tan, 1998[5,a]	MD/PT	of no benefit. Inquire about the time of injury (i.e., within the past
	P	Judovich, 1952[3,b]	MD	72 hours) and evaluate if area is swollen, hot, and red (i.e., inflamed).[1,9]
	CI	Hooker, 2002[8,c]	PT/ATC	
	CI	Weisberg and Schmidt, 2006[9,c]	PT	

a, Soft tissue inflammation (i.e., whiplash); b, Cervical torticollis or myositis; c, Acute sprain or strain.

Y70-Y82 MEDICAL DEVICES

Issue	LOC	Expert	Affil	Rationale/Comment
Dentures	P Not rated	Cameron, 2003[1] Shore, 1979[22,a]	PT DDS	**For cervical traction**. Do not remove dentures during treatment. Removing them can alter alignment and forces through the TMJ if a mandibular halter is used. Alternatively, use an occipital halter to protect TMJ, teeth, and dentures.[1] Shore et al[22] suggest use of an occlusion splints for missing back molars like those used by prize fighters. **In a case report, Franks[23] described a 35-year-old woman with cervical OA and missing teeth who experienced early right TMJ OA as a result of joint loading during cervical traction.**
Hazardous traction belts— cervical or lumbar-thoracic	P CI	Cameron, 2003[1] Weisberg and Schmidt, 2006[9,b]	PT PT	Belts can compress vulnerable, regions (pregnant uterus, carotid artery, femoral arteries, inguinal hernia, cardiopulmonary disorders). Consider self-traction or manual traction, or adjust belts away from compromised vessels.[1] **In a case report, Simmers et al[24] describe a 49-year-old woman with neck and back pain who presented with a right internal jugular vein thrombus 3 days after receiving Glisson cervical axial traction. The thrombus was possibly due to trauma-induced venous status during cervical traction.**

a, Shore et al did not offer a set of guidelines and therefore was not included in the descriptive statistics; b, Also individuals with skin sensitivity (diabetes).

Issue	LOC	Source	Affil	Rationale/Comment
Any condition that worsens with traction	CI CI	Hooker, 2002[8] Weisberg and Schmidt, 2006[9]	PT/ATC PT	Increased numbness, sensory loss, or pain radiation with traction in individuals with spinal dysfunction can indicate a worsening of the condition.[9]
Inadequate expertise/training	CI CI	Tan, 1998[5] Geiringer and deLateur, 1990[6]	MD/PT MD	Treatment failure may be due to insufficient force or improper patient positioning.[5]
Motion—when contraindicated	CI CI	Cameron, 2003[1] Weisberg and Schmidt, 2006[9,a]	PT PT	An unstable spine can worsen with traction (movement) forces. Inquire about recent spinal surgery, spinal compression, spinal fractures, or use of corsets and braces to immobilize the spine.[1] Low continuous force loads to immobilize area may be indicated.[9]
Old age	CI P	Hinterbuchner, 1985[4] Yates, 1972[11,b] Tan, 1998[5]	MD MD MD/PT	Most concerns for traction apply to older people (i.e., comorbidities).[5]
Positioning—marked hyperextension	P	Judovich, 1952[3]	MD	**For cervical traction.** The halter's side straps can compress the jugular vein during traction.
Poor tolerance of position for procedure	P CI	Cameron, 2003[1] Weisberg and Schmidt, 2006[9,c]	PT PT	The patient may not be able to relax, which may work against any potential benefits of traction.[9] Mechanical traction is typically administered in supine or prone positions. Inquire about problems such as reflux esophagitis. Alternatively, consider the sitting position for cervical traction and using self-traction for lumbar traction.[1]
Steroids—systemic (prolonged use)	P	Cameron, 2003[1]	PT	Steroid use over time may affect spine structurally.

a, CI unless continuous traction; b, Lumbar traction; c, Not position-specific.

ADVERSE EVENTS

Source	Background	Therapy	Outcome	Follow-up/Interpretation
Eie, 1962[12] **Herniation, root compression, and lumbar traction** Case series (from the 12 cases) J Oslo City Hosp	A 23-year-old female with an L4-5 lateral herniation and six lumbar vertebrae presented with lumbar pain and sciatic irradiation due to strain.	Lumbar traction was attempted following conservative treatment. On the third session, pain increased and then suddenly disappeared. Traction was discontinued.	She noted left foot numbness, bladder paresis, a more marked scoliosis, and an inability to dorsiflex her left foot. Myelograph revealed an enlarged herniation. Surgery revealed an almost complete rupture.	Fifteen months after surgery, she reported occasional pain in her left leg, discomfort in her spine, difficulties voiding, but no paresis.
	A 36-year-old presented with chronic low back pain and acute irradiation into the toes of the left foot.	Lumbar traction resulted in foot weakness after a few sessions and drop foot after 13 sessions (pain relief was reported during sessions but became worse at completion).	Myelography revealed a large L4 interspace herniation with 5th lumbar root compression and sacral root 1 and 2 displacement. The individual underwent surgery 1 week following the paralysis.	Four years later, only slight dorsiflexion foot paresis remained.
	A 29-year-old female presented with pain and scoliosis.	Lumbar traction was administered twice a day for about 1 month despite worsening symptoms.	Paresis of the right big toe dorsiflexors occurred. Surgery revealed a large lateral disk herniation compressing on the 5th lumbar root.	No complaints noted over a year following surgery.

	A 40-year-old man presented with a 4-year history of lumbar pain and bilateral sciatica that worsened with coughing.	Following conservative treatment, lumbar traction was attempted. Pain was relieved during sessions but weakness occurred 1 hour later (he required a taxi to return home). He became bedridden with bowel and bladder problems after the 17th session.	Weakness was noted in left dorsiflexion. Surgery revealed a large herniation with detached extradural disk material at the 5th lumbar interspace.	Follow-up was not reported.
	A 48-year-old female with a 9-year history of recurrent lumbago experienced acute pain radiation to her right heel.	Following conservative treatments, she received lumbar traction, which initially relieved symptoms but recurred 2 weeks later. She became bedridden with weakness of the right dorsiflexors.	Myelography revealed a very large herniation with loose cartilage in the 4th midline interspace.	Over 3 years later, the patient reported no problems.
Franks, 1965[23] **Incomplete dentition, TMJ pain, and cervical traction** Case report Ann Phys Med	A 35-year-old woman presented with a history of neck fibrositis and a diagnosis of cervical vertebrae OA.	She was treated with a course of cervical traction. Analgesics were required for facial pain after each session. This acute pain gradually progressed to a continuous dull ache over the right TMJ.	Dx: Early OA of the right TMJ due to joint loading during traction. Examination revealed incomplete dentition, crepitus, tenderness of the right TMJ, limited opening/lateral movements, and a right deviation on closing. Radiographs were negative. Treatment included rest, analgesics,	The author states forces of cervical traction are usually tolerated in normal occlusion of teeth. "Undoubtedly in the case reported here the lack of posterior tooth support had allowed overloading of the

Continued

Source	Background	Therapy	Outcome	Follow-up/Interpretation
			the termination of traction, and partial restoration of her dentition. Symptomatic relief occurred 2 weeks after the appliance was given.	temporomandibular joints during the cervical traction." The author recommended that dentition be restored before administering cervical traction to reduce the risk of iatrogenic injury.
Frazer, 1954[13] Review **Traction and complications** Med J Aust	Frazer reviewed the literature on traction and suggested care in recommending tractions for probable contraindications: • Active peptic ulcer • Unduly high blood pressure • Hernia • Cardiac disturbances • Gross hemorrhoids	Six complications are reported: • Dislocation of one apophyseal articulation • Cardiovascular reaction in mitral disease • Leg paresis following the disappearance of sciatica • Three cases of hyperalgic reactions		"In 25,000 tractions reported in Europe, only six untoward sequelae resulted." Note: No citations or evidence provided with regard to the origin of these six reported complications.
Haskvitz and Hanten, 1986[18] **Retinal tear and inversion traction** Experiment Phys Ther	60 women, ages 20-30, without cardiovascular history were randomly assigned to an experimental or control group.	The experimental group assumed an inverted position for 2 minutes.	Both systolic and diastolic blood pressure significantly increased ($P < .05$).	The authors caution to avoid inversion in persons with hypertension, those with borderline hypertension, and in those unaware of their blood pressure status.

Kobet, 1985[14] **Retinal tear and inversion** Case report Ann Ophthalmol	A 44-year-old highly myopic photographer with no past medical history of retinal disease used an inversion device.	The device was used for 3 consecutive days as directed in the manual, progressing to a head-down position. On day 3, the individual remained upside-down for 4 to 5 minutes. Within several hours, photopsia and floaters in the right eye were noted.	Ophthalmoscope examination revealed a large horseshoe retinal tear located at the 6 o'clock meridian (inferior retinal break) with the posterior edge of the tear at the equator. Treatment consisted of same-day prophylactic cryopexy. Six weeks later, an excellent chorioretinal adhesion surrounded the tear.	The author states that the temporal sequence of events along with the location of the retinal tear suggested the injury was precipitated by the inverted posture.
LaBan et al, 1992[25] **Fibrotic lumbar root and cervical traction** Case series Arch Phys Med Rehabil	12 subjects (7 female; 5 male) ages 33 to 66 years presented with cervical radiculopathy. These patients also all had either congenital lumbar spinal anomalies or associated osteoarthrosis.	PT suburban community hospital. Intermittent cervical traction, seated, neck 30 degrees flexed, start 15 lb, graduating up to 30 lb (10 sec on—3 sec off).	The patients experienced increased lumbar pain and sciatica with traction that was not relieved by LE flexion positional changes.	After 3 weeks, marked improvement of sciatica was noted in all patients, suggesting that tension was transmitted via the dural covering from the cervical spine to the tethered, fibrotic lumbar roots. The authors consider this situation a CI for cervical traction.

Source	Background	Therapy	Outcome	Follow-up/Interpretation
LaBan and Meerschaert, 1977[10] **Tumor, quadriparesis, and cervical traction** Case series APMR	A 77-year-old man presented with severe paravertebral, cervical, bilateral shoulder and anterior chest pain.	He underwent intermittent heavy overhead cervical traction at 12 lb (5.5 kg); details not reported.	The following day, pain was less. On day 2, gait instability, LE weakness, hyperalgesia in the C7-T3 dermatome distribution, and absent abdominal cutaneous reflexes were noted. In the morning of day 3, he had difficulty voiding and tested positive for a left Babinski reflex. Myelogram revealed a complete block at T3 to retrograde flow. Radiographs revealed a severe degenerative spondylosis. The patient underwent a total laminectomy at C7-T3 with partial removal of an extradural prostatic adenocarcinoma; his quadriparesis progressed.	The authors stress the importance of recognizing early signs/symptoms of spinal cord tumor: • Hx primary malignancy • Inappropriate response to conservative treatment • New or progressive motor signs Low cervical distraction may potentiate quadriplegia by compromising blood supply, overstretching a pathological cord, and increasing ligament instability.
Lehmann and Brunner, 1958[26] **Respiration and harness straps** Descriptive Arch Phys Med Rehabil	Study of upright heavy traction to the lumbar area.	Traction forces between 300 and 400 pounds were assessed.	The authors report a complication of obese patients undergoing lumbar traction.	"The most difficult complication was that some obese persons exhibited a tendency to faint under heavy traction of this type. This was

Quain and Tecklin, 1985[19] **Respiration and lumbar traction** Within subjects Phys Ther	The respiratory status of 30 healthy volunteers, age 21-35, were monitored under three lumbar traction conditions.	These conditions were: supine, supine with a harness, and supine with a garment and lumbar traction.	RR increased and VC and TL decreased under the third condition. Mean respiration rate increased from 14 to 16 rpm. Mean vital capacity decreased from 4.21 to 3.17 L and mean tidal volume decreased from 0.88 to 0.70 L.	partially explained on the basis of the pressure applied to the chest and abdomen by the harness and the pelvic belt; this, in turn, probably decreased the venous return and made breathing difficult. However, none of our volunteers or patients actually fainted since the hydraulic device permitted smooth and fast release of the heavy traction." The authors suggest that if lumbar traction is administered to persons with respiratory disease, one should closely monitor for respiratory distress during the first few treatment sessions.

Continued

Source	Background	Therapy	Outcome	Follow-up/Interpretation
Simmer et al, 1997[26] **Thrombus and cervical traction** Case report J Intern Med	A 49-year-old woman presented with a long history of neck and back ache. She was taking oral contraceptives and had no infection or malignancy in the area.	A physiotherapist administered Glisson traction for eight sessions biweekly for 15 min duration to decrease neck pain. (Note: This device involves cervical axial traction using weight attached to a pulley, and straps encompassing the head.)	Three days after treatment, right neck pain and swelling along the sternocleidomastoid muscle was noted. Ultrasonography revealed a right internal jugular vein thrombus.	The patient was hospitalized and given intravenous heparin. Pain and swelling subsided in 8 days, suggesting trauma-induced venous stasis and vascular injury, that resulting in a thrombus.
Vehr et al, 1988[17] **Hypertension and inversion traction** Experiment (nonrandomized) Arch Phys Med Rehabil	19 healthy, moderately active male students trained for 5 weeks three times a week using inversion traction.	The experimental and control groups were composed of 10 and 9 subjects, respectively. Traction durations gradually increased from 10 minutes to 30 minutes under passive conditions or while exercising.	Significant increases in systolic and diastolic blood pressure (average BP = 146/97) and decreases in heart rate were recorded during inversion. In addition, no training effects were noted.	The authors state a need to carefully screen people for gravity inversion devices because the increased blood pressures may be dangerous.

FDA[2] REPORTS FOR MECHANICAL TRACTION

Date	Device	Event	Outcome
7/28/00	Hydrocollator Tx traction unit	A patient underwent traction for 13-15 minutes. A sudden release of tension occurred as the traction rope unwound.	The patient sustained a sudden jerk.

Date	Device	Description	Outcome/Cause
3/8/96	Triton Chatt	Cervical traction started at 2 lb, gradually increasing up to 17 lb (four steps up and four steps down, 10 sec hold and 10 sec release).	At 4 minutes, the patient stopped traction due to discomfort. Force recorded: 56 lbs.
7/19/90	TXE 7	A cervical traction force cycled beyond its maximal treatment setting of 40 lb. The abort switch was beyond the patient's reach.	Report type: serious injury (no details).
1/25/88	Tru tract	A patient s/p whiplash underwent traction. After treatment, the machine turned on after being turned off. The traction release switch was broken (based on an investigation).	Report type: serious injury (no details).
1/25/88	Tru tract	The unit "clicked" and began winding up before the patient could stop the unit. He complained of headaches in the suboccipital region and went to the ER.	A microswitch was not correctly adjusted. A repair technician readjusted the switch and calibrated the unit. The cause of the problem could not be determined.
1/25/88	Tru tract	The unit allegedly pulled past the prescribed poundage, overstressing soft tissue or aggravating the existing condition.	A technician found loose screws on a switch arm/plate. The item was tightened and the unit calibrated.
1/25/88	Tru tract	A traction table dropped from a high to a low position while the patient was on it. The patient complained of pain, but no injury was noted by the physician.	
1/5/88	Tru tract	While receiving cervical traction set at 12 lb in a static mode, the poundage allegedly increased to 35 lb. The patient complained of TMJ pain.	Possible user error. The manufacturer found the unit to function properly.
2/19/85	Tru tract	The unit fell from a stand, striking a female patient on her head and shoulder. She sustained a contusion to her scalp and went to the ER.	The clamp and bracket attaching the traction unit to a portable traction stand broke.

Note: FDA Reports do not necessarily establish cause-effect relationships between equipment and injury. Incidences may be due to equipment or user error. Also, some reports are alleged by attorneys.

LITIGATION

Year, State	Background	Treatment	Adverse event	Verdict
1997, Virginia[21] **TMJ and cervical traction**	A woman had TMJ surgery 8 years previously and was taking pain medication for a back injury.	A physical therapist administered cervical traction using chin strap.	The chin strap on the head halter traction device aggravated a preexisting TMJ problem.	The patient claimed a special occipital harness used to avoid TMJ injury should have been used. She failed to inform the therapist of her prior surgery but also voiced no complaints of TMJ problems just prior traction. The TMJ problems may have been masked by her back pain and the medication she was taking. $600,000 verdict

Note: Awards and settlements do not necessarily prove a cause-effect relationship between equipment or therapy and injury.

REFERENCES

1. Cameron MH: Physical agents in rehabilitation: from research to practice. St Louis: Saunders; 2003.
2. U.S. Food and Drug Administration: Web page. Available at: http://www.fda.gov/cdrh/mdr/. Accessed: November 7, 2005.
3. Judovich BD: Herniated cervical disc; a new form of traction therapy. Am J Surg 84:646, 1952.
4. Hinterbuchner C: Traction. In Basmajian JV, editor: Manipulation, traction, and massage, ed 3. Baltimore: Williams & Wilkins; 1995.
5. Tan JC: Practical manual of physical medicine and rehabilitation: diagnostics, therapeutics, and basic problems. St Louis: Mosby; 1998.
6. Geiringer SR, deLateur BJ: Physiatric therapeutics 3. Traction, manipulation, and massage. Arch Phys Med Rehabil 71(4-S):S264-S266, 1990.
7. Pellechia GL: Lumbar traction: a review of the literature. J Orthop Sports Phys Ther 20(5):262-267, 1994.
8. Hooker DN. Spinal traction. In: Prentice WE, editor: Therapeutic modalities for physical therapists, ed 2. New York: McGraw-Hill; 2002.
9. Weisberg J, Schmidt TA. Spinal traction. In: Hecox B, Mehreteab TA, Weisberg J, eds: Integrating physical agents in rehabilitation. Upper Saddle River (NJ): Pearson Prentice Hall; 2006.

10. LaBan MM, Meerschaert JR: Quadriplegia following cervical traction in patients with occult epidural prostatic metastasis. Arch Phys Med Rehabil 56(10):455-458, 1975.
11. Yates DAH: Indications and contra-indications for spinal traction. Physiotherapy 58(2):55-57, 1972.
12. Eie N: Complications and hazards of traction in the treatment of ruptured lumbar intervertebral disks. J Oslo City Hosp Board 12:5-12, 1962.
13. Frazer EH: The use of traction in backache. Med J Aust 41,694-697, 1954.
14. Kobet KA Retinal tear associated with gravity boot. Ann Ophthalmol 17(5):308-310, 1985.
15. Goodman CC: The cardiovascular system. In: Goodman CC, Boissonnault WG, Fuller KS, eds: Pathology: implications for the physical therapist, ed 2. Philadelphia: Saunders; 2003.
16. Jensen FE: Cerebrovascular disease. In Loscalzo J, Creager MA, Dzau VJ, eds: Vascular medicine: a textbook of vascular biology and diseases, ed 2. Boston: Little, Brown; 1996.
17. Vehr PR, Plowman SA, Fernhall B: Exercise during gravity inversion: acute and chronic effects. Arch Phys Med Rehabil 69(11):950-954, 1988.
18. Haskvitz EM, Hanten WP: Blood pressure response to inversion traction. Phys Ther 66:1361-1364, 1986.
19. Quain MB, Tecklin JS: Lumbar traction. Its effect on respiration. Phys Ther 65:1343-1346, 1985.
20. Goodman CC: The gastrointestinal system. In: Goodman CC, Boissonnault WG, Fuller KS, eds: Pathology: implications for the physical therapist, ed 2. Philadelphia: Saunders; 2003.
21. Medical malpractice verdicts, settlements, and experts, November 1997, p 41, loc 1.
22. Shore NA, Schaefer MG, Hoppenfeld S: Iatrogenic TMJ difficulty: cervical traction may be the etiology. J Prosthet Dent 41(5):541-542, 1979.
23. Franks AST: Temporomandibular joint dysfunction associated with cervical traction. Ann Phys Med 8(1):38-40, 1965.
24. Simmers TA, Bekkenk MW, Vidakovic-Vukic M: Internal jugular vein thrombosis after cervical traction. J Intern Med 241(4):333-335, 1997.
25. LaBan MM, Macy JA, Meerschaert JR: Intermittent cervical traction: a progenitor of lumbar radicular pain. Arch Phys Med Rehabil 73:295-296, 1992.
26. Lehmann JF, Brunner GD: A device for the application of heavy lumbar traction: its mechanical effects. Arch Phys Med Rehabil 39(11):696-700, 1958.

52   ACUPUNCTURE

OVERVIEW. Acupuncture, a traditional form of Chinese medicine, involves the insertion of fine needles through the skin and into strategic body points along meridians, for a desired therapeutic or preventive effect. Some of its uses include pain relief and anesthesia induction.[1]

SUMMARY: CONTRAINDICATIONS AND PRECAUTIONS. Three sources cited a total of 37 concerns for acupuncture. Concerns ranged from 3 to 24 per source, with the World Health Organization (WHO) citing the largest number. The largest proportion of concerns is related to puncturing vulnerable biological tissue (31%) or introducing infections (procedural issues). The most frequently cited concerns (two or more) involved bleeding disorders, pregnancy (miscarriages), and penetrating vulnerable body regions such as the supraclavicular fossa area where lung puncture and pneumothorax can occur.

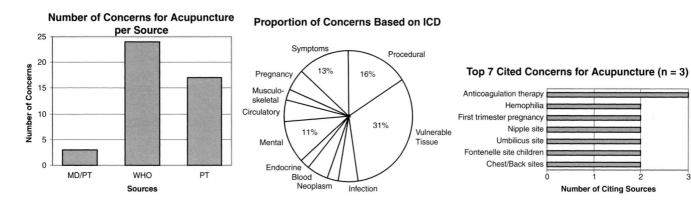

Number of Concerns for Acupuncture per Source

Proportion of Concerns Based on ICD

Top 7 Cited Concerns for Acupuncture (n = 3)

CONTRAINDICATIONS AND PRECAUTIONS

A00-B99 CERTAIN INFECTIONS AND PARASITIC DISEASES

Issue	LOC	Sources	Affil	Rationale/Comment
Infection—at needle site	CI	Tan, 1998[2]	MD/PT	Infection at site of needle insertion.
Infection (active)—blood-borne	CI			

C00-C97 NEOPLASMS

Issue	LOC	Sources	Affil	Rationale/Comment
Malignant tumors—at needling site	CI	WHO, 1999[3]	Org	Avoid needling at the cancer site. Acupuncture has been used as an adjunct for pain management or symptom relief of chemotherapy or radiation.

D50-D89 DISEASES OF BLOOD AND BLOOD-FORMING ORGANS AND CERTAIN DISORDERS

Issue	LOC	Sources	Affil	Rationale/Comment
Anticoagulant therapy	CI/Caution	Pearce, 2000[4]	PT	Do not use deep needling.[4] **In a 2001 prospective survey by White et al,[5] 78 acupuncturists reported 982 events of bleeding over a 21-month period.**
	CI	Tan, 1998[2]	MD/PT	
	CI	WHO, 1999[3]	Org	
Hemophilia	CI	Pearce, 2000	PT	There is a danger of intraarticular bleeding.
	CI	WHO, 1999[3]	Org	

E00-E90 ENDOCRINE, NUTRITIONAL, AND METABOLIC DISEASES

Issue	LOC	Sources	Affil	Rationale/Comment
Diabetics	Caution	Pearce, 2000[4]	PT	Caution due to poor circulation, impaired sensation, and the ability of some points to raise blood sugar levels in this population. **Saw et al[6] described a 55-year-old diabetic woman who developed a life-threatening needle-transmitted necrotizing fasciitis of the right knee with multiple discharging sinuses following an acupuncture treatment. The wound required extensive débridement. (Also see Sterile procedures.)**

F00-F99 MENTAL AND BEHAVIORAL DISORDERS

Issue	LOC	Sources	Affil	Rationale/Comment
Children (small)—moving	CI	Pearce, 2000[4]	PT	Small children may not be able to remain still during needling. Consider acupressure.
Needle—phobic	CI			

Continued

Issue	LOC	Sources	Affil	Rationale/Comment
"Strong reactors"	Caution			Some patients may experience profound relaxation, or report sensations traveling in directions consistent with meridian charts. **Ogata et al[7] reported a 29-year-old man with bronchial asthma who died from a severe asthma attack after receiving Chinese acupuncture and moxibustion treatment for the first time, possibly set off by the emotional stress of the initial treatments.**
Uncooperative	CI	Pearce, 2000[4]		Uncooperative/lack of understanding, i.e., cognitively disabled.

I00-I99 DISEASES OF THE CIRCULATORY SYSTEM

Issue	LOC	Sources	Affil	Rationale/Comment
Circulation—poor (in area)	P	WHO, 1999[3]	Org	Increased risk of infection developing in areas of poor circulation.
Varicose veins	P			

M00-M99 DISEASES OF THE MUSCULOSKELETAL SYSTEM AND CONNECTIVE TISSUE

Issue	LOC	Sources	Affil	Rationale/Comment
Muscle tone—needed for stability	CI	Pearce, 2000[4]	PT	Local orthopedic condition where area relies on the presence of muscle tone for stability.

O00-O99 PREGNANCY, CHILDBIRTH, AND PUERPERIUM

Issue	LOC	Sources	Affil	Rationale/Comment
Pregnancy—first trimester (with strong-acting acupuncture points)	CI CI	Pearce, 2000[4,a] WHO, 1999[3]	PT Org	Avoid strong-acting acupuncture points during the first trimester of pregnancy because of the potential for miscarriage. Points may also induce labor. Avoid abdominal and lumbosacral area during first trimester. After the third month, avoid upper abdomen, lumbosacral, ear acupuncture points, and points that have a strong sensation.

a, Some conditions treated depending on care and experience level.

R00-R99 SYMPTOMS, SIGNS, AND ABNORMAL CLINICAL AND LABORATORY FINDINGS (NOT ELSEWHERE CLASSIFIED)/MISCELLANEOUS

Issue	LOC	Sources		Rationale/Comment
Drug withdrawal therapy	Caution	Pearce, 2000[4]	PT	Adjust drug dosage in patient on a drug withdrawal therapy.
Hunger	CI			Blood chemistry may be altered.
Moles or lumps	CI			Avoid needling directly into moles or lumps of unknown origin.
Pain—undiagnosed	CI			
Weak—very	CI			Blood chemistry may be altered.

Vulnerable Biological Tissue

Issue	LOC	Sources	Affil	Rationale/Comment
Abdomen, back—kidney, liver, spleen	P	WHO, 1999[3]	Org	Avoid kidney, liver, spleen. For chest, back, and abdomen, insert needles obliquely or horizontally to avoid vital organs.
Carotid artery—near	P			ST 9 renying.
Cervical vertebral region	P			Avoid CNS CV 15 yamen; GV 16 fengfu. Needling may puncture the medulla oblongata.
Chest, back, supraclavicular fossa—lung and pleura	P Caution	WHO, 1999[3] Pearce, 2000[4] (for thorax)	Org PT	For chest, back, and abdomen, insert needles obliquely or horizontally to avoid vital organs such as the lung and pleura and to reduce risk of traumatic pneumothorax. **In 2004, Peuker[8] reported a slender woman who sustained a tension pneumothorax after receiving acupuncture at points LU1 (subacromial area) and BL13 (near T3) from a medical acupuncturist.** **In 1995, Halvorsen et al[9] described a 40-year-old woman with fibromyalgia and congenital sternal foramen who died from a perforated right ventricle 2 hours after an acupuncture needle was inserted at the 4th intercostal space (ac pt Ren 17).**
Eye—near	P	WHO, 1999[3]	Org	BL 1 jingming; ST 1 chenqi points.
Eyeballs	Do not puncture			
External genitalia	Do not puncture			
Femoral artery—near	P			SP 11 jimen; SP 12 chongmen.

Fontanelles of children	CI	Pearce, 2000[4]	PT	Forbidden points.
	Do not puncture	WHO, 1999[3]	Org	
Nipple	CI	Pearce, 2000[4]	PT	Forbidden points: nipple. **In 1965, Schiff[10] described an 82-year-old white woman, found dead in her apartment from cardiac tamponade. A sewing needle projected from her precordial area 2 inches to right and 1½ inches below her left nipple, and another needle puncture was noted 3 inches below this site.**
	Do not puncture	WHO, 1999[3]	Org	
Radial artery—near	P	WHO, 1999[3]	Org	LU 9 taiyuan.
Umbilicus—for acupuncture	CI	Pearce, 2000[4]	PT	Forbidden points: umbilicus; moxibustion allowed.
	Do not puncture	WHO, 1999[3]	Org	

PROCEDURAL CONCERNS

Issue	LOC	Sources	Affil	Rationale/Comment
Aseptic technique	Required	WHO, 1999[3]	Org	Do not touch the shaft of the needle prior to inserting it.
Clean hands	Required			Prevent infection. Wash hands immediately before the procedure; sterile surgical gloves or individual finger stalls also recommended. If operator has infected hand lesions, wait until healed before practicing.
Clean needling site	Required			The needle site should be free of cuts or infections. Clean area with 70% alcohol.
Medical emergencies	CI			Acupuncture is CI during medical emergencies.

Continued

Issue	LOC	Sources	Affil	Rationale/Comment
Sterilized needles	Required			Disposable sterile acupuncture needles are strongly recommended. Discard disposable needles in a special container immediately. All needles require proper sterilization and storage. (Improper storage can lead to loss of sterility.) Sterile filiform needles should be used for puncture only once. **In 1982, Pierik[11] reported a 58-year-old housewife with a diagnosis of rheumatoid arthritis who received home acupuncture, developed increased joint swelling and fever, was hospitalized, and died 14 days later, possibly from sepsis.**
Surgeries—necessary	CI			CI if surgery is required for the condition.

Electroacupuncture

Issue	LOC	Sources	Affil	Rationale/Comment
Pacemakers	CI	Pearce, 2000[4]	PT	Electroacupuncture can inhibit demand pacemakers. **(Also see Electrotherapy.)**

ADVERSE EVENTS

Source	Background	Therapy	Outcome	Follow-up/Interpretation
White et al, 2001[5] **Adverse effects and acupuncture**	Surveys collected from June 1998 to February 2000 (21 months) from	Of 31,822 consultations, 2178 events were reported (684 per 10,000 consultations).	43 significant events included administrative (forgetting patient, needle), site (cellulites, blister, allergy, pain), cardiovascular	The authors believe the risk of adverse events following acupuncture is minimal.

Prospective survey (questionnaire) Acupunct Med	78 acupuncturists (doctors and physiotherapists) identified from two organizations in the UK. Two forms were completed: minor adverse events and significant events.	Common events included bleeding (982), needling pain (364), and aggravation (306). Other events included faintness (93), drowsiness (93), bent/stuck needle (40), headache (34), and sweating (33).	(fainting), gastrointestinal, neurological/ psychiatric (panic, headache, seizure, slurred speech, euphoria, sensory changes), and exacerbation of symptoms (back pain, fibromyalgia, shoulder pain, vomiting, migraine).	Some events are preventable. Some of the acupuncturists' recommendations included: • Counting the needles • Ask about allergies and anxiety • Don't treat edematous limb • Don't treat in sitting (i.e., fainting) • Advice about driving after treatment (if "spaced out") • Discontinue if symptoms increase • Reminders of patients (i.e., alarm)
Halvorsen et al, 1995[9] **Intercostals needle insertion and death** Case report Lancet	A 40-year-old woman with fibromyalgia was treated by a professional acupuncturist.	A needle was inserted at the 4th intercostal space (ac pt Ren 17). She shook, complained of chest pain, and demanded needle be removed.	She was taken by ambulance but died about 2 hours after needle insertion. Necropsy revealed a distended pericardial cavity (320 ml of blood), and a perforated lesion in the anterior wall of the right ventricle.	Avoid serious heart injuries in this common acupuncture point. A congenital sternal foramen is found in 9.6% of men and 4.3% of women.

Continued

Source	Background	Therapy	Outcome	Follow-up/Interpretation
Ogata et al, 1992[7] **Asthma, acupuncture and death** Case report Am J Forens Med Pathol	A 29-year-old Japanese man with branchial asthma (since age 20) in increasing frequency and duration presented with severe attacks 2 months prior to seeking acupuncture/moxibustion.	He received Chinese acupuncture and moxibustion treatment for the first time. After two needles (3.5 cm length; 0.1 cm diameter) were inserted in the nuchal area and three moxibustion applications were performed, the man suddenly collapsed.	He died en route to the hospital secondary to a severe asthma attack. Dx: status asthmaticus. Immunohistochemical examination revealed hypoxic brain damage (laminar necrosis) and pulmonary surfactant (unusual distribution). Also, minor right semispinal muscle intramuscular hemorrhage (1.3 × 0.5 cm wide) and round bruises (2 cm diameter) were noted from the treatment.	The authors speculate on whether emotional stress while undergoing Chinese acupuncture and moxibustion for the first time may have played a role. Ischemic changes in the brain may have been due to a severe attack occurring 4 to 6 days before his death.
Pierik, 1982[11] **Needle-induced sepsis and immunosuppressed patient** Case series (1 case reported here) R I Med J	A 58-year-old housewife presented with a diagnosis of rheumatoid arthritis, hypercortisonism due to steroid therapy, and a history of low compliance for Gold salt and thyroid medication (had received no treatment for 7 years).	In 1977, she received home acupuncture (practitioner type and needle sites not recalled but may have included knees and ankles). Following treatment, increased joint swelling and fever were noted.	She was febrile, confused, and malnourished (marked anasarca) with petechiae and purpura on dorsum of UEs, low blood pressure (80/60 mmHg), sacral decubiti, and congested lung bases. She was on bed rest due to flexion deformities and active RA. Cultures were positive for knee, ankle, and blood for hemolytic *Staphylococcus aureus*. Although she received antibiotics and metabolic derangement, she died on the 14th day of hospitalization.	The author argues for the need of a complete medical workup. The author calls attention to evidence of needle-induced sepsis that is "too strong to ignore."

Schiff, 1965[10] **Cardiac tamponade and self-administered acupuncture** Case report Med Times	An 82-year-old white woman (Hungarian emigrant) was found dead in her apartment with a sewing needle projecting from her precordial area.	The $1\frac{7}{8}$-inch long sewing needle penetrated ($\frac{1}{3}$) into thorax 2 inches to right and $1\frac{1}{2}$ inches below her left nipple. Another needle puncture was noted 3 inches below and 2 inches to left of this site.	Dx: Cardiac tamponade. Autopsy revealed that the needle pierced the pericardium and produced a $\frac{1}{8}$-inch laceration of the distal branch of the anterior descending coronary artery. The pericardial cavity was filled with 250 cc of partially clotted blood.	The patient was known to practice acupuncture. The author speculates that she self-administered acupuncture to treat angina.

REFERENCES

1. Eisenberg MG: Dictionary of rehabilitation. New York: Springer; 1995.
2. Tan JC: Practical manual of physical medicine and rehabilitation: diagnostics, therapeutics, and basic problems. St Louis: Mosby; 1998.
3. World Health Organization: Guidelines on basic training and safety in acupuncture, WHO/EDM; 1999. Available at: http://www.who.int/medicine/en. Accessed December 4, 2005.
4. Pearce L: Acupuncture and related therapies. In Charman RA, editor: Complementary therapies for physical therapists. Oxford: Butterworth-Heinemann; 2000.
5. White A, Hayhoe S, Hart A, et al: Survey of adverse events following acupuncture (SAFA): a prospective study of 32,00 consultations. Acupunct Med 19(2):84-92, 2001.
6. Saw A, Kwan MK, Sengupta S: Necrotising fasciitis: a life-threatening complication of acupuncture in a patient with diabetes mellitus. Singapore Med J 45(4):180-182, 2004.
7. Ogata M, Kitamura O, Kubo S, et al: An asthmatic death while under Chinese acupuncture and moxibustion treatment. Am J Forens Med Pathol 13(4):338-341, 1992.

8. Peuker E: Case report of tension pneumothorax related to acupuncture. Acupunct Med 22(1):40-43, 2004.

9. Halvorsen TB, Anda SS, Naess AB, et al: Fatal cardiac tamponade after acupuncture through congenital sternal foramen. Lancet 345:1175, 1995.

10. Schiff AF: A fatality due to acupuncture. Med Times 93(6):630-631, 1965.

11. Pierik MG: Fatal staphylococcal septicemia following acupuncture: report of two cases. R I Med J 65:251-253, 1982.

53   AROMATHERAPY

OVERVIEW. Aromatherapy is the application of essential aromatic plant oils (highly concentrated, pure extract), applied internally or externally to address health problems. Essential oils are plant or tree products (i.e., leaves, berries, bark, roots) derived from *one species* using a physical process (e.g., distillation). In its external application, aromatherapy incorporates the use of essential oils with massage to address tension headaches, treat depression, or induce a sedative effect.[1,2]

Precautions or advice below is generally based on concerns for adverse reactions leading to toxicity, skin and mucous membrane irritation, sensitization (allergies), photosensitization, or for use in specified populations (pregnancy, epilepsy, hypertensive or hypotensive conditions).[1] Other concerns relate to some novel (not adequately tested) and potentially toxic essential oils and herbal oils (i.e., phytols or infused oils) used in aromatherapy.[2]

Note: In 1999, Burkhard et al[3] reported two adults who exhibited generalized tonic-clonic seizures and one child who suffered a generalized tonic status seizure, all associated with the absorption of oils (several) for therapeutic purposes. These plant-related toxic seizures were attributed to highly reactive monoterpene ketones such as camphor or thujone contained in the oils. In 1981, Millet et al[4] reported eight cases of human intoxication (tonic-clonic convulsions) with sage, hyssop, thuja, and cedar. These researchers also demonstrated the convulsive-related toxic properties of commercialized sage and hyssop essential oils in rats using electrocortical recordings.

CONTRAINDICATIONS AND PRECAUTIONS

PRECAUTIONS WITH OILS

Issue	LOC	Sources	Affil	Rationale/Comment
Arnica	Novel and potentially toxic	Lis-Balchin, 1999[2]	Chem	Poisonous if taken internally.
Basil	Extra care	Campbell and Jones, 2000[1]	PT	Strongly emmenagogic oils (promote menstruation).
Bergamot				
Calendula	Novel and potentially toxic	Lis-Balchin, 1999[2]	Chem	Possibly abortigenic.
Carvacrol	P	Campbell and Jones, 2000[1]	PT	May cause inflammation of skin and mucous membranes.
Centella	Novel and potentially toxic	Lis-Balchin, 1999[2]	Chem	Photosensitizer, pruritic.
Clary Sage	Extra care	Campbell and Jones, 2000[1]	PT	Low blood pressure.
Comfrey	Novel and potentially toxic	Lis-Balchin, 1999[2]	Chem	Hepatotoxic, carcinogenic.
Devil's claw	Novel and potentially toxic			Hypoglycemic and oxytocic.
Dragon's blood	Novel and potentially toxic			A dermal sensitizer.
Echinacea	Novel and potentially toxic			Dermatitic, possibly hepatotoxic.
Eugenol	Extra care	Campbell and Jones, 2000[1]	PT	May cause inflammation of skin and mucous membranes.
Fenugreek	Novel and potentially toxic	Lis-Balchin, 1999[2]	Chem	Hypoglycemic and oxytocic.
Hyssop	Extra care	Campbell and Jones, 2000[1]	PT	May precipitate a seizure.
				Avoid these strongly emmenagogic oils (promote menstruation).
Juniper	Extra care	Campbell and Jones, 2000[1]	PT	Avoid these strongly emmenagogic oils (promote menstruation).
Kanuka	Caution	Lis-Balchin, 1999[2]	Chem	Toxicity not studied.

Continued

Issue	LOC	Sources	Affil	Rationale/Comment
Lavender	Extra care	Campbell and Jones, 2000[1]	PT	Low blood pressure.
Lemon	Extra care	Lis-Balchin, 1999[2]	Chem	Low blood pressure; photosensitization.
Lime blossom	Novel and potentially toxic	Campbell and Jones, 2000[1]	PT	Cardiotoxic.
		Lis-Balchin, 1999[2]	Chem	
Mandarin	Extra Care	Campbell and Jones, 2000[1]	PT	High blood pressure.
Manuka	Caution			Toxicity not studied.
Marjoram	Extra care	Lis-Balchin, 1999[2]	Chem	Low blood pressure.
				Avoid these strongly emmenagogic oils (promote menstruation).
Melissa	Extra care			Low blood pressure.
Molle	Novel and potentially toxic	Campbell and Jones, 2000[1]	PT	Dermal irritant, sensitizer.
Muna	Caution			Toxicity not studied.
Myrrh	Extra care	Lis-Balchin, 1999[2]	Chem	Avoid these strongly emmenagogic oils (promote menstruation).
Novel essential oils	Possible danger			Never tested for toxicity.
Pampa muna	Novel and potentially toxic			Hepatotoxicant.
Pennyroyal	Possible danger			Fatal in high doses.
Peru balsam	Novel and potentially toxic			Dermal sensitizer.
Phenols	P	Campbell and Jones, 2000[1]	PT	Phenols (also ketones) may cause toxicity at higher dosages (does-dependent).
Rosemary	Extra care	Campbell and Jones, 2000[1]	PT	Avoid. These may precipitate a seizure.
				High blood pressure.
				Low blood pressure.

Sweet fennel	Extra care			These may precipitate a seizure.
Sage	Extra care	Lis-Balchin, 1999[2]	Chem	Avoid. These may precipitate a seizure.
				Avoid. High blood pressure.
				Avoid these strongly emmenagogic oils (promote menstruation).
St John's wort	Novel and potentially toxic	Campbell and Jones, 2000[1]	PT	Photodermatitis.
Thyme	Extra care			High blood pressure.
				Avoid these strongly emmenagogic oils (promote menstruation).
Thymol	P	Campbell and Jones, 2000[1]	PT	May cause inflammation of skin and mucous membranes.
Toxicity risks	P			The greater the dosage, the higher the risk. Note: Phenols and ketones.
Wormwood	P	Lis-Balchin, 1999[2]	Chem	Neurotoxin/renal failure.
Ylang ylang	Extra care	Campbell and Jones, 2000[1]	PT	Low blood pressure.

Note: Lis-Balchin lists novel and potentially toxic essential oils and herbal oils (phytols; infusion oils); affiliation unclear.

REFERENCES

1. Campbell T, Jones E: Aromatherapy. In Charman RA, editor: Complementary therapies for physical therapists. Oxford: Butterworth-Heinemann; 2000.
2. Lis-Balcin M: Possible health and safety problems in the use of novel plant essential oils and extracts in aromatherapy. J R Soc Health 119(4):240-243, 1999.
3. Burkhard PR, Burkhardt K, Haenggeli CA, et al: Plant-induced seizures; reappearance of an old problem. J Neurol 246(8):667-670.
4. Millet Y, Jouglard J, Steinmetz MD, et al: Toxicity of some essential plant oils. Clinical and experimental study. Clin Toxicol 18(12):1485-1498, 1981.

54 CRANIOSACRAL THERAPY

OVERVIEW. Craniosacral therapy (CST) is a noninvasive light touch therapy that explores skull and pelvis mobility, facial integrity, and a craniosacral rhythm with the aim of normalizing body structures and promoting healing. The belief is that an absence of these movements suggests a diminished expression of health. The approach involves locating and feeling a rhythm (using 5 grams of touch), finding facial distortions, and then following the tissue movement in order to facilitate a release.[1]

SUMMARY: CONTRAINDICATIONS AND PRECAUTIONS. Three sources cited a total of 10 concerns for CST. Concerns ranged from four to seven per source, with osteopaths citing both the largest and smallest numbers of concerns. The largest proportion of concerns is related to neurological and circulatory diseases. The most frequently cited concerns were increased acute intracranial hemorrhage and a history of skull fracture.

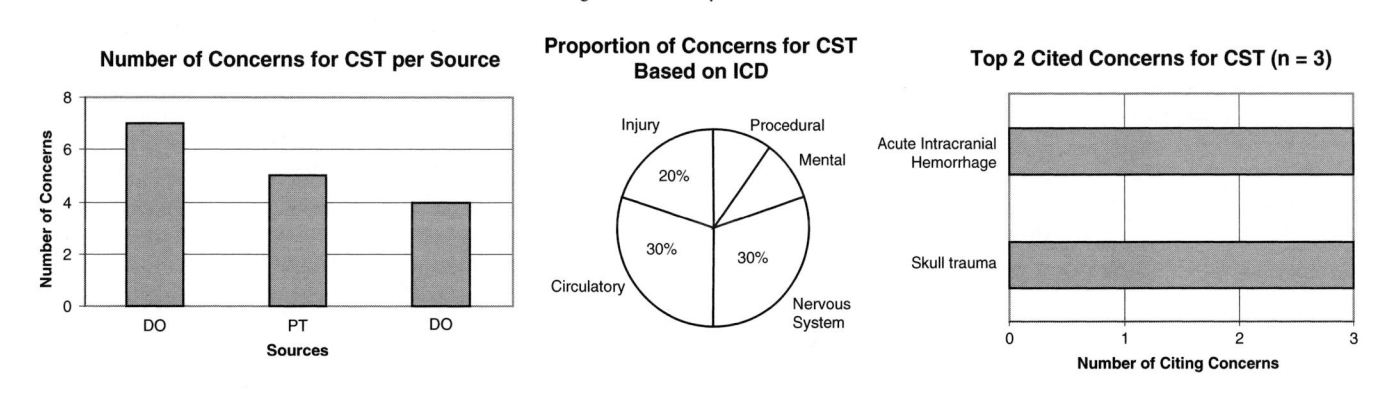

CONTRAINDICATIONS AND PRECAUTIONS

F00-F99 MENTAL AND BEHAVIORAL DISORDERS

Issue	LOC	Sources	Affil	Rationale/Comment
Psychiatric or psychological problems	Care	Greenman, 2003[2]	DO	Technique can affect emotions.

G00-G99 DISEASES OF THE NERVOUS SYSTEM

Issue	LOC	Sources	Affil	Rationale/Comment
Herniation—medulla oblongata through	CI	Harries, 2000[1]	PT	This is a life-threatening event where any altered fluid pressure to the CNS must
foramen magnum	CI	Upledger, 1983[3]	DO	be avoided.
Intracranial pressure—increased	CI	Greenman, 2003[2]	DO	The concern is for any condition where change in intracranial pressure would be
	CI	Harries, 2000[1]	PT	dangerous.[1] The patient should be properly evaluated before treating.
Seizures	RCI	Greenman, 2003[2]	DO	The technique can influence membranous tension within the system and exacerbate seizures/neurologic symptoms depending on the patient's status (i.e., are seizures controlled?).[4]

I00-I99 DISEASES OF THE CIRCULATORY SYSTEM

Issue	LOC	Sources	Affil	Rationale/Comment
Aneurysm—intracranial	CI	Harries, 2000[1]	PT	CST may change the intracranial fluid pressure dynamics sufficient enough to
	CI	Upledger, 1983[3]	DO	cause a rupture or leak in an existing (weakened) intracranial aneurysm.
Intracranial hemorrhage (acute)	CI	Greenman, 2003[2,a]	PT	By changing intracranial fluid pressure dynamics during therapy, an enhanced
	CI	Harries, 2000[1]	DO	intracranial circulation may exacerbate bleeding (i.e., interrupting clot
	CI	Upledger, 1983[3]		formation).
Intracranial hemorrhage (acute)—suspicion	CI	Greenman, 2003[2]	DO	

a, Subarachnoid hemorrhage.

S00-T98 INJURY, POISONING, AND CERTAIN OTHER CONSEQUENCES OF EXTERNAL CAUSES

Issue	LOC	Sources	Affil	Rationale/Comment
Skull trauma—history of	CI	Greenman, 2003[2,b]	DO	Any increased bone motion during CST may cause a bleed or membrane tear in an already
	CI	Harries, 2000[1,a]	PT	traumatized skull. You must rule out fracture of cranial base or depressed vault fractures or
	CI/caution	Upledger, 1983[3]	DO	subarachnoid hemorrhage. **In a 1995 case series, Greenman and McPartland[4] reported three cases (5% of patients seen within a 6-year period) with a history of traumatic brain injury (skull fracture history unclear) and who subsequently experienced increased symptoms following CST.**
Traumatic brain injury	Care	Greenman, 2003[2]	DO	Difficult to predict outcome in this group.

a, Especially unstable; b, Fracture of cranial base; depressed fracture of the vault.

PROCEDURAL CONCERNS

Issue	LOC	Sources	Affil	Rationale/Comment
Technique—improper, aggressive	Advice	Greenman, 2003[2]	DO	Symptoms may worsen with an overly aggressive technique or improper temp rocking (of a synchronous and asynchronous nature). The vestibular system is very sensitive to temporal balances or imbalances, and symptoms such as headaches, dizziness, tinnitus, vertigo, and nausea can occur.[2]

ADVERSE EVENTS

Source	Background	Therapy	Outcome	Follow-up/Interpretation
Greenman and McPartland, 1995[4] **CST and brain injury patients** Case series (5% incidence rate); three cases from a review of 55 patients with	A 33-year-old man s/p 30 months fall 15 feet, injuring occipital area with complaints of severe headaches, dizziness, memory deficits, and ataxic gait presented with severe anterior sphenobasilar compression and vomer restriction of motion.	He was treated with a two-person decompression craniosacral technique, with increased headache, nausea, vomiting, diarrhea, cardiac palpitation, and anxious respirations 6 hours following treatment.	The following day, the patient no longer experienced new symptoms. Head pain was decreased.	Alterations may have precipitated the adverse reaction in these three patient with major skull trauma and sphenobasilar compression with low rate/amplitude cranial rhythmic impulse.

Continued

Source	Background	Therapy	Outcome	Follow-up/Interpretation
traumatic brain injury seen in an outpatient clinic from 1987 to 1992. J Am Osteopath Assoc	A 22-year-old white man s/p 9 months after motor vehicle accident presented with left parietal occipital lobe involvement and marked compression of the right condylar (of occiput), severe ant post sphenobasilar compression, and restricted cranial motions.	After a second craniosacral treatment, the patient experienced acute head pain that was treated with acetaminophen with Vicodin.	On follow-up, the patient had episodes of paranoia ("somebody was watching him") and difficulty controlling emotions. CST was discontinued and he obtained psychiatric care.	
	A 27-year-old white man s/p 11 months fall 4 feet landing on left shoulder and back of head presented with cooccipital headache, but no organic cause was identified. He had previously experienced "severe total body muscle spasm" following cervical manipulation under anesthesia. Marked anterior-posterior sphenobasilar compression was noted with a low-amplitude cranial rhythmic impulse (cri) of 8 c/min. Perceptual, cognitive, and motor deficits were also noted.	A two-person decompression technique was employed to reduce sphenobasilar compression and later to restore temporal bone mobility/balance. Following treatment, opisthotonos developed with Cheyne-Stokes respirations despite administration of IV Valium. He was later hospitalized, intubated, mechanically ventilated, and treated with Pavulon.	No organic cause was found. He was discharged 4 days later with Dilantin. Another episode occurred following a minor MVA 2 weeks later.	

REFERENCES

1. Harries RA: Craniosacral therapy. In Charman RA, editor: Complementary therapies for physical therapists. Oxford: Butterworth-Heinemann; 2000.
2. Greenman PE: Principles of manual medicine, ed 3. Philadelphia: Lippincott Williams & Wilkins; 2003.
3. Upledger JE. Craniosacral therapy, Chicago: Eastland Press; 1983.
4. Greenman PE, McPartland JM: Cranial findings and iatrogenesis from craniosacral manipulation in patients with traumatic brain syndrome. J Am Osteopath Assoc 95(3):182-192, 1995.

55 HIPPOTHERAPY

OVERVIEW. Hippotherapy is an intervention that uses equine (horse) movement to improve a patient's neurological function. The patient engages in controlled, enjoyable, and challenging activity while riding on a horse. The intent is not to improve horse riding skills.[1] Horses provides sensory input through their movement. The movements are thought to mimic movements occurring during human gait.

SUMMARY: CONTRAINDICATIONS AND PRECAUTIONS. Two sources cited a total of 17 concerns for hippotherapy. Lelong et al[2] cited one concern (for horse allergies), whereas Strauss[3] listed 17. The largest proportion of concerns was for persons with neurological diseases (35%) and included issues such as the riding-related risks with epilepsy, spasticity-related sitting difficulties, or the concern of aggravating an existing condition (e.g., increased spasticity; fatigue-related deterioration). Horse allergy concerns were cited by both sources. Lelong et al[2] advised that children be monitored for sensitivity.

CONTRAINDICATIONS AND PRECAUTIONS

D50-89 DISEASES OF BLOOD AND BLOOD-FORMING ORGANS AND CERTAIN DISORDERS

Issue	LOC	Sources	Affil	Rationale/Comment
Allergies to horses	Advice	Lelong et al, 1992[2]	—	Be aware of clinical signs of allergies during horse contact. If noted, terminate
	CI	Strauss, 1995[3,a]	—	future contact with horses. **Lelong et al[2] observed 56 children with eye, nose, and breathing allergies from horse contact.**
Anticoagulation therapy	CI	Strauss, 1995[3]	—	

a, Or any allergy linked to the riding environment; b, Source affiliations are uncertain.

F00-F99 MENTAL AND BEHAVIORAL DISORDERS

Issue	LOC	Sources	Affil	Rationale/Comment
Fear—unconquered	CI	Strauss, 1995[3]	—	

G00-G99 DISEASES OF THE NERVOUS SYSTEM

Issue	LOC	Sources	Affil	Rationale/Comment
Epilepsy	Advice	Strauss, 1995[3]	—	Even when seizures are controlled with medication, the risk is not eliminated completely. Obtain informed consent to accept a degree of risk.

Hypertonicity—severe	CI			Tendency for a blood pressure crisis.
Motor control—head and sitting	CI			Inability to sit independently or control head (in adults).
Neurologic symptoms— aggravated	CI			If horse movements aggravate neurologic symptoms.
Parkinson's disease	Care			Impulses from horse movements may "overtax" these individuals and aggravate symptoms.
Spasticity that interferes with ability to straddle the horse	CI			

I00-I99 DISEASES OF THE CIRCULATORY SYSTEM

Issue	LOC	Sources	Affil	Rationale/Comment
Circulatory insufficiency	CI	Strauss, 1995[3]	—	
Thrombophlebitis; thrombosis	CI			Embolism danger.

M00-M99 DISEASES OF THE MUSCULOSKELETAL SYSTEM AND CONNECTIVE TISSUE

Issue	LOC	Sources	Affil	Rationale/Comment
Hip—structural bone/joint changes	CI	Strauss, 1995[3]	—	If the deformity precludes the possibility of relaxed sitting on a horse or if it increases the risk of hip dislocation.
Spine—structural abnormalities or changes in the physiologic curves	CI			Structural abnormalities will interfere with goals of righting responses and trunk control. Also, inadequate cushioning between vertebrae may endanger the spinal cord. Examples include: • Spondylolisthesis • Intravertebral disc surgery • Gibbous formation • Kyphosis • Scoliosis • Pins, rods, or plates in posttraumatic individual

Q00-Q99 CONGENITAL MALFORMATIONS, DEFORMITIES, AND CHROMOSOMAL ABNORMALITIES

Issue	LOC	Sources	Affil	Rationale/Comment
Down syndrome	CI	Strauss, 1995[3]	—	Atlantoaxial instability would be regarded as a CI. Note: 15% of persons with Down syndrome have atlantoaxial instability.[4]
Dystrophia musculorum progressive	CI			Disease progression and strength may be affected by the physical demands of riding.
Spina bifida with a shunt	Monitor			Note: Any behavioral changes related to shunt malfunction such as headaches or nausea.

R00-R99 SYMPTOMS, SIGNS INVOLVING A SYSTEM

Issue	LOC	Sources	Affil	Rationale/Comment
Secondary conditions	—	Strauss, 1995[3]	—	Negative impact on secondary condition.

ADVERSE EVENTS

Source	Background	Therapy	Outcome
Lelong et al, 1992[2] (from foreign abstract) **Allergies and horses** Descriptive Pediatrie	56 children observed over an 11-year period.	Contact with horses.	Allergies observed included ocular, asthma, and rhinopharyngitis.

REFERENCES

1. American Hippotherapy Association: www..americanhippotherapyassociation.org, accessed September 20, 2004
2. Lelong M, Castelain MC, Bras C, et al: An outbreak of allergy to horses in children: a review of 56 recent cases. Pediatrie 47:55-58, 1992 (from French abstract).
3. Strauss I: Hippotherapy: neurophysiological therapy on the horse. Thornhill, Ontario: Ontario Therapeutic Riding Association; 1995.
4. Harris SR, Lundgren BD: Joint mobilization for children with central nervous system disorders: indications and precautions. Phys Ther 71(12):890-896, 1991.

56   HYPNOSIS

OVERVIEW. Hypnosis (i.e., under hypnosis) is a state resembling sleep but induced by suggestion whereby the individual is responsive to imaginative experiences. During a session, the individual is guided to respond to suggestions for changes in thoughts, behaviors, sensations, perceptions, or subjective experiences.[1]

Abreaction is a specific technique that involves the reliving (dramatic) of traumatic events under hypnosis for the treatment of trauma victims (e.g., child abuse cases; posttraumatic stress disorder). Patients may present with massive psychogenic amnesia, or loss of a single functional system such as limb paralysis or psychogenic blindness. The technique serves to release repressed material that must then be followed up with psychotherapy to process the material.[2]

SUMMARY: CONTRAINDICATIONS AND PRECAUTIONS. Four sources cited a total of 11 concerns for hypnosis. Concerns ranged from two to four per source with a psychologist and a nurse citing the largest number and a physician, the fewest. The largest proportion of concerns was procedural (over 70%) and related to appropriateness of treatment and skill level. The most frequently cited concerns were working with an incorrect diagnosis and poor patient selection for abreaction.

Note: Health care providers should probably be informed if their patients are undergoing hypnosis so that a patient's induced behaviors don't become confused with a real deterioration in medical status. In 1984, Smith and Kamitsuka[3] reported a 13-year-old girl who used self-hypnosis to treat anxiety/tension headaches and confused health care workers into thinking that subsequent hypnotic-induced myopathies had an organic basis.

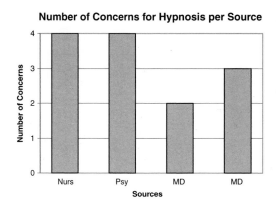

Number of Concerns for Hypnosis per Source

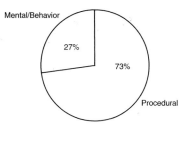

Proportion of Concerns for Hypnosis Based on ICD

Mental/Behavior 27%

73% Procedural

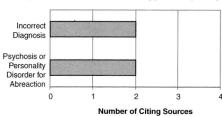

Top 2 Cited Concerns for Hypnosis (n = 4)

CONTRAINDICATIONS AND PRECAUTIONS

F00-F99 MENTAL AND BEHAVIORAL DISORDERS: FOR ABREACTION (SPECIFIC)

Issue	LOC	Sources	Affil	Rationale/Comment
Abreaction—anxiety or depressed without bizarre coloration	CI	Putnam, 1992[2]	MD	These patient types are not good candidates for therapeutic abreactions, especially persons with antisocial disorders and paranoid disorders.[2]

Continued

Issue	LOC	Sources	Affil	Rationale/Comment
Abreaction—exaggerated startle reactions	CI			
Abreaction—psychosis or personality disorders	CI	Putnam, 1992[2]	MD	
	CI	Wickramasekera, 1999[4,a]	Psychiatry	

a, Baseline personalities, major dissociative disorders, paranoid.

PROCEDURAL CONCERNS

Issue	LOC	Sources	Affil	Rationale/Comment
Aggressiveness—triggering traumatic memories	CI	Valente, 1991[5]	Nurs	
Physical basis	CI			Hypnosis is contraindicated if there is a physical basis for a problem. If it can endanger the patient (i.e., pain from a fracture or appendicitis).
Incorrect diagnosis	CI	Valente, 1991[5]	Nurs	Working with an incorrect diagnosis.
	CI	Wickramasekera, 1999[5]	Psychiatry	
Medications—contraindicated (hypnotic-related)	CI	Wickramasekera, 1999[5]	Psychiatry	Check medications that are medically contraindicated to induce abreaction in a particular patient (e.g., barbiturates).
Most appropriate treatment	CI	Valente, 1991[5]	Nurs	If alternative treatment is more appropriate.

| Overmanipulative parents Performing embarrassing behaviors | Misuse of hypnosis in children | Podoll, 1981[6] | MD | Allowing children to perform embarrassing behaviors. Use on children by overmanipulative parents can lead to anxieties and phobias, affect creative ability, and "make the child into a zombie." |
| Psychotherapeutic skills—poor | CI | Wickramasekera, 1999[5] | Psychiatry | Poor psychodiagnostic skills. The issue concerns countertransference problems in the therapist since changes occur rapidly during hypnotherapy. |

EVIDENCE

Source	Background	Therapy	Outcome	Follow up//Interpretation
Smith and Kamitsuka, 1984[3] **Misinterpretation of CNS deterioration** Case report Am J Clin Hypn	13-year-old girl was taught self-hypnosis to treat anxiety, tension headaches (symptom control) associated with a lymphoblastic leukemia cancer regimen (involving prednisone, vincristine [antineoplastic agent], and L-asparaginase).	After learning the technique, she was hospitalized with complaints of diplopia, headaches, LE weakness, inability to walk, perioral and distal extremity paresthesia, absent Achilles tendon reflexes, alopecia, and mild cachexia (she was able to move her limbs on command but refused to bear weight on legs due to perceived weakness).	Her hospital course fluctuated and she had two episodes where she was unresponsive to verbal commands. Her psychotherapist discovered she had been using self-hypnosis and the patient was not sure how to "come back" to her normal state. She recovered following a posthypnotic suggestion.	The patient's failure to communicate her use of the technique in the clinical setting resulted in anxiety and confusion with the health care providers. Note that L-asparaginase is associated with CNS deterioration, prednisone can lead to myopathies, and vincristine toxicity can cause headaches and weakness.

REFERENCES

1. American Psychology Association Executive Committee, Division of Psychological Hypnosis: Web page. Available at: http://www.apa.org. Accessed: November 30, 2005.
2. Putnam FW: Using hypnosis for therapeutic abreaction. Psychiatr Med 10(1):51-65, 1992.
3. Smith MS, Kamitsuka M: Self-hypnosis misinterpreted as CNS deterioration in an adolescent with leukemia and vincristine toxicity. Am J Clin Hypn 26(4):280-282, 1984.
4. Wickramasekera I: Hypnotherapy. In Jonas WB, Levin JS, eds: Essentials of complementary and alternative medicine. Philadelphia: Lippincott Williams & Wilkins; 1999.
5. Valente SM: Using hypnosis with children for pain management. Oncol Nurs Forum 18(4):699-704, 1991.
6. Podoll E: The use and misuse of hypnosis in children. J Am Soc Psychosom Dent Med 28(2):57-62, 1981.

57   QIGONG

OVERVIEW. Qigong is a Chinese form of physical training and method of harnessing energy for mental and physical well-being. The approach involves slow, controlled movements, static postures, postural awareness, relaxation, visualization, and breath and mental control.[1] Energy that normally flows through energy channels (meridians) is thought to be blocked and result in physical and emotional problems. By harmonizing the mind, the nervous system (autonomic) is believed to function more efficiently.[1]

SUMMARY: CONTRAINDICATIONS AND PRECAUTIONS.   Three sources cited a total of 11 concerns for qigong. Concerns ranged from 1 to 6 per source with a physical therapist citing the greatest number and a qigong master the fewest. The largest proportion of concerns was procedural and included issues related to the manner in which qigong is performed (e.g., rate of progression, intensity, temperature, meals).

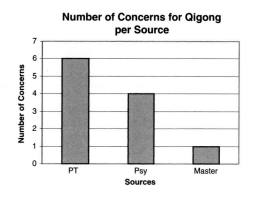

Number of Concerns for Qigong per Source

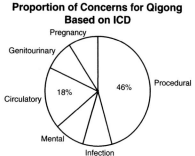

Proportion of Concerns for Qigong Based on ICD

CONTRAINDICATIONS AND PRECAUTIONS

A00-B99 CERTAIN INFECTIONS AND PARASITIC DISEASES

Issue	LOC	Sources	Affil	Rationale/Comment
Infection—active	CI/P	Mokone, 2000[1]	PT	Circulation may further spread infection.

F00-F99 MENTAL AND BEHAVIORAL DISORDERS

Issue	LOC	Sources	Affil	Rationale/Comment
Anxiety	CI	Lee and Lei, 1999[2]	Psy	Techniques that concentrate (focus) on the forehead may increase sympathetic tone in persons with anxiety.

I00-I99 DISEASES OF THE CIRCULATORY SYSTEM

Issue	LOC	Sources	Affil	Rationale/Comment
Angina	CI	Lee and Lei, 1999[2]	Psy	Techniques that concentrate (focus) on forehead may increase sympathetic tone in persons with angina or hypertension.
Hypertension	CI			

N00-N99 DISEASES OF THE GENITOURINARY SYSTEM

Issue	LOC	Sources	Affil	Rationale/Comment
Menstruating	CI/P	Mokone, 2000[1]	PT	Do not strain downward or hold "low" postures. Caution not to visualize flow of energy below the waist as it may increase blood flow.

O00-O99 PREGNANCY, CHILDBIRTH, AND PUERPERIUM

Issue	LOC	Sources	Affil	Rationale/Comment
Pregnancy—straining	CI	Mokone, 2000[1]	PT	Do not strain downward or hold "low" postures.

PROCEDURAL CONCERNS

Issue	LOC	Sources	Affil	Rationale/Comment
Intensity—appropriate	CI/Advice	Lee and Lei, 1999[2]	Psy	Qigong should be adapted to the needs and condition of the individual. Vigorous, consistent use of qigong may be inappropriate.
Tired	CI/P	Mokone, 2000[1]	PT	Avoid qigong when very tired.
Meals—immediately after	CI/P			Avoid qigong immediately after meal.
Cold weather	CI/P			Avoid qigong outside in the cold. Illness can result.
				Maintain a warm, protective environment.
Progression	P	Cohen, 1996[3]	Qigong Master	Study qigong in stages. Avoid advancing in the technique too quickly because one may experience adverse affects (physical and emotional illness).

REFERENCES

1. Mokone S: Qigong and Taichi in physical therapy. In: Charman RA, editor: Complementary therapies for physical therapists. Oxford: Butterworth-Heinemann; 2000.

2. Lee C-T, Lei T: Qigong. In: Jona WB, Levin JS, eds: Essentials of complementary and alternative medicine: Philadelphia: Lippincott Williams & Wilkins; 1999.

3. Cohen K: The way of qigong: the art and science of Chinese energy healing. London: Bantam; 1996.

58   SHIATSU

OVERVIEW.   Shiatsu is a Japanese finger pressure technique used primarily for musculoskeletal (neck, shoulder, low back, arthritic) and psychological (depression, stress, anxiety) problems. The belief is that during illness, qi energy is either excessive, deficient, or in a state of imbalance. The goal is to stimulate the free flow of qi energy through the meridians or energy channels. In shiatsu, the practitioner's body weight is used to apply bilateral finger pressure along the client's meridians and acupuncture points in order to access qi energy.[1,2]

SUMMARY: CONTRAINDICATIONS AND PRECAUTIONS.   Two sources cited a total of 30 concerns for shiatsu. Battermann[1] cited 24 concerns, whereas Bereford-Cooke[2] cited 14. The largest proportion of concerns was related to circulation (26%) and pregnancy (16%). Modification of technique (lighter pressure) was recommended over lymphatic tissue,[1] during pregnancy,[1] and in people with hypertension.[2] Remarkably, no pressure-related concerns were mentioned for work over superficial nerves (see Herskovitz et al[3] and Mumm et al[4] below).

OTHER ISSUES: OVERLY AGGRESSIVE TECHNIQUE. In a 1992 case report, Herskovitz et al[3] reported a 61-year-old who sustained an adductor pollicis brevus nerve compression following strong digital shiatsu pressure of the palm and thenar muscle. In 1993, Mumm et al[4] reported a 64-year-old woman with a prior history of severe varicella as a child and who presented with vesicular zoster over the 8th cervical dermatome following very vigorous shiatsu massage.

Note: In 2002, Elliott and Taylor[5] reported a case of an ICA dissection associated with a "shiatsu massager." Note that this injury was machine-induced and not attributed to a practitioner's manual technique of shiatsu.

CONTRAINDICATIONS AND PRECAUTIONS

A00-B99 CERTAIN INFECTIONS AND PARASITIC DISEASES

Issue	LOC	Sources	Affil	Rationale/Comment
Infection—systematic/contagious	CI	Battermann, 2000[1]	PT	

C00-C97 NEOPLASM

Issue	LOC	Sources	Affil	Rationale/Comment
Cancer	CI	Beresford-Cooke, 1996[2]	Lic Ac[a]	Cancer may spread with enhanced venous and lymphatic flow. The decision is left to the advanced practitioner.

a, Licensed acupuncturist.

D50-D89 DISEASES OF BLOOD AND BLOOD-FORMING ORGANS AND CERTAIN DISORDERS

Issue	LOC	Sources	Affil	Rationale/Comment
Hemorrhage	CI	Battermann, 2000[1]	PT	

E00-E90 ENDOCRINE, NUTRITIONAL AND METABOLIC DISEASES

Issue	LOC	Sources	Affil	Rationale/Comment
Diabetic coma	CI	Battermann, 2000[1]	PT	

I00-I99 DISEASES OF THE CIRCULATORY SYSTEM

Issue	LOC	Sources	Affil	Rationale/Comment
Atherosclerosis—severe	CI	Battermann, 2000[1]	PT	In 2001, Tsuboi and Tsuboi[6] reported an 80-year-old man with carotid stenosis who developed a retinal artery embolism and sustained infarcts to the right frontoparietal lobe following shiatsu massage to the neck.

Issue	LOC	Sources	Affil	Rationale/Comment
Cerebral vascular accident—if not stabilized	CI			
High blood pressure	CI	Beresford-Cooke, 1996[2]	Lic Ac	The concern is damage to vessels. Beresford-Cooke recommend lighter
	CI	Battermann, 2000[1,a]	PT	pressures.
Myocardial infarct—not stabilized	CI	Battermann, 2000[1]	PT	
Shock	CI			
Thrombosis	CI			
Varicose veins: do not work directly on	P	Battermann, 2000[1]	PT	Apply pressure elsewhere.
	Avoid	Beresford-Cooke, 1996[2]	Lic Ac	

a, Severe unstable.

J00-J99 DISEASES OF THE RESPIRATORY SYSTEM

Issue	LOC	Sources	Affil	Rationale/Comment
Asthma attack—severe	CI	Battermann, 2000[1]	PT	
Pneumothorax	CI			

K00-K93 DISEASES OF THE DIGESTIVE SYSTEM

Issue	LOC	Sources	Affil	Rationale/Comment
Appendicitis and peritonitis—acute	CI	Battermann, 2000[1]	PT	
Chronic organ disease—for abdominal treatment	P			Use light touch to the abdominal area if severely ill or advanced/complicated chronic organ disease.

L00-L99 DISEASES OF THE SKIN AND SUBCUTANEOUS TISSUE

Issue	LOC	Sources	Affil	Rationale/Comment
Scar tissue	P	Battermann, 2000[1,a]	PT	Do not work directly on a scar.
	Avoid	Beresford-Cooke, 1996[2,b]	Lic Ac	
Skin rashes	P	Battermann, 2000[1]	PT	Do not work directly over a skin rash.

a, New; b, Operations.

M00-M99 DISEASES OF THE MUSCULOSKELETAL SYSTEM AND CONNECTIVE TISSUE

Issue	LOC	Sources	Affil	Rationale/Comment
Inflammatory arthrides—acute	CI	Battermann, 2000[1]	PT	e.g., rheumatoid arthritis, ankylosing spondylitis.
	Avoid	Beresford-Cooke, 1996[2]	Lic Ac	

Osteoporosis and if had chemotherapy—except with lightest pressure	CI	Beresford-Cooke, 1996[2]	Lic Ac	Fear of damaging bone.

O00-O99 PREGNANCY, CHILDBIRTH, AND PUERPERIUM

Issue	LOC	Sources	Affil	Rationale/Comment
Acupuncture points in pregnancy:	P/Avoid	Battermann, 2000[1]	PT	
GB 21	CI	Beresford-Cooke, 1996[2]	Lic Ac	
LI 4				
SP 6				
Acupuncture points in pregnancy:	P/Avoid	Battermann, 2000[1]	PT	
BL 60				
LIV 3				
Low back and sacrum	P	Battermann, 2000[1]	PT	Care in pregnancy—gentle work on.
Pregnancy—direct pressure to abdomen	CI	Beresford-Cooke, 1996[2]	Lic Ac	
Pregnancy—first 3 months	CI	Beresford-Cooke, 1996[2]	Lic Ac	This is more of a litigation issue since miscarriages often occur during this time—do not treat, or leave to an experienced practitioner.

R00-R99 SYMPTOMS, SIGNS, AND ABNORMAL CLINICAL AND LABORATORY FINDINGS (NOT ELSEWHERE CLASSIFIED)

Issue	LOC	Sources	Affil	Rationale/Comment
Debilitated, frail, persons with chronic fatigue syndrome	CI	Beresford-Cooke, 1996[2]	Lic Ac	
Fever	CI	Beresford-Cooke, 1996[2]	Lic Ac	To avoid overloading the client's system. Certain points may help speed
	CI	Battermann, 2000[1,a]	PT	recovery. Apply judiciously or avoid during acute illness with fever.[2]
Inflammation	CI/P	Battermann, 2000[1,b]	PT	Apply pressure elsewhere.
	Avoid	Beresford-Cooke, 1996[2]	Lic Ac	

a, Fever; b, CI if acute.

S00-T98 INJURY, POISONING, AND CERTAIN OTHER CONSEQUENCES OF EXTERNAL CAUSES

Issue	LOC	Sources	Affil	Rationale/Comment
Fractures	Avoid	Beresford-Cooke, 1996[2]	Lic Ac	Apply pressure elsewhere.
Wounds	P	Battermann, 2000[1]	PT	
	Avoid	Beresford-Cooke, 1996[2,a]	Lic Ac	

a, Locally.

VULNERABLE BIOLOGICAL TISSUE

Issue	LOC	Sources	Affil	Rationale/Comment
Lymphatic areas	P	Battermann, 2000[1]	PT	Use light touch (i.e., throat, below ear, groin, armpits). **In a 1995 animal study, Eliska and Eliskova[7] showed that forceful massage with external pressure using two fingers in direction of lymph flow (70-100 mmHg) resulted in lymphatic damage after 10 minutes in dogs.**

ADVERSE EVENTS

Source	Background	Therapy	Outcome	Follow-up/Interpretation
Herskovitz et al, 1992[3] **Nerve compression and shiatsu** Case report Muscle Nerve	Physician.	Professional shiatsu practitioner applied shiatsu with strong digital pressure to the base of client's palm and the thenar muscles for at least 30 sec with transient discomfort.	• The next day, there was painless weakness of the left adductor pollicis brevis (thumb) but no sensory symptoms. • Week 1: needle EMG revealed mild active denervation and reduced mu recruitment with reduced action potentials from thenar muscles. • Week 3: A significant improvement in strength was noted.	"Overzealous massage" can result in compression injury to recurrent motor branch of median nerve.

Continued

Source	Background	Therapy	Outcome	Follow-up/Interpretation
Mumm et al, 1993[4] **Vesicular zosters and shiatsu** Case report Lancet	A 64-year-old woman with a history of severe varicella at age 11.	She received shiatsu massage that was described as "overly vigorous."	She experienced the following: • Pain left pericervical and suprascapular area • 7th hour paresthesia in the left back, chest, and arm • The next morning, radiating pain • Day 6 (onset day 3-4), rash in area of numbness	• Day 7, typical vesicular zoster over the 8th cervical dermatome
Tsuboi and Tsuboi, 2001[6] **Neck, and cerebral/retinal artery embolism (stroke) and shiatsu** Case report Stroke	An 80-year-old man presented with a recent history of TIA, right frontal lobe small infarct, and bilateral internal carotid artery stenoses. Following anticoagulation, he was free of neurologic symptoms.	That evening, he received shiatsu massage on his neck while prone for 10 minutes because of a mild headache with neck/shoulder stiffness.	After the massage, he noted right visual field impairment (nasal half). At the hospital, slight left UE hemiparesis was noted. Retinal edema with multiple emboli in central retinal artery branches and small infarctions of right frontoparietal lobe were found.	The patient's left paresis recovered with urokinase after 1 week, but ocular symptoms improved only minimally. The authors postulated that direct pressure at extracranial carotid artery (at the neck) may have led to the embolic event in this high-risk patient.

REFERENCES

1. Battermann A: Shiatsu with physiotherapy—an integrative approach. In: Charman RA, editor: Complementary therapies for physical therapists. Oxford: Butterworth-Heinemann; 2000.

2. Beresford-Cooke C: Shiatsu theory and practice: a comprehensive text for the student and professional. New York: Churchill Livingstone; 1996.

3. Herskovitz S, Strauch B, Gordon MJ: Shiatsu massage-induced injury of the median recurrent motor branch. Muscle Nerve 15(10):1215, 1992.

4. Mumm AH, Morens DM, Elm JL, et al: Zoster after shiatsu massage. Lancet 341(8842):447, 1993.

5. Elliott MA, Taylor LP: "Shiatsu sympathectomy": ICA dissection associated with a shiatsu massager. Neurology 58(8):1302-1304, 2002.

6. Tsuboi K, Tsuboi K: Retinal and cerebral artery embolism after "shiatsu" on the neck [letter]. Stroke 32(10):2441-2442, 2001.

7. Eliska O, Eliskova M: Are peripheral lymphatics damaged by high pressure manual massage? Lymphology 28(1):1-3, 1995.

59 | THERAPEUTIC TOUCH

OVERVIEW. Therapeutic touch (TT) is a form of energy field work that is believed to access a patient's energy field by having the practitioner's hands placed over (above) the patient's body. The practitioners attempt to direct some of their own energy (which they have an excess of) to the patient, who is viewed as having some less optimal level. The aim of TT is to treat health problems such as pain or anxiety, or to help the patient relax.[1,2]

Ironically, therapeutic touch does not involve touch. The technique involves five steps that includes (1) centering (getting into a meditative state); (2) assessing by tuning into the patient (with hands 5-15 cm above the patient's body surface to detect energy fields); (3) clearing (facilitate the flow of energy in patient areas that are sluggish by sweeping the hands over the patient's body from head to toe); (4) redirecting areas of accumulated tension to areas sensed as depleted; and then (5) evaluating the patient's energy flow.[1]

SUMMARY: CONTRAINDICATIONS AND PRECAUTIONS. Five sources (four nurses, one physical therapist) cited a total of 11 concerns for therapeutic touch. Concerns ranged from one to four per source, with a nurse citing the largest number and a physical therapist citing the fewest. The largest percentage of concerns related to procedures (36%) and mental disorders (18%). The most frequently cited concerns were the need to modify the technique when working with very young, very old, or debilitated patients.

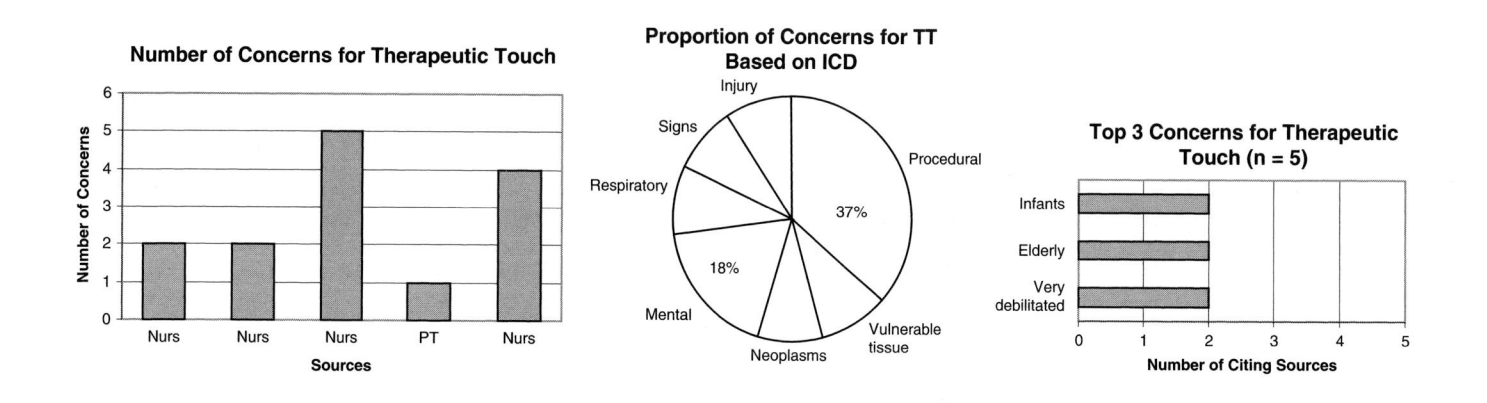

CONTRAINDICATIONS AND PRECAUTIONS

C00-C97 NEOPLASMS

Issue	LOC	Sources	Affil	Rationale/Comment
Tumor area	Advice	Cownes, 1996[3]	Nurs	Focusing ("sending") energy to tumor area may serve to make disease more virulent.

F00-F99 MENTAL AND BEHAVIORAL DISORDERS

Issue	LOC	Sources	Affil	Rationale/Comment
Emotional instability	CI	Cotter et al, 2000[4]	Nurs	No rationale provided.
Psychosis	CI			

J00-J99 DISEASES OF THE RESPIRATORY SYSTEM

Issue	LOC	Sources	Affil	Rationale/Comment
Colds	Advice	Cownes, 1996[3]	Nurs	The technique may trigger waste product elimination and intensify symptoms.

R00-R99 SYMPTOMS, SIGNS

Issue	LOC	Sources	Affil	Rationale/Comment
Signs of overload	Advice	Krieger, 1993[5]	Nurs	Watch for signs of overload. Signs may include increased restlessness, irritability, anxiety, or expressions of hostility.

S00-T98 INJURY, POISONING, AND CERTAIN OTHER CONSEQUENCES OF EXTERNAL CAUSES

Issue	LOC	Sources	Affil	Rationale/Comment
Burn patients	Advice	Krieger, 1993[5]	Nurs	Burn patients are very sensitive to energy overload, so administer treatment very gently at site of burn tissue for short periods of 2-3 minutes at a time. Keep hands moving so energy is not focused too intensely at the burn site.

VULNERABLE BIOLOGICAL TISSUE

Issue	LOC	Sources	Affil	Rationale/Comment
Head—directing energy	P	Wytias, 1994[6]	Nurs	Directing energy to the head. Note: No rationale provided.

PROCEDURAL CONCERNS

Issue	LOC	Sources	Affil	Rationale/Comment
Infants	P	Wytias, 1994[6]	Nurs	Keep process brief with no more than 2-3 minutes in children, very old people, and
	Advice	Krieger, 1993[5]	Nurs	very debilitated individuals.[5]
Elderly	P	Wytias, 1994[6]		
	Advice	Krieger, 1993[5]		
Very debilitated patients	P	Wytias, 1994[6]		
	Advice	Krieger, 1993[5]		
Informed consent	CI	Ramsey, 1997[2]	PT	Not obtaining informed consent.

REFERENCES

1. Childs A: Therapeutic touch. In: Charman RA, editor: Complementary therapies for physical therapists. Oxford: Butterworth; 2000.
2. Ramsey SM: Holistic manual therapy techniques. Primary Care 24(4):759-786, 1997.
3. Cownes D: A gift for healing: how you can use therapeutic touch. New York: Crown; 1996.
4. Cotter AC, Bartoli L, Schulman RA: An overview of massage and touch therapies. Phys Med Rehabil State Art Rev 14(1):43-64, 2000.
5. Krieger D: The therapeutic touch: how to use your hands to help or to heal. Englewood Cliffs (NJ): Prentice-Hall; 1979.
6. Wytias CA: Therapeutic touch in primary care. Nurs Pract Forum 5(2):91-97, 1994.

60 TRAGER (PSYCHO-PHYSICAL INTEGRATION)

OVERVIEW. Trager is a technique that combines gentle hands-on movement, relaxation exercise, and education, and is thought to address deep-seated psycho-physiological patterns in the mind (patterns that disrupt function, cause pain, and inhibit free movement) with the intent of interrupting their influence on the body. The goal is to achieve increased vitality, mental clarity, creativity, and relaxation. The approach involves both table work (patient is horizontal) and gentle exercise while the patient is vertical (for self-care) and incorporates procedures of tissue elongation, stretching, compression, rocking, jiggling, and vibration.[1]

SUMMARY: CONTRAINDICATIONS AND PRECAUTIONS. Two sources cited a total of 11 concerns for Trager. Russell (nurse) cited four concerns, whereas Ramsey (physical therapist) cited eight. The largest proportion of concerns are circulatory and pregnancy. Shared concerns included cancer and pregnancy.

Note: Few rationales are provided. Because this technique incorporates stretching, compression, and vibration, it may share similar theoretical concerns with other manual techniques.

CONTRAINDICATIONS AND PRECAUTIONS

C00-C97 NEOPLASM

Issue	LOC	Sources	Affil	Rationale/Comment
Cancer	CI	Russell, 1994[2]	Nurs	The effects are unknown.
	CI	Ramsey, 1997[3]	PT	Concern about metastatic cancer.[2]

D50-D89 DISEASES OF BLOOD AND BLOOD-FORMING ORGANS AND CERTAIN DISORDERS

Issue	LOC	Sources	Affil	Rationale/Comment
Anticoagulant therapy	CI	Ramsey, 1997[3]	PT	

F00-F99 MENTAL AND BEHAVIORAL DISORDERS

Issue	LOC	Sources	Affil	Rationale/Comment
Mind-altering drugs	CI	Russell, 1994[2]	Nurs	

G00-G99 DISEASES OF THE NERVOUS SYSTEM

Issue	LOC	Sources	Affil	Rationale/Comment
Nerve impingement—acute	CI	Ramsey, 1997[3]	PT	

I00-I99 DISEASES OF THE CIRCULATORY SYSTEM

Issue	LOC	Sources	Affil	Rationale/Comment
Carotid artery disease—severe	CI	Ramsey, 1997[3]	PT	
Deep vein thrombosis	CI	Russell, 1994[2]	Nurs	

M00-M99 DISEASES OF THE MUSCULOSKELETAL SYSTEM AND CONNECTIVE TISSUE

Issue	LOC	Sources	Affil	Rationale/Comment
Disk—rupture	CI	Ramsey, 1997[3]	PT	

O00-O99 PREGNANCY, CHILDBIRTH, AND PUERPERIUM

Issue	LOC	Sources	Affil	Rationale/Comment
Pregnancy—first trimester	CI	Russell, 1994[2]	Nurs	The effects are unknown.
Pregnancy—high risk	CI	Ramsey, 1997[3]	PT	

R00-R99 SYMPTOMS, SIGNS, AND ABNORMAL CLINICAL AND LABORATORY FINDINGS (NOT ELSEWHERE CLASSIFIED)

Issue	LOC	Sources	Affil	Rationale/Comment
Vertigo; seasickness.	CI	Ramsey, 1997[3]	PT	

S00-T98 INJURY, POISONING, AND CERTAIN OTHER CONSEQUENCES OF EXTERNAL CAUSES

Issue	LOC	Sources	Affil	Rationale/Comment
Injury—acute	CI	Ramsey, 1997[3]	PT	

REFERENCES

1. Mid-Atlantic Trager Association: Web page. Available at: http://www.tragermata.com. Accessed: November 30, 2005.
2. Russell JK: Bodywork: the art of touch. Nurs Pract Forum 5(2):85-90, 1994.
3. Ramsey SM: Holistic manual therapy techniques. Primary Care 24(4):759-786, 1997.

61 **YOGA**

OVERVIEW. Yoga is an India-based system of exercises that involves breathing techniques and the assumption of various postures with the goal of achieving well-being, health, and mental and bodily control.[1]

SUMMARY: CONTRAINDICATIONS AND PRECAUTIONS. Two sources cited a total of 14 concerns for yoga. Cameron, a nurse, cited one concern, whereas Brosnan, a yoga instructor, cited 13. The largest proportion of concerns was musculoskeletal (37%). Most concerns were phrased with the term "avoid" and often related to issues of overexertion, stressing vulnerable joints, or assuming an inverted posture that could lead to breathlessness or other problems with select populations.

SUMMARY: ADVERSE EVENTS. Vertebral artery obstruction with neurologic sequela[2,3] and peripheral[4] nerve injuries have been reported during yoga that either involved extreme head postures or prolonged positioning. See case descriptions below.

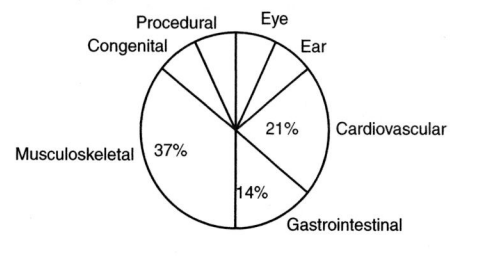

**Proportion of Concerns for Yoga
Based on ICD**

CONTRAINDICATIONS AND PRECAUTIONS

H00-H59 DISEASES OF THE EYE

Issue	LOC	Sources	Affil	Rationale/Comment
Eye trouble	Advice/Avoid	Brosnan, 1982[5]	Yoga instr	Avoid inverted postures. Note: **In a case report, Kobet[6] describes a 44-year-old highly myopic photographer with no past medical history of retinal disease who sustained a retinal tear during inversion (from using an inversion device for 3 consecutive days for up to 5 minutes).**

H00-H95 DISEASES OF THE EAR AND MASTOID PROCESS

Issue	LOC	Sources	Affil	Rationale/Comment
Ear troubles	Advice/Avoid	Brosnan, 1982[5]	Yoga instr	Avoid inverted postures. Note: No rationale provided, but if the source was referring to inner ear problems, perhaps the concern was balance/vertigo related.

I00-I99 DISEASES OF THE CIRCULATORY SYSTEM

Issue	LOC	Sources	Affil	Rationale/Comment
Cardiac problems	Advice/avoid	Brosnan, 1982[5]	Yoga instr	The concern is breathlessness. The supine position may be difficult to tolerate. Inverted postures should be avoided.

Continued

Issue	LOC	Sources	Affil	Rationale/Comment
High blood pressure	Advice/Avoid			Avoid inverted postures. Note: **In 1988, Vehr et al[7] showed significant increases in systolic and diastolic blood pressures (average BP = 146/97) and no training effect in healthy male students who exercised while inverted (using inversion traction). In a randomized experiment in 1986, Haskvitz and Hanten[8] demonstrated significantly increased systolic and diastolic blood pressure in a group of young women without cardiovascular history while in an inverted posture (inversion traction).**
Low blood pressure	Advice/Avoid			Perform all work on the floor and take care when changing positioning.

K00-K93 DISEASES OF THE DIGESTIVE SYSTEM

Issue	LOC	Sources	Affil	Rationale/Comment
Diaphragmatic hernia—head to floor in standing	Advice/Avoid	Brosnan, 1982[5]	Yoga instr	All inverted postures must be avoided. Avoid compressing the gut. Note: In diaphragmatic (hiatal) hernias, the stomach slides into the thoracic cavity, resulting in regurgitation and heartburn. Avoid bending over.[9]
Gastric or duodenal ulcer	Advice/Avoid			Avoid inverted postures when ulcer is active. Avoid dynamic postures and breath holding.

Issue	LOC	Sources	Affil	Rationale/Comment
Ankylosing spondylitis	Advice/avoid	Brosnan, 1982[5]	Yoga instr	Caution with the spine (fragility). Also, if the patient is taking cortisone (long term), bones may be fragile.[5] Note: **In a 1978 review of 64 cases of ankylosing spondylitis with osteoporotic spines, Hunter and Dubo[10] reported 30 sustained spinal fractures due to minor falls. The lower cervical area is a common site. In one case, a cervical fracture occurred in a patient while supine when the head was unsupported. If minor trauma is suspected in this population, manage as a fracture initially.**
Arthritis—of knees and hips	Advice/avoid			Avoid forcing of knees to floor level.
Disc—cervical	Advice/avoid			Avoid backward extension of the head.
Osteoporosis	Advice/avoid			Perform everything cautiously. Minimal movements; involve the whole spine or limb.
Prolapsed disc—severe	Advice/avoid			Avoid hyperextension of spine; never raise both legs off ground together in any posture.

Q00-Q99 CONGENITAL MALFORMATIONS, DEFORMITIES, AND CHROMOSOMAL ABNORMALITIES

Issue	LOC	Sources	Affil	Rationale/Comment
Muscular dystrophy	Advice/avoid	Brosnan, 1982[5]	Yoga instr	As in all neuromuscular disorders, caution not to fatigue.

PROCEDURAL CONCERNS

Issue	LOC	Sources	Affil	Rationale/Comment
Straining to achieve postures	P	Cameron, 2002[1]	Nurs	Do gently and in moderation; develop an attitude of noncompetitiveness. In 1971, Chusid[4] described a lean 22-year-old man who sustained a common peroneal nerve injury during hatha yoga that involved heel sitting for 6-hour durations. In 1973, Nagler[2] reported a 28-year-old female yoga enthusiast who sustained a cerebellar infarct during a bridging posture that involved a hyperextension maneuver. In 1977, Hanus et al[3] reported a 25-year-old man who had strained his neck 3 weeks earlier when diving into a pool and subsequently suffered a lateral medullary lesion due to a left vertebral artery occlusion after yoga (involving neck hyperrotation, extension, and inverted standing with neck flexion).

ADVERSE EVENTS

Source	Background	Therapy	Outcome	Follow-up/Interpretation
Hanus et al, 1977[3] **Yoga, neck posture, and brain lesion** Case report Arch Neurol	A 25-year-old right-handed man strained his left neck 3 weeks earlier while diving in pool.	He participated in yoga for 20 minutes (for past 18 months) involving hyperrotation and extension of neck to his left and then right for 3 minutes. He then assumed inverted standing with head and neck in flexion against floor for 5 minutes.	Within 2 hours, he was unable to walk (even with assistance). He presented with rotary nystagmus, with hypalgesia and hypesthesia (supply to left trigemina nerve); left extremities were weak and dysmetric. Dx: Left lateral medullary lesion due to occlusion of the left vertebral artery (self-inflicted).	At 2 months, he walked with cane and had difficulty with fine movements of the left hand.
Nagler, 1973[2] **Bridging and cerebellar infarct** Case series (1 case reported here) Arch Phys Med Rehabil	A 28-year-old female yoga enthusiast had no significant past medical history.	She performed a bridging (back push up) posture by extending her cervical spine and using her head as one side of a support with the floor. The position was maintained for 30 seconds.	She experienced a sudden throbbing headache and was unable to walk without assistance (tended to fall to the left). She presented with left nystagmus, LUE dysmetria, and left Horner's syndrome. Dx: Cerebellar infarct due to a vertebral artery obstruction during a hyperextension maneuver (self-inflicted).	Two years later, she walked with wide base gait, exhibited LUE dysmetria and L Horner's syndrome.

Continued

Source	Background	Therapy	Outcome	Follow-up/Interpretation
Chusid, 1971[4] **Hatha yoga, sitting, and nerve injury** Case report JAMA	A 22-year-old tall, lean, college male presented with progressive difficulty walking over past 5 months.	He had engaged in yoga exercises that involved sitting on his heels with an erect spine over the past 18 months but increased the intensity of the practice (i.e., kneeling pose durations up to 6 hours daily) in the preceding 2 months.	The man presented with moderate to severe motor impairment of the dorsiflexors and evertors (L > R), and a steppage gait with bilateral foot drop. Electrodiagnostics noted partial, bilateral involvement of the common peroneal nerve. It was coined "yoga drop foot" (self-inflicted).	Nine weeks later, findings were normal (he discontinued yoga and took thiamine). The common peroneal nerve is vulnerable when sitting cross legged or heel sitting, particularly if person is lean or has weight loss.

REFERENCES

1. Cameron ME: Yoga. In: Snyder M, Lindquist R, eds: Complementary/alternative therapies in nursing, ed 4. New York: Springer; 2002.
2. Nagler W: Vertebral artery obstruction by hyperextension of the neck: report of three cases. Arch Phys Med Rehabil 54(5):237-240, 1973.
3. Hanus SH, Homer TD, Harter DH: Vertebral artery occlusion complicating yoga exercise. Arch Neurol 34(9):574-575, 1977.
4. Chusid J: Yoga foot drop. JAMA 217:827-828, 1971.
5. Brosnan B: Yoga for handicapped people. London: Souvenir Press; 1982.
6. Kobet KA: Retinal tear associated with gravity boot. Ann Ophthalmol 17(5):308-310, 1985.
7. Vehr PR, Plowman SA, Fernhall B: Exercise during gravity inversion: acute and chronic effects. Arch Phys Med Rehabil 69(11):950-954, 1988.
8. Haskvitz EM, Hanten WP: Blood pressure response to inversion traction. Phys Ther 66:1361-1364, 1986.
9. Goodman CC: The gastrointestinal system. In: Goodman CC, Boissonnault WG, Fuller KS, eds: Pathology: implications for the physical therapist, ed 2. Philadelphia: Saunders; 2003.
10. Hunter T, Dubo H: Spinal fractures complicating ankylosing spondylitis. Ann Intern Med 88(4):546-569, 1978.

62 INJECTION THERAPY

OVERVIEW. Joint and soft tissue injection may be administered to differentially diagnose (i.e., identify the pain source), treat soft tissue pain, reduce inflammation (e.g., corticosteroid injections), or assist in the physical therapy of inflamed joints.[1] Three sources (all physicians) mentioned 39 concerns for injection therapy. Concerns ranged from 10 to 31; many are corticosteroid related. The largest proportion of concerns was procedural (e.g., excessive cortisone treatments, poor technique) or musculoskeletal (e.g., some arthritic conditions). The most frequently cited injection therapy concerns were septicemia, coagulation defects, local infection, dosage restrictions with corticosteroids, and the need for aseptic technique.

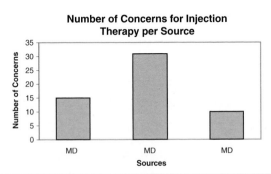

Number of Concerns for Injection Therapy per Source

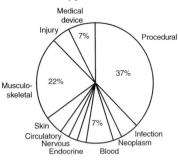

Proportion of Concerns for Injection Therapy Based on ICD

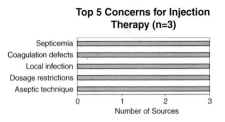

Top 5 Concerns for Injection Therapy (n=3)

CONTRAINDICATIONS AND PRECAUTIONS

INJECTION PROCEDURES (ANY)

A00-B99 CERTAIN INFECTIONS AND PARASITIC DISEASES

Issue	LOC	Sources	Affil	Rationale/Comment
Septicemia	ACI	Walsh and Rogers, 2005[2,c,d]	MD	Corticosteroid injections may accelerate the infection and/or complicate the diagnosis in an early septic joint.[1]
	CI	Rifat and Moeller, 2001[3,a]	MD	
	CI	Pfenninger, 1991[1,b]	MD	
Local infection	ACI	Walsh and Rogers, 2005[2,c]	MD	

a, Bacteremia; b, Also septic effusion, bacteremia; c, For any injection technique; d, Bacteremia for intraarticular injections.

C00-C97 NEOPLASTIC CONCERNS

Issue	LOC	Sources	Affil	Rationale/Comment
Tumor at injection site	ACI	Walsh and Rogers, 2005[2,a]	MD	

a, For any injection technique.

D50-D89 DISEASES OF BLOOD AND BLOOD-FORMING ORGANS AND CERTAIN DISORDERS

Issue	LOC	Sources	Affil	Rationale/Comment
Blood thinners—taking	CI	Rifat and Moeller, 2001[3]	MD	If without evaluation and control.
	RCI	Pfenninger, 1991[1]	MD	
Coagulation abnormalities (minor)	RCI	Walsh and Rogers, 2005[2,a,b]	MD	I.e., mini dosage heparin.
Coagulation defect—gross	ACI	Walsh and Rogers, 2005[2,b]	MD	If without medical evaluation and control.
	CI	Rifat and Moeller, 2001[3]	MD	
	CI	Pfenninger, 1991[1]	MD	

a, Minor; b, For any injection technique.

E00-E90 ENDOCRINE, NUTRITIONAL AND METABOLIC DISEASES

Issue	LOC	Sources		Rationale/Comment
Diabetes—for corticosteroids	RCI	Walsh and Rogers, 2005[2,a]	MD	A diabetic condition may worsen with corticosteroid injections, with
	Advice	Pfenninger, 1991[1]	MD	the possibility of hyperglycemia, glycouria, electrolyte imbalance, and increased risk of infection.[2]

a, For any injection technique.

G00-G99 NEUROLOGICAL CONCERNS (EPIDURAL PROCEDURES)

Issue	LOC	Sources	Affil	Rationale/Comment
Intracranial pressure—increased (for epidurals)	ACI	Walsh and Rogers, 2005[2,a]	MD	This concern is specific for epidural procedures.

a, For any injection technique.

I00-I99 DISEASES OF THE CIRCULATORY SYSTEM

Issue	LOC	Sources	Affil	Rationale/Comment
Hypovolemia (severe)	ACI	Walsh and Rogers, 2005[2,a]	MD	

a, For any injection technique.

L00-L99 DISEASES OF THE SKIN AND SUBCUTANEOUS TISSUE

Issue	LOC	Sources	Affil	Rationale/Comment
Cellulitis: signs shown	CI	Rifat and Moeller, 2001[3]	MD	
on overlying skin	CI	Pfenninger, 1991[1]	MD	
Dermatological conditions	ACI	Walsh and Rogers, 2005[2,a]	MD	If condition prevents adequate skin preparation.

a, For any injection technique.

M00-M99 DISEASES OF THE MUSCULOSKELETAL SYSTEM AND CONNECTIVE TISSUE

Issue	LOC	Sources	Affil	Rationale/Comment
Avascular necrosis	CI	Walsh and Rogers, 2005[2,a]	MD	
Arthritis—traumatic, and steroid injections	CI			I.e., a fracture through the joint. The benefits are short lived.
Arthritis, septic	CI			
Charcot's joint and steroid injections	CI			Such treatment is correlated with avascular necrosis in this patient population. Also, treatment will not provide long-term relief.
Neurotropic joint	CI			
Osteonecrosis	CI			
Osteoporosis (severe) and steroid injections	CI			I.e., at/around joint area.
Soft tissue sepsis, overlying	CI			
Unstable joint	CI			Unless corrective surgery or bracing are planned.

a, For intraarticular injections.

S00-T98 INJURY, POISONING, AND CERTAIN OTHER CONSEQUENCES OF EXTERNAL CAUSES

Issue	LOC	Sources	Affil	Rationale/Comment
Acute injury	Advice	Walsh and Rogers, 2005[2,a]	MD	Injections not recommended immediately before acute injury.
Broken skin over the injection site	CI	Rifat and Moeller, 2001[3]	MD	

a, For intraarticular injections.

Y70-Y82 MEDICAL DEVICES

Issue	LOC	Sources	Affil	Rationale/Comment
Joint prosthesis	CI	Pfenninger, 1991[1]	MD	
Surgical implant—injection into	RCI	Walsh and Rogers, 2005[2,a]	MD	Implanted joints are prone to infection, not synovitis.

a, For intraarticular injections.

PROCEDURAL CONCERNS

Issue	LOC	Sources	Affil	Rationale/Comment
Aseptic preparation	Advice	Walsh and Rogers, 2005[2]	MD	Strict aseptic procedures of all injections.
	Advice	Rifat and Moeller, 2001[3]	MD	
	Advice	Pfenninger, 1991[1]	MD	
Athletic events	Advice	Walsh and Rogers, 2005[2,f]	MD	Injections not recommended immediately before an athletic event.
Allergy to local anesthetic	ACI	Walsh and Rogers, 2005[2,e]	MD	In some patients, an allergic reaction to anesthetic can occur.[1]
	Advice	Pfenninger, 1991[1]	MD	
Dosage limitations—corticosteroid injections	CI	Pfenninger, 1991[1,c,d,g]	MD	Repeated steroid injections can lead to osteoporosis and cartilage damage in weight-bearing joints. Tendon ruptures have been reported when more than three injections are administered. (See footnotes g, h, j.)
	CI	Walsh and Rogers, 2005[2,f,h]	MD	
	CI	Rifat and Moeller, 2001[3,j]	MD	
Heavy activity—inability to avoid heavy activity at injection site for 2-3 days following procedure	Advice	Walsh and Rogers, 2005[2,f]	MD	Following injection: Rest, immobilize joint, and protect it from additional injury.
	P	Pfenninger, 1991[1,b,d]	MD	Duration of rest depends on the joint.[1]

Informed consent	Advice	Walsh and Rogers, 2005[2]	MD	
	Advice	Rifat and Moeller, 2001[3]	MD	
Inaccessible joints	CI	Pfenninger, 1991[1]	MD	
	CI	Walsh and Rogers, 2005[2,f]	MD	
Lack of response after 2-4 injections	CI	Pfenninger, 1991[1]	MD	As a precaution for corticosteroid complications (i.e., avoiding excessive treatment).
Quick aspiration—avoid	Advice	Rifat and Moeller, 2001[3]	MD	To avoid joint injury.
Patient refusal	ACI	Walsh and Rogers, 2005[2,i]	MD	
Pertendinous injection instead of direct tendon injection	P	Pfenninger, 1991[1,d]	MD	To avoid injuring and therefore predisposing the tendon to rupture.
Provider education/training/skill of physician—lack of	RCI	Walsh and Rogers, 2005[2,i]	MD	
Technique—avoid moving needle side to side in joint	Advice	Rifat and Moeller, 2001[3]	MD	To avoid joint injury and cartilage trauma during injection.[1]
	P	Pfenninger, 1991[1,a,d]	MD	
Uncooperative patients	CI	Walsh and Rogers, 2005[2,f]	MD	
Universal precautions	P	Walsh and Rogers, 2005[2]	MD	
	P	Pfenninger, 1991[1]	MD	

a, Avoid cartilage trauma during injection; b, Withhold treatment if unable to rest; c, Also limit injections if not providing relief; d, For corticosteroid injection therapy; e, History of allergy; f, For intraarticular injections; g, More than three corticosteroid injections/year in weight-bearing joints is CI; h, For large joints, inject not more than 3-4×/year or 10 times cumulatively; for small joints, inject no more than 2-3×/year or 4 times cumulatively; for inflamed weight-bearing joints, inject not more than every 3-4 months to minimize damage to ligaments and cartilage; i, For any injection technique; j, Inject no more than three times per location per year.

REFERENCES

1. Pfenninger JL: Injection of joints and soft tissue: part I, general guidelines. Am Fam Phys 44(4):1196-1202, 1991.
2. Walsh NE, Rogers JN: Injection procedures. In: Delisa JA, editor: Physical medicine and rehabilitation: principles and practice, ed 4, vol 1. Philadelphia: Lippincott Williams & Wilkins; 2005.
3. Rifat SF, Moeller JL: Basics of joint injection: general techniques and tips for safe, effective use. Postgrad Med 109(1):157, 2001.

63   TRIGGER POINT INJECTION

OVERVIEW. Trigger point therapy involves needling or repeated insertion and withdrawal of a needle[1] into muscle tissue[2] with the goal of mechanically breaking up pockets of fibrotic tissue that entrap nerve endings and a sensitizing substance in order to interrupt a pain cycle.[1] Trigger point therapy includes both injection therapy and noninjection modalities such as spray and stretch (i.e., vapocoolants; **see Cryotherapy**).[1] This section will cover injection therapy for trigger points.

SUMMARY: CONTRAINDICATIONS AND PRECAUTIONS. Three sources list 15 concerns for trigger point therapy that ranged from six to nine per source. The largest proportion of concerns was blood or procedurally related. The most frequently cited concerns were gross coagulation defects and local infections.

In general, except for pregnancy and some psychiatric concerns, issues listed here are also mentioned under concerns for injection therapy (**see Injection therapy**). Because trigger points are regarded as a problem of reflex irritability rather than inflammation, corticosteroids are not typically recommended during trigger point therapy.[1]

CONTRAINDICATIONS AND PRECAUTIONS

A00-B99 CERTAIN INFECTIONS AND PARASITIC DISEASES

Issue	LOC	Sources	Affil	Rationale/Comment
Systemic infection	CI	Rachlin, 1994[3]	MD	
		Walsh and Rogers, 2005[2,a]	MD	

a, Septicemia.

C00-C97 NEOPLASMS

Issue	LOC	Sources	Affil	Rationale/Comment
Tumor	ACI	Walsh and Rogers, 2005[2]	MD	At the site of injection.

D50-D89 DISEASES OF BLOOD AND BLOOD-FORMING ORGANS AND CERTAIN DISORDERS

Issue	LOC	Sources	Affil	Rationale/Comment
Blood thinners—taking	CI	Rachlin, 1994[3]	MD	If without evaluation and control.
	CI	Tan, 1998[1,a]	MD/PT	

Continued

Issue	LOC	Sources	Affil	Rationale/Comment
Coagulation defect—gross	CI	Rachlin, 1994[3]	MD	If without medical evaluation and control.
	CI	Tan, 1998[1,a]	MD/PT	
	ACI	Walsh and Rogers, 2005[2]	MD	
Immunosuppressed	CI	Tan, 1998[1]	MD/PT	

a, Also thrombocytopenia; all listings are injection therapy concerns mentioned under trigger point therapy.

F00-F99 MENTAL/BEHAVIORAL DISORDERS

Issue	LOC	Sources	Affil	Rationale/Comment
Certain psychiatric disorders Anxiety; paranoia, schizophrenia	CI	Tan, 1998[1]	MD/PT	

L00-L99 DISEASES OF THE SKIN AND SUBCUTANEOUS TISSUE

Issue	LOC	Sources	Affil	Rationale/Comment
Local infection[a]	CI	Rachlin, 1994[3]	MD	
	CI	Tan, 1998[1]	MD/PT	
	ACI	Walsh and Rogers, 2005[2]	MD	
Skin conditions preventing skin preparation	ACI	Walsh and Rogers, 2005[2]	MD	

a, Involved local tissue not specified.

O00-O99 PREGNANCY, CHILDBIRTH, AND PUERPERIUM

Issue	LOC	Sources	Affil	Rationale/Comment
Pregnant	CI	Rachlin, 1994[3]	MD	

R00-R99 SYMPTOMS, SIGNS

Issue	LOC	Sources	Affil	Rationale/Comment
Patient feels or appears ill	CI	Rachlin, 1994[3]	MD	

PROCEDURAL CONCERNS

Issue	LOC	Sources	Affil	Rationale/Comment
Allergies, history of	ACI	Walsh and Rogers, 2005[2]	MD	Allergies to local anesthetics.
Heavy activity—inability to avoid heavy activity at injection site for 2-3 days following procedure	CI	Tan, 1998[1]	MD/PT	

Continued

Issue	LOC	Sources	Affil	Rationale/Comment
Informed consent	Advice	Walsh and Rogers, 2005[2]	MD	
Uncooperative patients	ACI			
Universal precautions	P/Advice			

REFERENCES

1. Tan JC: Practical manual of physical medicine and rehabilitation: diagnostics, therapeutics, and basic problems. St Louis: Mosby; 1998.
2. Walsh NE, Rogers JN: Injection procedures. In: Delisa JA, editor: Physical medicine and rehabilitation: principles and practices, ed 4, vol 1. Philadelphia: Lippincott Williams & Wilkins; 2005.
3. Rachlin ES: Trigger point management. In Rachlin ES, editor: Myofascial pain and fibromyalgia. St Louis: Mosby; 1994.

64 POTENTIAL DRUG INTERACTIONS IN PHYSICAL MEDICINE

Potential interactions of 22 medications commonly prescribed in physical rehabilitation are based on two studies.[1,2] Read the table from left to right. For example, the drug under column A interacts with the drugs under column B, C, D, E, and F. Consult a PDR for contraindications and associated complications. Also, note the FDA (2002)[3] warning about the abrupt discontinuation of intrathecal baclofen; in rare cases, the practice has led to death.

| Column A | Column B | Column C | Column D | Column E | Column F | | |
Drug interaction of	with Drug	with Drug	with Drug	with Drug	with Drug	Comment	Source
Acetaminophen/codeine	Chlorozoxazone						Braverman, 1996[1]
ASA	Atenolol	Salsalate	Fiorinal	Ibuprofen	Warfarin		
Atenolol	ASA	Clonidine	Ibuprofen	Tolmetin	Diclofenac		
Chlorzoxazone	Acetaminophen/ codeine						
Clonidine	Atenolol	Hydralazine	Prazosin	Enalapril			
Deconomine	Atropine	Albuterol					
Diabetic	Beta blockers					Monitor to avoid asymptomatic hypoglycemia.	Parrish, 1995[2]
Digoxin	Diuretics					Monitor for hypokalemia to avoid digoxin intoxication	

Continued

Column A	Column B	Column C	Column D	Column E	Column F		
Drug interaction of	with Drug	with Drug	with Drug	with Drug	with Drug	Comment	Source
Doxepin	Oxycodone	Fiorinal					Braverman, 1996[1]
Enalapril	Clonidine	Chlorthalidone	Triamterene/ HCTZ				
Fiorinal	ASA	Doxepin	Amitriptyline	Ibuprofen	Choline Also magnesium trisalicylate, warfarin		
Fluoroquinolones	Methylxanthine						Parrish, 1995[2]
Ibuprofen	ASA	Piroxicam	Fiorinal	Inderal	Atenolol Also tolmetin, choline magnesium trisalicylate		Braverman, 1996[1]
Pirozicam	Ibuprofen						
Prednisone	Insulin	Warfarin					
Salsalate	ASA	Warfarin					
Seligiline or MOI	Meperidine					Monitor to prevent hypertensive crisis.	Parrish, 1995[2]
Tolmetin	Atenolol	Ibuprofen					Braverman, 1996[1]
Triamterene/HCTZ	Triamcinolone	Enalapril					
Trisalicylate	Fiorinal	Ibuprofen					
Warfarin	ASA	Phenytoin	Salsalate	Fiorinal	Prednisone Also ranitidine		
Warfarin	Theophylline					Common.	Parrish, 1995[2]

Note: Parrish[2] also noted specific excessive dose/duration concerns for Ciprofloxacin, histamine-2-antagonists, phenytoin, benzodiazepines.

FDA DRUG WARNING: INTRATHECAL BACLOFEN

Studies of Interactions in Physical Rehabilitation

Source	Background	Outcome	Details	Comments
FDA, 2002[3] **Abrupt discontinuation of intrathecal baclofen**	Abrupt discontinuation of intrathecal baclofen in rare cases has led to death. The sequelae include fever (high), altered mental status, rebound spasticity (exaggerated), muscle rigidity, rhabdomyolysis and multiple organ-system failure.	The FDA reports 27 cases of withdrawal with death in six patients in the first 9 years of (postmarketing) experience.	Common reasons for interruption of baclofen include disconnection or malfunction of the catheter, low volume in reservoir, end of pump battery life, and human error.	Rapid and accurate diagnosis and treatment are important. Attention to proper programming and monitoring of infusion system, refill schedule, pump alarms, keeping refill visits. Educated to early symptoms of withdrawal such as pruritus, paresthesias, return spasticity to baseline levels, or hypotension. Know patients at risk, including persons with SCI T-6 or above, communication problems, or a history of withdrawal from baclofen.
Braverman et al, 1996[1] **Potential drug interactions in rehabilitation** Descriptive Am J Phys Med Rehabil	The prevalence of potential drug-drug interactions (PDDI) in a tertiary care outpatient PM&R clinic of a U.S. Army hospital was examined to evaluate MDs' ability to correctly identify	A total of 121 subjects (60 female; 61 male) aged 18 to 78 years participated. CSDISS identified 46 level II PDDIs in 27 patients (22% prevalence rate). No level 1 computer-identified	Medications commonly identified as interactions are included in the table above.	Note: Level II interactions may lead to deterioration in a patient's status. Authors note some error may be attributed to MD disagreement with CSDISS-identified PDDI pairs. Not to be generalized to all PM&R outpatient clinics (i.e., patients on PVD/cardiac/ hypoglycemic medications).

Continued

Source	Background	Outcome	Details	Comments
	PDDI in 121 consecutive new patient referrals over a 1-month period. Questionnaires were completed by patients regarding medications, confirmed by the physicians, and then entered to the hospital's computer software drug interaction screening system (CSDISS).	interactions (i.e., life threatening) were identified; 63% of the PDDIs were not identified by MDs, and they falsely identified 28 drug combinations which were not level 1 or II PDDIs. Outpatient clinics (subspecialty) had the most PDDIs, possibly due to a more varied patient population.		Authors believe a high rate of PDDI is occurring in PM&R outpatient populations and MDs are "inadequately prepared to identify these PDDI." Suggest physician education on class-specific PDDI.
Parrish, 1995[2] **Pharmacotherapy practice in rehabilitation** Descriptive Hospital pharmacy	Log sheets for 2-year period (Feb 1991-Feb 1993) collected in a physical rehabilitation hospital (40 beds; mostly stroke, orthopedic, multiple trauma, deconditioned patients) by chart review,	120 medication-related problems: Medication-induced problem ($n = 30$) Excessive dose or duration ($n = 21$) In need of medication ($n = 13$)	Most frequent problem was drug induced ($n = 30$). B&B, K balance, tachyarrhythmias, elevated blood pressure, mood/cognition, leukocyte, thrombocyte production, liver function: affected by meds	Activities most frequently affected by medication were (1) bowel and bladder training, (2) cognitive retraining, and (3) gait and strengthening.

| prospective medication review, nurse reports, and patient interviews. | Unnecessarily medicated ($n = 13$)
Interaction ($n = 11$)
Inadequate dosage ($n = 7$)
Ineffective ($n = 6$)
No patient died or transferred out to acute care. | The most serious problem was dose/duration of med too great ($n = 21$).
Specific excessive dose/duration medication were:
Ciprofloxacin
Histamine-2 antagonists
Phenytoin
Benzodiazepines
Drug interactions (included in table) |

REFERENCES

1. Braverman SE, Howard RS, Bryant PR, et al: Potential drug interactions in a physical medicine and rehabilitation clinic. Am J Phys Med Rehabil 75(1):44-49, 1996.
2. Parrish RH II: Pharmacotherapy practice in a rehabilitation hospital. Hosp Pharm 30(9):783-785, 1995.
3. U.S. Food and Drug Administration: MedWatch 2002 safety alert—Lioresal (baclofen injection). Available at: http://www.fda.gov/medwatch/SAFETY/2002/safety02.htm#drugs. Accessed December 7, 2005.

65   POSITIONING

OVERVIEW. Positioning is the act of placing or arranging.[1] In physical rehabilitation, it pertains to the adequate arrangement of patients for a treatment (e.g., postural drainage; pressure ulcer treatment), prevention (e.g., prevention of contractures or pressure ulcers), or function (e.g., optimal wheelchair placement for independent locomotion).

Positioning must be monitored to reduce complications. Complications may be pressure related (ulcer development, nerve palsies), joint position related (contractures, dislocations), fall related (falls off support surfaces), and body fluid related (orthopnea) **(also see Restraints; Postural drainage; Yoga).** Positioning concerns listed below are organized by diagnosis and then by position.

CONTRAINDICATIONS AND PRECAUTIONS

DIAGNOSIS—BODY PART

Issue	LOC	Sources	Affil	Rationale/Comment
Amputation—above knee Avoid prolonged hip flexion, hip abduction, prolonged sitting	Advice	Pierson and Fairchild, 2002[2]	PT	Patient may experience problems fitting or using a prosthesis for ambulation if flexion or abduction contractures develop. Stump should not be elevated on a pillow while supine for more than few minutes each hour, and sitting should be limited to no more than 40 min each hour.[2]

Amputation—below knee	Avoid			As above, if limb is elevated, the knee should be maintained in extension.
Prolonged hip and knee flexion, or sitting				
Burns: Avoid "positions of comfort"[3]	Avoid	Helm et al, 1982[3]	MD	Use anticontracture positions for burn patients in the acute and subacute phases.[3]
• Anterior neck burns—"avoid pillows"[3]		Pierson and Fairchild, 2002[3]	PT	Split-thickness burns and grafted burn areas: Avoid positions of comfort, which are positions that do not produce stress or tension to the wound or graft. Prolonged flexion or adduction of the peripheral joints should be avoided when burn is noted on flexor or adductor surface of these joints.[2]
• Cubital fossa burns—"avoid medial elbow pressure"[3]				
• Perineal burns—"avoid flexion and external rotation of hip"[3]				
Hemiplegia—upper limb	Avoid	Pierson and Fairchild, 2002[2]	PT	Muscle spasticity can lead to soft tissue flexion contractures in the upper limb. Positions to be avoided in this population include prolonged shoulder adduction; internal rotation; elbow flexion; forearm supination or pronation; wrist, finger, or thumb flexion; and finger thumb adduction in the upper limbs and prolonged hip flexion and external rotation, knee flexion, ankle plantar flexion, and foot inversion in the lower limbs.[2]
Prolonged flexion postures if upper extremity is involved				
Rheumatoid arthritis				Prolonged immobilization of the affected extremity (especially flexion) should be avoided in this population.[2]
THR				**(See supine, side-lying, sitting, also ROM sections.)**

PRONE

Issue	LOC	Sources	Affil	Rationale/Comment
Anterior ankle support	Caution	Pierson and Fairchild, 2002[2]	PT	A support under the ankle while prone relieves stress on hamstrings and low back, but prolonged use may contribute to contracture formation.[2]
Chest tubes	P	Crane, 1981[4]	PT	Avoid placing pressure directly over chest tubes, as it can occlude tube drainage.
Contracture-related concerns— potential	Advice	Pierson and Fairchild, 2002[2]	PT	Monitor: Neck rotators; shoulder extensors, adductors, rotators; ankle plantar flexors.[2]
Knee to chest posture— in pregnancy	P	Kisner and Colby, 1996[5]	PT	Air embolisms can occur when patients assume a knee-to-chest position with buttocks elevated above the chest level in this population (especially in postpartum clients). The uterus moves superiorly in this position and the pressure change causes air to be sucked into the vagina and uterus, where it can enter the circulatory system through the open placental wound.[5]
Nasal CDAP	ACI	Crane, 1981[4]	PT	
Pneumothorax—untreated	ACI			**(See postural drainage, bronchial drainage.)**
Pressure ulcer–related concerns—potential	Advice	Pierson and Fairchild, 2002[2]	PT	Monitor the following body areas: forehead, ear (lateral), acromion (tip), sternum, pelvis (anterior superior iliac crest), humerus (anterior head), patella, tibia (ridge), foot (dorsum).[2]

REVERSE TRENDELENBURG

Issue	LOC	Sources	Affil	Rationale/Comment
See Postural Drainage	ACI	Crane, 1981[4]	PT	**Trendelenburg**

SIDE LYING

Issue	LOC	Sources	Affil	Rationale/Comment
Contracture sites—related concerns (potential)	Advice	Pierson and Fairchild, 2002[2]	PT	Monitor: Hip flexors, adductors, and internal rotators; knee flexors; shoulder adductors and internal rotators.[2]
Direct pressure over greater trochanter	Guideline/avoid	AHCPR, 1992[6]	Agency	Place body in a slightly reclined position (when side-lying) to remove pressure from the trochanter area. Interface pressures are higher and transcutaneous oxygen tensions are lower when side-lying directly over the trochanter compared to positioning on an off angle.[6]
Instability during bed mobility	Caution	Pierson and Fairchild, 2002[2]	PT	Side-lying is an unstable position. When moving dependent patient to a side-lying position, be cautious and roll the patient toward you, guarding the edge of the bed/mat (i.e., with your thigh). The concern also applies to position changes such as supine-to-prone and prone-to-supine transitions.[2]
Pressure ulcer-related concerns—potential	Advice			Monitor: <u>Lower side:</u> ear, ribs, acromion (lateral), humeral head (lateral), humeral epicondyle, femur (greater trochanter), femur (condyles), malleoli; and <u>Upper side:</u> humeral epicondyle (medial), femoral condyle (medial), tibia malleolus.[2]
THR	Advice	Pierson and Fairchild, 2002[2]	PT	The operated hip should be uppermost when side-lying; supported with pillows, powder board, or bolsters and maintained in hip abduction and neutral rotation. One must not cross the ankle of the operated limb over the opposite extremity or allow patient to lie on the surgically replaced hip.[2]
	Advice	Kisner and Colby, 1996[5]	PT	

Continued

Issue	LOC	Sources	Affil	Rationale/Comment
				For posterior lateral approaches, suggest that patients sleep with an abduction pillow and avoid sleeping on that side for at least 8 to 12 weeks postoperatively.[5]

SITTING

Also See Wheelchair—Manual; Bath Chair

Issue	LOC	Sources	Affil	Rationale/Comment
Contracture-related concerns—potential	Advice	Pierson and Fairchild, 2002[2]	PT	Monitor: Hip flexors, adductors, and internal rotators; knee flexors; shoulder adductors, extensors, and internal rotators.
Pressure ulcer–related concerns—potential	Advice			Monitor: Ischial tuberosities; vertebral spinous processes; scapular processes; humeral epicondyle (medial).
THR	Advice			For posterior or posterolateral surgical approach, do not sit erect in wheelchair or bed (i.e., supported on flat surface with fully upright trunk). Avoid excessive trunk flexion while sitting; use elevated toilet seat and elevated chair seats for most patients. Avoid internal hip rotation or hip flexion beyond 60 to 90 degrees.
	Advice	Kisner and Colby, 1996[5]	PT	For posterolateral incisions, avoid sitting on soft low chairs.
				Suggest a raised toilet seat. Do not bend the trunk excessively over the operated hip when rising from a chair or when picking up objects from the floor. Do not let patient cross legs.[5]

Ring cushions	Guideline	AHCPR, 1992[6]	Agency	Do not use ring cushions (donuts) if patient is chair-bound. Ring cushion may cause edema and venous congestion and are more prone to cause an ulcer than to prevent one from occurring.[6]
Syncope and chair (sitting) massage	Advice	Palmer, 2000[7]	Massage	Screen patients and be aware of signs of syncope. **In 2000, Palmer[7] describes a caller on a radio show who described a client in the gym who received a massage in a sitting position and was caught just before she collapsed (fainted) to the floor.** Massage clients are less likely to faint while on a massage table, as they are already lying down.[7]
Uninterrupted sitting	Guideline	AHCPR, 1992[6]	Agency	Avoid uninterrupted sitting (i.e., chair; wheelchair) in those at risk for pressure ulcers. Reposition at least every hour. Use foam, gel, air, or combination.[6]

STANCE

Issue	LOC	Sources	Affil	Rationale/Comment
Assisted standing		—		**See Gravity-assisted compression devices; also see Gait training.**
Peripheral vascular disease— lower limb dependency	Advice	Kisner and Colby, 1996[5]	PT	Avoid prolonged periods of time standing still and sitting with dependent legs.[5]
Pregnancy—one-legged stance	Unsafe			Weight-bearing activities on one leg can result in SI joint or pubic symphysis irritation (avoid if preexisting SI symptoms). Also, one-legged balancing may be affected due to increased weight and changes in the patient's center of gravity during pregnancy.[5]

SUPINE (ALSO SEE PROCEDURAL CONCERNS BELOW)

Issue	LOC	Sources	Affil	Rationale/Comment
Contracture-related concerns—potential	Advice	Pierson and Fairchild, 2002[2]	PT	Hip flexors and external rotators; knee flexors; ankle plantar flexors; shoulder extensors, adductors, and internal rotators.[2]
Heels	Guideline	AHCPR, 1992[6]	Agency	Dependent patients (completely immobile) need "extra protection" for their heels while in bed.[6]
Knees—support under	Advice	Pierson and Fairchild, 2002[2]	PT	Avoid support under knees for prolonged periods of time as it encourages hip (iliopsoas) and knee flexion (hamstrings) contractures.
Orthopnea	FYI	Thomson et al, 1991[8]	PT	In persons with chronic lung disease and congestive heart disease, breathlessness that is aggravated when the patient lies flat (supine) and relieved with sitting or standing may be observed.[9] In supine, (excess) fluid moves from the LEs to the heart and lungs, interfering with lung perfusion and ventilation in this population. Also, the abdominal organs push up on the diaphragm and increase lung congestion in this position.[8]
Preterm or neonates, sick	Advice	Gardner and Lubchenco, 1998[10]	—	Acutely ill preterm infants are often positioned supine to accommodate ventilators and umbilical catheters. Unfortunately, supine does not promote flexion and may be stressful to acutely ill infants. With prolonged positioning, increased startle and sleep disturbances may occur.[10]
Pregnancy—supine	Avoid/Advice	Kisner and Colby, 1996[5]	PT	After the 4th month of pregnancy, the weight of the uterus can compress the vena cava. Avoid supine for more than 5 minutes at a time. Turning the patient slightly toward the left will reduce the effects of uterine compression on abdominal vessels and improve cardiac output.[5]

Pressure ulcer–related concerns—potential	Advice	Pierson and Fairchild, 2002[2]	PT	Monitor: Occipital tuberosity, scapula (spine, inferior angle); vertebral spinous processes; pelvis (posterior iliac crest); sacrum, humeral epicondyle (medial); calcaneus (posterior); hip (greater trochanter), fibula (head), malleolus (lateral).[2]
THR	Advice			Maintain operated hip in neutral and slightly abducted (avoid adduction past neutral).

TRENDELENBURG—INVERTED POSITIONS (ALSO SEE MECHANICAL TRACTION—INVERSION)

Issue	LOC	Sources	Affil	Rationale/Comment
See Postural drainage	ACI	Crane, 1981[4]	PT	

PROCEDURAL CONCERNS—GENERAL

Issue	LOC	Sources	Affil	Rationale/Comment
Bony prominences	Guideline	AHCPR, 1992[6]	Agency	Prevent bony prominences from touching to avoid ulcer development.[6]
Changing positioning	Guideline			Avoid friction and shear forces. Use proper transfer technique. Also consider lubricants, protective films, dressings, and padding to reduce friction injuries.[6]
Head of bed—angle	Guideline			Keep the head of the bed at its lowest level of elevation permitted for the patient's medical condition. Also, minimize the duration of time with head elevated. Shear forces increase with head elevation, leading to ischemic and necrotic tissue changes

Continued

Issue	LOC	Sources	Affil	Rationale/Comment
				in the skin. Under these conditions, underlying tissue shifts relative to stationary skin, diminishing blood supply to the skin (blood vessels become distorted), causing ischemia, necrosis, and tissue ulcers (e.g., sacral ulcer).[6]
Extended periods— positioned	Advice	Pierson and Fairchild, 2002[2]	PT	Avoid positioning for an extended period of time in any position that promotes excessive stress of various structures (skin), promotes soft tissue contractures, or increases patient discomfort.
Repositioning patients at risk for pressure ulcer	Guideline	AHCPR, 1992[6,11]	Agency	Reposition patients at risk for pressure ulcer at least every 2 hours when consistent with overall patient management. This strategy is based on the inverse relationship between spontaneous movements in bed-bound elderly and pressure ulcer incidence.[6]
Pressure ulcer—positioned on	Avoid			Avoid positioning over a pressure ulcer. Healing may be delayed because pressure of sufficient duration and intensity can cause ischemia and necrosis. Use positioning devices (not ring cushions) to raise pressure ulcer off the support surface.[11]
Projecting body parts	Advice	Pierson and Fairchild, 2002[2]	PT	Patient body parts should not project beyond support (mat) surface. For example, projecting feet can be struck by passing equipment.

ADVERSE EVENTS

Source	Background	Therapy	Outcome	Follow-up/Interpretation
Nagler, 1973[12] **Strained posture** Case series Arch Phys Med Rehabil	A 18-year-old male gymnast.	He performed a handstand in the parallel bars, forcefully extending his head to maintain balance.	His legs and arms suddenly weakened and he fell to floor. He was hospitalized with complete flaccid paralysis (motor C5, sensory T4) His diagnosis was acute myelopathy due to an anterior spinal artery occlusion (self-inflicted).	At 2 months, spasticity developed; at 18 months, he was quadriplegic and using a wheelchair.
	A 54-year-old cigar-smoking man with a sedentary lifestyle experienced headaches and some giddiness when he turned his head quickly.	He started exercising prone on a table, flexed down at the lumbar area. He then attempted to raise his back to a horizontal position with maximal neck extension.	He experienced sudden dizziness, limbs became weak; radiographs revealed C1-C2 abnormality with OA changes and a small foramen magnum. His diagnosis was acute myelopathy (motor C5, sensory C4) due to anterior spinal artery occlusion (self-inflicted). He underwent cervical laminectomy.	One year later, he was ambulating with platform crutches.
Preston and Grimes, 1985[13] **Poor positioning and neuropathy** Case series Arch Neurol	A 72-year-old woman presented with a 6-year history of PD.	Over the previous 2 years, she spent all her time in either a bed or a wheelchair.	She developed left wrist drop that led to a fixed flexion deformity.	The authors believe bradykinesia along with improper positioning in bed or wheelchair led to nerve compression at the UE site where
	A 76-year-old woman presented with 10-year history of PD stage 5 for 3 years.	She spent most of her day sleeping in a wheelchair.	She developed a left radial motor neuropathy, but completely recovered in 3 months.	

Continued

Source	Background	Therapy	Outcome	Follow-up/Interpretation
	A 63-year-old woman presented with a 22-year history of PD. A 75-year-old woman with 8-year history of PD; had been wheelchair dependent for the past 2 years.	She was in bed 10 days during a drug holiday. She was taking thioridazine hydrochloride for agitation.	A right wrist drop with preservation of triceps was noted that recovered in 1 month. The medication led to decreased mobility. Wrist drop was later noted. The medication was discontinued, and she recovered in 4 months.	the radial nerve pierces the lateral intermuscular septum. Prevention includes frequent position changes, avoidance of sleeping in wheelchairs, and if nerve compression occurs, use a wrist splint to avoid the development of a fixed wrist deformity.

LITIGATION

Year, State	History	Location	Complication	Comments Award
1999, New York[14] **Fall from table**	A 57-year-old warehouseman presented with a leg injury.	He was treated with physical therapy. In 1995, the patient fell from PT examining table.	The patient was startled and fell off the table, suffering a trimalleolar fracture of his left ankle. He wore a long leg cast for 13 weeks.	The patient claimed he was totally incapacitated. He also claimed he was "hit" by a physical therapist, which startled him and resulted in the fall. $170,000 settlement.

Note: Awards and settlements do not necessarily prove a cause-effect relationship between equipment or therapy and injury.

REFERENCES

1. Webster's third new international dictionary. Springfield (MA): Merriam-Webster; 1981.
2. Pierson FM, Fairchild SL: Principles and techniques of patient care, ed 3. Philadelphia: Saunders; 2002.
3. Helm PA, Kevorkian CG, Lushbaugh M, et al: Burn injury: rehabilitation management in 1982. Arch Phys Med Rehabil 63:6-16, 1982.
4. Crane L: Physical therapy for neonates with respiratory dysfunction. Phys Ther 61(12):1764-1773, 1981.
5. Kisner C, Colby LA: Therapeutic exercise: foundations and techniques, ed 3. Philadelphia: FA Davis; 1996.
6. AHCPR: Pressure ulcers in adults: prediction and prevention, clinical practice guideline no. 3, AHCPR Pub. No. 92-0047, May 1992.
7. Palmer D: What just happened? Massage Bodywork 15(3):76-81, 2000.
8. Thomson A, Skinner A, Piercy J: Tidy's physiotherapy, ed 12. Oxford: Butterworth-Heinemann; 1991.
9. Goodman CC: The cardiovascular system. In: Goodman CC, Boissonnault WG, Fuller KS, eds: Pathology: implications for the physical therapist, ed 2. Philadelphia: Saunders; 2003.
10. Gardner SL, Lubchenco LO: The neonate and the environment: impact on development. In: Merenstein GB, Gardner SL, eds: Handbook of neonatal intensive care, ed 4. St Louis: Mosby; 1998.
11. AHCPR: Treatment of pressure ulcers, clinical guideline no. 15. AHCPR Publication No. 95-0652, December 1994.
12. Nagler W: Vertebral artery obstruction by hyperextension of the neck: report of three cases. Arch Phys Med Rehabil 54(5):237-240, 1973.
13. Preston DN, Grimes JD: Radial compression neuropathy in advanced Parkinson's disease. Arch Neurol 42:695-696, 1985.
14. Medical malpractice verdicts, settlements, and experts, December 1999, p 43, loc 3.

66   DRAPING

OVERVIEW. Draping (drape = cloth) means to cover or adorn with cloth.[1] In physical rehabilitation, it pertains to the procedure of allowing exposure of some body part(s) for a treatment while covering other parts for modesty, comfort (warmth), and protection from soiling patient's clothing (e.g., conduction gels).

PROCEDURAL CONCERNS

Issue	LOC	Sources	Affil	Rationale/Comment
Assistance—appropriate	Advice	Pierson and Fairchild, 2002[2]	PT	Depending on gender of caregiver and patient, it may be necessary for the caregiver to request another person to assist patient in undressing, draping, and redressing.
Consent—obtain patient's consent to remove draping	Advice			If garments need to be removed, explain and receive patient's permission.
Clothing (patient) for draping	Advice			Do not use patient clothing for draping. Clothing may be soiled with perspiration, lubricants, and wound drainage.
Exposure—avoid exposure of sensitive body parts	Advice			Avoid unnecessary exposure of sensitive areas of patient body—breast and perineum. Be aware of personal, cultural, or religious factors affecting modesty in patients.
Linen—clean, unused	Advice			To prevent transmission of disease/infection, linen should be clean, unused on patients, and unsoiled.
Linen—folds or wrinkles	Advice			Wrinkles may cause localized pressure problems. Remove or reduce folds or wrinkles in linen beneath patient.
Room temperature—burn patients	Advice	Staley and Richard, 2001[3]	PT	Burn patients lose heat in normal ambient room temperatures. Keep room temperature at 86 °F (30 °C).

REFERENCES

1. Webster's third new international dictionary. Springfield (MA): Merriam–Webster; 1981.

2. Pierson FM, Fairchild SL: Principles and techniques of patient care, ed 3. Philadelphia: Saunders; 2002.

3. Staley MJ, Richard RL: Burns. In O'Sullivan SB, Schmitz TJ, eds: Physical rehabilitation: assessment and treatment, ed 4. Philadelphia: FA Davis; 2001.

CARDIAC REHABILITATION SCREENING

Note: The following issues are considered a concern (advice, precaution, contraindication, or warning) from one or more published sources. If you check any item, consult page 94 for information

E00–E90 Endocrine, Nutritional, and Metabolic Diseases

- ☐ Diabetes (uncontrolled)
- ☐ Hyperkalemia
- ☐ Hypokalemia
- ☐ Hypovolemia
- ☐ Thyroiditis (acute)
- ☐ Other metabolic conditions

I00–I99 Circulatory System

- ☐ Angina (unstable)
- ☐ Aortic stenosis (critical)
- ☐ Atrial or ventricular arrhythmia (uncontrolled)
- ☐ Congestive heart failure (uncompensated)
- ☐ Diastolic BP (resting >110 mm Hg)
- ☐ Embolism (recent)
- ☐ Orthostatic BP drop >20 mm Hg with symptoms
- ☐ Pericarditis or Myocarditis (acute)
- ☐ Sinus tachycardia (uncontrolled)
- ☐ ST segment displacement (resting) 2 mm
- ☐ Systolic BP (resting) >200 mm Hg
- ☐ Third-degree AV Block
- ☐ Thrombophlebitis

M00–M99 Musculoskeletal System

- ☐ Severe orthopedic conditions, prohibiting exercise

R00–R99 Symptoms & Signs

- ☐ Systemic fever (acute)

COLD LASER SCREENING

Note: The following issues are considered a concern (advice, precaution, contraindication, or warning) from one or more published sources. If you check any item, consult page 643 for information.

C00-C97 Neoplasms
- ☐ Cancer (near)

D50-D89 Blood
- ☐ Hemorrhagic region (over)

F00-F99 Mental & Behavioral
- ☐ Confused

G00-G99 Nervous System
- ☐ Sensation impaired

I00-I99 Circulatory System
- ☐ Cardiac patients

L00-L99 Skin
- ☐ Dry skin, extra (over)
- ☐ Eschar, thick (over)
- ☐ Infected skin (over)
- ☐ Photosensitive skin (over)
- ☐ Photosensitized from medication
- ☐ Scar tissue (over)

O00-O99 Pregnancy
- ☐ Pregnant women

R00-R99 Symptoms & Signs
- ☐ Fever
- ☐ Infection

Vulnerable tissue
- ☐ Cornea
- ☐ Endocrine glands
- ☐ Epiphysial area (children)
- ☐ Fontanels, unclosed (over)
- ☐ Testicular region

Procedural Concerns
- ☐ Age (extreme)
- ☐ Medicated heavily
- ☐ Syncope lasting >5 minutes
- ☐ Within 4-6 months after radiotherapy

CONTINUOUS PASSIVE MOTION SCREENING

Note: The following issues are considered a concern (advice, precaution, contraindication, or warning) from one or more published sources. If you check any item, consult page 714 for information.

D50-D89 Blood

☐ Anticoagulation

G00-G99 Nervous System

☐ Sensation loss

M00-M99 Musculoskeletal

☐ Arthrosis (acute)
☐ Joint infection
☐ Joint instability
☐ Translation of opposing bone (unwanted)

Y70-Y82 Medical Devices

☐ Dressing - restrictive
☐ Strap & carriage - rubbing

S00-T98 Injuries

☐ Fractures - rigid fixation not attained

Vulnerable tissue

☐ Peripheral nerves - excessive pressure

Procedural

☐ Use only as an adjunct
☐ Tension in wound (if swelling) during ranging

CRYOTHERAPY SCREENING

Note: The following issues are considered a concern (advice, precaution, contraindication, or warning) from one or more published sources. If you check any item, consult page 578 for information.

A00-B99 Certain Infections
- ☐ Infection

D50-D89 Blood
- ☐ Cryoglobulinemia
- ☐ Paroxysmal cold hemoglobinuria

F00-F99 Mental & Behavioral
- ☐ Cold aversion
- ☐ Mentation, Poor

G00-G99 Nervous System
- ☐ Regenerating nerve, peripheral
- ☐ Sensation - Poor
- ☐ Thermoregulation

I00-I99 Circulatory System
- ☐ Cardiac - Left shoulder
- ☐ Circulation impaired
- ☐ Hypertension
- ☐ PVD, affecting arterial circulation
- ☐ Raynaud's phenomenon

L00-L99 Skin
- ☐ Cold hypersensitivity
- ☐ Cold intolerance
- ☐ Cold urticaria
- ☐ Skin conditions

M00-M99 Musculoskeletal
- ☐ Rheumatoid arthritis

R00-R99 Symptoms & Signs
- ☐ Cold Pressor Response, Severe

S00-T98 Injury
- ☐ Frostbite, history
- ☐ Wound, healing

Vulnerable Tissue
- ☐ Ear, behind (repetitive icing)
- ☐ Facial (above lips)
- ☐ Midline trunk (over)
- ☐ Peripheral nerve, superficial

Procedural Concerns
- ☐ Age
- ☐ Stretching (after cold application)
- ☐ Quick movement (after cold application)
- ☐ Direct skin contact
- ☐ Blood pressure- monitor

Vapocoolant Spray
- ☐ Dropping bottle, do not
- ☐ Eyes, avoid spraying
- ☐ Flammable, highly
- ☐ Skin, avoid frosting
- ☐ Vapors, minimize inhalation

DIATHERMY SCREENING

Note: The following issues are considered a concern (advice, precaution, contraindication, or warning) from one or more published sources. If you check any item, consult page 598 for information.

C00-C97 Neoplasm
- ☐ Malignancy, area

D50-D89 Blood
- ☐ Hemophilia
- ☐ Hemorrhage

E00-E90 Endocrine
- ☐ Obesity

F00-F99 Mental & Behavioral
- ☐ Mentation impaired

G00-G99 Nervous System
- ☐ Sensation impaired
- ☐ Thermoregulation

I00-I99 Circulatory System
- ☐ Angina, unstable
- ☐ Blood pressure, unstable
- ☐ Circulation impaired (ischemia)
- ☐ Thrombophlebitis
- ☐ Cardiac insufficiency

L00-L99 Skin
- ☐ Atrophic skin
- ☐ Blisters
- ☐ Infected skin
- ☐ Scar, immature

M00-M99 Musculoskeletal
- ☐ Infection, joint

N00-N99 Genitourinary
- ☐ Menstruating

O00-O99 Pregnancy
- ☐ Pregnancy
- ☐ Vaginal electrodes, in pregnancy

R00-R99 Symptoms & Signs
- ☐ Edema
- ☐ Fever
- ☐ Inflammation (acute)

S00-T98 Injury
- ☐ Injury (acute)
- ☐ Wounds, open

Y70-Y82 Medical Devices
- ☐ Contact lenses
- ☐ Electric/magnetic equipment
- ☐ IUD with copper
- ☐ Leads, implanted
- ☐ Metal implants
- ☐ Pacemakers, cardiac
- ☐ Stimulators, neural (any)
- ☐ Pumps, implanted

Vulnerable Tissue
- ☐ Epiphyses
- ☐ Eyes
- ☐ Fluid-filled joints
- ☐ Gonads
- ☐ Space-occupying lesions

Procedural concerns
- ☐ Dressings or clothing, moist
- ☐ Edema, dependent (limb)
- ☐ Hazards, therapist
- ☐ Perspiration
- ☐ Synthetic material
- ☐ Training, personnel
- ☐ Counterirritants, topical
- ☐ Pregnant, therapist

ELECTROTHERAPY SCREENING

Note: The following issues are considered a concern (advice, precaution, contraindication, or warning) from one or more published sources. If you check any item, consult page 538 for information. Note: Some concerns may be specific to a type of ES.

A00-B99 Certain Infections
- ☐ Tuberculosis

C00-C97 Neoplasm
- ☐ Tumors, malignant

D50-D89 Blood
- ☐ Hemorrhage (active)
- ☐ Hemorrhage (prone)

E00-E90 Endocrine
- ☐ Obese patients

F00-F99 Mental & Behavioral
- ☐ Incompetent patient
- ☐ Mentation impaired
- ☐ Psychological states
- ☐ Unreliable

G00-G99 Nervous
- ☐ Cell body pathology
- ☐ CNS disorders
- ☐ Epilepsy/Seizure disorder
- ☐ Muscle - nerve junction pathology
- ☐ Myelin sheath pathology
- ☐ Peripheral neuropathy
- ☐ Sensation impaired

I00-I99 Circulatory
- ☐ Arrhythmias
- ☐ Cardiac disease/history
- ☐ Hypertension
- ☐ Hypotension
- ☐ Thrombosis/phlebitis
- ☐ Varicose veins

L00-L99 Skin
- ☐ Allergies, skin
- ☐ Skin, conditions
- ☐ Skin, fragile

N00-N99 Genitourinary
- ☐ Menstruating uterus

O00-O99 Pregnancy
- ☐ Birth, TENS
- ☐ Pregnancy
- ☐ Pregnancy, abdomen/lumbar

Q00-Q99 Congenital
- ☐ Muscular dystrophy

R00-R99 Signs & Symptoms
- ☐ Infected area
- ☐ Inflamed area
- ☐ Swollen (over)

S00-T98 Injury
- ☐ Fracture
- ☐ Skin damage

Y70-Y82 Medical Devices
- ☐ Bladder stimulators (near)
- ☐ Cardiac pacemakers, demand
- ☐ Cardioverter defibrillators, implantable
- ☐ Diathermy devices (near)
- ☐ Metal, superficial (pins, plates, hardware)

Vulnerable tissue
- ☐ Carotid sinus
- ☐ Cerebral (trans)
- ☐ Cranial/cervical (trans) in CVA, TIA,
- ☐ Seizures
- ☐ Eye (over)
- ☐ Heart, cardiac patient
- ☐ Internal use
- ☐ Mouth (over)
- ☐ Neck, anterior
- ☐ Phrenic nerve (near)
- ☐ Thoracic (trans)
- ☐ Thoracic region (over)

Procedural (multiple issues)
- ☐ See chapter 41

EXERCISE TESTING SCREENING

Note: The following issues are considered a concern (advice, warning, precaution, contraindication, or absolute contraindication) from one or more published sources. If you check any item, consult page 21 for information.

A00–B99 Certain Infections

- ☐ Infections (acute)
- ☐ Infections (chronic)

E00–E90 Endocrine

- ☐ Electrolyte abnormalities
- ☐ Metabolic disease (uncontrolled)

F00–F99 Mental & Behavioral

- ☐ Mental impairment

I00–I99 Circulatory

- ☐ Aneurysm, dissecting (suspected or known)
- ☐ Aneurysm, ventricular
- ☐ Angina (if unstable)
- ☐ Aortic stenosis (severe)
- ☐ Aortic stenosis (uncontrolled and symptomatic)
- ☐ Arterial hypertension (severe)
- ☐ Atrial fibrillation
- ☐ Atrioventricular block, high degree
- ☐ Bradyarrhythmias
- ☐ Cardiac arrhythmias, unstable
- ☐ Coronary stenosis, left main artery

I00–I99 Circulatory cont'd

- ☐ Endocarditis (active)
- ☐ Hypertrophic cardiomyopathy
- ☐ MI (acute) (within 2 days)
- ☐ Myocarditis or pericarditis (acute)
- ☐ Other outflow tract obstructions
- ☐ Pulmonary embolus or infarction (acute)
- ☐ Resting ECG shows recent significant change
- ☐ Tachyarrhythmias
- ☐ Valvular heart disease, stenotic (moderate)

N00–N99 Genitourinary

- ☐ Renal failure

R00–R99 Symptoms & Signs

- ☐ Physical impairments

Procedural

- ☐ Disorders, exacerbated by exercise
- ☐ Informed consent
- ☐ Mental impairments
- ☐ Physical impairments

FUNCTIONAL ELECTRICAL STIMULATION SCREENING

Note: The following issues are considered a concern (advice, precaution, contraindication, or warning) from one or more published sources. If you check any item, consult page 569 for information.

E00-E90 Metabolic Disease
- ☐ Metabolic disturbance
- ☐ Obesity

F00-F99 Mental & Behavioral
- ☐ Alcohol/Drug abuse
- ☐ Educational/mental level inadequate
- ☐ Motivation level
- ☐ MMPI score - high

G00-G99 Nervous System
- ☐ Flaccid paraplegia
- ☐ High lesion
- ☐ Sitting balance - inadequate
- ☐ Spasticity - severe

H00-H59 Eye
- ☐ Vision - Poor

H60-H95 Ear
- ☐ Hearing - Poor

I00-I99 Circulatory System
- ☐ Cardiac pathology
- ☐ Hypertension (uncontrolled)

J00-J99 Respiratory System
- ☐ Respiratory infection
- ☐ Respiratory pathology

L00-L99 Skin
- ☐ Cutaneous disorder

M00-M99 Musculoskeletal System
- ☐ Contractures
- ☐ Degenerative joint disease
- ☐ Heterotopic ossification
- ☐ Osteoporosis
- ☐ Short extremities
- ☐ Spinal deformity
- ☐ Spinal mobility - Poor

N00-N99 Genitourinary
- ☐ Urinary tract infection

O00-O99 Pregnancy
- ☐ Pregnancy

R00-R99 Symptoms & Signs
- ☐ General state - Poor

S00-T98 Injury
- ☐ Pressure ulcer

Procedural Concerns
- ☐ Age
- ☐ Attendant support
- ☐ Hypersensitivity (electric current)
- ☐ Vital signs (monitor)

HYDROTHERAPY SCREENING

Note: The following issues are considered a concern (advice, precaution, contraindication, or warning) from one or more published sources. If you check any item, consult page 620 for information. Also see Debridement and Aquatic therapy.

A00-B99 Certain Infections
- ☐ Infectious conditions
- ☐ Tuberculosis

C00-C97 Neoplasm
- ☐ Malignancy

D50-D89 Blood
- ☐ Hemorrhage, danger

F00-F99 Mental & Behavioral
- ☐ Alcohol ingestion
- ☐ Confusion / Disorientation
- ☐ Fear of water
- ☐ Mental disorder
- ☐ Mentation impaired
- ☐ Suicidal

G00-G99 Nervous
- ☐ Epilepsy (severe; uncontrolled)
- ☐ Multiple sclerosis, warm
- ☐ Sensation impaired
- ☐ Thermoregulation impaired (very warm or hot water)

I00-I99 Circulatory
- ☐ Blood pressure, unstable
- ☐ Cardiac dysfunction
- ☐ Cardiac instability
- ☐ Hypertensive
- ☐ Medication, cardiac
- ☐ Peripheral vascular disease
- ☐ Thrombophlebitis

J00 -J99 Respiratory
- ☐ Pulmonary disease
- ☐ Upper respiratory infection
- ☐ Vital capacity <1000 ml

K00-K93 Digestive
- ☐ Incontinence, bowel

L00-L99 Skin
- ☐ Atrophic, skin
- ☐ Conditions, skin (some)
- ☐ Hypersensitivity, thermal
- ☐ Ichthyosis, senile, winter pruritus
- ☐ Infection, skin
- ☐ Maceration (around wound)
- ☐ Scar
- ☐ Skin, graft
- ☐ Tissue flaps

M00-M99 Musculoskeletal
- ☐ Musculoskeletal impairments
- ☐ Rheumatoid arthritis (acute)

N00-N99 Genitourinary
- ☐ Incontinence, urinary
- ☐ Sperm count reduced

O00-O99 Pregnancy
- ☐ Very warm or hot water, pregnancy

R00-R99 Symptoms & Signs
- ☐ Edema
- ☐ Febrile episode (acute)
- ☐ Inflammation (acute)

S00-T98 Injury
- ☐ Injury (acute)
- ☐ Wound, open

Y70-Y82 Medical Devices
- ☐ Metal (in area)

Procedural
- ☐ Counterirritants, topical
- ☐ Elderly
- ☐ UE dependent

JOINT MOBILIZATION SCREENING

Note: The following issues are considered a concern (advice, precaution, contraindication, or warning) from one or more published sources. If you check any item, consult page 285 for information.

A00-B99 Certain Infections
- ☐ Infection
- ☐ Tuberculosis

C00-C97 Neoplasm
- ☐ Neoplasm
- ☐ History (non spinal)

F00-F99
- ☐ Developmental delay
- ☐ Neurosis, severe
- ☐ Pain, psychologic with hypotonia

G00-G99 Nervous System
- ☐ Cauda equina lesion (with bowel / bowel disturbance)
- ☐ Cerebral palsy (Athetoid, Ataxia)
- ☐ Spasticity, in children
- ☐ Spinal cord involvement
- ☐ Neurologic signs

I00-I99 Circulatory
- ☐ Circulatory disturbance
- ☐ Dizziness, aggravated by neck rotation or extension

M00-M99 Musculoskeletal
- ☐ Arthroses
- ☐ Connective tissue weakness
- ☐ Hypermobility (or associated joint)
- ☐ Internal derangement
- ☐ Joint effusion / inflammation
- ☐ Autoimmune disease (RA: AS)
- ☐ Bone disease
- ☐ Deformity, operative
- ☐ Laxity, ligament
- ☐ Osteomyelitis

M00-M99 Musculoskeletal cont'd
- ☐ Polymyalgia rheumatica
- ☐ Prolapse, disk with neurological changes
- ☐ Proplapse/Herniated, disk
- ☐ Scoliosis
- ☐ Vertebral ligament necrosis, rheumatoid collagen

O00-O99 Pregnancy
- ☐ Pregnancy, first trimester
- ☐ Pregnancy, last stage

Q00-Q99 Congenital
- ☐ Deformity, congenital
- ☐ Down syndrome
- ☐ Prader-Willi syndrome

R00-R99 Symptoms & Signs
- ☐ Debilitation, general
- ☐ Elderly
- ☐ Inflammation
- ☐ Neurologic signs
- ☐ Pain, excessive

S00-T98 Injury
- ☐ Fracture (recent)
- ☐ Ligament rupture

Y70-Y82 Medical Devices
- ☐ Joint replacements, total

Procedural concerns
- ☐ Spasms, protective
- ☐ Temporary soreness from treatment (warn)

PERCUSSION AND VIBRATION SCREENING

Note: The following issues are considered a concern (advice, precaution, contraindication, or warning) from one or more published sources. If you check any item, consult page 471 for information.

A00-B99 Certain Infections
- ☐ Tuberculosis, pulmonary (active)

C00-C97 Neoplasm
- ☐ Bone metastases
- ☐ Tumors, obstructing airway

D50-D89 Blood
- ☐ Coagulopathy
- ☐ Hemorrhage, active
- ☐ Platelet count <200,000 per mm^3

F00-F99 Mental & Behavioral
- ☐ Anxious / Nervous
- ☐ Confused / combative

G00-G99 Nervous
- ☐ ICP elevated
- ☐ Seizure disorder
- ☐ Spinal anesthesia, epidural (recent)

I00-I99 Circulatory
- ☐ Hemodynamics, unstable
- ☐ Pulmonary embolism

J00-J99 Respiratory
- ☐ Bronchopleural fistula
- ☐ Bronchospasm
- ☐ Empyema
- ☐ End-stage lung disease
- ☐ Hemoptysis
- ☐ Pleural effusion (large)
- ☐ Pleuritic pain (acute)
- ☐ Pneumothorax, untreated
- ☐ Pulmonary contusion
- ☐ Pulmonary edema

J00-J99 Respiratory cont'd
- ☐ Subcutaneous emphysema
- ☐ Therapy-induced hypoxemia

L00-L99 Skin
- ☐ Myocutaneous flap, thorax (recent)
- ☐ Skin graft (recent)
- ☐ Skin infection, thorax

M00-M99 Musculoskeletal
- ☐ Bone disease, degenerative
- ☐ Flail chest
- ☐ Osteomyelitis
- ☐ Osteoporosis of ribs
- ☐ Spinal surgery (recent)

R00-R99 Symptoms
- ☐ Pain, chest wall

S00-T98 Injury
- ☐ Burns
- ☐ Rib fractures
- ☐ Soft tissue injury, thorax
- ☐ Spinal injury, unstable
- ☐ Wound, open
- ☐ Wound, surgical

Y70-Y82 Medical Device
- ☐ Pacemaker

Procedural
- ☐ Aged
- ☐ Anterior lobe, pediatrics
- ☐ If positions contraindicated (Trendelenburg; reverse)
- ☐ Unnecessary service

POSTURAL DRAINAGE SCREENING

Note: The following issues are considered a concern (advice, precaution, contraindication, or warning) from one or more published sources. If you check any item, consult page 494 for information.

D50-D89 Blood

☐ Hemorrhage (severe hemoptysis)

E00-E90 Endocrine

☐ Obesity, massive

F00-F99 Mental & Behavioral

☐ Confused
☐ Nervous patient

G00-G99 Nervous System

☐ Cerebral edema
☐ ICP >20 mm Hg

H00-H59 Eye

☐ Eye surgery, post

I00-I99 Circulatory System

☐ Aneurysm, aortic
☐ Arrhythmia, cardiac
☐ Cardiovascular instability
☐ Cerebral vascular accident
☐ Hemorrhage
☐ Hypertension, severe
☐ Pulmonary embolism

J00-J99 Respiratory

☐ Asthma (acute)
☐ Bronchopleural fistula
☐ Emphysema (severe)
☐ Empyema

J00-J99 Respiratory cont'd

☐ Hemoptysis
☐ Pleural effusion (large)
☐ Pneumothorax
☐ Pulmonary edema

K00-K93 Digestive

☐ Ascites (massive)
☐ Esophagectomy, post-op
☐ Gastric reflux, esophageal
☐ Hernia, diaphragm

M00-M99 Musculoskeletal

☐ Laminectomy, recent
☐ Spinal fusion

N00-N99 Genitourinary

☐ Peritoneal dialysis, during filling cycle

S00-T98 Injury

☐ Burns
☐ Head trauma (recent)
☐ Neck injury
☐ Rib fracture
☐ Spinal injury
☐ Wound, surgical

Procedural Concerns

☐ Aged

SPINAL MANIPULATION SCREENING

Note: The following issues are considered a concern (advice, precaution, contraindication, or warning) from one or more published sources. If you check any item, consult page 298 for information.

C00-C97 Neoplasms
- ☐ Carcinoma, metastatic

D50-D89 Blood
- ☐ Anticoagulation
- ☐ Hemophilia

E00-E90 Endocrine
- ☐ Diabetes (severe)

F00-F99 Mental & Behavioral
- ☐ Compensation
- ☐ Neurosis, non organic
- ☐ Obsessive fixation, pain

G00-G99 Nervous System
- ☐ Cauda equine syndrome
- ☐ CNS disease
- ☐ Compression of 4th sacral root
- ☐ Myelopathy
- ☐ Neurologic signs
- ☐ Radiculopathy, multiple adjacent
- ☐ Root pain

I00-I99 Circulatory System
- ☐ Aneurysm, local
- ☐ Atherosclerosis
- ☐ Graft, aortic
- ☐ Vertebral artery disease

M00-M99 Musculoskeletal
- ☐ Abnormality, bony
- ☐ Aseptic necrosis
- ☐ Bone disease
- ☐ Deformity, spinal

M00-M99 Musculoskeletal cont'd
- ☐ Degenerative joint disease
- ☐ Gout
- ☐ Hypermobility
- ☐ Hypermobility adjacent
- ☐ Infection, vertebral
- ☐ Inflammatory joint disease (RA, AS)
- ☐ Irritability, adjacent
- ☐ Joint instability
- ☐ Joint irritability
- ☐ Lumbago (hyper-acute)
- ☐ Osteomalacia
- ☐ Osteoporosis
- ☐ Paget's disease
- ☐ Rheumatologic disease (inactive)
- ☐ Spondylosis

O00-O99 Pregnancy
- ☐ Pregnancy, last months

Q00-Q99 Congenital
- ☐ Genetic Disorders
- ☐ Laxity syndromes
- ☐ Odontoid, agenesis

R00-R99 Symptoms & Signs
- ☐ No pain-free direction
- ☐ Pain, Undiagnosed
- ☐ Spasm, protective

Procedural
- ☐ Forceful manipulation if root signs
- ☐ Relax, inability to
- ☐ Skill, inadequate
- ☐ Work-up, inadequate

SPINAL TRACTION SCREENING

Note: The following issues are considered a concern (advice, precaution, contraindication, or warning) from one or more published sources. If you check any item, consult page 723 for information.

C00-C97 Neoplasms
- ☐ Malignancy

D50-D89 Blood
- ☐ Bleeding disorders

F00-F99 Mental & Behavioral
- ☐ Anxious
- ☐ Disoriented
- ☐ Claustrophobic

G00-G99 Nervous
- ☐ Complete resolution of
- ☐ Cord compression
- ☐ Peripheralization of symptoms
- ☐ Sacral 4th root compression severe pain
- ☐ Spondylotic myelopathy

H00-H59 Eye
- ☐ Glaucoma

I00-I99 Circulatory
- ☐ Aneurysm, aortic
- ☐ Cardiovascular disease
- ☐ Carotid/vertebral arteries, arteriosclerotic obstruction
- ☐ Hypertension
- ☐ Vertebral basilar arterial disease

J00-J99 Respiratory
- ☐ Restrictive lung disease

K00-K93 Digestive
- ☐ Hemorrhoids
- ☐ Hernia, abdominal
- ☐ Hernia, hiatal
- ☐ Hernia, other
- ☐ Peptic ulcer

M00-M99 Musculoskeletal
- ☐ Annular fragment, displacement
- ☐ C1-C2 subluxation

M00-M99 Musculoskeletal cont'd
- ☐ Dislocation, previous
- ☐ Herniated disc, midline protrusion
- ☐ Inflammatory spondylitis
- ☐ Joint hypermobility/ instability
- ☐ Ligamentous instability, cervical
- ☐ Lumbago (acute)
- ☐ Osteoporosis
- ☐ Rheumatoid arthritis
- ☐ Spinal infection
- ☐ Structural spinal disease
- ☐ TMJ problems

O00-O99 Pregnancy
- ☐ Pregnancy

Q00-Q99 Congenital
- ☐ Down syndrome
- ☐ Marfan's syndrome
- ☐ Spinal deformity, congenital

R00-R99 Symptoms & Signs
- ☐ Inflammation (acute)

S00-T98 Injury
- ☐ Injury (acute)
- ☐ Fracture

Y70-Y82 Medical Devices
- ☐ Dentures
- ☐ Traction belts, hazardous

Procedural
- ☐ Elderly
- ☐ Expertise, inadequate
- ☐ Hyperextension, marked
- ☐ If motion is contraindicated
- ☐ Prone/Supine, poorly tolerated
- ☐ Steroid use, prolong
- ☐ Worsening with traction

THERAPEUTIC MASSAGE SCREENING

Note: The following issues are considered a concern (advice, precaution, contraindication, or warning) from one or more published sources. If you check any item, consult page 260 for information.

A00-B99 Certain Infections
- ☐ Infected tissue

C00-C99 Neoplasms
- ☐ Malignancy (over)

D50-D89 Blood
- ☐ Anticoagulant therapy
- ☐ Bleeding disorder, bleeding
- ☐ Immune system, compromised

E00-E90 Endocrine
- ☐ Nutritional status of skin, compromised

F00-F99 Mental & Behavioral
- ☐ Medication; Alcohol, Recreational Drugs
- ☐ Pain, chronic

G00-G99 Nervous
- ☐ Hyperesthesia
- ☐ Sensation reduced
- ☐ Spasticity

I00-I99 Circulatory
- ☐ Arrhythmia or Carotid brut
- ☐ Arteriosclerosis
- ☐ Cardiac disease, compromised
- ☐ Hypertension (severe)
- ☐ Hypotension
- ☐ Lymphangitis
- ☐ Pulmonary embolism (acute)
- ☐ Stroke
- ☐ Thrombophlebitis / DVT
- ☐ Varicose veins
- ☐ Vascular response, impaired

L00-L99 Skin
- ☐ Allergies to lotions
- ☐ Cellulitis
- ☐ Radiation or surgery
- ☐ Scar tissue (new)
- ☐ Skin graft
- ☐ Skin infection
- ☐ Skin inflamed (acute)
- ☐ Skin, fragile

M00-M99 Musculoskeletal
- ☐ Calcified tissue
- ☐ Dermatomyositis
- ☐ Osteoporosis
- ☐ Spinal fusion (recent)
- ☐ Fragile ribs
- ☐ Synovitis

O00-O99 Pregnancy
- ☐ Abdominal massage, in pregnancy

R00-R99 Symptoms & Signs
- ☐ Distress, severe
- ☐ Edema, several forms
- ☐ Inflamed, acutely

S00-T98 Injury
- ☐ Burns
- ☐ Foreign body
- ☐ Fractured rib / flail chest
- ☐ Surgeries, recent
- ☐ Trauma, acute
- ☐ Wound, open

Y70-Y82 Medical Devices
- ☐ Contact lenses
- ☐ Prosthetic devices; Stents

Vulnerable tissue
- ☐ Abdomen
- ☐ Abnormal structures
- ☐ Axilla
- ☐ Elbow
- ☐ Eye
- ☐ Inguinal
- ☐ Kidney
- ☐ Major vessels/veins, of limbs
- ☐ Neck
- ☐ Popliteal
- ☐ Thoracic cage
- ☐ Umbilicus
- ☐ Vertebral column

Procedural
- ☐ Deep abdominal massage
- ☐ Condition worsens with massage
- ☐ Edema, worsens with massage
- ☐ Technique, excessively vigorous

THERAPEUTIC ULTRASOUND SCREENING
(includes ultrasound and phonophoresis)

Note: The following issues are considered a concern (advice, precaution, contraindication, or warning) from one or more published sources. If you check any item, consult page 664 for information.

A00-B99 Certain Infections
- ☐ Infectious conditions

C00-C97 Neoplasm
- ☐ Tumor

D50-D89 Blood
- ☐ Bleeding disorders
- ☐ Hemorrhage

E00-E90 Endocrine
- ☐ Diabetes

F00-F99 Mental & Behavioral
- ☐ Inability to communicate

G00-G99 Nervous
- ☐ Pain/temperature sensation impaired
- ☐ Thermoregulation impaired

I00-I99 Circulatory
- ☐ Blood vessels, poor condition
- ☐ Cardiac disease
- ☐ Circulation impaired
- ☐ Thrombophlebitis (near)

L00-L99 Skin
- ☐ Grafts
- ☐ Scar, immature
- ☐ Skin, atrophy
- ☐ Skin infection

M00-M99 Musculoskeletal
- ☐ Bone sepsis (acute)
- ☐ Osteoporosis
- ☐ Soft tissue sepsis (acute)
- ☐ Tendon / ligament repair

O00-O99 Pregnancy
- ☐ Pregnant uterus

R00-R99 Symptoms & Signs
- ☐ Edema
- ☐ Fever
- ☐ Inflammation (acute)

S00-T98 Injury
- ☐ Fracture
- ☐ Trauma (acute)

Y70-Y82 Medical Devices
- ☐ Breast implant
- ☐ Cardiac pacemaker (over)
- ☐ Cement, joint, or plastic components, prosthetic
- ☐ Metal implant

Vulnerable tissue
- ☐ Cervical & stellate ganglia
- ☐ CNS tissue (over)
- ☐ Epiphyseal area (over)
- ☐ Eyes (over)
- ☐ Heart (over)
- ☐ Reproductive organs

Procedural Concerns
- ☐ Deep X-rays
- ☐ Transducer technique (see chapter)

Specific to Phonophoresis
Allergies and sensitivities to substances
- ☐ Hydrocortisone/Novocain
- ☐ Iodine
- ☐ Mecholyl
- ☐ Metals
- ☐ Salicylates

THERMOTHERAPY SCREENING

(Includes hot packs, Paraffin wax, infrared lamps)

(excludes ultraviolet and hydrotherapies)

Note: The following issues are considered a concern (advice, precaution, contraindication, or warning) from one or more published sources. If you check any item, consult page 678 for information.

A00-B99 Certain Infections
- ☐ Infected area (over)

C00-C97 Neoplasm
- ☐ Malignancy

D50-D89 Blood
- ☐ Hemorrhage (recent or potential)

F00-F99 Mental & Behavioral
- ☐ Mentation impaired

G00-G99 Nervous System
- ☐ Sensation impaired
- ☐ Thermoregulation impaired

I00-I99 Circulatory System
- ☐ Angina, unstable
- ☐ Blood pressure, unstable
- ☐ Cardiac insufficiency
- ☐ Circulation impaired
- ☐ Thrombophlebitic area

L00-L99 Skin
- ☐ Scar, immature
- ☐ Skin disorders (some)
- ☐ Skin graft, superficial
- ☐ Skin, atrophic

M00-M99 Musculoskeletal
- ☐ Repaired tendon or ligament
- ☐ Rheumatoid arthritis

O00-O99 Pregnancy
- ☐ Pregnancy

R00-R99 Symptoms & Signs
- ☐ Edema
- ☐ Inflammation, acute

S00-S98 Injury
- ☐ Injury (acute)
- ☐ Wounds, open

Y70-Y82 Medical Devices
- ☐ Metal, in area

Vulnerable tissue
- ☐ Eyes (infrared lamps)

Procedural Concerns
- ☐ Counterirritant, topical
- ☐ Drain excessive water, hot pack
- ☐ Edema, in dependent limb
- ☐ Falling asleep
- ☐ Insulating pack, not wet
- ☐ Weight, of hot pack
- ☐ Visually inspect area

Paraffin (additional)
- ☐ Blisters (in burn patient)
- ☐ Contagious skin disease
- ☐ Fragile & atrophic skin
- ☐ Grafts
- ☐ Hypersensitive skin
- ☐ Inflamed, acutely
- ☐ Paraffin + sustained stretch
- ☐ Sensation impaired
- ☐ Skin infection (over)
- ☐ Wax temperature, check
- ☐ Wounds, open (over) (burns)

ULTRAVIOLET THERAPY SCREENING

Note: The following issues are considered a concern (advice, precaution, contraindication, or warning) from one or more published sources. If you check any item, consult page 653 for information.

A00-B99 Certain Infections
- ☐ Tuberculosis, Pulmonary

C00-C97 Neoplasm
- ☐ Cancer

E00-E90 Endocrine
- ☐ Diabetes
- ☐ Hyperthyroidism
- ☐ Porphyria

F00-F99 Mental & Behavioral
- ☐ Alcoholism

I00-I99 Circulatory
- ☐ Arteriosclerosis (advanced)
- ☐ Cardiac disease

K00-K93 Digestive
- ☐ Hepatic insufficiency

L00-L99 Skin
- ☐ Dermatitis (acute)
- ☐ Eczema
- ☐ Herpes simplex
- ☐ Lupus erythematosus
- ☐ Pellagra
- ☐ Photosensitivity
- ☐ Premature aging
- ☐ Psoriasis (acute)
- ☐ Sarcoidosis
- ☐ Scars

L00-L99 Skin cont'd
- ☐ Skin cancer or history
- ☐ Skin, atrophic
- ☐ Xeroderma pigmentosum
- ☐ Dermatitis (generalized)

N00-N99 Genitourinary
- ☐ Renal insufficiency

R00-R99 Symptoms & Signs
- ☐ Complexion, fair
- ☐ Fever

S00-S98 Injury
- ☐ Burns; Redness

Vulnerable tissue
- ☐ Eyes, irradiation

Procedural
- ☐ Age–infant; elderly
- ☐ Chemotherapy; receiving
- ☐ Food ingestion, some
- ☐ Hazard, shock
- ☐ Photosensitive medications
- ☐ Previous treatment effects still apparent
- ☐ Protective (polarized) goggles (for both patient & therapist)
- ☐ Superficial heat prior to UV treatment
- ☐ X-rays to area (recent)

VASOPNEUMATIC COMPRESSION DEVICE SCREENING

Note: The following issues are considered a concern (advice, precaution, contraindication, or warning) from one or more published sources. If you check any item, consult page 699 for information.

C00-C97 Neoplasms
☐ Cancer

E00-E90 Metabolic
☐ Hypoproteinemia

F00-F99 Mental & Behavioral
☐ Mentation impaired

G00-G99 Nervous System
☐ Sensation impaired

I00-I99 Circulatory System
☐ Congestive heart failure
☐ Deep vein thrombosis
☐ Hypertension (uncontrolled)
☐ Lymphatic or venous obstruction

I00-I99 Circulatory System cont'd
☐ Peripheral artery disease
☐ Pulmonary embolism
☐ Vascular insufficiency or stroke

J00-J99 Respiratory System
☐ Pulmonary edema

L00-L99 Skin & Subcutaneous
☐ Skin infection

S00-T98 Injury
☐ Fracture (acute)
☐ Trauma (acute)

Vulnerable Tissue
☐ Peripheral nerve (superficial)

Figure E indicates the number of interventions listing some specific patient condition as a concern in physical rehabilitation. For example, although only six interventions list a concern for hernias (e.g., abdominal; hiatal) and 10 interventions list a concern for seizure disorders, more than 25 therapies express concerns for anticoagulated patients (or bleeding tendencies). Consult the index in Part V of this text for a complete list of interventions cross-referenced by disease categories.

The Number of Interventions With Some Common Condition-Specific Concerns

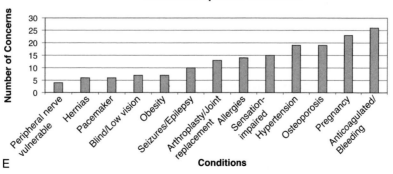

Figure F presents the number of vulnerable tissue-related concerns for some interventions. These are body parts that may be highly vulnerable to injury or unwanted stimulation during treatment. For example, acupuncture lists a dozen vulnerable tissue concerns including warnings to avoid nipple and eye (ball) areas during needle applications.

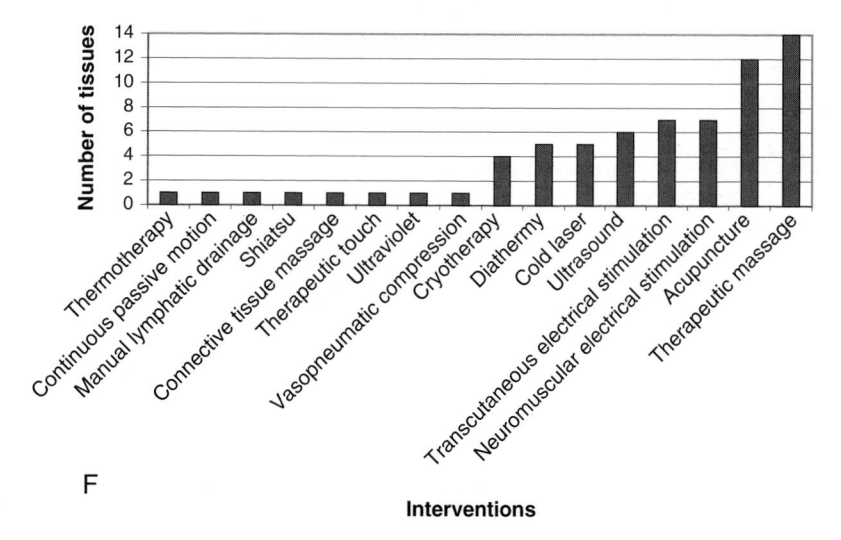

The Number of Vulnerable Tissue-Related Concerns for Common Interventions

F

Figure G illustrates the number of medical device-related concerns for a particular intervention. Examples of such devices that may be of concern during some therapies include metal implants, trachiostomies, and axillary-type crutches. The top four interventions with device-related concerns are diathermy, functional training (gait training), and two water therapies (hydrotherapy and aqua therapy).

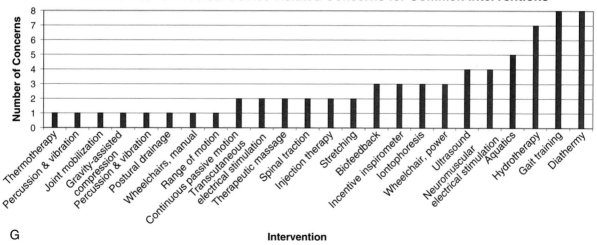

The Number of Medical Device-Related Concerns for Common Interventions

G

Intervention

Vasopneumatic compression device, 699-708
screening form, 856
VCD See Vasopneumatic compression device.
Veins
varicose
acupuncture and, 752
electrical stimulation and, 548
shiatsu and, 785
spinal traction and, 730
therapeutic massage and, 266
as vulnerable tissue in therapeutic massage, 273
Venous insufficiency, whirlpool for cleaning pressure ulcers and, 517
Venous return, obstructed, vasopneumatic compression device and, 702
Venous ulcer
compression supports and, 443, 444
whirlpool cleaning of, 517
Ventilation, mechanical, 451-452
Ventricular aneurysm, exercise testing and, 26
Ventricular arrhythmia, 95
Ventricular ectopy, complex, therapeutic aerobic exercise and, 72
Ventricular failure, aquatic therapy and, 93
Ventricular peritoneal shunt, Swiss ball and, 383
Ventricular tachycardia, exercise testing and, 28
Vertebral artery disease
spinal manipulation and, 304, 311
vigorous head/neck movements and, 282
Vertebral artery test, 282, 290
Vertebral body, dislocation or fracture of, spinal manipulation and, 308
Vertebral column See Spine.
Vertebrobasilar arterial disease, spinal traction and, 729
Vertigo
older drivers and, 236, 240
on post-trauma bed, 336
Trager and, 799
Vesicular zoster, shiatsu and, 790

Vestibular exercise, 101-104
Vibration and percussion of chest, 471-490
in premature infant, 471
screening form, 848
Vibratory device, 352-354
Viral infection, therapeutic massage and, 261 See Infection.
Visual impairment
communication and, 43
functional electrical stimulation and, 573
older drivers and, 235, 240
prosthetics and, 429
sport activities and, 231
wheelchairs and
manual, 360
power, 371
Visual issues in patient instruction, 58
Vital capacity
aquatic therapy and, 88
hydrotherapy and, 627
incentive respiratory spirometry and, 461
reduced due to age, Boomerang pillow and, 436
Vital sign monitoring
during functional electrical stimulation, 576-577
during tilt table therapy, 710
Vitamin B_3 deficiency, ultraviolet therapy and, 658
Vocal cord injury, airway suctioning and, 492
Vulnerable biologic tissues, 5, 7, 9-14
in acupuncture, 754-755
in cold laser, 648
in connective tissue massage, 258
in continuous passive motion, 718
in cryotherapy, 587
in diathermy, 610
in eccentric exercise, 164
in electrical stimulation, 554-555
in electrodiagnostic testing, 17
in infrared therapy, 687
in manual lymphatic drainage, 250
in progressive resistive exercise, 176